# Cardiovascular Disease in the Elderly Patient

**FUNDAMENTAL AND CLINICAL CARDIOLOGY**



1. *Drug Treatment of Hyperlipidemia*, edited by Basil M. Rifkind
2. *Cardiotonic Drugs: A Clinical Review. Second Edition, Revised and Expanded*, edited by Carl V. Leier
3. *Complications of Coronary Angioplasty*, edited by Alexander J. R. Black, H. Vernon Anderson, and Stephen G. Ellis
4. *Unstable Angina*, edited by John D. Rutherford
5. *Beta-Blockers and Cardiac Arrhythmias*, edited by Prakash C. Deedwania
6. *Exercise and the Heart in Health and Disease*, edited by Roy J. Shephard and Henry S. Miller, Jr.
7. *Cardiopulmonary Physiology in Critical Care*, edited by Steven M. Scharf
8. *Atherosclerotic Cardiovascular Disease, Hemostasis, and Endothelial Function*, edited by Robert Boyer Francis, Jr.
9. *Coronary Heart Disease Prevention*, edited by Frank G. Yanowitz
10. *Thrombolysis and Adjunctive Therapy for Acute Myocardial Infarction*, edited by Eric R. Bates
11. *Stunned Myocardium: Properties, Mechanisms, and Clinical Manifestations*, edited by Robert A. Kloner and Karin Przyklenk
12. *Prevention of Venous Thromboembolism*, edited by Samuel Z. Goldhaber
13. *Silent Myocardial Ischemia and Infarction: Third Edition*, Peter F. Cohn
14. *Congestive Cardiac Failure: Pathophysiology and Treatment*, edited by David B. Barnett, Hubert Pouleur, and Gary S. Francis
15. *Heart Failure: Basic Science and Clinical Aspects*, edited by Judith K. Gwathmey, G. Maurice Briggs, and Paul D. Allen

16. *Coronary Thrombolysis in Perspective: Principles Underlying Conjunctive and Adjunctive Therapy*, edited by Burton E. Sobel and Désiré Collen
17. *Cardiovascular Disease in the Elderly Patient*, edited by Donald D. Tresch and Wilbert S. Aronow

*Additional Volumes in Preparation*

*Systemic Cardiac Embolism*, edited by Michael Ezekowitz

*Low-Molecular-Weight Heparins in Prophylaxis and Therapy of Thromboembolic Diseases*, edited by Henri Bounameaux

*Valvular Heart Disease*, edited by Muayed Al Zaibag

# Cardiovascular Disease in the Elderly Patient

edited by


Donald D. Tresch

*Medical College of Wisconsin*
*Milwaukee, Wisconsin*

Wilbert S. Aronow

*Mount Sinai School of Medicine*
*and Hebrew Hospital Home*
*New York, New York*



Marcel Dekker, Inc. New York • Basel • Hong Kong

**Library of Congress Cataloging-in-Publication Data**

Cardiovascular disease in the elderly patient / edited by Donald D. Tresch, Wilbert S. Aronow.
p. cm. — (Fundamental and clinical cardiology ; 17)
Includes bibliographical references and index.
ISBN 0-8247-8864-8 (alk. paper)
1. Geriatric cardiology. I. Tresch, Donald D. II. Aronow, Wilbert S. III. Series: Fundamental and clinical cardiology ; v. 17.
[DNLM: 1. Cardiovascular Diseases—in old age. 2. Cardiovascular Diseases—physiopathology. W1FU538TD v. 17 / WG 100 C26728 1993]
RC669.C279 1993
618.97'612—dc20
DNLM/DLC
for Library of Congrress 93-25822
CIP

The publisher offers discounts on this book when ordered in bulk quantities. For more information, write to Special Sales/Professional Marketing at the address below.

This book is printed on acid-free paper.



Marcel Dekker, Inc.
270 Madison Avenue, New York, New York 10016

Current printing (last digit):
10 9 8 7 6 5 4 3 2 1

PRINTED IN THE UNITED STATES OF AMERICA

All beginnings are joyous.
Our elderly patients show us that endings
may also be joyous.
To them we dedicate this book.
They never fail to teach us that life,
even with the struggles of aging and disease,
may be full of meaning and joy.

# Series Introduction

Marcel Dekker, Inc. has focused on the development of various series of beautifully produced books in different branches of medicine. These series have facilitated the integration of rapidly advancing information for both the clinical specialist and the researcher.

My goal as editor of the Fundamental and Clinical Cardiology series is to assemble the talents of world-renowned authorities to discuss virtually every area of cardiovascular medicine. In the current monograph, *Cardiovascular Disease in the Elderly Patient,* Drs. Tresch and Aronow have edited a much needed and timely book. Future contributions to the series will include books on molecular biology, interventional cardiology, and clinical management of such problems as coronary artery disease and ventricular arrhythmias.

*Samuel Z. Goldhaber*

# Foreword

Fifty years ago it was widely held that the overall process of human aging was intimately related to, if not caused by, changes in the cardiovascular system—in particular, the heart. The idea that the heart was important to age changes was a by-product of emerging understanding of the role of circulation in human health and disease. Excluding malignant disease, most serious illnesses manifest themselves in the cardiovascular system, directly or indirectly, and ultimately result in death of the organism due to circulatory failure. Early studies by Bronfenbrenner and his associates (1), which demonstrated reduced cardiac output at rest in hospitalized older individuals compared to their younger counterparts, seemed to reinforce the notion that heart function declined with age. In retrospect, however, these changes likely reflected disease and inactivity rather than aging.

We now know that, without exercise conditioning, the normal individual free of heart disease has the ability to augment cardiac output during exercise or stress 2½- to 3-fold. With exercise conditioning, the cardiac output of the older individual during exercise can increase even further. This remarkable ability of the heart of the older individual free of disease to augment function undermines any theory or hypothesis that aging reflects the inadequacy of the heart to pump blood.

Fifty years ago it was also widely believed that the heart became dysfunctional with age because it received inadequate oxygen supply. According to this theory, progressive reduction in the coronary vascular tree size resulted in diminished blood flow delivery to each myocardial fiber, and increased resistance to the diffusion of oxygen from the capillary bed into the tissues existed due to altered ground substance and/or altered connective tissue. Thus decreased blood flow to contracting muscle and decreased oxygen delivery resulted in progressive destruction and dysfunction of myocardial cells, which, in turn, led to dysfunction of the heart, failure of the circulation, and aging of the organism.

One of my most striking experiences as a young investigator in Nathan Shock's laboratory some years ago was an attempt to test these hypotheses directly (2). I perfused hearts from old and young adult rats with oxygenated solution. The hearts were paced at a constant rate and were vented so that they developed no left ventricular pressure. Thus there was no hemodynamic impediment to coronary blood flow. Under these conditions, the hearts were subjected to progressively decreasing oxygen content of the perfusate. As anticipated, coronary blood flow increased due to active coronary vasodilation. I measured the magnitude of this increase as well as the percent oxygen extracted and the venous affluent oxygen content coming from the coronary tree. I found that under these conditions coronary flow increased almost identically in the old and young hearts and oxygen extraction and oxygen consumption were identical under the conditions of hypoxic stress. The extent to which these experiments undermined an entire theoretical construct did not impress me as much at the time as they have over the subsequent 20 years. Clearly, the coronary vasculature was adequate and well dilated. There was no problem with oxygen delivery and therefore diffusion.

Many experiments have shown that contractile function of heart muscle from older animals does not diminish (3,4). The velocity of contraction is slower, but the overall tension and, in fact, the ability to shorten are unchanged with age. In recent years, many studies have tended to confirm these basic observations in humans. That is to say, the intrinsic contractile ability of cardiac muscle is unchanged with age. There is a slowing of the velocity of shortening and relaxation but no change in the overall performance capabilities in terms of shortening ability or tension generation. Thus, the heart is not the seat of diminished functional capability with age and not a major fact in age-associated alterations in other organs or systems. In addition, the intrinsic contractile proteins of the heart, as well as their ability to extract oxygen, are also unchanged with age. Finally, the coronary vascular bed capacity does not limit the ability of the older heart to augment flow.

Beyond this fundamental physiological normalcy of the aging heart, there are significant age changes. These issues are addressed comprehensively in Chapter 1 by Steven Schulman. What has emerged as the important change in the cardiovascular system response to stress with aging is quite simply a decrease in the magnitude of the beta sympathetic response. Thus, the increase in heart rate with exercise and stress diminishes with age, as do the inotropic response to sympathetic stimulation or exercise and the central arterial vasodilating response.

A patient confronted with acute, severe mitral regurgitation from ruptured papillary muscle would have a decreased heart rate response to severe hemodynamic stress, an increase in impedance to ejection, and thus greater ventricular workload and greater valvular regurgitation. There would also be decreased inotropic response and thus decreased left ventricular contractile function. Such considerations would lead to an emphasis in treatment of heart failure states in the elderly on vasodilator therapy to reduce the high impedance to left ventricular ejection (5). Since there are also some suggestions that inotropic agents, such as digitalis, are less effective with aging, even more emphasis would be placed on a strategy to reduce afterload in treatment of heart failure. Finally, the older heart confronted with acute hemodynamic stress would appear to have decreased propensity to hypertrophy over time (6,7). The older patient developing aortic stenosis due to calcific aortic valve disease may have less time before symptoms appear than the younger individual who would have more robust left ventricular hypertrophy in response to an increase in afterload.

This volume emphasizes cardiac disease and its management in the context of the aging patient. It is not of importance for the clinical reader and physician to memorize a catalog of facts related to age-associated alterations in subcellular enzyme systems and/or individual drug responses. Rather, it is important to understand the principles. What are the major age-associated physiological changes that have impact on the response to the disease? How does an understanding of these principles relate to caring for an elderly patient? These discussions are dominated by the fact that frequency and severity of cardiovascular disease usually increase with age. Frequently, in the elderly patient, one is dealing with severe rather than mild disease, and with diffuse rather than localized disease. And very often there are multisystem problems rather than a single clinical problem in need of a definitive answer. In the older individual it is management rather than cure, and improvement in symptomatology rather than prolongation of life. False hypotheses and false theories need to be rejected. There is an optimistic picture here of well-maintained cardiovascular function throughout the normal life span if cardiovascular disease is avoided. In the presence of cardiovascular disease age changes make compensation less adequate and the job of the physician more important and more rigorous.

*Myron L. Weisfeldt, M.D.*
*Samuel Bard Professor of Medicine*
*Chair, Department of Medicine*
*Columbia University, College of Physicians & Surgeons*
*New York, New York*

## REFERENCES

1. Bronfenbrenner M, Landowne M, Shock NW. Changes in cardiac output with age. Circulation 1955; 12: 557.

2. Weisfeldt ML, Wright JR, Shreiner DP, Lakatta E, Shock NW. Coronary flow and oxygen extraction in the perfused heart of senescent male rats. J Appl Physiol 1971; 30(1): 44–49. 1971.
3. Alpert NR, Gale HH, Taylor N. The effect of age on contractile protein ATPase activity and the velocity of shortening. In Kavaler F, Tanz RD, Roberts J, eds. Factors Influencing Myocardial Contractility. New York: Academic, 1967: 127–133.
4. Weisfeldt ML, Loeven WA, Shock NW. Resting and active mechanical properties of trabeculae carneae from aged male rats. Am J Physiol 1971; 220(6): 1921–1927.
5. Weisfeldt ML, Lakatta GE, Gerstenblith G. Aging and the heart. In Braunwald E, ed. Heart Disease. Philadelphia: Saunders, 1992; 52: 1656–1669.
6. Isoyama S, Wei YJ, Izumo S, Fort P, Schoen FJ, Grossman W. Effect of age on the development of cardiac hypertrophy produced by aortic constriction in the rat. Circ Res 1987; 61: 337–345.
7. Isoyama S, Grossman W, Wei JY. Effect of age on myocardial adaptation to volume overload in the rat. Circ Res 1988; 81: 1850–1857.

# Preface

Heart disease is one of the most prevalent diseases in the elderly and, the number one cause of death in patients over 65 years of age. Because the percentage of persons over 65 years of age is continuing to increase rapidly, it is increasingly important that the practicing physician be well versed in both the diagnosis and treatment of heart disease in the elderly. Cardiac disease in the elderly often presents in an atypical manner because the presence of other disease processes may modify the symptoms and, thereby, skew the findings of the physical examination; as a result, cardiac disorders in this age group are frequently misdiagnosed, or may even go undiagnosed. Treatment choices, too, may become complicated because the elderly cardiac patient commonly has other diseases that affect drug or other therapeutic interventions.

This book provides all physicians involved in the care of elderly patients—family physicians, internists, cardiologists, surgeons, residents, and students—with an understanding of the pathophysiology of cardiac disorders in this age group; demonstrates the usual and atypical presentations of these disorders; and presents a logical approach to the treatment of the elderly patient with such cardiac disorders.

The contributors, all of whom have many years of experience in cardiology and have made valuable contributions to the cardiology literature, are particularly well qualified to discuss the subject of geriatric cardiology. The emphasis has been placed on those specific cardiac disorders most relevant to the physician who cares for the elderly. Special attention is given to how the disorders pertain to the elderly patient and to recognizing the differences in both clinical presentation and response to therapy, compared to the younger patient. We hope that the book will serve as a source of information that will be of continual use to the practicing physician in the daily care of elderly patients.

*Donald D. Tresch*
*Wilbert S. Aronow*

# Contents

# Contributors

**Wilbert S. Aronow, M.D.** Adjunct Professor of Geriatrics and Adult Development, Mount Sinai School of Medicine, New York; and Medical Director, Department of Medicine, Hebrew Hospital Home, Bronx, New York

**David A. Cesario, B.S.** Department of Medicine, University of California, Irvine, California

**Thomas C. Cesario, M.D.** Professor and Chair, Department of Medicine, University of California, Irvine Medical Center, Orange, California

**Deanna G. Cheung, M.D.** Clinical Instructor, Department of Medicine, University of California, Irvine, and Veterans Affairs Medical Center, Long Beach, California

**Dennis J. Esterbrooks, M.D., F.A.C.C.** Associate Professor of Medicine, Division of Cardiology, Creighton University School of Medicine, Omaha, Nebraska

**Kevin J. Ferrick, M.D.** Associate Professor of Medicine, Albert Einstein College of Medicine, and Arrhythmia Service, Division of Cardiology, Montefiore Medical Center, Bronx, New York

**John D. Fisher, M.D., F.A.C.C.** Professor of Medicine, Albert Einstein College of Medicine, and Director of Cardiology/Director, Arrhythmia Service, Department of Cardiology, Montefiore Medical Center, Bronx, New York

**Jerome L. Fleg, M.D.** Senior Investigator, Laboratory of Cardiovascular Science, Gerontology Research Center, National Institute on Aging; Associate Professor of Medicine, Johns Hopkins University School of Medicine, Baltimore, Maryland

**Robert Forman, M.D.** Professor of Medicine, Division of Cardiology, Albert Einstein College of Medicine and Montefiore Medical Center, Bronx, New York

**William H. Frishman, M.D.** Professor and Associate Chairman, Department of Medicine, Albert Einstein College of Medicine and Montefiore Medical Center, Bronx, New York

**Steven R. Gambert, M.D., F.A.C.P.** Professor of Medicine and Associate Dean for Academic Programs, New York Medical College, Valhalla, New York

**Julius M. Gardin, M.D.** Professor, Division of Cardiology, Department of Medicine, University of California, Irvine, California

**Donald B. Hunninghake, M.D.** Professor of Medicine and Pharmacology, and Director of the Heart Disease Prevention Clinic, University of Minnesota Hospital and Clinic, Minneapolis, Minnesota

**William B. Kannel, M.D., M.P.H.** Professor of Medicine and Public Health, Boston University School of Medicine; former Medical Director, Framingham Heart Study, Boston, Massachusetts

**Wishwa N. Kapoor, M.D., M.P.H.** Professor, Department of Medicine, University of Pittsburgh, Pittsburgh, Pennsylvania

**Thierry H. LeJemtel, M.D.** Professor of Medicine, Division of Cardiology, Albert Einstein College of Medicine, Bronx, New York

**Ross T. Lyon, M.D.** Assistant Professor of Surgery, Albert Einstein College of Medicine and Montefiore Medical Center, Bronx, New York

**Ben D. McCallister, M.D.** Consultant in Cardiovascular Disease, Mid America Heart Institute; and Clinical Professor of Medicine, University of Missouri, Kansas City, Missouri

**Anthony D. Mercando, M.D.** Clinical Associate Professor of Medicine, Columbia University, College of Physicians and Surgeons, New York, New York; Assistant Clinical Professor of Medicine, Albert Einstein College of Medicine and Montefiore Medical Center, Bronx, New York

**Chandra K. Nair, M.D.** Professor of Medicine, Division of Cardiology, Department of Medicine, Creighton University School of Medicine, Omaha, Nebraska

**Michele Nanna, M.D.** Assistant Professor, Department of Medicine, Albert Einstein College of Medicine, Bronx, New York

**Steven P. Rivers, M.D.** Associate Professor, Division of Vascular Surgery, Department of Surgery, Albert Einstein College of Medicine and Montefiore Medical Center, Bronx, New York

**William C. Roberts, M.D.** Executive Director, Baylor Cardiovascular Institute, Baylor University Medical Center, Dallas, Texas

**Steven P. Schulman, M.D.** Assistant Professor of Medicine, Division of Cardiology, Johns Hopkins University School of Medicine, Baltimore, Maryland

**James L. Sebastian, M.D.** Associate Professor of Medicine, Divisions of General Internal Medicine and Educational Affairs, Medical College of Wisconsin, Milwaukee, Wisconsin

**Thomas M. Shimshak, M.D.** Consulting Cardiologist, Mid-America Heart Institute; and Clinical Associate Professor of Medicine, University of Missouri, Kansas City, Missouri

**Edmund H. Sonnenblick, M.D.** Olson Professor of Medicine, and Chief, Division of Cardiology, Albert Einstein College of Medicine, Bronx, New York

**Paul D. Stein, M.D.** Director, Cardiovascular Research, Henry Ford Heart and Vascular Institute, Detroit, Michigan

**Ranjan K. Thakur, M.D.** Assistant Professor, Arrhythmia Service, University of Western Ontario, London, Ontario, Canada

**Donald D. Tresch, M.D.** Professor of Medicine, Departments of Cardiology and Geriatrics/Gerontology, and Director of Cardiology Fellowship Program, Medical College of Wisconsin; and Adjunct Professor, University of Wisconsin, College of Letters and Science, Milwaukee, Wisconsin

**Frank J. Veith, M.D.** Professor and Interim Chairman, Department of Surgery, Montefiore Medical Center; and Chief, Vascular Surgical Services, Albert Einstein College of Medicine, Bronx, New York

**Pantel S. Vokonas, M.D.** Professor of Medicine and Public Health, Boston University School of Medicine; and Director, Department of Veterans Affairs Normative Aging Study, Veterans Affairs Medical Center, Boston, Massachusetts

**Michael A. Weber, M.D.** Professor of Medicine, University of California, Irvine; and Director, Clinical Pharmacology and Hypertension Section, Veterans Affairs Medical Center, Long Beach, California

**Myron L. Weisfeldt, M.D.** Samuel Bard Professor of Medicine, Chair, Department of Medicine, Columbia University, College of Physicians and Surgeons, New York, New York

**Mark A. Williams, Ph.D., F.A.A.C.V.P.R., F.A.C.S.M.** Associate Professor of Medicine, Division of Cardiology, Creighton University School of Medicine, Omaha, Nebraska

**Philip A. Wolf, M.D.** Professor of Neurology, Research Professor of Medicine (Preventive Medicine & Epidemiology), Department of Neurology, Boston University School of Medicine, Boston, Massachusetts

# 1

# Normal Aging Changes of the Cardiovascular System

**Steven P. Schulman**
*Johns Hopkins University School of Medicine, Baltimore, Maryland*

## INTRODUCTION

Epidemiological trends demonstrate a continuing increase in the percentage of the U.S. population surviving to older age. Those Americans over the age of 75 years make up the fastest growing segment of the population (1). Although there has been a recent decline in mortality from coronary heart disease and stroke (2), cardiovascular disease is still the leading cause of morbidity and mortality in this age group. Therefore, it is important to distinguish alterations in cardiovascular function associated with disease from those associated with normal aging in the cardiovascular evaluation of the elderly patient.

There are several challenges to studying normal aging in humans. Foremost among these is that cardiovascular disease is so prevalent in the aging population that changes ascribed to aging are often due to underlying disease. Hypertension and coronary artery disease are the two most prevalent diseases affecting the elderly population. It is estimated that 40% of elderly Americans are hypertensive, and nearly that many have silent ischemia on exercise stress thallium scans (3,4). The prevalence of obstructive coronary artery disease at autopsy approaches 50% in elderly women and 70–80% in elderly men (5). This high prevalence of disease in the elderly makes it impossible to interpret any age-associated change in cardiac function unless subjects are rigorously screened for cardiac disease. Second, many secondary changes occur in the elderly that may affect cardiovascular function but are not necessarily inherent to the aging process. One such example is the increasingly sedentary life-style known to occur in the elderly, which may result in changes in cardiac function (6). Third, the distinction between age-associated and disease-associated changes in the cardiovascular system is not always clear (6). Examples include left ventricular mass and systolic blood pressure. Both left ventricular mass and systolic blood pressure increase with age in subjects free of disease (7,8). However, both are independent risk factors for developing future cardiovascular disease in previously asymptomatic subjects (9,10). At what point these markers of the "aging process" become markers of disease is often blurred.

## FUNCTION IN ANIMAL MODELS

Animal models have yielded a wealth of information about the cardiovascular changes that occur with aging and the potential mechanisms for these changes. Since coronary artery disease occurs with a low frequency in these models (11), the obvious difficulties just discussed are not encountered. Interestingly, there is a great deal of agreement across species (including humans) concerning cardiovascular function in elderly animals.

### Cardiac Function

Contractile function in isolated rat papillary muscle is unchanged with aging (12–14). Lakatta and coworkers (13) studied isometric performance of rat left ventricular trabeculae carneae from young (6 months) and old (25 months) animals. The resting tension, peak active isometric tension, and maximal rate of tension development were similar in young and old cardiac muscle. Similar to the isolated papillary muscle, contractile function in the intact dog heart does not change with age (15).

The most significant difference between young and senescent cardiac muscle demonstrated in these studies was an age-associated prolongation in contraction duration. This difference represents a prolongation in the time to peak developed tension and, more importantly, relaxation time (12,13). The active state of aged myocardium is prolonged in this preparation and accounts for the delayed relaxation since there was greater electromechanical dissociation at high pacing rates in the papillary muscles from senescent compared to young adult rats (13). These age differences were not abolished after myocardial catecholamine depletion. A similar prolongation in left ventricular relaxation has been noted in the intact senescent dog heart (16).

There are two likely mechanisms responsible for the prolongation of the active state in senescent cardiac muscle. First, there is a prolongation of the action potential duration (17,18). Second, as shown in Figure 1, the velocity of

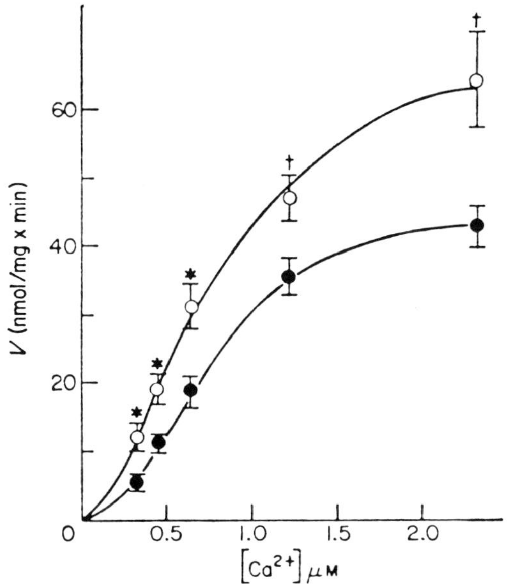


**Figure 1** Rates of calcium accumulation in microsomes from young adult (open circles) and senescent (closed circles) hearts. At all calcium concentrations tested, the rate of microsomal calcium uptake was significantly lower from the aged hearts. (From Ref. 19.)

calcium accumulation by sarcoplasmic reticulum from young adult rat myocardium is significantly greater than that from aged hearts (19). Since the active uptake of calcium by the sarcoplasmic reticulum from the myofibrils brings about relaxation, this decrease velocity of calcium uptake may explain the prolonged contraction duration found in senescent muscle.

Deconditioning may contribute to this age-associated prolongation in contraction duration and decline in sarcoplasmic reticulum calcium uptake. Spurgeon et al. measured twitch duration parameters of trabecula carneae from young adult and senescent rats that underwent 18–22 weeks of exercise training and compared them to age-matched untrained controls (20). Exercise training did not alter contraction duration and relaxation times in young myocardium. These parameters were significantly prolonged in aged muscle from sedentary rats. However, the contraction duration and relaxation time were significantly less in senescent myocardium from rats that underwent exercise training and similar to these parameters from young myocardium. Subsequent studies have demonstrated that the rate of sarcoplasmic reticulum calcium uptake increases with exercise training, which may account for the exercise-training effect on contraction duration (21). In addition to age-related changes in the active state properties affecting diastolic function, changes in passive properties may also play a role. Thus, the increase in left ventricular wall thickness and myocardial fibrosis in aged animals may increase left ventricular chamber stiffness and impair left ventricular filling (11). In summary, animal studies have demonstrated that the primary change that occurs in aged myocardium is a prolongation in active relaxation, likely due to a decrease in the rate of calcium uptake by the sarcoplasmic reticulum.

## Response to Stress

Mechanisms to increase cardiac output during exercise stress include the Frank-Starling mechanism and increases in heart rate and myocardial contractility (11). The use of the Frank-Starling mechanism remains intact in animal aging models: active length-tension curves from aged rat trabeculae are similar to those obtained from their younger counterparts (12). The exercise-related increase in heart rate and contractility rely on exercise-induced elaboration of catecholamines.

There is a marked age-related decrease in the chronotropic and inotropic response to catecholamines in animal models. There is a decrease heart rate response to isoproterenol in aged compared to younger dogs (22). Figure 2

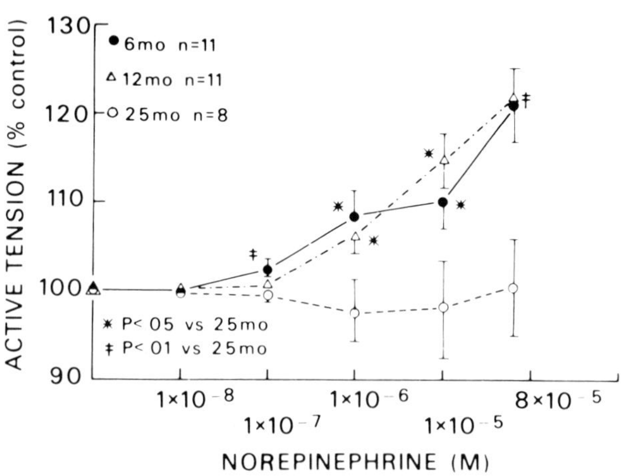


**Figure 2** The response of active tension development in isometric trabeculae carneae from young, middle-aged, and aged rats to increasing concentrations of norepinephrine. In contrast to the increase in active tension development to norepinephrine in the young and middle-aged muscle, there was no change in the aged muscle to catecholamines. (From Ref. 14.)

shows the active tension response of isometric trabeculae carneae from young adult, middle-aged, and aged rats to increasing concentrations of norepinephrine (14). Active tension increased significantly compared to baseline in young adult and middle-aged groups, but there was no change in active tension in the senescent muscle at any norepinephrine concentration. Similar age differences in this study were demonstrated to isoproterenol. This age difference in the inotropic response to catecholamines was also demonstrated when maximal rate of tension development was evaluated. Importantly, active tension and maximal rate of tension development were increased similarly in both young adult and aged trabeculae carneae to increasing concentrations of calcium, suggesting that myofibrillar contractile function is maintained in senescent cardiac muscle. The diminished inotropic response to catecholamines in aged myocardium suggests a specific defect in the ability of catecholamines to increase the amount of calcium delivered to the myofilaments (11,14). This decreased response to catecholamines in the aged rat model is not receptor mediated, because receptor density and affinity do not decrease with age (23).

## Ventricular–Vascular Coupling

The ability of the left ventricle to increase cardiac output with exercise is strongly coupled to the vascular load against which the heart ejects. For any level of left ventricular contractility, higher afterload would limit exercise cardiac output. Ventricular afterload can be partitioned into nonpulsatile and pulsatile components. The nonpulsatile component is quantified as the mean systemic vascular resistance, which relates mean aortic pressure to mean aortic flow and is determined by the size of the vascular bed and its arteriolar tone (11). The pulsatile component is determined by the degree of vascular stiffness and the magnitude and timing of pressure and flow waves reflected back to the aortic root (24). The stiffer the vascular tree and the larger the magnitude and more rapid the reflection of pressure waves, the greater is the pulsatile load against which the heart must eject blood. Various measurements help describe the pulsatile component of afterload, such as aortic characteristic impedance and pulse wave velocity (24). The vascular response to exercise, that is, vasodilation, is catecholamine mediated and in the animal model is another example of the age-associated decreased responsiveness to catecholamines. The smooth muscle vasodilating response to isoproterenol is significantly greater from young rabbit aortae compared to older rabbits (25). When the vasodilating response of rabbit aorta muscle strips to nitroprusside and nitroglycerin was evaluated, no age differences were noted, suggesting a selective decrease in the vascular responsiveness to $\beta$-adrenergic stimulation in older animals (25).

This age difference in catecholamine-mediated vasodilation has important implications in the cardiac response to exercise. Yin and coworkers (15) compared rest and exercise cardiac output, stroke volume, systemic vascular resistance, and aortic characteristic impedance in young (mean 2.4 years) and old (mean 10.5 years) chronically instrumented dogs. Resting hemodynamics were similar between the young and senescent dogs. During exercise, the younger animals had a stepwise increase in stroke volume with increasing levels of exercise. The senescent dogs had no increase in stroke volume, which resulted in a lower cardiac output at peak exercise. Both young and older animals had a decrease in systemic vascular resistance at mild exercise. However, the aortic characteristic impedance during exercise differed between the two. The older animals had a large increase in characteristic impedance from rest to exercise, whereas this measurement did not change from rest to exercise in the younger animals. This increased vascular load imposed on aged ventricles may contribute to the differences in exercise cardiac output and stroke volume between the young and old animals.

Yin and colleagues (15) then administered propranolol to measure the contribution of $\beta$-adrenergic stimulation to the age differences in the hemodynamic response to exercise. $\beta$-Adrenergic blockade abolished the age differences just noted. The young $\beta$-blocked animals did not increase the stroke volume from rest to exercise and had a large increase in aortic characteristic impedance, indistinguishable from that in the older group of animals. In summary, the limited inotropic, chronotropic, and vasodilatory response to exercise noted in older animals represents an age-associated decreased responsiveness to $\beta$-adrenergic stimulation.

## CARDIOVASCULAR FUNCTION IN HUMANS

Results of studies evaluating age-associated changes in cardiovascular function are difficult to interpret unless subjects are carefully screened for disease. Participants in the Baltimore Longitudinal Study of Aging are rigorously screened for cardiac disease by a detailed history and examination and a stress ECG thallium scan. Cardiovascular studies performed in this population have demonstrated age-associated changes that are predicted from the animal models.

### Resting Cardiac Function

Similar to the maintained contractility of senescent papillary muscle from animal models, resting systolic function in the human does not decline with increasing age. Noninvasive estimates of cardiac function in healthy subjects utilizing echocardiography and gated blood pool scintigraphy show normal resting left ventricular systolic function across a wide age range (26–28). This assessment includes fractional shortening, cardiac output, ejection fraction, and left ventricular volumes. Resting heart rate also does not change with increasing age in healthy subjects (27,28). Echocardiographic studies have demonstrated that left ventricular mass and wall thickness increase with age (26). This mild hypertrophy is due to the age-associated increase in vascular afterload (see later).

Similar to the prolonged contraction duration noted in senescent rat papillary muscle, there is slowed and delayed left ventricular relaxation in elderly healthy subjects (29,30). Thus, noninvasive studies of left ventricular filling have noted an age-associated decrease in the peak filling rate on gated blood pool scanning (31), a reduced early mitral valve closure slope on echocardiography (26), and decreased E to A velocity ratio on Doppler echocardiography (32). Although many hemodynamic and structural changes affect left ventricular filling (33), those associated with normal aging that could contribute to the decrease in early diastolic filling include prolonged relaxation (29), an increase in left ventricular wall thickness (26), an increase in chamber stiffness due to changes in left ventricular passive viscoelastic properties (11,34), an increase in afterload (35), and an increase in regional left ventricular diastolic asynchrony (36). Unlike the effects of exercise training on relaxation time in the animal model, endurance training does not appear to reverse the age-associated decrease in early left ventricular filling in humans (37). Importantly, since early diastolic filling is reduced in healthy elderly subjects, resting end-diastolic volume is maintained by an increase in the atrial contribution to left ventricular filling (38).

In summary, in healthy elderly subjects screened for coronary artery disease, left ventricular systolic function is maintained. Mild left ventricular hypertrophy occurs, which may contribute to an age-associated decline in early left ventricular filling. Resting end-diastolic volume is maintained because of an increase in atrial contribution to left ventricular filling in the elderly.

## Response to Stress

Exercise capacity, as indexed by maximal aerobic consumption, declines with age (39–41). This decline suggests an age-associated decrease in cardiac output and/or arteriovenous oxygen difference, the central and peripheral components of measured oxygen consumption, respectively. Although previous studies reported that exercise cardiac output declined with age as a result of a decrease in heart rate and stroke volume (41,42), in a population rigorously screened for coronary artery disease, exercise cardiac output is maintained with increasing age (27). Figure 3 shows the effect of age on cardiac output determined from upright bicycle exercise gated blood pool scans in a group of 61 participants aged 25–79 years in the Baltimore Longitudinal Study of Aging (27). All subjects were free of cardiac disease by history, physical examination, and normal

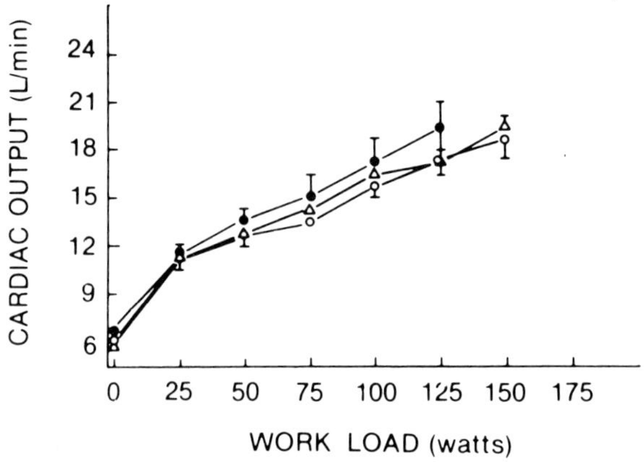


**Figure 3** Exercise cardiac output response to increasing work loads in young (aged 25–44 years, triangles), middle-aged (age 45–64 years, open circles), and elderly (age 65–80 years, closed circles) participants from the Baltimore Longitudinal Study of Aging. There were no age differences in resting or exercise cardiac output. (From Ref. 43.)

stress ECG thallium scans. The figure shows cardiac outputs were similar at rest and increasing work loads for the three age groups, young, middle-aged, and elderly.

Although cardiac output increased similarly with increasing work loads for each age group, young and older persons augmented cardiac output by different mechanisms (27). As shown in Figure 4A, young subjects had a large increase in heart rate from rest to exercise. Stroke volume increased with exercise in the younger subjects because of a large decrease in end-systolic volume compared to rest and only a small change in end-diastolic volume (Fig. 4). This exercise-induced increase in heart rate and decrease in end-systolic volume in young subjects is probably mediated via $\beta$-adrenergic stimulation. In contrast, older subjects had a much smaller increment in heart rate from rest to exercise compared to younger subjects at any level of cardiac output. Older subjects augmented their cardiac output with exercise by a greater increase in exercise stroke volume. This increase in stroke volume was due to cardiac dilatation during exercise (Frank-Starling mechanism), with a large increase in end-diastolic volume. This increase in end-diastolic volume during exercise suggests that the age-associated decrease in resting early diastolic filling does not persist during exercise.

Therefore, exercise cardiac output is maintained with age. Importantly, the mechanisms that account for the increase in exercise cardiac output differ according to age. Young subjects, through $\beta$-adrenergic stimulation, demon-

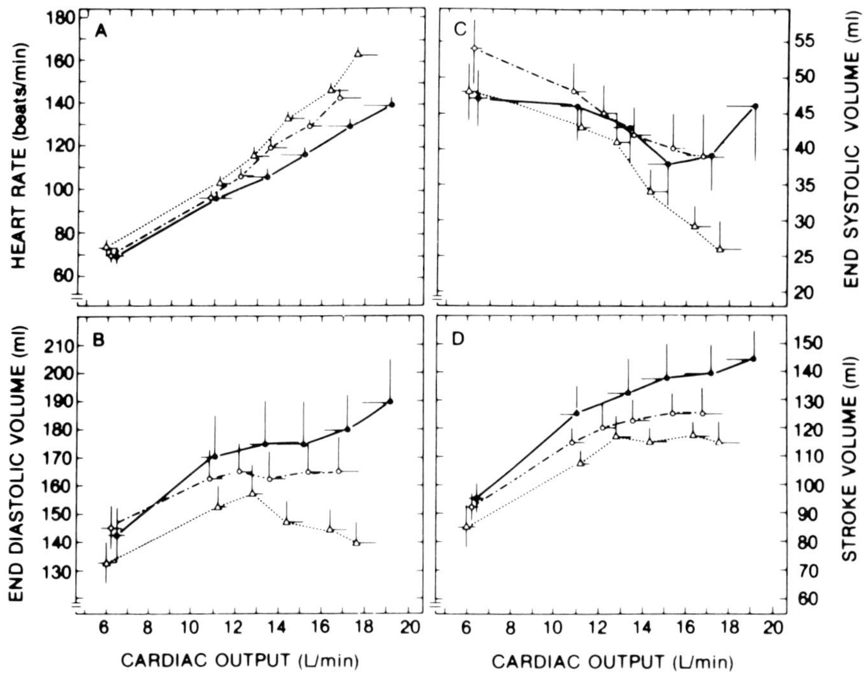


**Figure 4** The exercise related changes in heart rate (A), end-diastolic volume (B), end-systolic volume (C), and stroke volume (D) in the three age groups (see Fig. 3) according to increasing cardiac output. Older subjects had a large increase in end-diastolic volume and stroke volume with exercise (same symbols as Fig. 3). (From Ref. 43.)

strate a large increase in heart rate and decrease in end-systolic volume. Older subjects, likely because of the age-associated decreased responsiveness to catecholamines, show a failure of end-systolic volume to decrease and a less chronotropic response to exercise. End-diastolic volume increases in the older subject, with a consequent increase in exercise stroke volume. This shift to the Frank-Starling mechanism suggests some impairment of the exercise response in healthy elderly (43). Indeed, older subjects have less an increase in exercise ejection fraction compared to younger subjects.

The important role of $\beta$-adrenergic responsiveness in determining these age differences in the cardiac exercise response is suggested by studies in which young subjects were pretreated with intravenous propranolol before performing a bicycle exercise gated blood pool scan. The cardiac response of these $\beta$-blocked younger subjects is similar to that of older non–$\beta$-blocked subjects; that is, there is a large increase in end-diastolic volume to augment exercise cardiac output (44). Additional studies have demonstrated that the levels of norepinephrine and epinephrine at submaximal and maximal work loads in older subjects are similar to or greater than those in younger subjects (45). Therefore, this age-associated decrease in the $\beta$-adrenergic response during exercise is not due to a decrease in catecholamine levels but a decreased responsiveness to catecholamines likely due to alterations in $\beta$-receptor affinity for catecholamines (46,47).

The contribution of life-style to cardiovascular changes during exercise was highlighted by a recent study by Ehsani and coworkers (48). Healthy elderly subjects underwent 1 year of exercise conditioning. Maximum oxygen consumption improved significantly following training. Bicycle gated blood pool scans performed before and after training showed considerable changes in the cardiac response to exercise. Following training, exercise ejection fraction at maximal work load and the change in ejection fraction from rest to peak exercise were significantly greater than before training. Similar to the previous data, end-systolic volume did not change from rest to exercise in the initial study; however, it decreased significantly following training. This improvement led to a significantly greater exercise stroke volume and cardiac output. This decrease in end-systolic volume from rest to exercise following training (and thus an increase in exercise stroke volume, cardiac output, and ejection fraction) suggests an increased sensitivity to catecholamines and/or a decrease in arterial stiffness, which would decrease afterload and allow greater systolic emptying of the left ventricle.

## Ventricular–Vascular Coupling

The age differences in the cardiovascular response to exercise may relate not only to the decreased $\beta$-adrenergic responsiveness of senescent myocardium, but also to the vascular response to catecholamines. The human aorta undergoes changes in the composition and distribution of elastin and collagen that cause a stiffening of the central vessels (49). These pathological changes in the central arteries and arterioles lead to predictable hemodynamic changes, an increase in the afterload against which the left ventricle ejects.

Nichols and coworkers obtained invasive hemodynamic measurements in a group of 64 subjects without hypertension or coronary artery disease (50). Systemic vascular resistance increased progressively with increasing age. Characteristic impedance, a measurement of aortic stiffness, also increased with age. In a noninvasive study of arterial stiffness utilizing pulse wave velocity, Avolio et al. demonstrated a linear correlation between pulse wave velocity and age in a group of 524 rural Chinese subjects aged 2 months to 94 years (Fig. 5) (51). In this area of China there is a very low prevalence of atherosclerosis and hypertension, so the increase in vessel stiffness is likely a true age effect. The age-

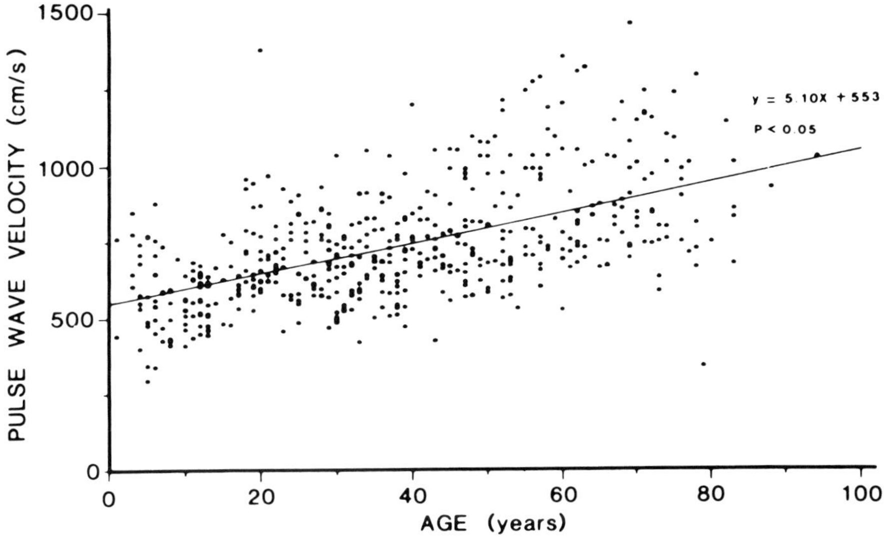


**Figure 5** The relationship of age and pulse wave velocity in rural China. Pulse wave velocity increased linearly with age. (From Ref. 51.)

associated increase in systolic blood pressure, pulse pressure (50), and left ventricular mass (26) are likely secondary to an increase in vascular stiffness.

This increase in afterload may have an important role in limiting the ability of older subjects to decrease end-systolic volume and increase ejection fraction with exercise. Similar to the animal model, it appears that arterial vasodilation to $\beta$-adrenergic stimulation is limited in older subjects. Van Brummelen et al. measured forearm blood flow and heart rate response to isoproterenol in a group of eight young and seven older subjects (52). The older subjects had a significantly lower chronotropic and vasodilator response to isoproterenol than the younger cohort. This diminished vasodilatation to catecholamines may result in a greater afterload to left ventricular ejection during exercise in older compared to younger subjects.

In conclusion, there is impressive agreement in animal models and humans on the age-associated changes in cardiovascular function. Both areas of research have demonstrated that there is not an inherent decline in the ability of senescent cardiac muscle to contract. The primary age-associated cardiovascular changes include prolonged relaxation, a decrease responsiveness of myocardium and vascular smooth muscle to $\beta$-adrenergic stimulation, and an increase in arterial stiffness with resultant increase in afterload. Whether these three changes are inherent to the aging process or due to a secondary change, such as the increasing sedentary life-style, are future areas of research. Healthy elderly appear to have adequate cardiac reserve, such as the Frank-Starling mechanism or the increase contribution of atrial contraction to end-diastolic volume, which maintain normal cardiac function at rest and exercise. However, these age-associated changes make the elderly more prone to develop symptoms in the setting of disease, such as hypertension, coronary artery disease, or atrial fibrillation. The manifestations and management of these common disorders in the elderly is the subject of the following chapters.

## REFERENCES

1. U.S. Bureau of the Census. Statistical Abstract of the United States, 101st ed. Washington, DC, 1980.
2. National Center for Health Statistics. Health, United States, 1984. DHHS Publication No. (PHS)85-1232, Hyattsville, MD,
3. Hypertension Detection Follow-up Group. Blood pressure studies in 14 communities: a two-stage screen for hypertension. JAMA 1977; 237:2385–2391.
4. Fleg JL, Gerstenblith G, Zonderman AB, Becker LC, Weisfeldt ML, Costa PT Jr, Lakatta EG. Prevalence and prognostic significance of exercise-induced silent myocardial ischemia detected by thallium scintigraphy and electrocardiography in asymptomatic volunteers. Circulation 1990; 81:428–436.
5. Elveback L, Lie JT. Continued high incidence of coronary artery disease at autopsy in Olmsted County, Minnesota, 1950 to 1979. Circulation 1984; 70:345–349.
6. Weisfeldt ML, Gerstenblith G. Cardiovascular aging and adaptation to disease. In: Hurst JW ed. The Heart, Arteries and Veins, 7th ed. New York: McGraw-Hill, 1900; 1488–1499.
7. Levy D, Anderson KM, Savage DD, Kannel WB, Christiansen JC, Castelli WP. Echocardiographically detected left ventricular hypertrophy: Prevalence and risk factors. The Framingham Study. Ann Intern Med 1988; 108:7–13.
8. Applegate WB. Hypertension in elderly patients. Ann Intern Med 1989; 110:901–915.
9. Levy D, Garrison RJ, Savage DD, Kannel WB, Castelli WP. Prognostic implications of echocardiographically determined left ventricular mass in the Framingham Heart Study. N Engl J Med 1990; 322:1561–1566.
10. Kannel WB, Gordon T, Schwartz MJ. Systolic versus diastolic blood pressure and risk of coronary artery disease. The Framingham Study. Am J Cardiol 1971; 27:335–346.
11. Gerstenblith G, Lakatta EG, Weisfeldt ML. Age changes in myocardial function and exercise response. Prog Cardiovasc Dis 1976; 19:1–21.
12. Weisfeldt ML, Loeven WA, Shock NW. Resting and active mechanical properties of trabeculae carneae from aged male rats. Am J Physiol 1971; 220:1921–1927.
13. Lakatta EG, Gerstenblith G, Angell CS, Shock NW, Weisfeldt ML. Prolonged contraction duration in aged myocardium. J Clin Invest 1975; 55:61–68.

14. Lakatta EG, Gerstenblith G, Angell CS, Shock NW, Weisfeldt ML. Diminished inotropic response of aged myocardium to catecholamines. Circ Res 1975; 36:262–269.
15. Yin FCP, Weisfeldt ML, Milnor WR. Role of aortic input impedance in the decreased cardiovascular response to exercise with aging in dogs. J Clin Invest 1981; 68:28–38.
16. Templeton GH, Platt MR, Willerson JT, Weisfeldt ML. Influence of aging on left ventricular hemodynamics and stiffness in beagles. Circ Res 1979; 44:189–194.
17. Capasso JM, Malhotra A, Remily RM, Scheuer J, Sonnenblick EH. Effects of age on mechanical and electrical performance of rat myocardium. Am J Physiol 1983; 245:H72–H81.
18. Wei JY, Spurgeon HA, Lakatta EG. Excitation-contraction coupling in rat myocardium: Alterations with adult aging. Am J Physiol 1984; 256:H784–H792.
19. Froelich JP, Lakatta EG, Beard E, Spurgeon HA, Weisfeldt ML, Gerstenblith G. Studies of sarcoplasmic reticulum function and contraction duration in young adult and aged rat myocardium. J Mol Cell Cardiol 1978; 10:427–438.
20. Spurgeon HA, Steinback MF, Lakatta EG. Chronic exercise prevents characteristic age-related changes rat cardiac contraction. Am J Physiol 1983; 244:H513–H518.
21. Penpargkul S, Repke DI, Katz AM, Scheuer J. Effect of physical training on calcium transport by rat cardiac sarcoplasmic reticulum. Circ Res 1977; 40:134–138.
22. Yin FCP, Spurgeon HA, Raizes GS, Greene HL, Weisfeldt ML, Shock NW. Age associated decrease in chronotropic response to isoproterenol. Circulation 1976; 54:II–167.
23. Guarnieri T, Filburn CR, Zitnik G, Roth GS, Lakatta EG. Contractile and biochemical correlates of beta-adrenergic stimulation of the aged heart. Am J Physiol 1980; 239:H501–H508.
24. Yin FCP. The aging vasculature and its effect on the heart. In: Weisfeldt ML, ed. The Aging Heart. New York: Raven Press, 1980: 137.
25. Fleisch JH, Hooker CS. The relationship between age and relaxation of vascular smooth muscle in the rabbit and rat. Circ Res 1976; 38:243–249.
26. Gerstenblith G, Frederiksen J, Yin FCP, Fortuin NJ, Lakatta EG, Weisfeldt ML. Echocardiographic assessment of a normal adult aging population. Circulation 1977; 56:273–278.
27. Rodeheffer RJ, Gerstenblith G, Becker LC, Fleg JL, Weisfeldt ML, Lakatta EG. Exercise cardiac output is maintained with advancing age in healthy human subjects: Cardiac dilatation and increased stroke volume compensate for a diminished heart rate. Circulation 1984; 69:203–213.
28. Port S, Cobb FR, Coleman RE, Jones RH. Effect of age on the response of the left ventricular ejection fraction to exercise. N Engl J Med 1980; 303:1133–1137.
29. Hirota Y. A clinical study of left ventricular relaxation. Circulation 1980; 62:756–763.
30. Harrison TR, Dixon K, Russell RO Jr, Bidwai PS, Coleman HN. The relation of age to the duration of contraction, ejection, and relaxation of the normal human heart. Am Heart J 1964; 67:189–199.

31. Miller TR, Grossman SJ, Schectman KB, Biello DR, Ludbrook PA, Ehsani AA. Left ventricular diastolic filling and its association with age. Am J Cardiol 1986; 58:531–535.
32. Migatake K, Okanoto M, Kinoshita N, Owa M, Nakasone I, Sakakibana H, Nimura Y. Augmentation of atrial contribution to left ventricular inflow with aging as assessed by intracardiac Doppler flowmetry. Am J Cardiol 1984; 53:586–590.
33. Fouad FM. Left ventricular diastolic function in hypertensive patients. Circulation 1987; 75:I-48–55.
34. Nixon JV, Hallmark H, Page K, Raven RP, Mitchell JH. Ventricular performance in human hearts aged 61 to 73 years. Am J Cardiol 1985; 56:932–937.
35. Bahler RC, Martin P. Effects of loading conditions and inotropic state on rapid filling phase of left ventricle. Am J Physiol 1985; 248:H523–H533.
36. Bonow RO, Vitale DF, Bacharach SL, Maron BJ, Green MV. Effects of aging on asynchronous left ventricular regional function and global ventricular filling in normal human subjects. J Am Coll Cardiol 1988; 11:50–58.
37. Schulman SP, Gerstenblith G, Fleg JL, Becker LC, Lakatta L, Drinkwater D, Lakatta EG. Vigorous exercise training does not prevent slowed and delayed early diastolic filling in healthy older men (abstr). Circulation 1988; 78(Suppl II):984.
38. Arora RR, Machac J, Goldman ME, Butler RN, Gorlin R, Horowitz SF. Atrial kinetics and left ventricular diastolic filling in the healthy elderly. J Am Coll Cardiol 1987; 9:1255–1260.
39. Hossack KF, Bruce RA. Maximal cardiac function in sedentary normal men and women: Comparison of age-related changes. J Appl Physiol 1982; 53:799–804.
40. Dehn MM, Bruce RA. Longitudinal variations in maximal oxygen intake with age and activity. J Appl Physiol 1972; 33:805–807.
41. Higginbotham MB, Morris KG, Williams RS, Coleman RE, Cobb FR. Physiologic basis for the age-related decline in aerobic work capacity. Am J Cardiol 1986; 57:1374–1379.
42. Julius A, Amery A, Whitlock LS, Conway J. Influence of age on the hemodynamic response to exercise. Circulation 1967; 36:222–230.
43. Gerstenblith G, Renlund DG, Lakatta EG. Cardiovascular response to exercise in younger and older men. Fed Proc 1987; 46:1834–1839.
44. Fleg JL, Schulman S, O'Connor F, Gerstenblith G, Clulow JF, Renlund DG, Lakatta EG. Effect of propranolol on age-associated changes in left ventricular performance during exercise (abstr). Circulation 1991; 84(Suppl II):187.
45. Fleg JL, Tzankoff SP, Lakatta EG. Age-related augmentation of plasma catecholamines during dynamic exercise in healthy males. J Appl Physiol 1985; 59:1033–1039.
46. Feldman RD, Limbird LE, Nadeau J, Robertson D, Wood AJJ. Alterations in leukocyte B-receptor affinity with aging. A potential explanation for altered B-adrenergic sensitivity in the elderly. N Engl J MEd 1984; 310:815–819.
47. Brodde OE, Kretsch R, Ikezono K, Zerkowski HR, Reidemeister JC. Human B-adrenoreceptors: Relation of myocardial and lymphocyte B-adrenoreceptor density. Science 1986; 231:1584–1585.

48. Ehsani AA, Agawa T, Miller TR, Spina RJ, Jilka SM. Exercise training improves left ventricular systolic function in older men. Circulation 1991; 83:96–103.
49. Hallock P, Benson IC. Studies of the elastic properties of human isolated aorta. J Clin Invest 1937; 16:595–602.
50. Nichols WW, O'Rourke MF, Avolio AP, Yaginuma T, Murgo JP, Pepine CJ, Conti CR. Effects of age on ventricular-vascular coupling. Am J Cardiol 1985; 55:1179–1184.
51. Avolio AP, Fa-Quan D, Wei-Qiang L, Yao-Fei L, Zhen-Dong H, Lian-Fen X, O'Rourke MF. Effects of aging on arterial distensibility in populations with high and low prevalence of hypertension: Comparison between urban and rural communities in China. Circulation 1985; 71:202–210.
52. Van Brummelen P, Buhler FR, Kiowski W, Amann FW. Age-related decrease in cardiac and peripheral vascular responsiveness to isoprenaline. Studies in normal subjects. Clin Sci 1981; 60:571–577.

# 2

# Morphological Features of the Elderly Heart

**William C. Roberts**
*Baylor Cardiovascular Institute, Baylor University Medical Center, Dallas, Texas*

## INTRODUCTION

As in any body tissue or organ, changes take place in the cardiovascular system as life progresses. Some of these changes allow easy identification of the very elderly heart when examining autopsy cardiac specimens as unknowns. The "normal" elderly heart has relatively small ventricular cavities and relatively large atria and great arteries. The ascending aorta and left atrium, in comparison with the relatively small left ventricular cavity, appear particularly large. The coronary arteries increase in both length and width; the former, particularly in association with the decreasing size of the cardiac ventricles, results in arterial tortuosity. (The young river is straight and the old one, winding.) The subepicardial adipose tissue increases in amount with aging. The leaflets of each of the four cardiac valves thicken with age, particularly the atrioventricular valves; these have a smaller area to occupy in the ventricles because of the diminished size of the latter. Histological examination discloses large quantities of lipofuscin pigment in myocardial cells; some contain mucoid deposits ("mucoid degeneration"). These changes appear to affect all population groups of elderly individuals irrespective of where they reside on the earth or their level of serum lipids. An elevated systemic arterial pressure appears to both accelerate and amplify these normal expected cardiac changes of aging.

Both the aorta and its branches and the major pulmonary arteries and their branches enlarge with age. Because the enlargement is in both the longitudinal and the transverse dimensions, the aorta, as the coronary arteries, tends to become tortuous. This process is further amplified as the vertebral bodies become smaller and the height, somewhat shorter. The major pulmonary arteries appear to be too short and to have too low a pressure to dilate longitudinally.

The amount of information at necropsy in very elderly persons is relatively sparse. In 1983, Waller and I (1) described some clinical and necropsy findings in 40 patients aged 90 years and over at death. Since that time 53 additional patients aged 90 or more years have been studied at necropsy in this laboratory (2). This chapter summarizes certain clinical and necropsy cardiac findings in the 93 patients aged 90 years or over.

## PATIENTS STUDIED

Certain clinical findings are summarized in Table 1. The ages at death ranged from 90 to 103 years (mean 93); 51 (55%) were men and 42 (45%) were women; 59 (63%) were white, 33 (36%) black, and 1 (1%) was Asian. Only 20

**Table 1** Clinical Findings in 93 Patients ≥ 90 Years of Age

| Variable | Number (%) |
|---|---|
| 1. Age, years | 90–103, mean 93 |
| 2. Male-female | 51 (55)–42 (45) |
| 3. Black-white-Asian | 33 (35)–59 (63)–1 (1) |
| 4. Systemic hypertension | 50 (54) |
| 5. Diabetes mellitus | 8 (9) |
| 6. Atrial fibrillation | 21/56 (38) |
| 7. Bundle branch block | 18/51 (35) |
| Right = 7 | |
| Left = 9 | |
| Both = 2 | |
| 8. Clinical evidence of myocardial ischemia | 20 (21) |
| Angina pectoris only = 3 | |
| Acute myocardial infarction only = 16 | |
| Both angina and acute infarction = 1 | |
| 9. Chronic congestive heart failure | 21 (23) |
| 10. Cause of death | |
| Cardiac | 29 (31) |
| Vascular, noncardiac | 17 (18) |
| Noncardiac, nonvascular | 47 (51) |

**Table 2** Cardiac Necropsy Findings in 93 Patients ≥ 90 Years of Age

| Variable | Number (%) |
|---|---|
| 1. Heart weight, g | 220–660, mean 418 |
| Men 260–660, mean 436 | |
| Women 220–630, mean 397 | |
| 2. Increased heart weight | 51 (55) |
| >400 g, men 29/51 (57) | |
| >350 g, women 22/42 (52) | |
| 3. One or more major coronary arteries narrowed >75% in cross-sectional area by plaque | 59 (63) |
| Men 33/51 (65) | |
| Women 26/42 (62) | |
| 4. Numbers of four major coronary arteries narrowed > 75% in cross-sectional area by plaque | 107/372 (29) |
| Men 57/204 (28) | |
| Women 50/168 (30) | |
| 5. Myocardial infarct | 35 (38) |
| Acute only = 10 (posterior = 4) | |
| Healed only = 21 (posterior = 14) | |
| Both = 4 | |
| 6. Calcium in | |
| Coronary arteries | 88 (95) |
| Mitral valve annulus | 39 (42) |
| $1^+$ = 20/39 (51) | |
| $2^+$ = 8/39 (21) | |
| $3^+$ = 11/39 (28) | |
| Aortic valve cusps | 59 (63) |
| $1^+$ = 43/59 (73) | |
| $2^+$ = 10/59 (17) | |
| $3^+$ = 6/59 (10) | |
| Papillary muscles | 22/25 (88) |
| 7. Dilated cardiac ventricle | 21/53 (40) |
| Right ventricle only = 3/53 (6) | |
| Left ventricle only = 1/53 (2) | |
| Both = 17/53 (32) | |
| 8. Cardiac amyloidosis | 16 (17) |
| Causing cardiac dysfunction = 9/16 (56) | |
| Not causing cardiac dysfunction = 7/16 (44) | |

of the 93 patients (21%) had clinical evidence of myocardial ischemia, either angina pectoris or acute myocardial infarction, or both. Although it is recognized that chronic congestive heart failure may be difficult to diagnose in elderly individuals, such was stated to be present in 21 patients (23%). A total of 50 patients (54%) had systemic hypertension by history, and 8 (9), diabetes mellitus. Death was attributed to a cardiac cause in 29 patients (31%), to a noncardiac but vascular cause in 17 patients (18%), and to a noncardiac and nonvascular cause in 47 patients (51%).

Certain necropsy findings are summarized in Table 2 and illustrated in Figures 1 through 19. The heart was increased in weight in 51 (55%) of the 93 patients. It averaged 397 g in the women and 436 g (9% more) in the men. Although only 20 patients (21%) were stated to have had evidence of myocardial ischemia during life, at necropsy 59 patients (63%) had 1 or more of the 4 major coronary arteries (left main, left anterior descending, left circumflex, and right) narrowed >75% in cross-sectional area by plaque. Of the 59 patients with significant (>75% cross-sectional area narrowing) narrowing of 1 or more major coronary arteries, 20 patients (34%) had only 1 artery so narrowed by plaque, 30 patients (51%) had 2 major arteries so narrowed, and 9 patients (15%) had 3 arteries so narrowed. No patient had all 4 major coronary arteries severely narrowed, and no patient had significant narrowing of the left main coronary artery. Of the 236 major coronary arteries in the 59 patients with significant coronary artery narrowing, 95 arteries (40%) were narrowed >75% in cross-sectional area by plaque, an average of 1.81 of 4 arteries per patient. Of the 51 men, 33 (65%) had 1 or more major coronary arteries significantly narrowed, and of the 42 women, 26 (62%) had significant narrowing. Of the 132 major coronary arteries in the 33 men, 57 arteries (37%; 1.72 per man) were significantly narrowed by plaque, and of the 104 major coronary arteries in the 26 women with significant coronary disease, 50 (40%; 1.92 per woman) were narrowed significantly by plaque.

**Figure 1** Tortuous and heavily calcified coronary arteries in a 95-year-old woman (SH #A80-74) who never had symptoms of cardiac dysfunction and who died from a perforated gastric ulcer. Top left: postmortem radiogram of the excised right (R), left main (LM), left anterior descending (LAD), and left circumflex (LC) coronary arteries. Top center: radiogram of a portion of the heart after removing the walls of the atria and most of the walls of the ventricles. MVA = mitral valve annulus. Top right and lower panels: photomicrographs of coronary arteries at sites of maximal narrowing by calcified atherosclerotic plaques. (Movat stains; magnification ×17, reduced 40%.) This case illustrates extensive calcific deposits in the coronary arteries without significant luminal narrowing.

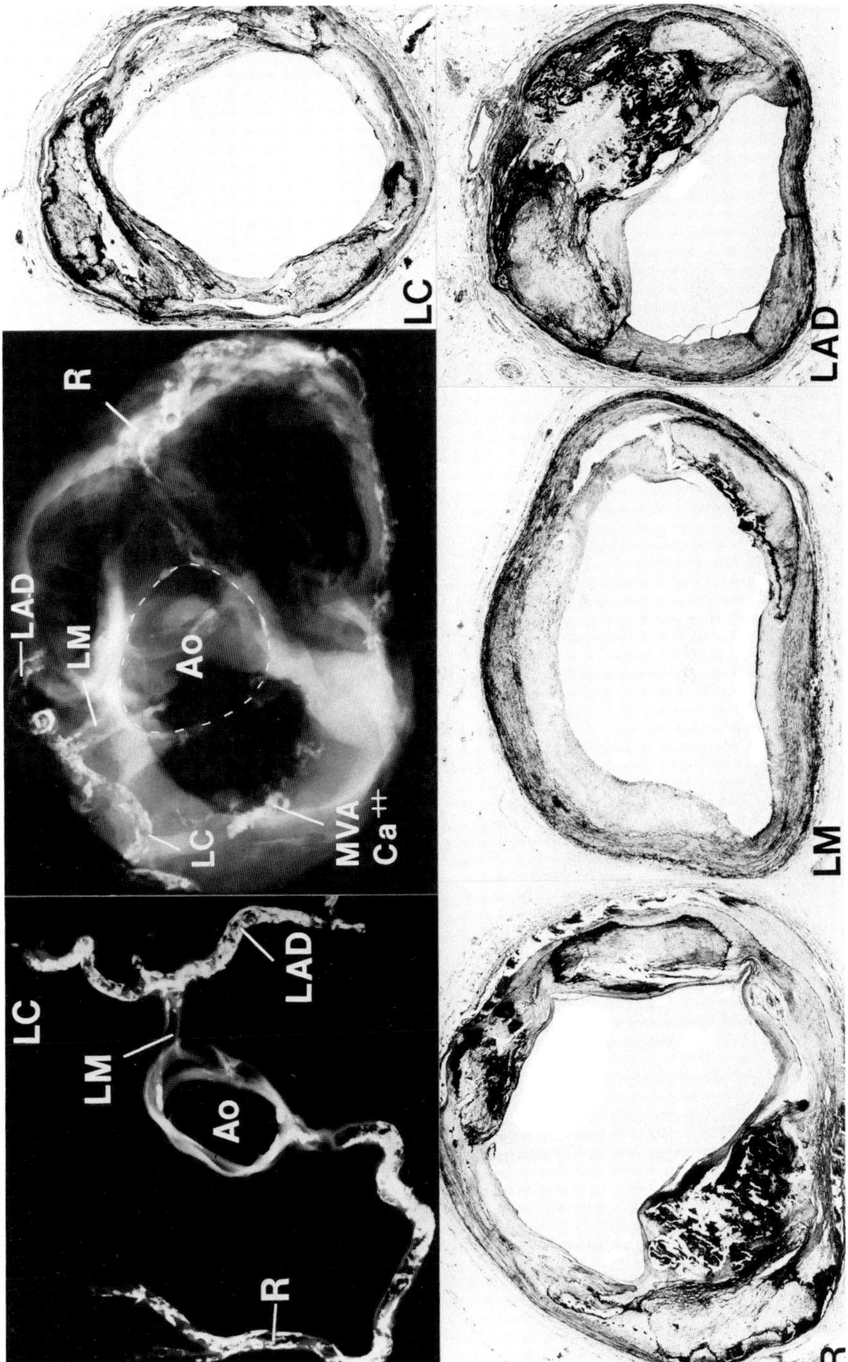
LC
LM
LAD
Ao
R
LAD
LM
Ao
R
LC
MVA
Ca++
LC
LAD
LM
R

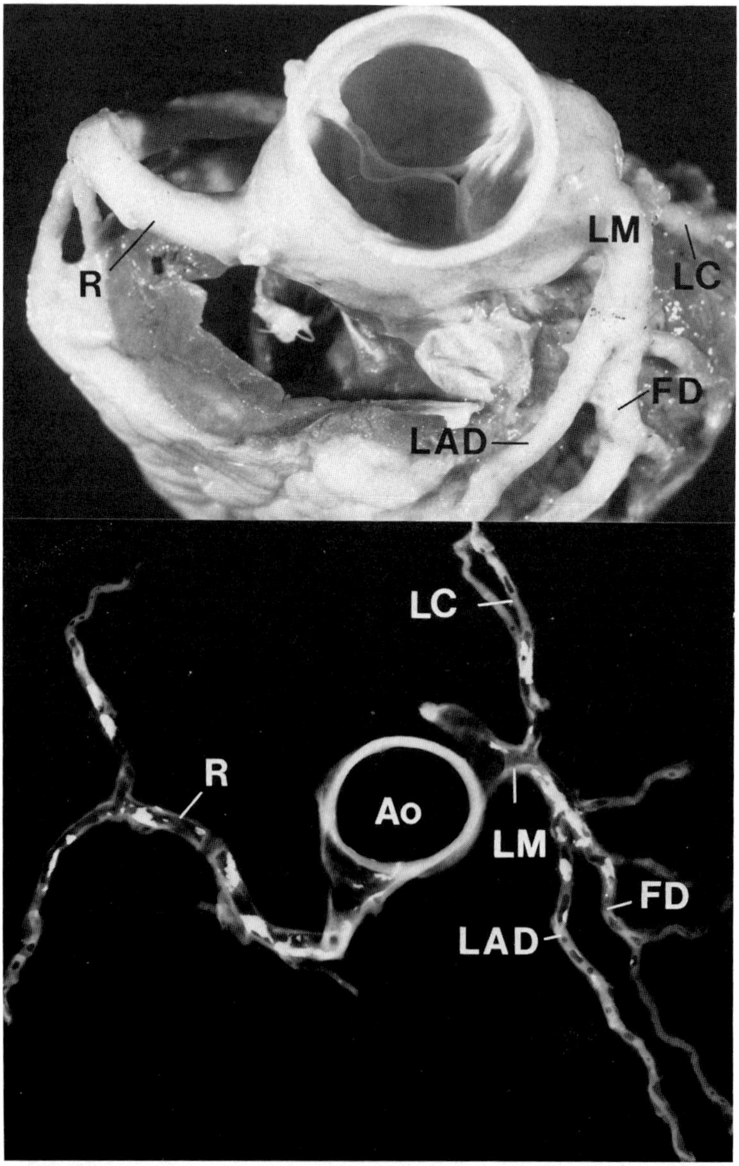


**Figure 2** Coronary arteries in a 95-year-old man (SH #A79-77) who never had symptoms of cardiac dysfunction and who died from cancer. Top: aorta and coronary arteries from above. Bottom: radiograms of aortic root (Ao) and excised coronary arteries that contain calcific deposits. FD = first diagonal, LAD = left anterior descending, LC = left circumflex, LM = left main, R = right.

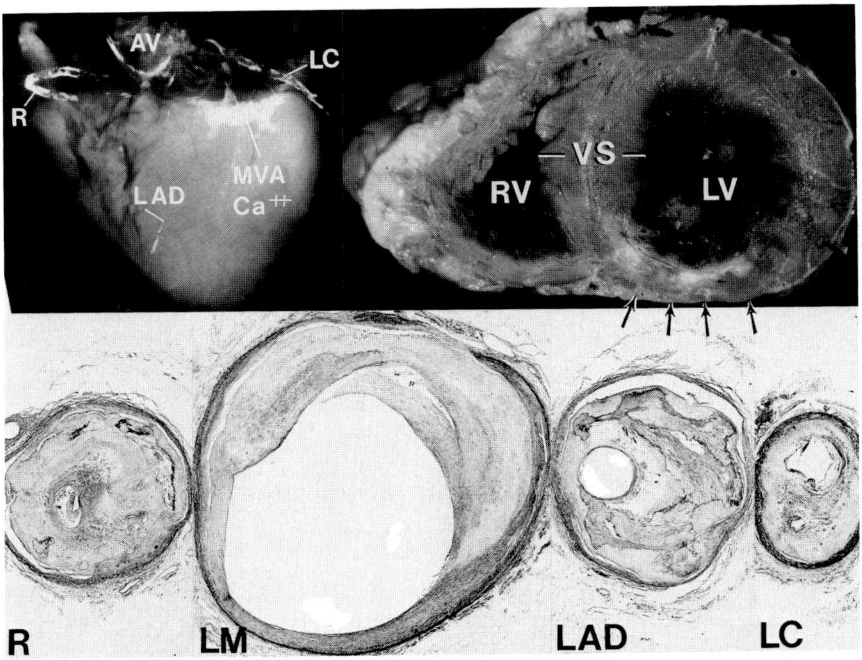


**Figure 3** Heart and coronary arteries in a 93-year-old woman (LRC #5) who was hospitalized with worsening chronic congestive heart failure. Top left: postmortem radiogram showing calcific deposits in the right (R), left anterior descending (LAD), and left circumflex (LC) coronary arteries and in the mitral valve annulus (MVA) and aortic valve. Top right: view of right (RV) and left (LV) ventricles and ventricular septum (VS) showing a transmural scar (arrows). Bottom: coronary arteries at sites of maximal narrowing. LM = left main. (Movat stains; magnification ×17, reduced 40%.)

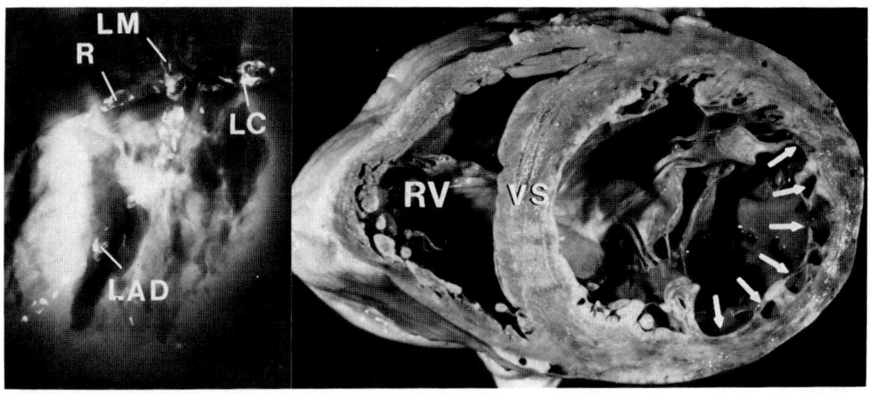


**Figure 4** This 91-year-old woman (LRC #3) had a "typical" clinical acute myocardial infarct, which was fatal. Left: postmortem radiogram showing calcific deposits in the right (R), left main (LM), left anterior descending (LAD), and left circumflex (LC) coronary arteries. Right: view of left and right (RV) ventricles showing transmural necrosis and fibrosis (arrows) and dilated ventricles. VS = ventricular septum.

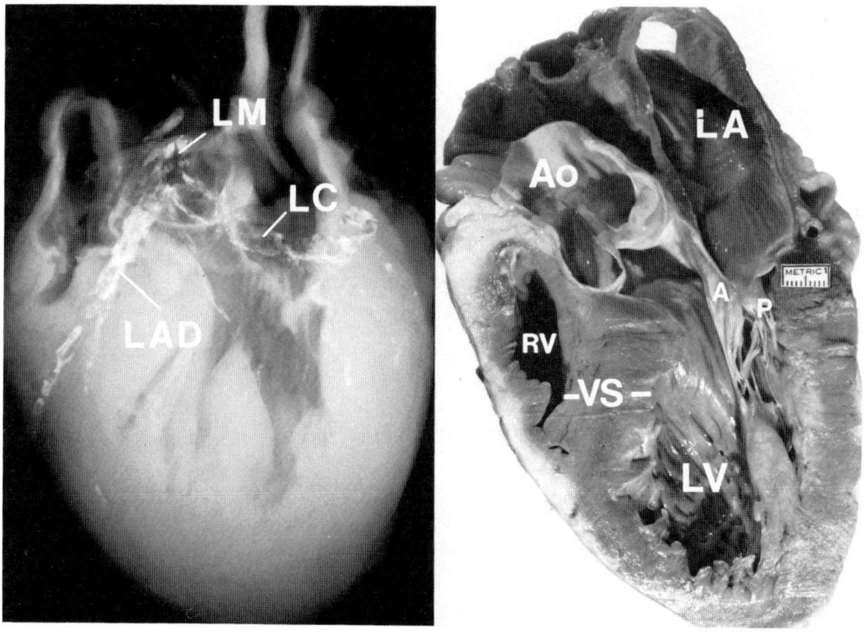


**Figure 5** This 90-year-old woman (SH #A82-1) had no symptoms of cardiac dysfunction and died from a ruptured fusiform abdominal aortic aneurysm. Left: postmortem radiogram of the entire heart showing calcific deposits in the left anterior descending (LAD), left circumflex (LC), and left main (LM) coronary arteries. Right: view of heart cut in an anteroposterior fashion (M-mode or long-axis two-dimensional echocardiographic view) showing a dilated left atrium (LA) and left ventricle (LV). A and P = anterior and posterior mitral valve leaflets; Ao = aorta; RV = right ventricle; VS = ventricular septum.

Myocardial infarction occurred in 35 patients (38% of the total), and all of them had significant narrowing by plaque of one or more major epicardial coronary arteries. Grossly visible acute infarcts without a grossly visible healed infarct occurred in 10 patients (29%), healed infarct only in 21 patients (60%), and both acute and healed infarcts in 4 patients (11%).

Calcific deposits were present at some site in the heart in nearly all patients. Of the 93 patients, 88 (95%) had calcific deposits in atherosclerotic plaques in the epicardial coronary arteries; 39 patients (42%) had grossly visible calcific deposits in the mitral annulus ($1^+$ in 20 patients, 51%; $2^+$ in 8 patients, 21%; and $3^+$ in 11 patients, 28%); 59 patients (63%) had grossly visible calcific deposits on the aortic aspects of the aortic valve cusps ($1^+$ in 43 patients, 73%; $2^+$ in 10 patients, 17%; and $3^+$ in 6 patients, 10%), and 22 (88%) of the 245

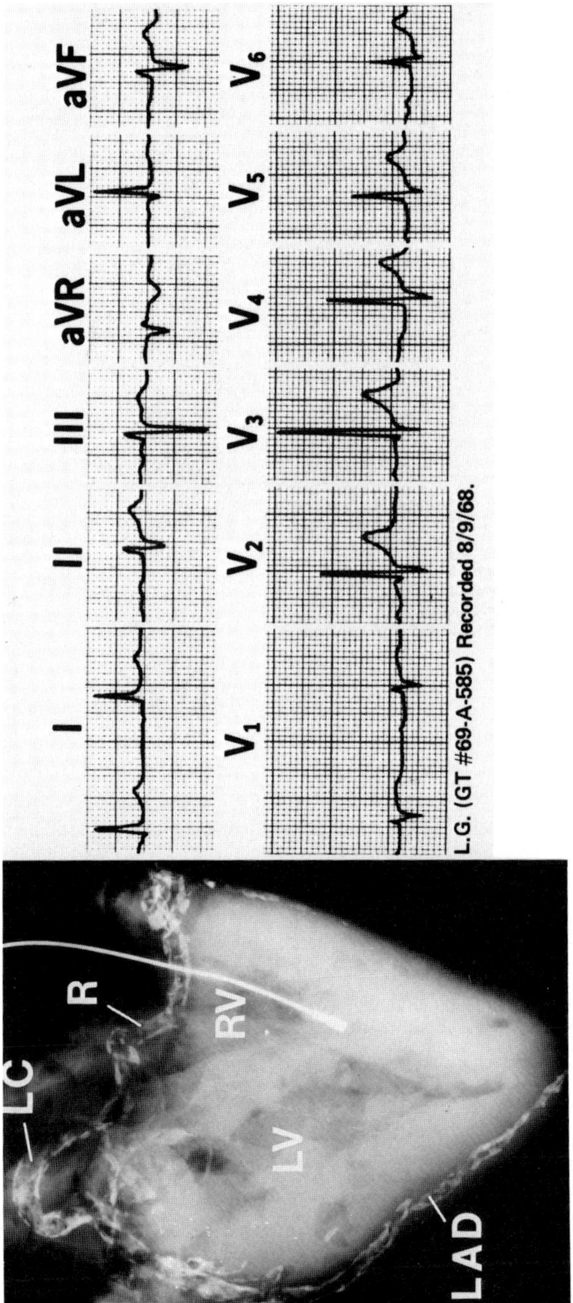


**Figure 6** This 97-year-old man (GT #69A-585) had complete heart block and had a pacemaker inserted when he was 91 years old. Left: radiogram of heart at necropsy showing calcific deposits in the left anterior descending (LAD), left circumflex (LC), and right (R) coronary arteries and a pacemaker wire in the right ventricle (RV). LV = left ventricle. Right: electrocardiogram.

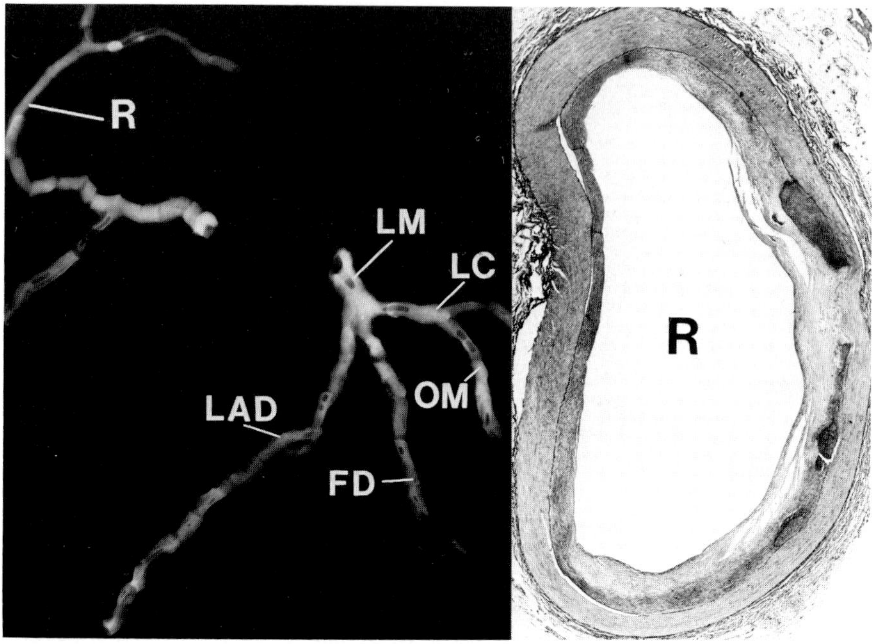


**Figure 7** This 96-year-old woman (DCGH #68A80) had chronic congestive heart failure from dilated cardiomyopathy. Her total serum cholesterol level was 108 mg/dl. Left: postmortem radiogram of the right (R), left main (LM), left anterior descending (LAD), left circumflex (LC), first diagonal (FD), and left obtuse marginal (OM) coronary arteries showing no calcific deposits. Right: right coronary artery section devoid of calcium or narrowing. (Movat stain; magnification $\times 16$, reduced 23%.)

patients examined specifically for calcific deposits in the left ventricular papillary muscles had these deposits in these locations. The 10 patients with $2^+$ and the 6 patients with $3^+$ calcium in the aortic valve cusps were considered to have sufficient amounts of calcium to prevent full opening of the orifices during ventricular systole, and therefore these 16 patients (17% of the 93 patients) actually had aortic valve stenosis.

Dilatation of either the right or left ventricle was present by gross inspection in 4 of 53 hearts examined specifically for cavity dilatation, and 17 patients (32%) had dilatation of both right and left ventricular cavities.

Cardiac amyloidosis was present in 16 of the 93 patients (17%): in 9 patients (56%) the deposits were large in amount and the cardiac amyloidosis caused cardiac dysfunction, fatal in 8; the other 7 patients (44%) had no grossly visible evidence of cardiac amyloid, which was found only on histological sections of the cardiac walls (3).

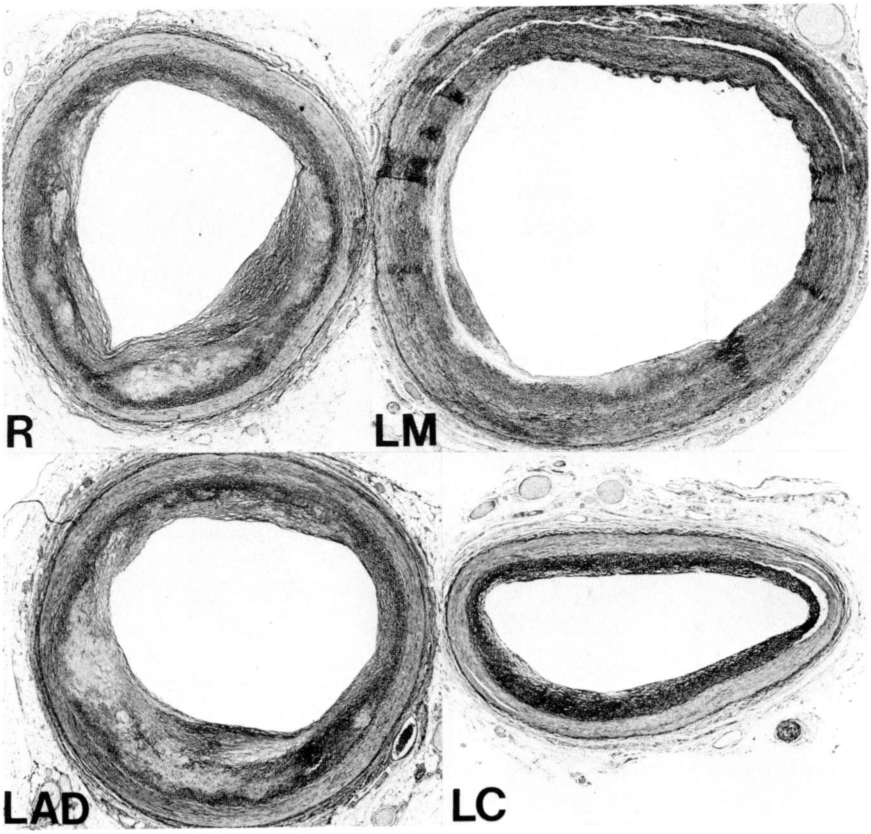


**Figure 8** Right (R), left main (LM), left anterior descending (LAD), and left circumflex (LC) coronary arteries at sites of maximal narrowing in a 103-year-old woman (GT #70A301). She never had evidence of cardiac dysfunction and died from complications of a duodenal ulcer. The coronary arteries are devoid of calcium and of significant narrowing. (Elastic-van Gieson's stain; magnification × 16, reduced 31%.)

## ELECTROCARDIOGRAPHIC FINDINGS

Information on electrocardiograms recorded at age 90 years or later was available in 30 of the 93 patients (1). Of the 30 patients, 3 had electrocardiograms recorded during acute myocardial infarction. The electrocardiograms in all 3, however, disclosed only atrial fibrillation and complete left bundle branch block, and these findings in all 3 patients were known to be present before the fatal acute myocardial infarction. The electrocardiograms in the other 27 patients were not recorded during periods of acute myocardial ischemia. Of the

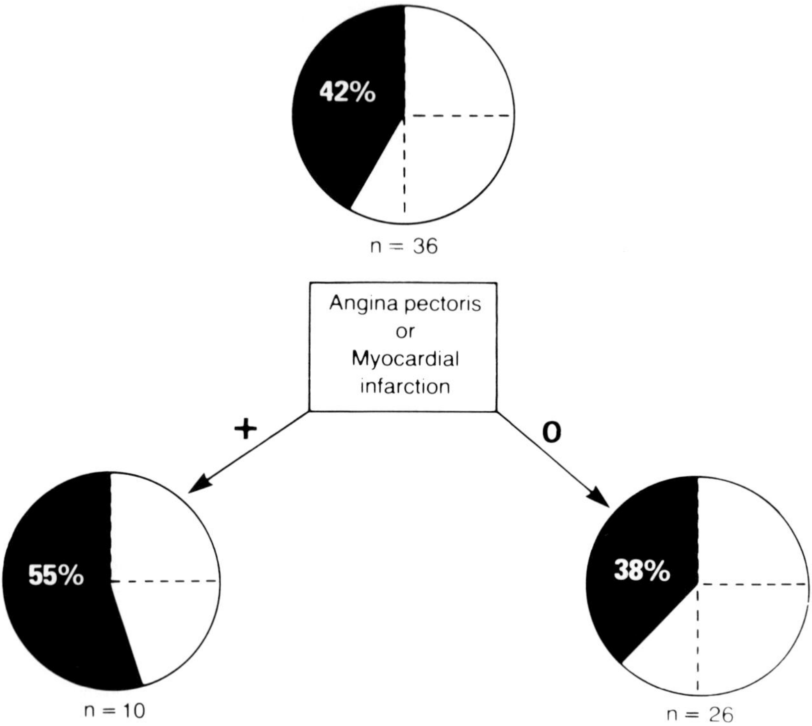


**Figure 9** Mean percentage cross-sectional area narrowing by atherosclerotic plaques in 1789 segments (5 mm) of the four major epicardial coronary arteries in 36 necropsy patients aged 90 years and older, 10 of whom had angina pectoris or acute myocardial infarction, or both, and 26 of whom did not. The mean percentage of narrowing for each 5-mm segment differs significantly in the group with clinical evidence of myocardial ischemia (55%) and the group without such evidence ($p < 0.05$).

30 patients on whom electrocardiographic information was available, 8 had clinical evidence of heart disease and 22 did not; the findings are summarized in Table 3. The total 12-lead QRS voltage ranged from 82 to 251 mm (mean 151; 10 mm = 1 mV). In the 19 women, the total voltage ranged from 82 to 251 mm (mean 158) and, in the 5 men, from 105 to 154 mm (mean 101; $p < 0.05$). The total 12-lead QRS voltage did not correlate with either heart ($r = -0.01$) or body weight ($r = -0.2$). The 24 patients in whom the total 12-lead QRS voltage was measured were separated into two groups: 8 patients in whom clinical evidence of cardiac dysfunction was present (coronary heart disease in 5, massive cardiac amyloid in 2, and aortic valve stenosis in 1) and 16 patients without

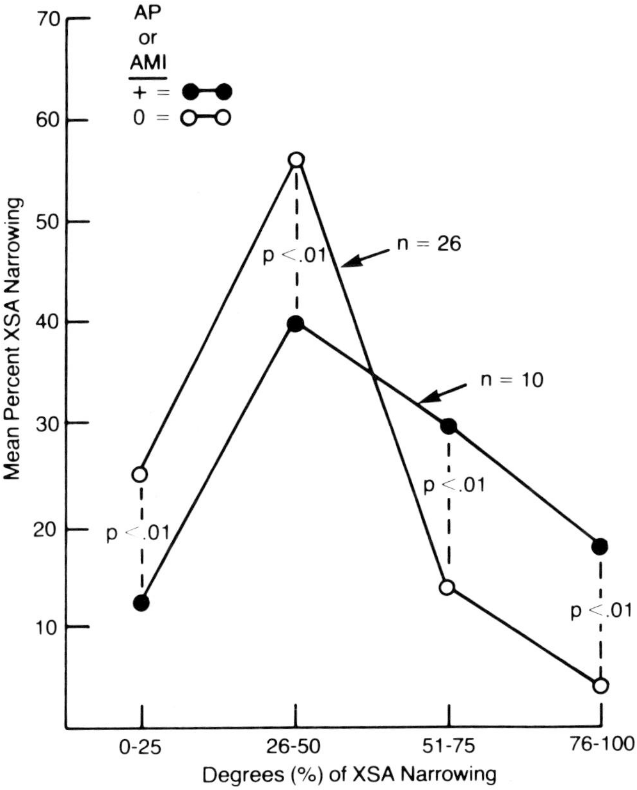


**Figure 10** Mean percentage cross-sectional area (XSA) narrowing by atherosclerotic plaques in the 5-mm segments of the right, left main, left anterior descending, and left circumflex coronary arteries in the 36 patients in whom the four major coronary arteries in their entirety were available for examination. The 36 patients were classified into 10 with and 26 without clinical evidence of myocardial ischemia. For each of the four categories of narrowing, a highly significant ($p < 0.01$) difference in the amount of narrowing was observed.

such evidence (Table 3). Comparison of the total QRS voltage in the 8 patients with and in the 16 patients without clinical evidence of heart disease disclosed no significant difference (mean 147 versus 152 mm). Breakdown on the 8 patients with cardiac dysfunction did show some differences: the total 12-lead QRS voltage in the 5 patients with angina pectoris or acute myocardial infarction ranged from 123 to 163 mm (mean 143); in the 2 patients with massive cardiac amyloidosis it was 102 and 117 mm (mean 109); and in the 1 patient with

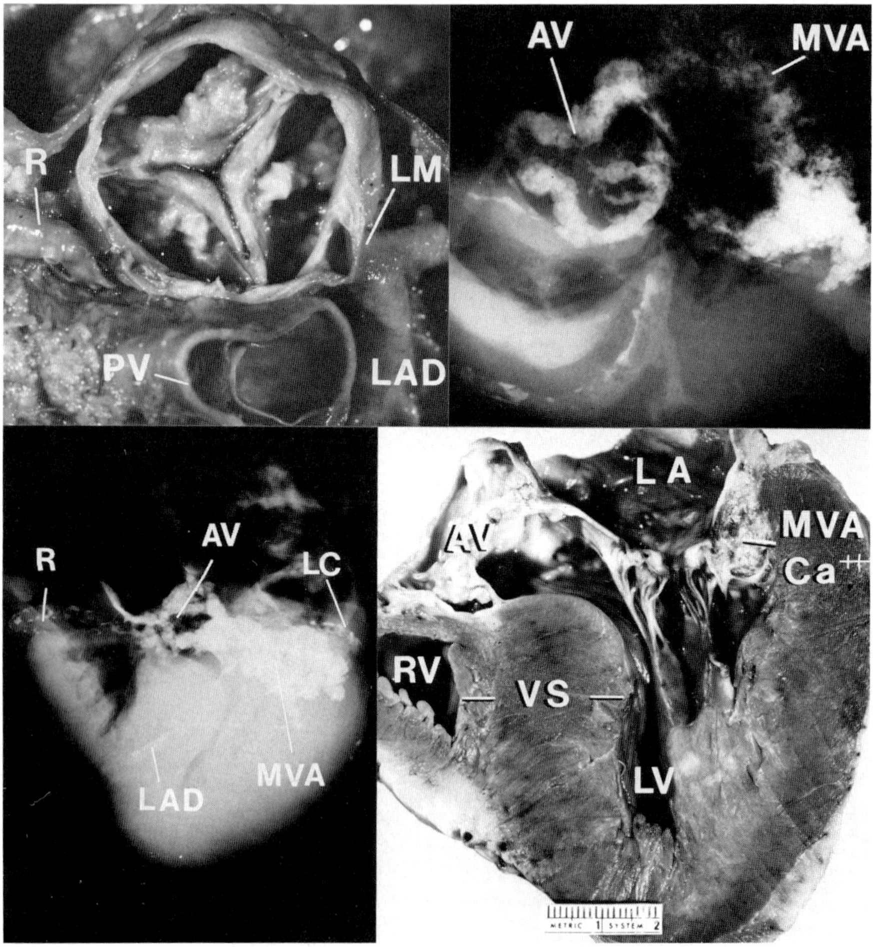


**Figure 11** A 92-year-old woman (GT #78A58) with clinically recognized and eventually fatal aortic valve stenosis. Top left: stenotic aortic valve from above. PV = pulmonic valve; R = right; LM = left main; LAD = left anterior descending coronary arteries. Top right: postmortem radiogram showing heavy calcific deposits in the aortic valve (AV) and in the mitral valve annular (MVA) region. Bottom left: radiogram of the heart at necropsy showing calcific deposits in the coronary arteries, in the aortic valve, and in the mitral annular region. Bottom right: long-axis view of heart (M-mode or two-dimensional long-axis view) showing a small left ventricular (LV) cavity, a thickened and "sigmoid-shaped" ventricular septum (VS), and the stenotic aortic valve just above the right ventricular (RV) outflow tract. LA = left atrium.

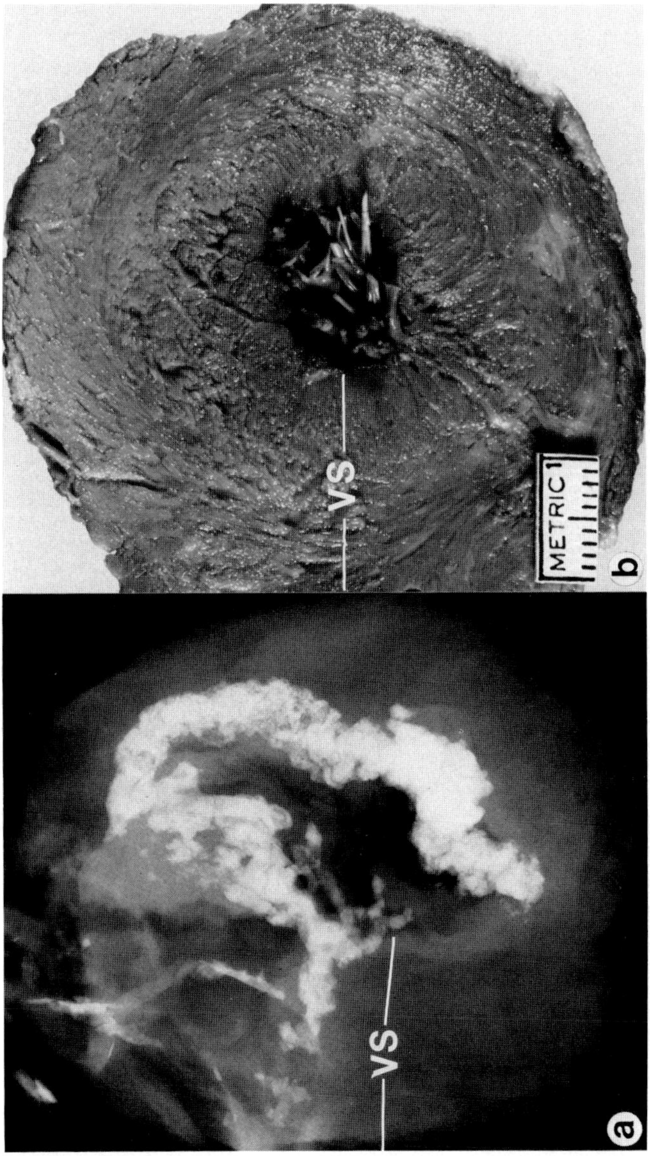


**Figure 12** A 90-year-old woman (GT #80A126) with heavy mitral valve annular calcific deposits that reduced the mitral valve orifice to <1 cm in diameter (a). The unusual feature of the mitral calcium in this patient was that it not only was located behind the posterior mitral leaflet (mitral annular region) but it also extended across the anterior mitral leaflet, nearly producing a letter O), as has been described previously. She died from rupture of a descending thoracic aortic aneurysm. VS = ventricular septum. (b) View of the left ventricle at the level of the tips of the mitral leaflets, showing a very small cavity.

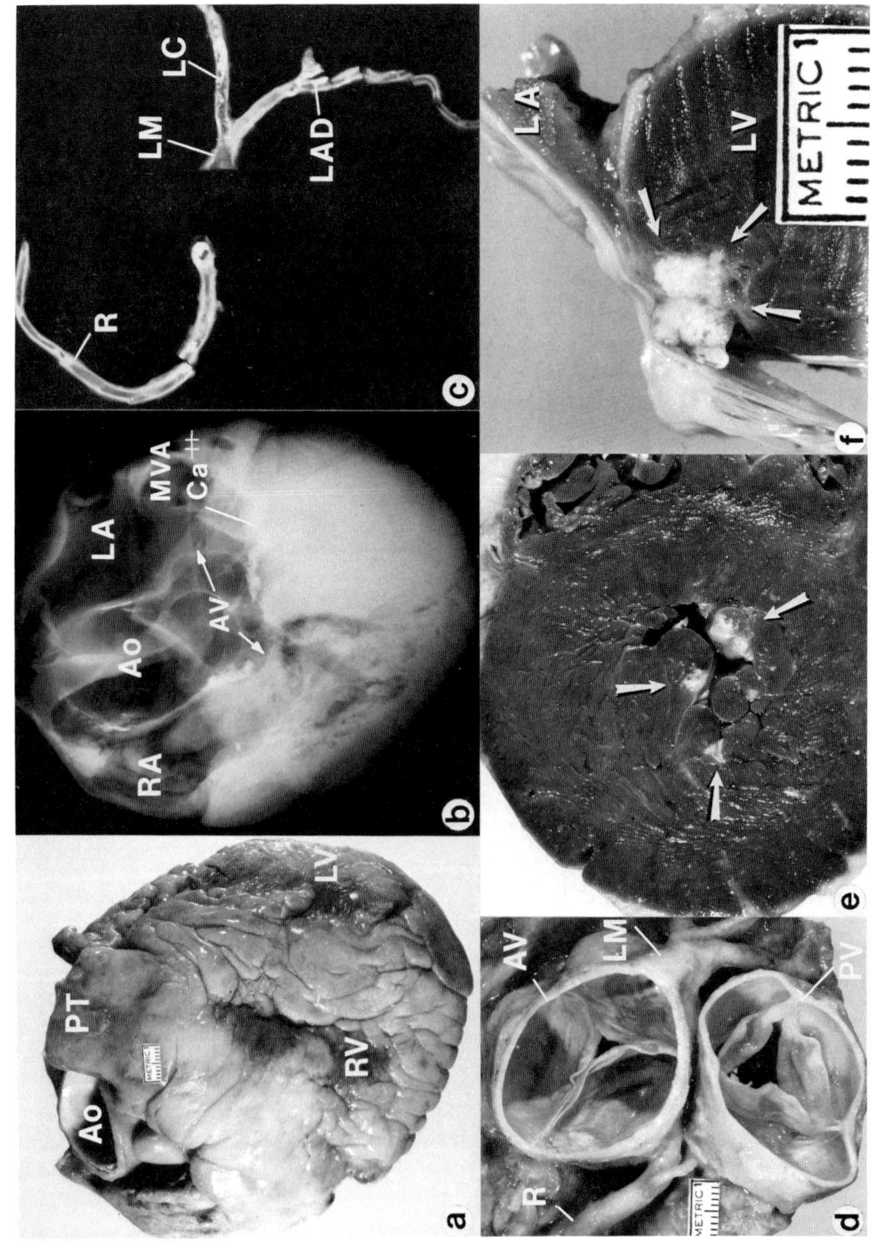
a
Ao
PT
RV
LV
b
RA
Ao
AV
LA
MVA
Ca++
c
R
LM
LC
LAD
d
R
AV
LM
PV
e
f
LA
LV
METRIC 1

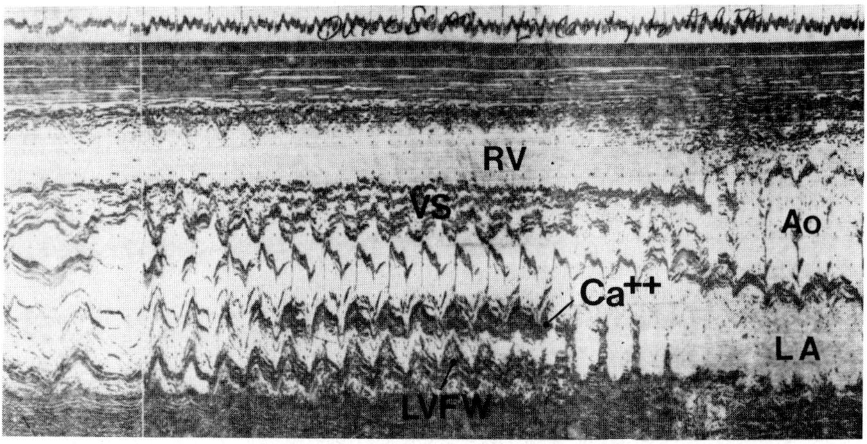


**Figure 14** M-mode echocardiogram obtained 10 months before death (SH #80-18). The ascending aorta (Ao) has a larger diameter than the left atrium (LA). The left ventricular (LV) cavity is small. Calcium is present in the mitral annular region. (I thank Dr. Robert Montgomery, Bethesda, Maryland, for allowing me to show this echocardiogram from his patient.)

aortic valve stenosis it was 238 mm. Of 29 patients on whom information was available, 18 (62%) received *digitalis* and only 2 appeared to have evidence of digitalis toxicity.

## COMMENTS

Although several reports have described cardiovascular findings at necropsy in aged persons, old age was defined as >55, >65, or >75 years (4–6), and consequently findings in those aged 90 years and over could not be separated from those occurring in the "younger" older persons. The study by Waller and

---

**Figure 13** A 97-year-old woman (SH #A81-62) who never had clinical evidence of cardiac dysfunction and who died from cancer. (a) External view of anterior surface of the heart showing an increased amount of subepicardial fat. Ao = aorta, LV = left ventricle, PT = pulmonary trunk, RV = right ventricle. (b) Postmortem radiogram showing calcific deposits in the mitral valve annulus (MVA) and aortic valve (AV). LA = left atrium, RA = right atrium. (c) Radiogram of the excised coronary arteries showing a few calcific deposits. LAD = left anterior descending, LC = left circumflex, LM = left main, R = right. (d) View of aortic valve (AV) and pulmonic valve (PV) from above. (e) View of left ventricle showing calcific deposits (arrows) in the papillary muscles. (f) Calcific deposits in the mitral annular region (arrows).

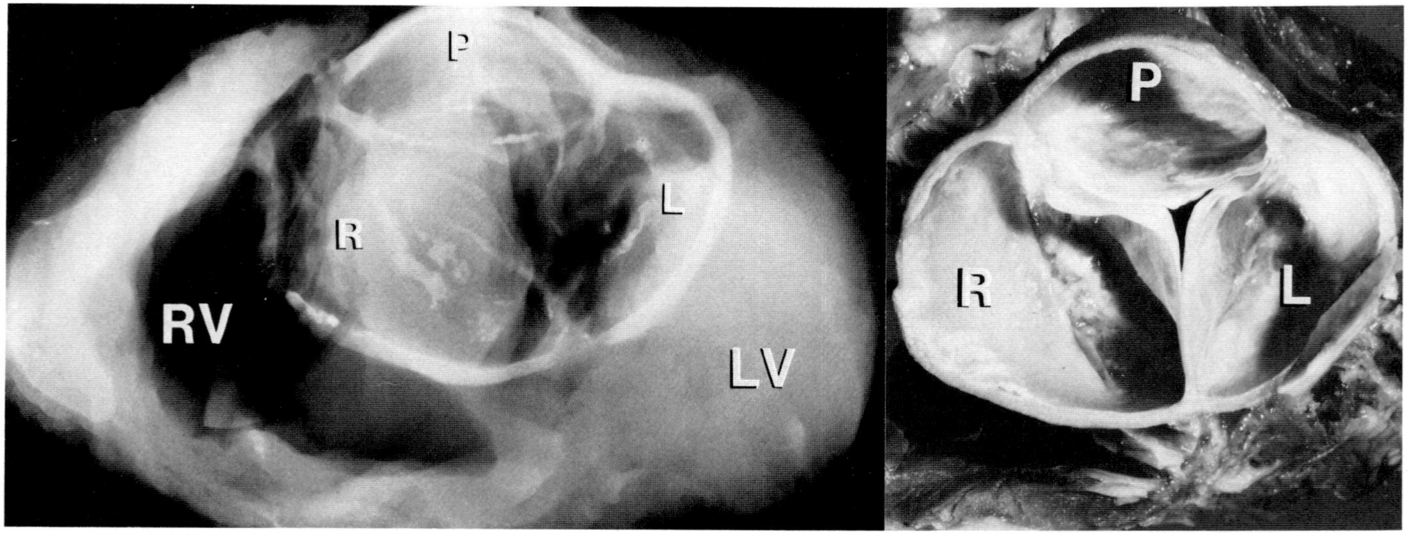


**Figure 15** A 95-year-old man (SH #79-77) who never had symptoms of cardiac dysfunction and died from sarcoma. The coronary arteries are shown in Figure 2. Left: radiogram of heart at necropsy showing considerable enlargement of the aorta in comparison to the ventricles. LV = left ventricle, RV = right ventricle, R = right, L = left, and P = posterior sinuses of Valsalva. Right: aortic valve from above. The coronary arteries were excised before the radiogram and photographs were taken.

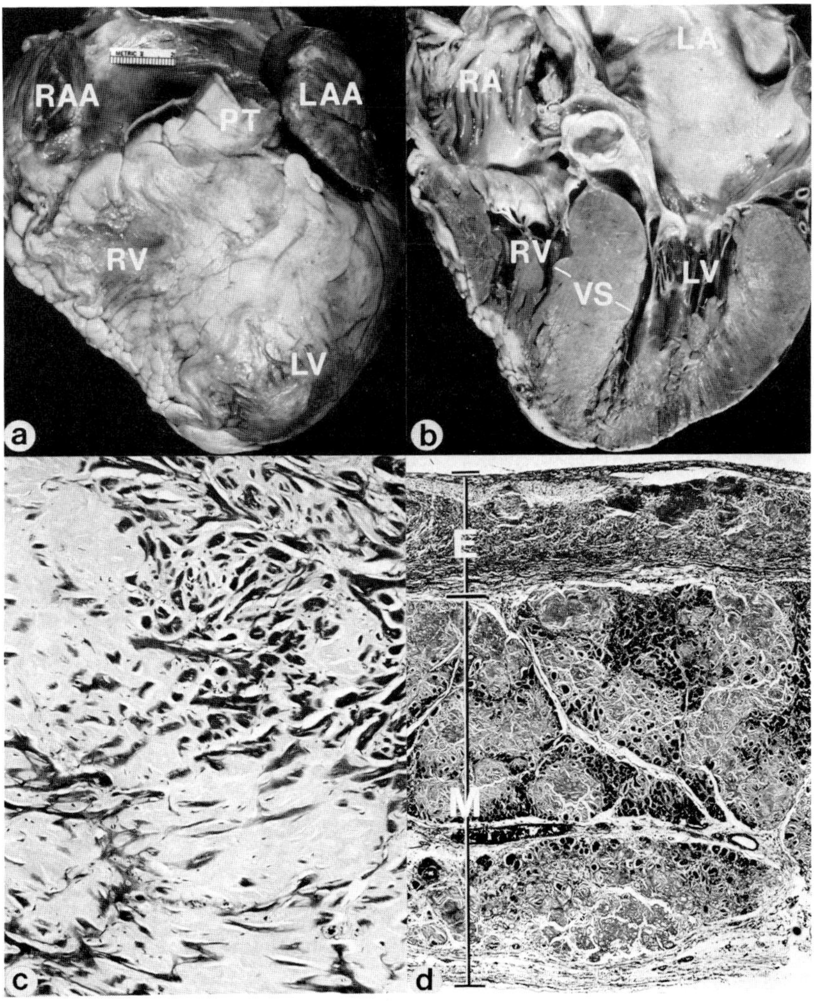


**Figure 16** A 90-year-old man (DCGH #69A391) with chronic, eventually fatal, congestive heart failure from clinically unrecognized cardiac amyloidosis. (a) External view of the heart showing a prominent left ventricle (LV) and left atrial appendage (LAA). PT = pulmonary trunk, RAA = right atrial appendage, RV = right ventricle. (b) Right-to-left longitudinal cut of the heart (four-chamber, two-dimensional echocardiographic view) showing thickened ventricular walls and dilated right (RA) and left (LA) atria. VS = ventricular septum. (c) Photomicrograph of a portion of the left ventricle showing extensive amyloid deposits. (d) Photomicrograph of LA wall showing amyloid deposits in endocardium (E) and in myocardium (M). (Hematoxylin and eosin; magnification ×100 (c) and ×25 (d), both reduced 35%.)

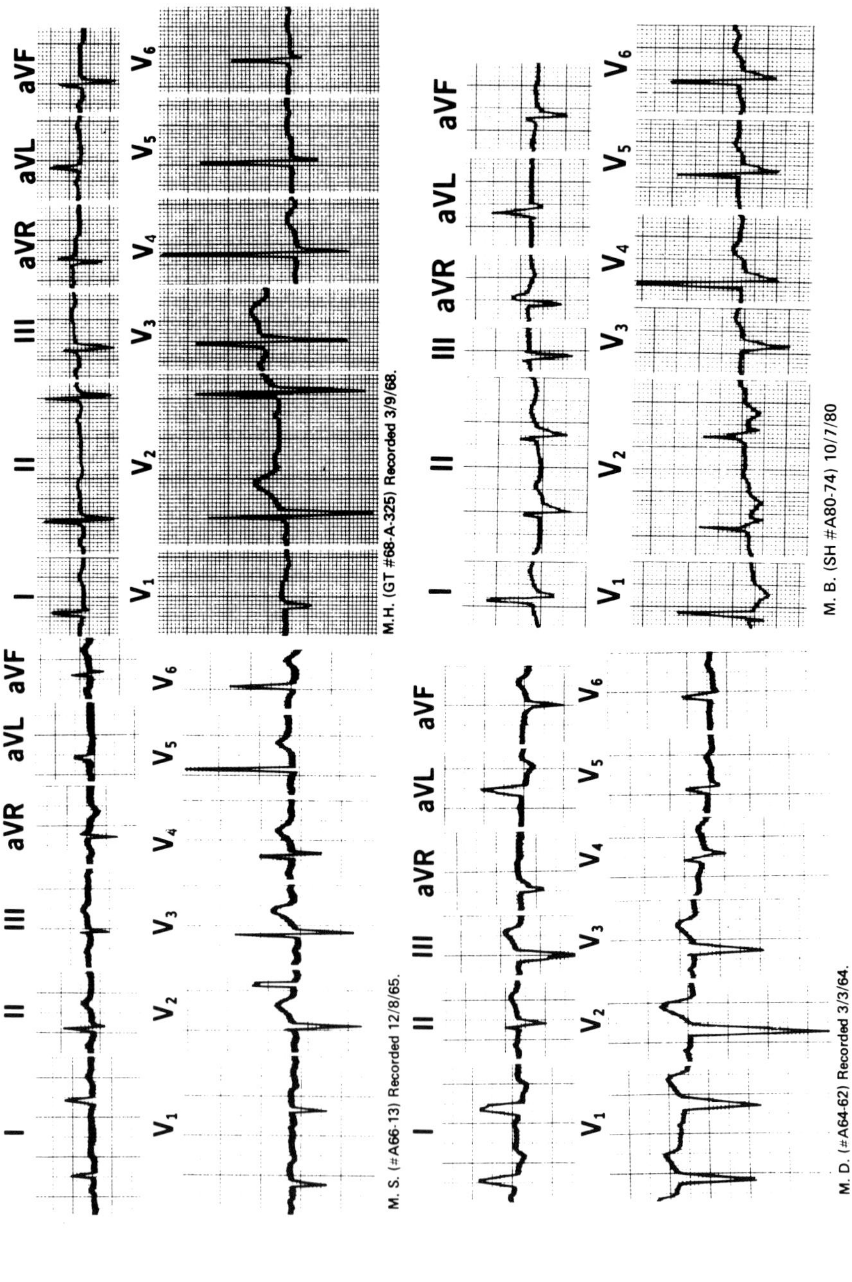
I II III aVR aVL aVF
V1 V2 V3 V4 V5 V6
M.H. (GT #68-A-325) Recorded 3/9/68.
M. B. (SH #A80-74) 10/7/80
M. S. (#A66-13) Recorded 12/8/65.
M. D. (#A64-62) Recorded 3/3/64.

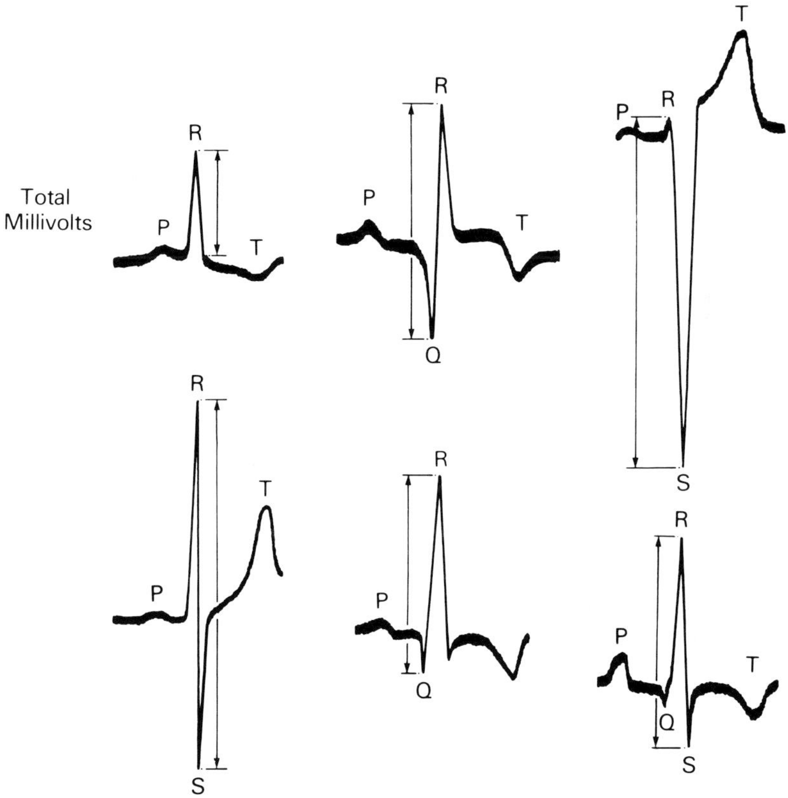


**Figure 18** Various QRS complexes, and how each was measured. (Reproduced with permission from Siegel RJ, Roberts WC. Electrocardiographic observations in severe aortic valve stenosis: Correlative necropsy study to clinical, hemodynamic, and ECG variables demonstrating relation of 12-lead QRS amplitude to peak systolic transaortic pressure gradient. Am Heart J 1982; 103:210–221.)

---

**Figure 17** Electrocardiograms in four patients, each recorded at age 90 years or older. None ever had symptoms of cardiac dysfunction, and each died from noncardiac conditions. Top left: The electrocardiogram was recorded 43 days before death (A66-13), and it is normal (heart weight 270 g). Top right: The electrocardiogram was recorded 11 days before death (GT #68A325), and it shows left QRS axis deviation and a slightly prolonged P-R interval (heart weight 400 g). Bottom left: This electrocardiogram was recorded 28 days before death (A64-62), and it shows left axis deviation and complete left bundle branch block (heart weight 320 g). Bottom right: This electrocardiogram was recorded 128 days before death (SH #A80-74), and it shows atrial fibrillation, left axis deviation, and complete right bundle branch block (heart weight 440 g).

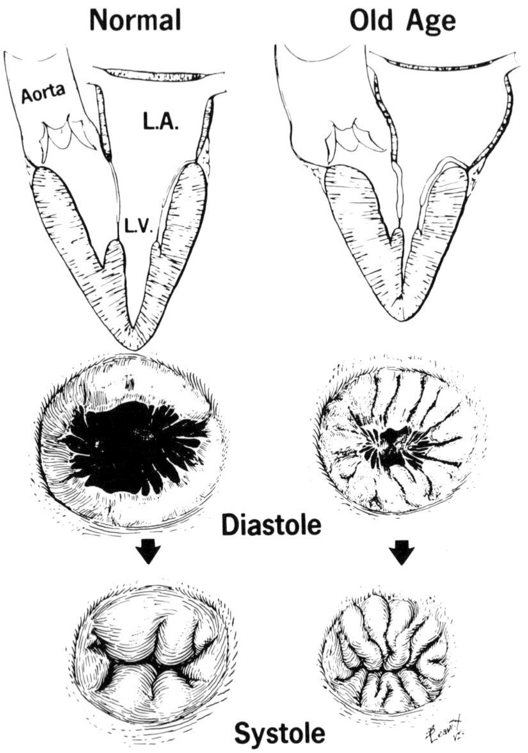


**Figure 19** Cardiac changes in the very elderly. The left atrial (LA) cavity enlarges, and the left ventricular (LV) cavity becomes smaller. The amount of space available for the mitral leaflets decreases with aging, and consequently the number of scallops in the leaflets appears to increase. (Reproduced from Roberts WC, Perloff JK. Mitral valvular disease. A clinicopathologic survey of the conditions causing the mitral valve to function abnormally. Ann Intern Med 1972; 77:939–975.)

Roberts (1) was the first to focus entirely on a group of necropsy patients aged 90 years or older, and this study was subsequently updated (2). A major finding in these studies was the high frequency of calcific deposits in the heart. Of the 93 patients, 88 (95%) had calcific deposits in the epicardial coronary arteries. In most, the deposits were extensive. Although the calcific deposits were located entirely in atherosclerotic plaques, which are located in the intima, the presence of calcific deposits in the coronary arteries in this very elderly population did not necessarily indicate the presence of significant (>75% cross-sectional area) luminal narrowing. In contrast, the presence of calcific deposits in epicardial coronary arteries in persons aged < 65 years generally indicates the presence of

**Table 3** Electrocardiographic Observations in 30 Patients Aged 90–103 Years

| Abnormality | Clinical heart disease: Present[a] ($n = 8$) | Clinical heart disease: Absent ($n = 22$) | Total: $n$ | Total: % |
|---|---|---|---|---|
| Atrial fibrillation | 5 | 7 | 12 | 40 |
| Abnormal QRS axis | | | 12 | 40 |
| Left (−30 to −90°) | 4 | 6 | | |
| Right (111–210°) | 1 | 1 | | |
| Complete (QRS ⩾ 0.12 s) BBB | | | 12 | 40 |
| Left | 6 | 1 | | |
| Right | 1 | 4 | | |
| Ventricular premature complexes | 4 | 6 | 10 | 33 |
| Atrial premature complexes | 1 | 2 | 3 | 10 |
| Heart block | | | 8 | 27 |
| P-R interval > 0.20 s | 3 | 3 | | |
| Second degree | 0 | 1 | | |
| Third degree (complete) | 1[b] | 0 | | |
| Q wave abnormality without BBB | | | 4 | 13 |
| QII, III, aVF | 0 | 1 | | |
| Q-$SV_1$-$V_3$ | 0 | 1 | | |
| Both | 0 | 2 | | |
| Left ventricular hypertrophy without BBB (R in $V_5$ or $V_6$ + S in $V_1 \geqslant 35$ mm) | 1 | 0 | 1 | 3 |
| Low voltage (QRS ⩽ 15 mm in I + II + III) | 0 | 1 | 1 | 3 |

[a] Coronary heart disease = 3; cardiac amyloidosis = 4; aortic valve stenosis = 1.
[b] Pacemaker inserted 6 years before death.
BBB = bundle branch block; s = seconds.

significant luminal narrowing. The calcific deposits tended to occur in each of the four major (right, left main, left anterior descending, and left circumflex) epicardial arteries and were always larger in the proximal than in the distal halves of the right, left anterior descending, and left circumflex arteries or, if small, limited to their proximal halves. The plaques consisted mainly (87 ± 8%) of fibrous tissue with calcific deposits forming 7 ± 6% of the plaques (7).

Calcific deposits also occurred with a high frequency (42 and 63%) in the aortic valve cusps and in the mitral annular region. The deposits in the aortic valve were located on the aortic aspects of one or more of the three cusps and usually were unassociated with commissural fusion. The presence or absence of aortic valve stenosis was determined by the quantity of calcium deposited. In 16 patients (17%), the extent of the calcific deposits imparted an immobility to the cusps, resulting in aortic valve stenosis. The mitral "annular" calcific deposits, of course, were not limited to the annulus but included the space between the ventricular aspect of the posterior mitral leaflet and the mural endocardium of left ventricular free wall behind posterior mitral leaflet. Often this annular calcium extended into the adjacent left ventricular myocardium. Most patients with aortic valve calcium had mitral annular calcium, and vice versa, and all with aortic valvular or mitral annular calcium had coronary arterial calcific deposits.

The presence of calcium in the three locations in the heart, namely, the coronary artery, the aortic valve, and the mitral annulus might be termed "the senile cardiac calcification syndrome" and strongly suggests that the etiology of the calcific deposits in each of the three locations is similar. It is well appreciated, as already mentioned, that the calcific deposits in the coronary arteries are located in atherosclerotic plaques and, therefore, that the calcific deposits in both aortic valve and mitral annular regions might be viewed as anatomical expressions of the atherosclerotic process. All three appear to occur only in populations in whom the total serum cholesterol level is >150 mg/dl per 700 ml. Calcific deposits in the coronary artery, aortic valve cusp, and mitral annulus are extremely rare in populations in whom total serum cholesterol levels are <150 mg per 100 ml, and, of course, clinical evidence of coronary artery disease in these population groups is extremely rare despite a high prevalence of systemic hypertension.

Of the 93 patients, 59 (63%) had narrowing > 75% in cross-sectional area in one or more of the four major epicardial coronary arteries. Of the 59 patients, 35 (38%) had transmural foci of left ventricular fibrosis or necrosis (myocardial infarction), and of the 34 with insignificant coronary narrowing, none had grossly visible acute or healed myocardial infarcts.

In 36 patients, each of the four major coronary arteries were divided into 5-mm-long segments and the degree of cross-sectional area narrowing by atherosclerotic plaque was determined for each segment. Of the 1789 segments (5 mm) in the 36 patients, the average amount of cross-sectional area narrowing by atherosclerotic plaques per segment was 42% (range 19–69). Of the 467 segments (5 mm) in the 10 patients with clinical evidence of coronary artery disease, the average amount of cross-sectional area narrowing per segment was 55% (range 43–69) and, of 1322 segments in the 26 patients without clinical evidence of coronary artery disease, 38% (range 19–40; $p < 0.01$). Among 129 patients aged 22–85 years (mean 56), the amount of cross-sectional area narrowing by atherosclerotic plaques per segment averaged 67%; in the control subjects, that is, those without symptomatic coronary artery disease, cross-sectional area narrowing averaged 32%. The mean percentage of 5-mm coronary segments narrowed 76–100% in cross-sectional area in the 36 patients was 13% (range 2–89); of the 10 patients with symptomatic coronary artery disease, the mean was 19% (range 10–34); and of the 26 patients without symptomatic coronary artery disease, the mean was 7% (range 2–28) ($p < 0.05$). The mean of 19% in patients with symptomatic coronary artery disease aged $\geqslant$ 90 was half that observed in patients aged $\leqslant$ 85 years (mean 56) with fatal coronary artery disease, and the mean of 7% was nearly three times that observed in the younger patients without fatal coronary artery disease (8).

These detailed morphological studies of the coronary arteries in these very elderly persons suggest that the degree of severe coronary narrowing necessary to have a fatal or nearly fatal coronary event is considerably less than that necessary to have a coronary event in younger patients. Moreover, these studies indicate that these very elderly patients without symptoms of coronary artery disease have distinctly more coronary luminal narrowing by atherosclerotic plaques than control subjects who are younger (mean age 52 years) (8). The latter observation suggests that coronary artery disease may be underdiagnosed clinically in the very elderly.

Clinical diagnosis of cardiac and other conditions in patients aged 90 years and over appears more difficult than in younger persons. Historical information may be difficult to obtain because of impaired intellect on the part of the patient and an impaired diagnostic pursuit on the part of the physician. Physicians caring for these very elderly persons may focus primarily on the prevention of suffering and only secondarily on accurate diagnosis or longer term therapy. Patients aged 90 years and over generally have outlived their spouses and private physicians and are often "inherited" by nursing home physicians, who may have limited access to earlier medical records.

Angina pectoris appears particularly difficult to diagnose in the very elderly because they may not be able to describe this symptom. Acute myocardial infarction is also difficult to diagnose clinically, but it is often fatal in the very elderly. Furthermore, the electrocardiogram is not as useful in diagnosis of acute myocardial infarction in the very elderly because left bundle branch block is frequent and, of course, it prevents the appearance of typical changes. Serial recordings of electrocardiograms also appear to be quite infrequent in the very elderly.

Physical examination in the very elderly may be both difficult and misleading. The lack of mobility may prevent proper positioning of the elderly patient for proper examining. Precordial murmurs, although common, infrequently indicate significant functional abnormality. Although calcific deposits in the aortic valve are common, actual aortic valve stenosis is not nearly as frequent. Likewise, although mitral annular calcific deposits are common, these calcific deposits rarely narrow the mitral orifice or produce significant mitral regurgitation.

Electrocardiographic abnormalities are common in elderly persons. Of my patients for whom electrocardiograms were available, all had one or more abnormalities recorded, the most frequent being abnormal axis, atrial fibrillation, and complete bundle branch block. Although 15 of the 30 patients had cardiomegaly (>350 g in women; >400 g in men) at necropsy, only 1 had voltage criteria for left ventricular hypertrophy shown by electrocardiogram. Likewise, only 1 had low voltage. Measurement of the QRS amplitude in each of the 12 leads was performed in 24 patients. The total QRS voltage was similar in the 8 patients with and in the 16 patients without clinical evidence of cardiac disease (mean 147 versus 152 mm; 10 mm = 1 mV).

## REFERENCES


1. Waller BF, Roberts WC. Cardiovascular disease in the very elderly. Analysis of 40 necropsy patients aged 90 or over. Am J Cardiol 1983; 51:403–421.
2. Roberts WC. The heart at necropsy in persons ⩾ 90 years of age. Analysis of 93 patients. Am J Cardiol 1993; 71:in press.
3. Roberts WC, Waller BF. Cardiac amyloidosis causing cardiac dysfunction. Analysis of 54 necropsy patients. Am J Cardiol 1983; 52:137–146.
4. Surglura M, Hiraoka K, Ohkawa S, Shimada H. A clinicopathologic study on the heart diseases in the aged. The morphologic classification of 1,000 consecutive autopsy cases. Jpn Heart J 1975; 16:526–537.
5. Pomerance A. Cardiac pathology in the elderly. In: Noble RJ, Rothbaum DA, eds. Geriatric Cardiology. Philadelphia: FA Davis, 1981: 9–54.
6. Pomerance A. Pathology of the heart with and without cardiac failure in the aged. Br Heart J 1965; 27:697–710.
7. Gertz SD, Malekzadeh S, Dollar AL, Kragel AH, Roberts WC. Composition of atherosclerotic plaques in the four major epicardial coronary arteries in patients ⩾ 90 years of age. Am J Cardiol 1991; 67:1228–1233.
8. Roberts WC. Qualitative and quantitative comparison of amounts of narrowing by atherosclerotic plaques in the major epicardial coronary arteries at necropsy in sudden coronary death, transmural acute myocardial infarction, transmural healed myocardial infarction and unstable angina pectoris. Am J Cardiol 1989; 64:324–328.

# 3

## Electrocardiographic Findings in Older Persons Without Clinical Heart Disease

**Jerome L. Fleg**
*Gerontology Research Center, National Institute on Aging; and Johns Hopkins University of School of Medicine, Baltimore, Maryland*

### INTRODUCTION

The dramatic aging of the U.S. population over the past several decades and the advent of Medicare have resulted in a tremendous increase in the utilization of health care services by older people. Although a large percentage of these services involves medical care for geriatric patients with acute or chronic cardiovascular disease, there has been an increasing use of routine health screening for relatively healthy older individuals. It has therefore become important to recognize how age-associated alterations in cardiovascular anatomy and physiology affect the results of commonly used diagnostic procedures.

Notwithstanding the introduction of numerous sophisticated cardiovascular techniques in the past 20 years, the resting electrocardiogram (ECG) remains our most widely applied diagnostic tool. This chapter therefore reviews the changes in the resting ECG that are thought to be secondary to age per se, as well as those that appear more often in older subjects but may indicate undetected heart disease. The striking age-associated increase in cardiac arrhythmias on ambulatory electrocardiography and exercise testing is also discussed. Whenever possible, the prognostic importance of these age-associated ECG changes is addressed.

## METHODOLOGICAL CONSIDERATIONS

The definition of what constitutes normative aging changes is strongly influenced by the criteria used to select the study population. In many early studies, the ECG findings in consecutive series of hospitalized elderly patients were tabulated. Although such studies provide prevalence data for specific ECG findings in the geriatric community, they do not provide insight regarding whether these findings are due to aging or disease. Thus "aging" changes delineated in a debilitated institutionalized geriatric population may differ greatly from aging changes in asymptomatic community-dwelling volunteers. Furthermore, even in apparently healthy populations, the use of additional screening procedures, such as echocardiography, exercise ECG, and thallium scintigraphy, may disclose covert heart disease that could warrant exclusion from a study of normative aging. Excessive screening, of course, will decrease the applicability of the results to the general population.

It should also be remembered that cross-sectional studies, which dominate the aging literature, are influenced by the selective survival of the older cohorts; subjects in their seventies and above represent the "survival of the fittest" and may not be comparable to the younger individuals to whom they are being compared. In addition, secular trends, such as the declines in smoking or cholesterol levels in the general population, over time may influence study results. Finally, the limits chosen for body weight, blood pressure, exercise habits, and other constitutional or life-style variables also influence the outcome of normative aging studies.

## SPECIFIC ECG CHANGES

### Sinus Node Function

Heart rate at rest is unrelated to age in most studies. However, the phasic variation in R-R interval known as respiratory sinus arrhythmia declines with age (1,2). Similarly, a reduced prevalence of sinus bradycardia on resting ECG is evident by the fourth decade (1). Because both sinus arrhythmia and sinus bradycardia are indices of cardiac parasympathetic activity, the age-associated reduction in parasympathetic function (2) may mediate both findings. Recently, spectral analysis of heart rate variability has confirmed an age-related reduction of high-frequency (0.15–0.45 Hz) oscillations indicative of vagal efferent activity (Fig. 1) (3). Given the strong influence of physical conditioning status on autonomic tone, it is probable that the deconditioning that usually accompanies the aging process is partially responsible for the lower prevalence of sinus arrhythmia and sinus bradycardia in older subjects.

Sinus bradycardia below 50 bpm was found in 4.1% of 1172 healthy non–endurance-trained unmedicated participants aged 40 and older from the Bal-

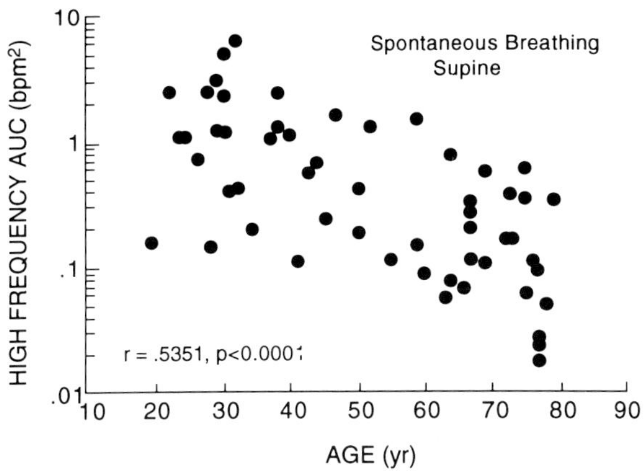


**Figure 1** Spectral analysis of heart rate variability as a function of age in the supine position. The area under the curve (AUC) for high-frequency components, indicative of vagal activity, declines with age. From Ref. 3 with permission.

timore Longitudinal Study of Aging (BLSA); the prevalence was similar in men (3.9%) and women (4.5%) (4). Although these 47 subjects (mean age 58 years) with unexplained sinus bradycardia had a significantly greater prevalence of associated conduction system abnormalities than nonbradycardic age- and sex-matched controls (Table 1), there was no difference in the incidence of future coronary events (angina pectoris, myocardial infarction, or cardiac death) over a 5.4 year mean follow-up period. Sinus bradycardia due to sick sinus syndrome is seen almost exclusively in old age and is probably due in part to the marked decline in the number of pacemaker cells in the SA node, which begins by age

**Table 1** Electrocardiographic Conduction Abnormalities in Healthy Volunteers ≥ 40 Years with Sinus Bradycardia < 50 Beats/Min and No Apparent Cause

| | Sinus bradycardia, $n = 47$ (%) | Control, $n = 47$ (%) |
|---|---|---|
| P-R interval greater than 0.20 s | 7 (15) | 2 (4) |
| Complete right bundle branch block | 5 (11) | 1 (2) |
| Incomplete right bundle branch block | 6 (13) | 5 (11) |
| Left axis deviation | 9 (19) | 5 (11) |
| Any of the above | 22 (47)[a] | 12 (26) |

[a] $p < 0.05$.
*Source*: Adapted from Ref. 4.

60. In the absence of organic heart disease, such bradycardia is not associated with increased cardiac mortality (5).

## P Waves

Although age-specific rates have not been reported, the prevalence of left atrial abnormality, defined by a negative p-terminal force in lead $V_1$ of at least 0.04 mm/s on the ECG, increases with age, paralleling the echocardiographic increase in left atrial size. Among 588 institutionalized elderly, such a p-terminal force was only 32% sensitive, although 94% specific, for echocardiographic left atrial enlargement (6). A small increment in p wave duration of about 8 ms from the third to seventh decades has been observed (7), presumably secondary to the modest increase in left atrial size. When subjects with significant chronic obstructive lung disease are excluded, there does not appear to be any increase in ECG evidence of right atrial enlargement with age.

## P-R Interval

There is general agreement that the P-R interval undergoes a slight but significant age-related prolongation, by approximately 0.01 s from the third to the sixth decades (8). An increase in P-R interval from 159 to 175 ms in men and from 156 to 165 ms in women was found between the ages of 30 and 72 years in BLSA volunteers (9). To ascertain whether this age-related slowing of A-V conduction was located proximal or distal to the His bundle, we performed high-resolution signal-averaged surface ECG on these subjects. The prolongation of A-V conduction was found to reside completely proximal to the His bundle deflection but within the P-R segment, presumably reflecting delay within the A-V junction (Fig. 2). In seven older men with first-degree A-V block, a similarly located but more pronounced delay was found. Given the age-associated slowing of A-V conduction, a value of 0.22 s has been proposed for the upper limit of normal P-R interval in persons over 50 years old (8). Using the conventional upper limit of 0.20 s, the prevalence of first-degree A-V block in healthy older men is usually 3–4%, a prevalence severalfold greater than in young men (8). Cross-sectional studies have generally found no correlation between first-degree A-V block and cardiac disease (10). Similarly, longitudinal studies have reported no association of first-degree A-V block with cardiac mortality (11).

## QRS Complex

Although the QRS duration shows no significant age relationship, the QRS axis shifts progressively leftward with age. In the extensive normative study of Simonson, the mean QRS axis shifted from 62.1 to 36.2° from the third to the sixth decades, with no gender difference (8). The corresponding lower normal limits shifted from 2.9 to −28.4°. The prevalence of left axis deviation < −30° therefore increases dramatically with age, with prevalence figures of 20% reported by the 10th decade (12). The etiology of this leftward QRS axis shift may be the age-related increase in left ventricular mass (13). Longitudinal studies have failed to demonstrate any increase in cardiac morbidity or mortality associated with this isolated ECG finding (14,15). In patients with known organic heart disease, however, the presence of left axis deviation combined with left or right bundle branch block portends a worse cardiovascular prognosis (16).

A decrease in R and S wave amplitudes with advancing age, evident by the fourth decade, has been shown in both cross-sectional (17) and longitudinal (18) studies. At first glance, this decrease in QRS amplitude seems paradoxical, given the age-related increase in left ventricular mass. It must be remembered, however, that the surface ECG is influenced by extracardiac as well as cardiac factors. The increasing distance between the heart and the chest wall due to senile kyphosis and lung hyperinflation in older individuals may be largely responsible for the decrease in QRS voltage.

Notwithstanding the age-related decline in mean QRS amplitude, electrocardiographic left ventricular hypertrophy (LVH) increases in prevalence with age (19), probably secondary to the high prevalence of hypertension, coronary artery disease, and degenerative valvular disease in the elderly. Echocardiographic studies have demonstrated that the standard ECG is quite insensitive, although very specific for anatomic LVH in older populations (20). Data from Framingham have shown convincingly that ECG evidence of LVH is strongly related to the presence of hypertension and is a potent independent risk factor for future cardiovascular morbidity and mortality (19–21). Thus, the prevalence of ECG criteria for LVH in an older individual should normally trigger further diagnostic assessment, particularly echocardiography.

Left and right bundle branch block (LBBB and RBBB) both increase in prevalence with age; nevertheless, these conduction defects should not be attributed to aging per se. In older populations LBBB occurs only about half as often as RBBB. In contrast to its right-sided counterpart, LBBB is uncommon in the absence of cardiovascular disease (22). The prognosis in LBBB therefore reflects that of the underlying heart disease. Although in men LBBB portends a more ominous prognosis than RBBB, the two conduction defects had similar prognostic significance in Framingham women (23,24). Nonspecific intraventricular conduction defects exceeding 120 ms occurred in only 1.9% of Framingham subjects aged 70 and older and, like LBBB, were strongly associated with clinical heart disease (25).

Complete RBBB was found in 39 of 1142 men (3.4%) in the BLSA (26). Among the 24 individuals (mean age 64 years) without evidence of heart disease

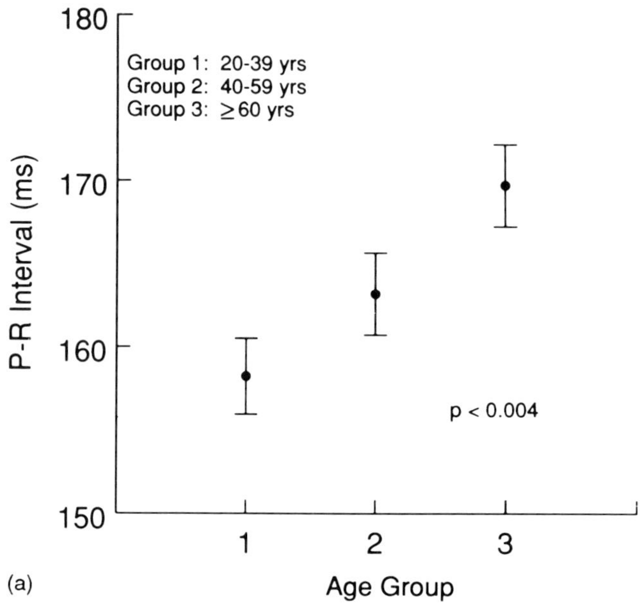


(a)

**Figure 2** Determining the basis for the normal age-associated prolongation of the P-R interval by noninvasive His bundle recording. (a) P-R interval as a function of age in 161 normal subjects without first-degree A-V block. (b) There is an increase in the interval from the P wave onset to the His bundle deflection (P-H interval) with age that mirrors the prolongation in PR interval. (c) In contrast to the P-H interval, the interval from His bundle deflection to ventricular activation (H-V interval) is not age related. From Ref. 9 with permission.

and for whom follow-up information was available, the incidence of angina, nonfatal myocardial infarction (MI), heart failure, advanced heart block, or cardiac death did not differ from those in age-matched control subjects over a mean observation period of 8.4 years (Fig. 3). At latest follow-up, maximal exercise capacity and chronotropic response were similar to those of controls, although a higher prevalence of left axis deviation was found in the RBBB group (46 versus 15%). These findings suggest that RBBB in the absence of clinical heart disease is not rare in older men and reflects a primary abnormality of the cardiac conduction system. In the Framingham study, women demonstrated a lower prevalence of RBBB than men but had a higher association of this conduction defect with cardiomegaly and congestive heart failure than their male counterparts (23).

The presence of Q waves in two or more contiguous ECG leads is generally considered evidence of prior myocardial infarction. In older as in younger populations, such Q waves are usually associated with clinical heart disease and

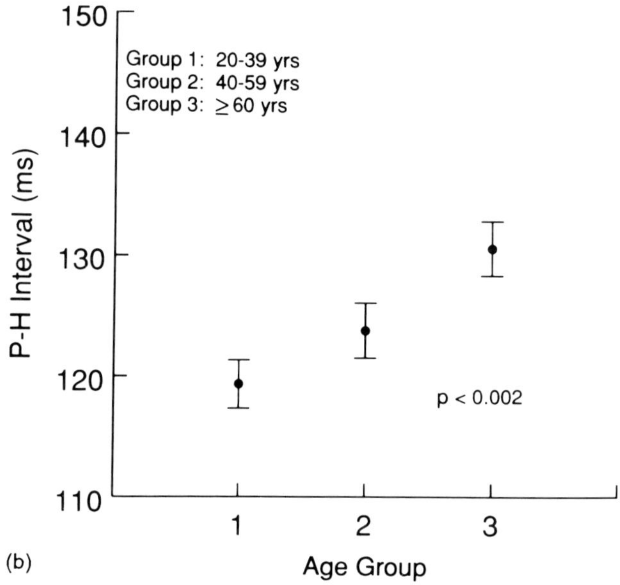
150
140
130
120
110
Group 1: 20-39 yrs
Group 2: 40-59 yrs
Group 3: ≥60 yrs
P-H Interval (ms)
p < 0.002
1
2
3
Age Group

(b)

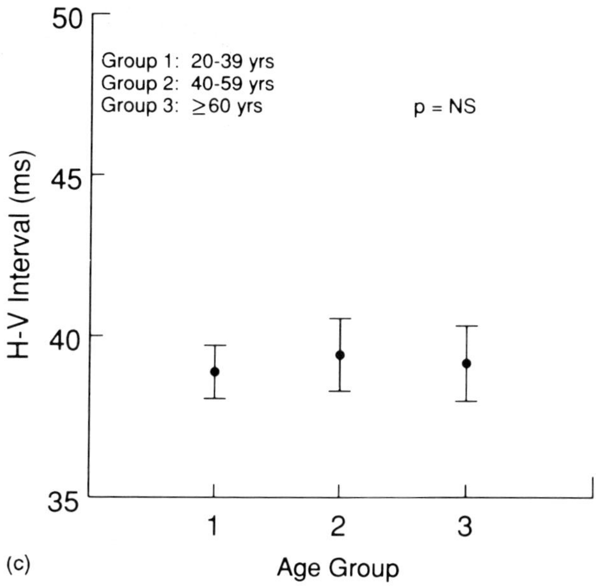
50
45
40
35
Group 1: 20-39 yrs
Group 2: 40-59 yrs
Group 3: ≥60 yrs
p = NS
H-V Interval (ms)
1
2
3
Age Group

(c)

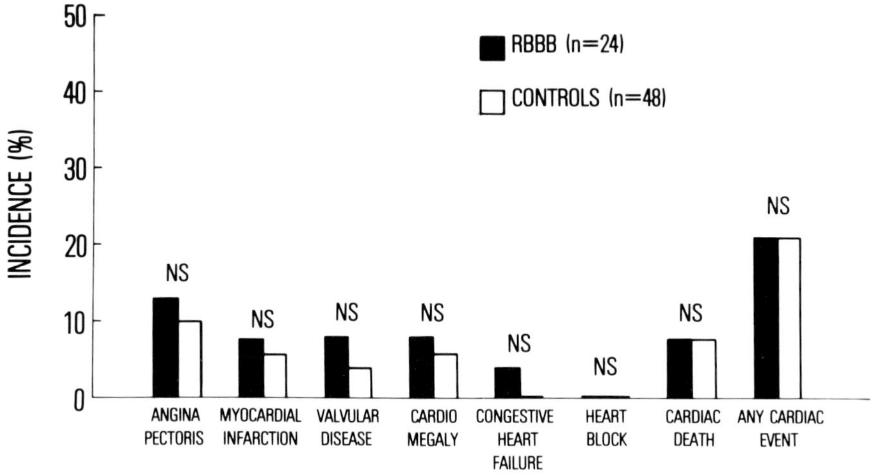


**Figure 3** Cardiac prognosis in male volunteers with complete right bundle branch block in the absence of apparent heart disease. Over a mean follow-up of 8.4 years, there was no increase in cardiac end points compared to age-matched control subjects. Adapted from Ref. 26.

increased cardiac mortality. Pathologic Q waves may in fact serve as the initial clue to the presence of coronary artery disease. Indeed, several studies have shown that 25–30% or more of acute infarctions are clinically silent (27–29). The incidence of these so-called "silent" MIs increases strikingly with age (Table 2). In geriatric chronic care facilities, rates of silent infarction as high as 68% have been reported (29). Despite the absence of symptoms, these silent infarctions portend a long-term risk of mortality similar to their symptomatic counterparts.

Q waves in the elderly not uncommonly occur in the absence of coronary artery disease. A QS complex in leads 3 and a VF may occasionally result from marked left axis deviation. A pattern of poor R wave progression in leads $V_1$–$V_3$ is a normal age trend, because of the decrease in the initial 20 ms anterior QRS vector with age (8). Such a pattern may also result from obesity, chronic obstructive lung disease, and LVH, all of which are common in older populations. Hypertrophic cardiomyopathy is also frequently associated with significant Q waves in the absence of coronary disease.

## Repolarization

Abnormalities involving the ST segment and T wave are perhaps the most prevalent age-associated ECG finding. For example, nonspecific ST-T changes were the most common ECG abnormalities seen in 671 subjects aged 70 years and

**Table 2** 10-Year Incidence (per 1000 Subjects) of Unrecognized Myocardial Infarctions in the Framingham Study

| | Men | | Women | |
|---|---|---|---|---|
| Age | Unrecognized infarcts | All infarcts | Unrecognized infarcts | All infarcts |
| 30–34 | 2.6 | 12.9 | 0.0 | 2.2 |
| 35–44 | 6.5 | 38.2 | 2.6 | 5.2 |
| 45–54 | 16.6 | 71.2 | 2.9 | 13.0 |
| 55–64 | 28.2 | 107.9 | 17.9 | 47.1 |
| 65–74 | 53.8 | 141.0 | 21.3 | 55.7 |
| 75–84 | 60.2 | 112.8 | 34.0 | 128.3 |

*Source*: Adapted from Ref. 27.

older in one study, occurring in 16% of subjects (22). In this series and others, repolarization abnormalities were generally associated with clinical heart disease. Such an association may stem in part from the frequent use of digitalis and various antiarrhythmic drugs by elderly cardiac patients. Thus, much of the reported increased risk attached to these nonspecific repolarization changes is undoubtedly due to the underlying heart disease that necessitated use of these cardiac medications. Even among clinically healthy older subjects, however, minor ST segment sagging or straightening is relatively common, although of questionable prognostic significance.

The T wave amplitude begins to decrease with age by the fourth decade (8,17). The spatial T wave vector shifts leftward with age in concert with the leftward shift in QRS axis. Obesity magnifies these changes in the T wave direction and amplitude, particularly in men (8). The isolated presence of flattened T waves, especially in lead a VL, does not portend increased cardiovascular risk, at least in middle-aged subjects (30). Definite T wave inversion, in contrast, usually occurs in patients with organic heart disease and is therefore associated with increased mortality. The heart rate-corrected Q-T interval increases by about 10 ms from the third to the sixth decade (31).

## Arrhythmias

Probably the most easily recognized ECG change associated with normative human aging is an increase in the prevalence and complexity of both supraventricular and ventricular arrhythmias, whether detected by resting ECG, ambulatory monitoring, or exercise testing. Isolated premature atrial ectopic beats (AEB) appear on resting ECG in 5–10% of subjects older than 60 years and are generally not associated with heart disease (22). Such isolated AEB were detected in 6% of healthy BLSA volunteers older than 60 years at rest, in 39% during exercise testing, and in 88% during ambulatory 24 h monitoring (32). Over a 10-year mean follow-up period, isolated AEB, even if frequent, were not predictive of increased cardiac risk in these individuals (33).

Atrial fibrillation (AF) is found in approximately 4% of subjects over age 60 years, a rate 10-fold higher than in the general population (34). Chronic AF is most commonly due to coronary and hypertensive heart disease, mitral valvular disorders, thyrotoxicosis, and sick sinus syndrome. The association between hyperthyroidism and AF occurs almost exclusively in the elderly (35); in fact, this arrhythmia may be the sole clinical manifestation of so-called apathetic hyperthyroidism in geriatric patients. In the Framingham population, atrial fibrillation without identifiable cause (so-called lone AF) represented 16.8% of men and 6.0% of women with AF, with mean ages of 70.6 and 68.1 years, respectively (36). During long-term follow-up, individuals with lone AF suffered over four times as many strokes as control subjects, although their rates of coronary events or congestive heart failure were similar to those of controls (Table 3). Atrial flutter is a rare arrhythmia in any age group and is usually associated with organic heart disease. Short bursts of paroxysmal supraventricular tachycardia (PSVT) on resting ECG are found in 1–2% of normal individuals older than 65 years. Ambulatory monitoring studies (24 h) have demonstrated short runs of this arrhythmia (usually three to five beats) in 13% of clinically healthy elderly subjects (32). Although the presence of nonsustained PSVT did not predict an increase in risk of a future coronary event in these subjects (33), 2 of 13 with PSVT later developed de novo atrial fibrillation, compared with only 1 of the 85 subjects without PSVT.

Exercise-induced PSVT has been observed in 3.5% of over 3000 maximal treadmill tests on apparently healthy BLSA volunteers (37). The arrhythmia

**Table 3** Age-Adjusted Cardiovascular Event Rates in Framingham Subjects with Lone Atrial Fibrillation

| | Cases | | | Controls | | |
|---|---|---|---|---|---|---|
| Event | No. at risk | No. of events | Age adjusted % | No. at risk | No. of events | Age adjusted % |
| Coronary heart disease | 34 | 4 | 11.2 | 1179 | 154 | 11.7 |
| Cardiac failure | 34 | 1 | 2.9 | 1179 | 35 | 2.8 |
| Stroke[a] | 30 | 8 | 28.2 | 998 | 51 | 6.8 |

[a] Significant difference between cases and controls, $p < .01$.
*Source*: From Ref. 36.

demonstrated a striking increase in incidence with age, from 0% in the twenties to approximately 10% in the eighties; like PSVT on ambulatory ECG, the vast majority of these episodes were asymptomatic three- to five-beat salvos. The prevalence of coronary risk factors and ECG or thallium scintigraphic evidence of ischemia in the 85 volunteers with exercise-induced PSVT resembled those in age- and sex-matched control subjects. Similarly, no increase in subsequent coronary events was observed over a 5.5-year mean follow-up period. However, 10% of the group with PSVT later developed a spontaneous atrial tachyarrhythmia compared with only 2% of the control group, analogous to the results of the ambulatory 24 h ECG.

An exponential increase in the prevalence of ventricular ectopic beats (VEB) with advancing age has been found both in unselected populations and in those clinically free of heart disease. Pooled data from nearly 2500 ECG from hospitalized patients older than 70 years revealed VEB in 8% (38). Among apparently healthy BLSA volunteers with a normal ST segment response to treadmill exercise, isolated VEB occurred at rest in 8.6% of men over age 60 compared to only 0.5% in those 20–40 years old (Table 4). In women, interestingly, the prevalence of resting VEB was not age related.

The prognostic significance of VEB detected on the resting ECG in the general elderly population is controversial. Studies in Busselton (39) and Manitoba (40) detected significant increases in cardiac mortality in such populations, with risk ratios of 3.3 and 2.4, respectively, compared with arrhythmia-free cohorts. In the Framingham community (41), however, no increase was found in the age-adjusted risk ratio for cardiac events. Data from the MRFIT study suggest that the prognostic significance of resting VEB may vary according to age; asymptomatic white men under 50 years with frequent or complex VEB on a 2

**Table 4** Prevalence of Ventricular Ectopic Beats on Resting ECG in Asymptomatic Volunteers with Normal Exercise Test

| | Men | | Women | |
|---|---|---|---|---|
| Age decade | *n* | % | *n* | % |
| 20–29 | 62 | 1.6 | 52 | 1.9 |
| 30–39 | 133 | 0 | 79 | 3.8 |
| 40–49 | 98 | 2.0 | 54 | 3.7 |
| 50–59 | 116 | 2.6 | 64 | 1.6 |
| 60–69 | 111 | 7.2 | 71 | 4.2 |
| 70–79 | 72 | 9.7 | 39 | 2.6 |
| $\geq$80 | 26 | 11.5 | 13 | 0 |
| Totals | 618 | 3.9 | 372 | 3.0 |

min resting rhythm strip suffered a 14-fold relative risk of sudden cardiac death, but in older men the risk was not significantly increased (42).

Ambulatory 24 h ECG recordings have demonstrated the presence of VEB in up to 96% of asymptomatic elderly subjects (43). Furthermore, not only the prevalence but the density and complexity of VEB increase with age. Among 101 subjects aged 10–69 who were free of heart disease by rigorous screening, including coronary angiography, both the prevalence and absolute number of VEB in 24 h increased with age; however, only 12 individuals in this series were older than 60 years (44). A study of 50 subjects, predominantly females, older than 80 years reported VEB in 96%, including multifocal VEB in 18%, couplets in 8%, and nonsustained ventricular tachycardia (VT) in 2% (43). Among 106 predominantly healthy patients aged 75 and above, Camm et al. noted VEB in 69% of subjects (45). VEB were multiform in 22%, paired in 4%, and in short runs in 4%. Among 98 carefully screened asymptomatic BLSA participants older than 60 years, 35% had multiform VEB, 11% VEB couplets, and 4% short runs of ventricular tachycardia on 24 h monitoring (32). These figures are all much lower in series of healthy younger subjects. Over a 10-year mean follow-up period, 14 of these 98 BLSA volunteers developed coronary events. The prevalence and complexity of VEB were virtually identical in the group who experienced an event and the group who did not (33). In the series of Camm et al., 92% of the 5-year survivors who were initially free of VEB remained without VEB on the 5-year follow-up recording (46). In contrast to the BLSA results, an almost doubled crude mortality was found among individuals with $\geqslant$ 10 VEB/h versus those with fewer VEB. It should be pointed out, however, that 83% of this series were taking medications, including several patients with known heart disease.

Exercise testing, like the ambulatory ECG, elicits a striking increase in the prevalence and complexity of VEB with advancing age. In apparently healthy BLSA volunteers, isolated VEB during or after maximal treadmill exercise increased in prevalence fivefold, from 11 to 57%, between the third and ninth decades. Asymptomatic exercise-induced runs of VT, all six beats or more in duration, were found in 4% of apparently healthy individuals aged 65 and older, a rate 25 times that of younger subjects (47). Perhaps more important, over a mean follow-up of about 2 years, none of these elderly subjects with nonsustained VT during exercise testing developed angina, myocardial infarction, syncope, or cardiac death.

In a more recent BLSA analysis, 80 of 1160 subjects developed frequent VEB ($\geqslant$10% of beats in any minute) or nonsustained VT during maximal treadmill exercise testing (an average of 2.4 tests per individual were performed) (48). These 80 individuals were older than those free of such arrhythmia (64 versus 50 years). Of note is that the striking age-associated increase in the prevalence of these complex exercise-induced VEB was limited to men (Fig. 4). The

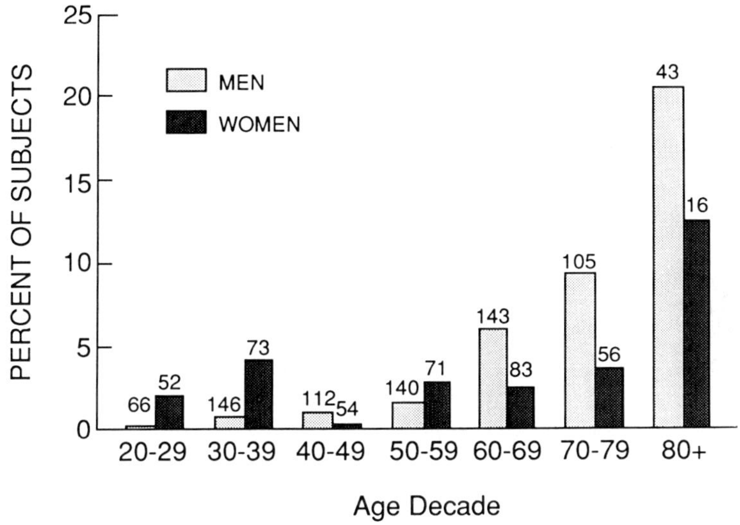


**Figure 4** Prevalence of exercise-induced complex ventricular ectopic beats as a function of age and sex in apparently healthy individuals during maximal treadmill testing. A striking age-associated increase is present in men but not women. From Ref. 48 with permission.

prevalence of coronary risk factors and exercise-induced ischemia by ECG and thallium scanning did not differ between the 80 cases and a group of 80 age- and sex-matched controls. Furthermore, the incidence of cardiac events (angina pectoris, nonfatal infarction, cardiac syncope, or cardiac death) was nearly identical in cases and controls (10 and 12.5%, respectively) over a mean follow-up of 5.6 years without antiarrhythmic drug therapy. Thus, the limited data available in older subjects without apparent heart disease support a striking age-related increase in the prevalence and complexity of exercise-related VEB; however, even frequent or repetitive VEB induced by exercise do not appear to increase cardiac morbidity or mortality in these older volunteers.

A critical factor in determining the prognostic significance of VEB in the elderly is the milieu in which they occur. For example, among 467 patients aged 62–101 years in a long-term care facility, complex VEB occurred in 21% (49). In the subset without clinical heart disease, future coronary events developed in an identical 4% of those individuals with or without complex VEB; among patients with coronary heart disease, however, such events developed in 46% with complex VEB versus only 23% of those without them. A similar doubling of risk was seen in patients with hypertension, valvular disease, or cardiomyopathy who demonstrated complex VEB. These data extend those of Hinkle et al., which documented increased coronary death rates in middle-aged men with suspected coronary heart disease and frequent VEB but not in their healthy age peers with similar VEB frequency (50).

## CONCLUSION

Several noteworthy aging changes in the ECG occur in apparently healthy subjects and have no known prognostic significance. Among these are a decrease in the prevalence of sinus bradycardia and sinus arrhythmia, an increase in the prevalence and density of supraventricular and ventricular ectopic beats, a mild P-R interval prolongation, and a leftward shift of the QRS axis. Although increased QRS voltage, Q waves, and ST-T wave abnormalities may appear in older persons without evident heart disease, these findings are generally associated with increased cardiac risk. Certain abnormalities, such as LBBB, definite LVH, or AF, are uncommon in healthy older individuals and are strongly predictive of subsequent cardiac morbidity and mortality. Of greatest practical importance is the concept that the prognosis associated with a given ECG abnormality in the elderly is largely dependent on the presence and severity of any underlying heart disease.

## ACKNOWLEDGMENTS

The secretarial assistance of Sharon Thomas and Miriam Glaser is gratefully acknowledged.

## REFERENCES

1. Hiss RG, Lamb LE. Electrocardiographic findings in 122,043 individuals. Circulation 1962; 25:947–961.
2. Pfeifer MA, Weinberg CR, Cook D, Best JD, Reenan A, Halter JR. Differential changes of autonomous nervous system function with age in men. Am J Med 1983; 75:249–258.
3. Schwartz J, Gibb WJ, Tran T. Aging effects on heart rate variation. J Gerontol 1991; 46:M99–106.
4. Tresch DD, Fleg JL. Unexplained sinus bradycardia: Clinical significance and long-term prognosis in apparently healthy persons older than 40 years. Am J Cardiol 1986; 58:1009–1013.
5. Gann D, Tolentino A, Samet P. Electrophysiologic evaluation of elderly patients with sinus bradycardia. Ann Intern Med 1979; 90:24–29.
6. Aronow WS, Schwartz KS, Koenigsberg M. Prevalence of enlarged left atrial dimension by echocardiography and its correlation with atrial fibrillation and an abnormal P terminal force in lead $V_1$ of the electrocardiogram in 588 elderly persons. Am J Cardiol 1987; 59:1003–1004.
7. Pipberger HV, Goldman MJ, Littmann D, Murphy GP, Cosma J, Snyder JR.

Correlations of the orthogonal electrocardiogram and vectorcardiogram with constitutional variables in 518 normal men. Circulation 1967; 35:536–551.
8. Simonson E. The effect of age on the electrocardiogram. Am J Cardiol 1972; 29:64–73.
9. Fleg JL, Das DN, Wright J, Lakatta EG. Age-associated changes in the components of atrioventricular conduction in apparently healthy volunteers. J Gerontol 1990; 45:M95–100.
10. Rodstein M, Brown M, Wolloch L. First-degree atrioventricular heart block in the aged. Geriatrics 1968; 23:159–165.
11. Mymin D, Mathewson FAL, Tate RB, Manfreda J. The natural history of primary first-degree atrioventricular heart block. N Engl J Med 1986; 315:1183–1187.
12. Golden GS, Golden LH. The "nona" electrocardiogram: findings in 100 patients of the 90 age group. J Am Ger Soc 1974; 22:329–331.
13. Gerstenblith G, Frederiksen J, Yin FC, Fortuin NJ, Lakatta EG, Weisfeldt ML. Echocardiographic assessment of a normal adult aging population. Circulation 1977; 56:273–278.
14. Ostrander LD. Left axis deviation: Prevalence, associated conductions and prognosis. An epidemiologic study. Ann Intern Med 1971; 75:23–28.
15. Yano K, Peskoe SM, Rhoads GG, Moore JO, Kagan A. Left axis deviation and left anterior hemiblock among 8,000 Japanese and American men. Am J Cardiol 1975; 35:809–815.
16. Pryor R, Blount SG. Clinical significance of true left-axis deviation. Am Heart J 1966; 72:391–413.
17. Hiss RG, Lamb LE, Allen MF. Electrocardiographic findings in 67,375 asymptomatic subjects. 10. Normal values. Am J Cardiol 1960; 6:200–231.
18. Harlan WR Jr, Graybiel A, Mitchell RE, Oberman A, Osborne RK. Serial electrocardiograms: Their reliability and prognostic validity during a 24-yr period. J Chron Dis 1967; 20:853–867.
19. Kannel WB, Gordon T, Offutt D. Left ventricular hypertrophy by electrocardiogram: Prevalence, incidence and mortality in the Framingham study. Ann Intern Med 1969; 71:89–105.
20. Levy D, Garrison RJ, Savage DD, Kannel WB, Castelli WP. Left ventricular mass and incidence of coronary heart disease in an elderly cohort. The Framingham Heart Study. Ann Intern Med 1989; 110:101–107.
21. Kannel WB, Gordon T, Castelli WP, Margolis JR. Electrocardiographic left ventricular hypertrophy and risk of coronary heart disease. The Framingham study. Ann Intern Med 1970; 72:813–822.
22. Mihalick NJ, Fisch C. Electrocardiographic findings in the aged. Am Heart J 1974; 87:117–128.
23. Schneider JF, Thomas HE Jr, Kreger BE, McNamara PM, Sorlie P, Kannel WB. Newly acquired right bundle branch block: The Framingham study. Ann Intern Med 1980; 92:37–44.
24. Schneider JF, Thomas HE Jr, Kreger BE, McNamara PM, Kannel WB. Newly acquired left bundle branch block: The Framingham study. Ann Intern Med 1979; 90:303–310.

25. Kreger BE, Anderson KM, Kannel WB. Prevalence of intraventricular block in the general population: The Framingham Study. Am Heart J 1989; 117:903–910.
26. Fleg JL, Das DN, Lakatta EG. Right bundle block: Long-term prognosis in apparently healthy men. J Am Coll Cardiol 1983; 1:387–392.
27. Kannel WB, Abbott RD. Incidence and prognosis of unrecognized myocardial infarction. An update on the Framingham study. N Engl J Med 1984; 311:1144–1147.
28. Rodstein M. The characteristics of non-fatal myocardial infarction in the aged. Ann Intern Med 1956; 98:84–90.
29. Aronow WS, Starling L, Etienne F, D'Alba P, Edwards M, Lee NH, Parungao RF. Unrecognized Q-wave myocardial infarction in patients older than 64 years in a long-term health-care facility. Am J Cardiol 1985; 56:483.
30. Higgins ITT, Kannel WB, Dawber TR. The electrocardiogram in epidemiological studies. Reproducibility, validity and international comparison. Br J Prev Soc Med 1965; 19:53–68.
31. Simonson E, Cady L, Woodbury M. The normal Q-T interval. Am Heart J 1962; 63:747–753.
32. Fleg JL, Kennedy HL. Cardiac arrhythmias in a healthy elderly population: Detection by 24-hour ambulatory electrocardiography. Chest 1982; 81:302–307.
33. Fleg JL, Kennedy HL. Prognostic significance of Holter monitoring in apparently healthy older subjects (abstr). J Am Coll Cardiol 1991; 17:330A.
34. Kannel WB, Abbott RD, Savage DD, McNamara PM. Epidemiologic features of chronic atrial fibrillation. N Engl J Med 1982; 306:1018–1022.
35. Staffurth JS, Gibberd MC, Ng Tang Fui S. Arterial embolism in thyrotoxicosis with atrial fibrillation. Br Med J 1977; 2:688–690.
36. Brand FN, Abbott RD, Kannel WB, Wolf PA. Characteristics and prognosis of lone atrial fibrillation. 30-Year follow-up in the Framingham Study. JAMA 1985; 254:3449–3453.
37. Maurer MS, Fleg JL, Shefrin EA. Exercise-induced supraventricular tachycardia in apparently healthy volunteers (abstr). J Am Coll Cardiol 1992; 19:35A.
38. Fisch C. Electrocardiogram in the aged. An independent marker of heart disease? Am J Med 1981; 70:4–6.
39. Cullen KJ, Stenhouse NS, Wearne KL, Cumpston GN. Electrocardiograms and thirteen year cardiovascular mortality in Busselton study. Br Heart J 1982; 47:209–212.
40. Rabkin SW, Mathewson FAL, Tate RB. Relationship of ventricular ectopy in men without apparent heart disease to occurrence of ischemic heart disease and sudden death. Am Heart J 1981; 101:135–142.
41. Kannel WB, Doyle JT, McNamara PM, Quickenton P, Gordon T. Precursors of sudden death: Factors related to the incidence of sudden death. Circulation 1975; 57:606–613.
42. Abdalla ISH, Prineas RJ, Neaton JD, Jacobs DR, Crow RS. Relations between ventricular premature complexes and sudden cardiac death in apparently healthy men. Am J Cardiol 1987; 60:1036–1042.
43. Kantelip J-P, Sage E, Duchene-Marullaz P. Findings on ambulatory electrocar-

diologic monitoring in subjects older than 80 years. Am J Cardiol 1986; 57:398–401.
44. Kostis JB, McCrone K, Moreyra AE, Gotzoyannis S, Aglitz NM, Netarejan N, Kuo PT. Premature ventricular complexes in the absence of identifiable heart disease. Circulation 1981; 63:1351–1356.
45. Camm AJ, Evans KE, Ward DE, Martin A. The rhythm of the heart in active elderly subjects. Am Heart J 1980; 99:598–603.
46. Martin A, Benbow LJ, Butrous GS, Leach C, Camm AJ. Five-year follow-up of 106 elderly subjects by means of long-term ambulatory cardiac monitoring. Eur Heart J 1984; 5:592–596.
47. Fleg JL, Lakatta EG. Prevalence and prognosis of exercise-induced nonsustained ventricular tachycardia in apparently healthy volunteers. Am J Cardiol 1984; 54:762–764.
48. Busby MJ, Shefrin EA, Fleg JL. Significance of exercise-induced frequent or repetitive ventricular ectopic beats in apparently healthy volunteers. J Am Coll Cardiol 1989; 14:1659–1665.
49. Aronow WS, Epstein S, Koenigsberg M, Schwartz KS. Usefulness of echocardiographic abnormal left ventricular ejection fraction, paroxysmal ventricular tachycardia, and complex ventricular arrhythmias in predicting new coronary events in patients over 62 years of age. Am J Cardiol 1988; 61:1349–1351.
50. Hinkle LE, Carver ST, Argyrus DC. The frequency of asymptomatic disturbances of cardiac rhythm and conduction in middle-aged men. Am J Cardiol 1969; 24:629–650.

# 4

# Echocardiographic Measurements in Elderly Patients Without Clinical Heart Disease

**Julius M. Gardin**
*University of California, Irvine, California*

## INTRODUCTION

The ability to image cardiac structures and to evaluate left ventricular function noninvasively has made echocardiography extremely useful in the evaluation of individuals with known or suspected heart disease. The noninvasive character of the ultrasound technique has made it particularly applicable to an older population. The goals of this chapter are (1) to discuss the effect of aging on left ventricular systolic and diastolic function by M-mode and Doppler echocardiography, and (2) to present normative M-mode and Doppler echocardiographic measurement data that can serve as a basis for evaluating cardiac structure and function in elderly individuals.

## BASIC PRINCIPLES OF ECHOCARDIOGRAPHY

Echocardiography involves the application of reflected ultrasound, that is, sound waves of frequency above the normally audible range, to the evaluation of the heart. Pulsed ultrasound waves in the frequency range of 1.6–5 MHz are emitted from a transducer that also acts as a receiver of reflected waves. Since ultrasound is reflected at interfaces having different acoustical impedances, internal structures of the heart possessing different densities, such as myocardium, valves, or cardiac chambers, can be readily imaged.

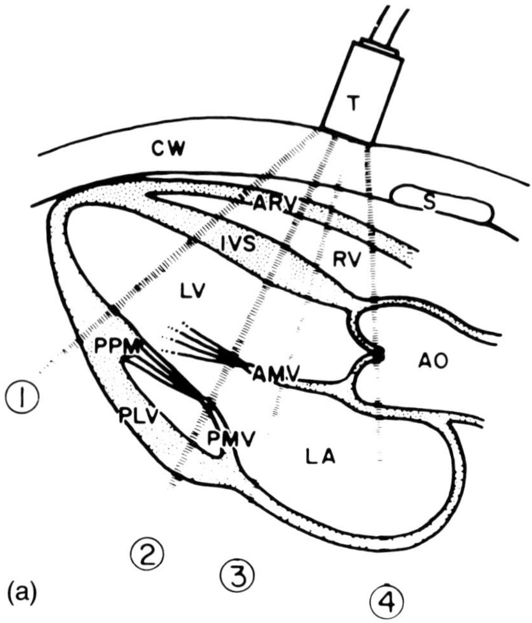
T
CW
ARV
S
IVS
RV
LV
PPM
AO
AMV
1
PLV
PMV
LA
2
3
4

(a)

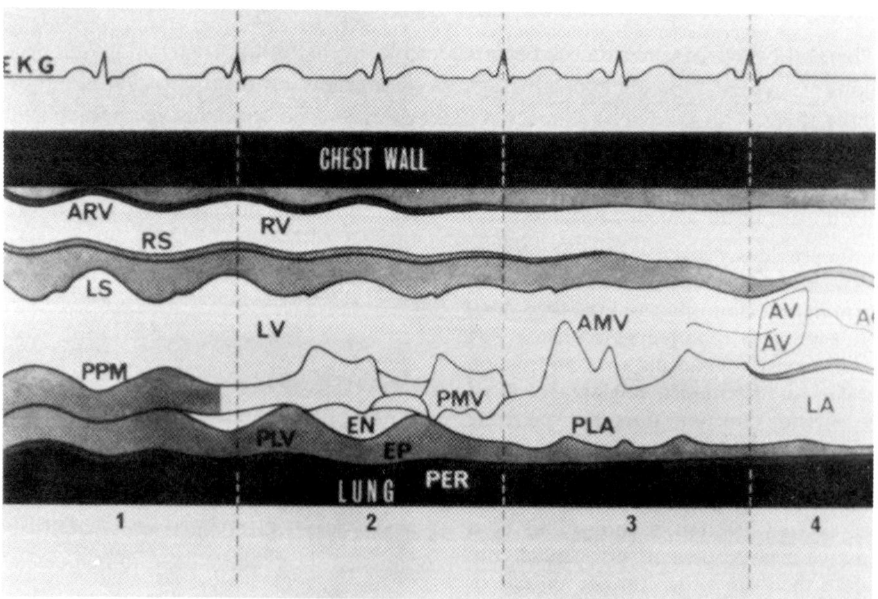
EKG
CHEST WALL
ARV
RV
RS
LS
LV
AMV
AV
AV
PPM
PMV
LA
EN
PLA
PLV
EP
PER
LUNG
1
2
3
4

(b)

The two basic cardiac ultrasound imaging modalities in clinical use are M-mode and two-dimensional echocardiography. The M-mode (time-motion) technique utilizes a single beam of ultrasound that begins at the chest wall and traverses identifiable cardiac structures at various depths. The reflected ultrasound waves ("echoes") can be displayed on an oscilloscope or television monitor (1) in proportion to the depth and density of the tissues from which they are reflected (on the vertical axis), and (2) as a function of time (on the horizontal axis). Structures can then be identified by the intensity and motion of the reflected echoes as well as by the characteristic anatomical relationships of the various structures to each other. In transthoracic echo cardiography, the transducer is usually placed in the second to fourth intercostal spaces to the left of the sternum, and a "sweep" is performed from the region of the ventricles to the interface of the left atrium and the aorta (Figs. 1 and 2). Additional views of the heart may be obtained from the apical, subcostal, and suprasternal positions (1,2).

Two-dimensional echocardiography is an attempt to provide a two-dimensional image, rather than the single dimension (over time) afforded by the M-mode technique. Various methods have been developed to produce a continuous (virtually real-time) display of cardiac function in up to a 90° arc (sector). The two most popular two-dimensional methods for cardiac imaging involve mechanical and electronic ("phased-array") sector scanning. In mechanical sector scanning, one or a few ultrasound crystals are mechanically rotated directly on the chest wall or within a housing in contact with the chest wall. A simultaneous display of echoes from each position in up to a 90° arc is possible with this approach. In phased-array sector scanning, a small transducer with multiple crystals, for example, 64–128 individual elements, is held stationary on the chest while the ultrasound beam is steered back and forth electronically by con-

---

**Figure 1** (a) A diagram of the heart in longitudinal section, depicting structures through which the ultrasound beam passes as it is directed from the apex toward the base of the heart. Numbers 1–4 refer to standard positions for recording the M-mode echocardiogram. CW = chest wall, T = transducer, S = sternum, ARV = anterior right ventricle, RV = right ventricular cavity, IVS = interventricular septum, LV = left ventricle, PPM = posterior papillary muscle, PLV = posterior left ventricular wall, AMV = anterior mitral valve leaflet, PMV = posterior mitral valve leaflet, AO = aorta, LA = left atrium. (b) M-mode echocardiogram as transducer is directed from cardiac apex (position 1) to base (position 4). Areas between the dotted lines correspond to the transducer positions as depicted in a. AV = aortic valve, EN = endocardium of left ventricle, LS = left septum, PER = pericardium, PLA = posterior left atrial wall, RS = right (side of ventricular) septum; other abbreviations as in a. (Reprinted from Feigenbaum H. Clinical applications of echocardiography. Prog Cardiovasc Dis 1972; 14:531, with permission.)

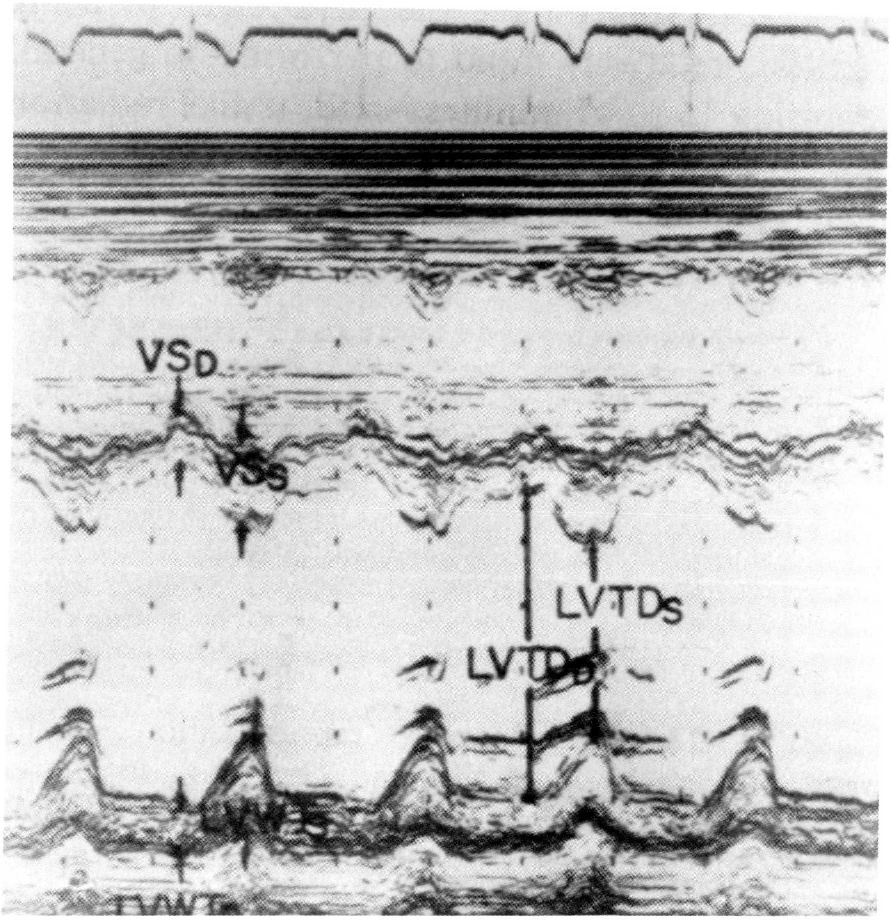


**Figure 2** Echocardiographic recording of the left ventricle indicating measurements of parameters of left ventricular muscle mass and percentage fractional shortening. $VS_D$ = interventricular septal thickness measured during diastole, $VS_S$ = ventricular septal thickness measured during systole, $LVWT_D$ = left ventricular posterior wall thickness measured during diastole, $LVWT_S$ = left ventricular posterior wall thickness measured during systole, $LVTD_D$ = left ventricular transverse dimension measured during diastole, $LVTD_S$ = left ventricular transverse dimension measured during systole. (Reprinted from Drayer J, Gardin JM, Weber MA, Aronow WS. Changes in cardiac anatomy and function during therapy with alpha-methyldopa: An echocardiographic study. Curr Ther Res 1982; 32:856–865, with permission.)

trolling the sequence of firing of the individual elements. Imaging in an arc of up to 90° is also possible with this technique. With both the mechanical and phased-array approaches, imaging in multiple views, including longitudinal, short-axis, apical, subcostal, and suprasternal, usually allows visualization of most areas of the heart and proximal great arteries (Fig. 3). Both M-mode and two-dimensional echocardiography have the advantages of being painless, relatively rapid to perform—in general requiring 15–45 min—and, unlike radiation exposure, without known biologic ill effects as used clinically in humans. Consequently, both techniques can be utilized repetitively in a given patient for serial evaluation of cardiac anatomy and function.

Cardiac ultrasound can also be used to display and measure characteristics of blood flow in the heart using the Doppler principle. Briefly, the Doppler principle dictates that the shift in frequency of ultrasound reflected from moving targets (e.g., red blood cells) is directly proportional to the velocity of these targets in the direction of the ultrasound beam. This principle is expressed by the Doppler equation,

$$V = \frac{\Delta Fc}{2f \cos \phi},$$

where $\Delta F$ corresponds to the shift in frequency between the transmitted and reflected ultrasound beam, $\cos \phi$ is the cosine of the angle between the ultrasound beam and the major axis of blood flow, $F$ is the fundamental (transmitted) frequency of the ultrasound transducer, and $c$ corresponds to the velocity of ultrasound in tissues (approximately 1540 m/s) (1,2).

Doppler echocardiography combines Doppler flow velocity recording with M-mode or two-dimensional echocardiographic imaging. The Doppler component uses such modalities as continuous wave, pulsed wave, and color flow Doppler. The continuous wave technique involves one (or more) transducers that are continually transmitting and one (or more) transducers that are continuously receiving the reflected ultrasound. This technique has proven particularly useful in evaluating cardiac lesions that produce high-velocity jets, such as valvular stenosis, regurgitation, and intracardiac shunts. Pulsed Doppler recording has proven useful generally (but not exclusively) in evaluating lower velocity events associated with nondisturbed flow across the cardiac valves. For example, pulsed Doppler recordings of aortic and transmitral flow have been used to evaluate left ventricular systolic and diastolic function. Color Doppler echocardiography ("flow mapping") is a multigated pulsed Doppler approach in which mean flow velocities in many "pixels" (picture elements) along each ultrasound line in the sector are displayed in intensities of red (flow toward transducer) and blue (flow away from transducer) corresponding to their respective frequency shifts. This technique has been particularly helpful in the evaluation of valvular stenosis and regurgitation, as well as in intracardiac shunt lesions (1,2).

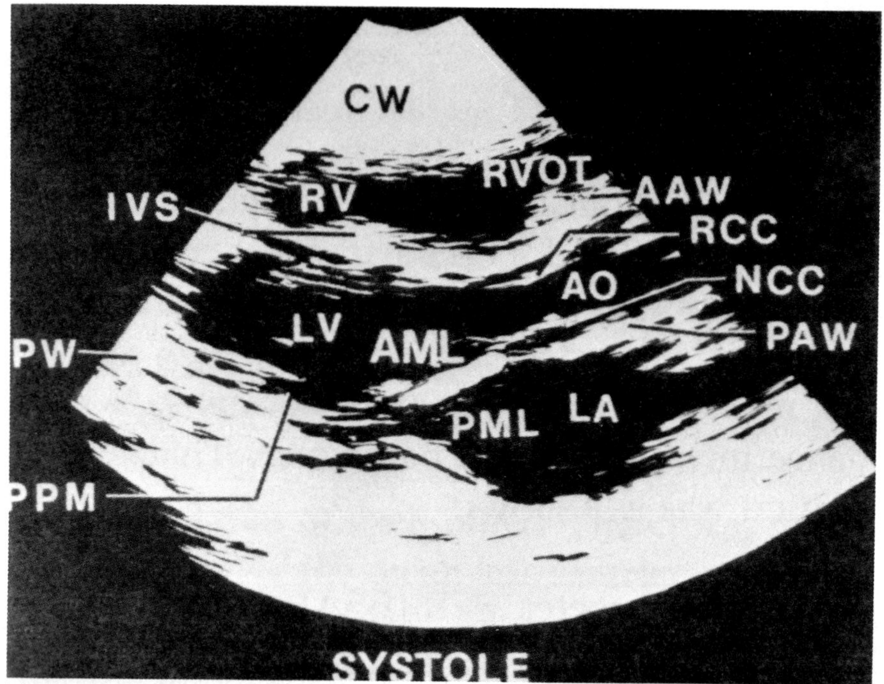
CW
RVOT
AAW
IVS
RV
RCC
AO
NCC
LV
AML
PAW
PW
LA
PML
PPM
SYSTOLE

(a)

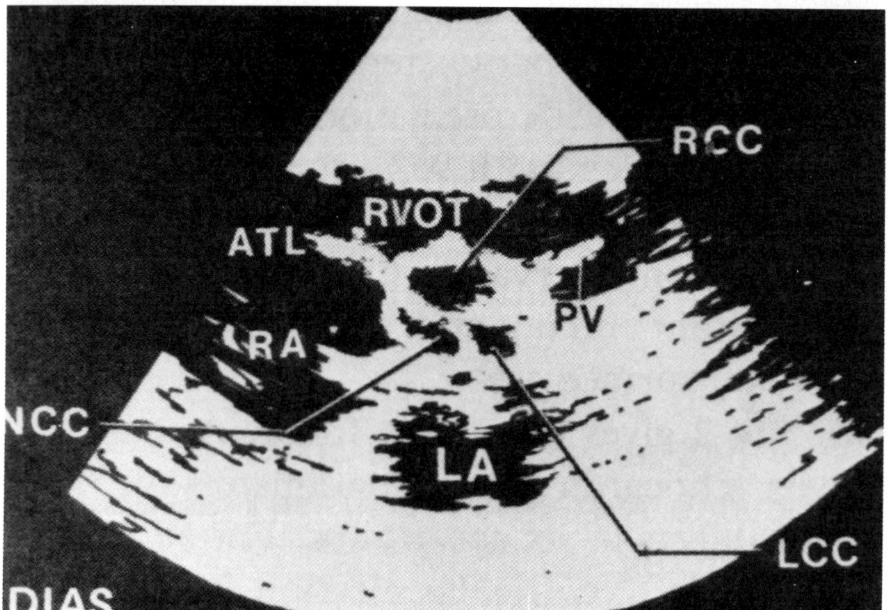
RCC
RVOT
ATL
PV
RA
NCC
LA
LCC
DIAS

(b)

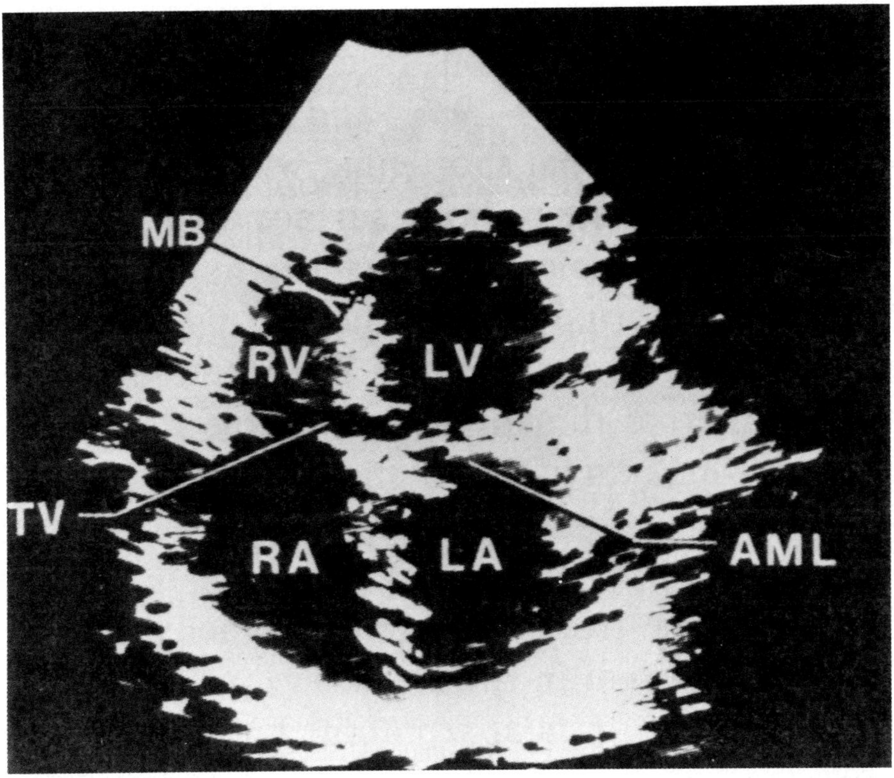


(c)

**Figure 3** (a) Drawing of the heart in systole, in the parasternal long-axis view. P = posterior, I = inferior, S = superior, AAW = anterior aortic wall, AO = aortic root, PAW = posterior aortic wall, LA = left atrium, RCC = right coronary cusp, NCC = noncoronary cusp, AML = anterior mitral leaflet, PML = posterior mitral leaflet, LV = left ventricle, PW = posterior left ventricular wall, PPM = posterior papillary muscle, IVS = interventricular septum, RV = right ventricle, RVOT = right ventricular outflow, CW = chest wall. (b) The heart at the level of the great arteries in the parasternal short-axis view. ATL = anterior tricuspid leaflet, PV = pulmonic valve, LCC = left coronary cusp, RA = right atrium, DIAS = diastole. (c) The heart in systole in the apical four-chamber view. MB = moderator band, TV = tricuspid valve. (Reprinted from Koenigsberg D, Ganote C. Cardiac anatomy. In: Talano JV, Gardin JM, eds. Textbook on Two-Dimensional Echocardiography. New York: Grune & Stratton, 1983, with permission.)

In this chapter we present data derived from (1) Doppler measurements of aortic flow velocity, used to evaluate left ventricular systolic performance at rest and during exercise, and (2) transmitral flow velocity measurements, used to assess left ventricular diastolic function at rest.

## RELATIONSHIP OF AGE TO NORMAL M-MODE ECHOCARDIOGRAPHIC MEASUREMENTS

To determine the relationship between age and M-mode echocardiographic measurements in normal subjects, we studied 136 adults (78 men and 58 women, 20–97 years of age) without evidence of cardiovascular disease (3). These subjects, whose ages ranged from 20 to 97 years, all underwent history taking and physical examination, chest roentgenography, electrocardiography, and M-mode echocardiography. In no subject did this evaluation reveal the presence of heart disease, hypertension, other serious illness, or obesity. Furthermore, all subjects had a normal electrocardiogram (ECG), normal chest film, and no evidence of mitral valve prolapse or pericardial effusion on M-mode echocardiogram. M-mode echocardiography was performed in the left lateral decubitus position, and the following measurements were made: left ventricular internal dimensions at end diastole ($LVID_d$) and end systole ($LVID_s$); ventricular septal ($VS_d$) and posterobasal left ventricular free-wall thicknesses ($LVPW_d$) at end diastole; aortic root and left atrial dimensions; and mitral valve E-F slope, which corresponds to the rate of early diastolic closure of the anterior mitral valve leaflet (see Figs. 1 and 2). In addition, LV mass, ejection fraction, and fractional shortening were derived from the following formulas (4):

$$\text{LV mass} = (1.05)[(LVID_d + VS_d + LVPW_d)^3 - (LVID_d)^3] \quad (1)$$

$$\text{LV ejection fraction} = \frac{(LVID_d)^3 - (LVID_s)^3}{(LVID_d)^3} \times 100\% \quad (2)$$

$$\text{LV \% fractional shortening} = \frac{(LVID_d - LVID_s)}{LVID_d} \times 100\% \quad (3)$$

In the absence of localized disorders of left ventricular function like those that may be present in coronary artery disease, M-mode echocardiographic estimates have been reported to correlate well with two-dimensional echocardiographic and angiographic measurements of left ventricular volume and ejection fraction (4). Also, under these conditions, LV percentage fractional shortening gives information similar to that obtained from LV ejection fraction. Although ejection fraction does not perfectly characterize the functional state of the left ventricle, this measurement is accepted as providing an overall assessment of pump performance. Furthermore, ejection fraction is thought to be a more sensitive measurement of myocardial contractile state than are either cardiac output or left ventricular end-diastolic pressure.

Echocardiographic measurements were analyzed for the influence of age, sex, and body surface area. When the data for each echocardiographic parameter were analyzed separately for men and women as a function of body surface area, statistically significant differences between men and women were found for three parameters: (1) ventricular septal thickness, (2) posterobasal free-wall thickness, and (3) estimated left ventricular mass. However, since the sex differences for these three parameters were relatively small (range 6.2–7.2%), we chose for the sake of simplicity to combine data for men and women in our calculation of regression equations and prediction intervals (3,5,6).

When patients were subdivided into six age groups, progressive changes were found in mean normal values for various M-mode echocardiographic parameters (Fig. 4). Specifically, when the oldest group (over 70 years) was compared with the youngest group (21–30 years), significant ($p < 0.01$) increases in aortic root (22%) and left atrial (16%) dimensions, in ventricular septal (20%) and left ventricular free-wall (18%) thicknesses, and in estimated

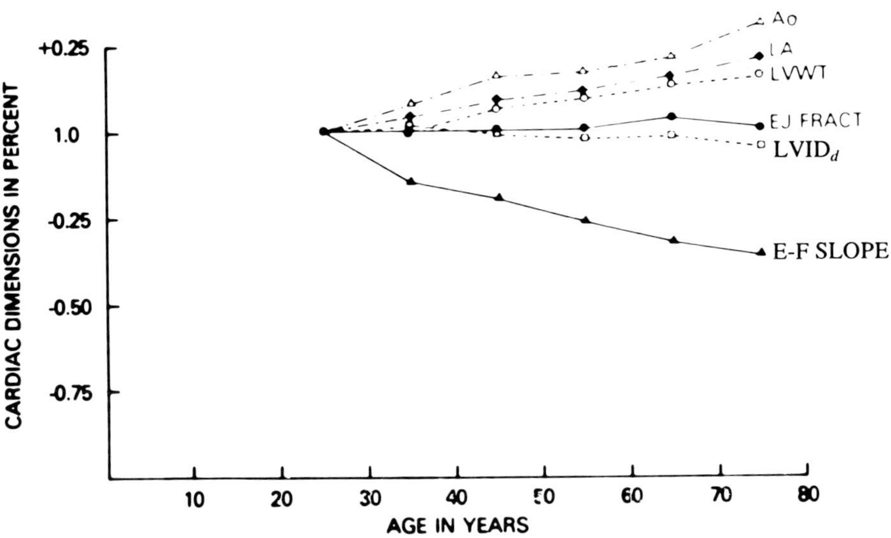


**Figure 4** Percentage change in M-mode echocardiographic measurements in the five older age groups compared with the 21–30 year age group. Data are displayed for aortic root dimension (AO), left atrial dimension (LA), LV posterobasal free-wall thickness in diastole (LVWT), LV ejection fraction (EJ FRACT), left ventricular internal dimension in diastole (LVID$_d$), and mitral E-F SLOPE.

left ventricular mass (15%) were noted (3,5,6). In addition, a significant ($p < 0.01$) decrease in mean mitral E-F slope (43%) and slight decreases in mean left ventricular systolic and diastolic internal dimensions (5 and 6%, respectively, $p < 0.05$) were noted. Left ventricular ejection fraction and percentage fractional shortening were found to be independent of age. These data were used to derive regression equations related to both age and body surface area (BSA). The regression equations can be used to calculate mean normal values and 95% prediction intervals for echocardiographic measurements in adults.

We analyzed our data according to the general regression equation

$$\text{Echo parameter} = B(\text{BSA}) + A \pm C$$

where $A$ represents the intercept, $B$ represents a slope unique for each parameter, and $C$ represents the width of the 95% prediction interval, that is, the interval into which, with 95% confidence, a new normal observation would fall (3). When subjects were grouped into six age groups, the slope of the regression relationship was found to be independent of age for every parameter ($p > 0.05$), whereas the intercept showed significant variation with age for every parameter ($p < 0.05$). Therefore, we assumed that the intercept $A$, but not the slope $B$, was influenced by age and that the width of the 95% prediction interval $C$ was constant and not appreciably influenced by age or BSA. The values of $A$ derived from our data for each age group are given in Table 1, which also includes the values of $B$ and $C$ for each parameter (3).

Figures 5 through 9 depict the relationships between age and aortic root dimension, left atrial dimension, left ventricular diastolic and systolic dimension, left ventricular posterior wall thickness, and left ventricular mass. For each figure, the regression equations in Table 1 have been utilized to adjust the values to three common body surface area values (1.4, 1.8, and 2.2 $m^2$) (3).

Our echocardiographic findings are compatible with information derived from previous studies using other methods. Roberts and Perloff noted that hearts of older individuals studied at necropsy appear to have small ventricular chambers and thicker walls than those of their younger counterparts (7). Although the magnitude of the decrease was small, we also noted that the internal dimensions of the left ventricle decreased as age increased. We also noted progressive increases in the thicknesses of the ventricular septum and the left ventricular free wall with increasing age. The magnitudes and rates of increase were similar for septum and free wall, so that there was no change in the septum-free wall ratio with increasing age. Estimated left ventricular mass showed a small but progressive increase from the 21–30 age group to the over 70 age group. This increase reflected an increase in wall thickness that was relatively greater than the decrease in left ventricular diastolic dimension. Since the mean systolic and diastolic blood pressures varied by less than 15 mm Hg

**Table 1** Regression Equations of Echocardiography Measurements Versus Age

| Equation | | Intercepts (age dependent) | | | | | | Prediction interval |
|---|---|---|---|---|---|---|---|---|
| | | 21–30 | 31–40 | 41–50 | 51–60 | 61–70 | ≥ 70 | |
| $LVID_d$ | = 6.94(BSA) + | 35.5 | 36.2 | 34.4 | 34.1 | 34.8 | 32.7 | ± 5.60 |
| $LVID_s$ | = 4.24(BSA) + | 22.4 | 22.6 | 21.5 | 21.1 | 21.7 | 20.8 | ± 5.81 |
| Septum | = 2.53(BSA) + | 5.27 | 5.47 | 6.27 | 6.53 | 6.84 | 7.20 | ± 1.75 |
| LVPW | = 2.18(BSA) + | 6.11 | 6.02 | 6.94 | 6.97 | 7.34 | 7.81 | ± 1.43 |
| LV mass | = 124(BSA) + | 9.87 | −1.98 | 8.56 | 10.8 | 26.8 | 22.2 | ±57.6 |
| Ao | = 8.31(BSA) + | 12.3 | 13.1 | 14.7 | 15.6 | 16.4 | 18.5 | ± 5.76 |
| LA | = 9.98(BSA) + | 16.3 | 16.7 | 17.6 | 18.0 | 19.3 | 21.7 | ± 7.01 |
| E-F slope | = 20.1(BSA) + | 99.9 | 90.2 | 78.3 | 66.6 | 62.2 | 43.5 | ±62.2 |

Abbreviations: Ao = aortic root dimension, BSA = body surface area, LA = left atrial dimension, LVID = left ventricular internal dimension, *d* = diastole, *s* = systole.

*Source*: Reprinted from Gardin et al., J Clin Ultrasound 1979, with permission, Ref. 3.

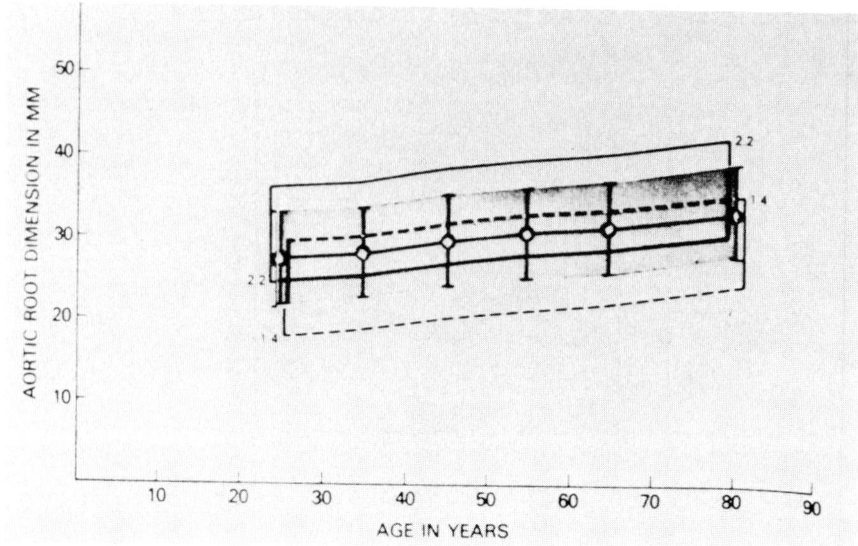


**Figure 5** Aortic root dimension in late diastole is plotted in millimeters versus age in years. In Figures 5–9, the mean value for each age group is depicted by a circle plotted at the mean age in the age group. The bracketed and shaded area on either side of the circle represents the 95% prediction interval for normal values for a subject with a BSA of 1.8 $m^2$. The 95% prediction intervals are also shown for subjects with BSA values of 1.4 $m^2$ (dotted lines) and 2.2 $m^2$ (solid lines). (Reprinted from Gardin et al., J Clin Ultrasound 1979; 7:439–447. Copyright 1979 John Wiley & Sons, Inc., with permission.)

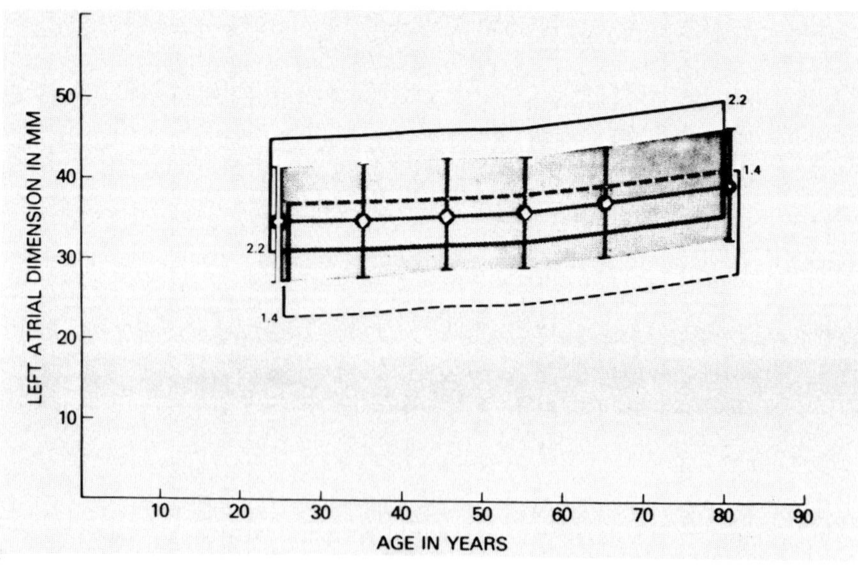


**Figure 6** Left atrial dimension in late diastole in millimeters versus age in years. For each age group, the mean and 95% prediction interval for normal values are depicted. (Reprinted from Gardin et al., J Clin Ultrasound 1979; 7:439–447. Copyright 1979 John Wiley & Sons, Inc., with permission.)

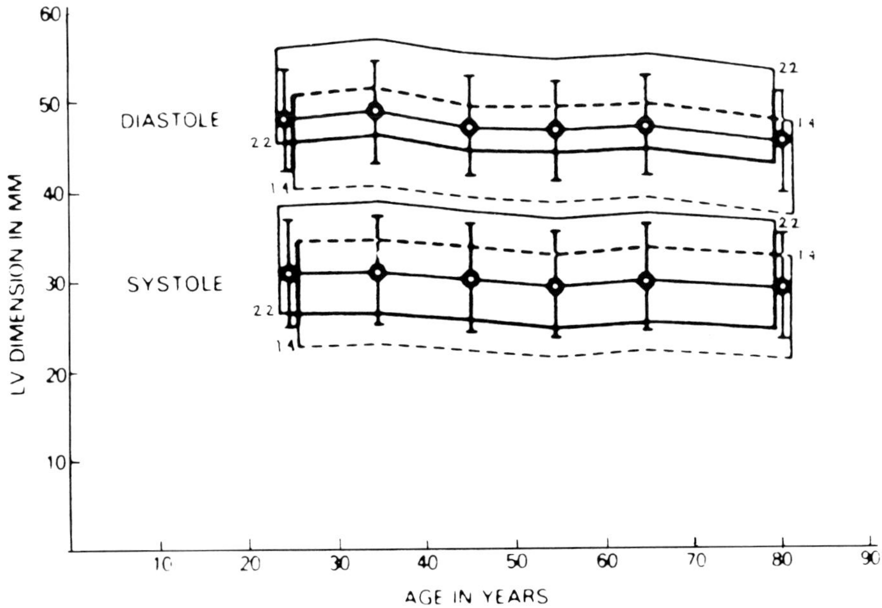


**Figure 7** Left ventricular end-diastolic and end-systolic dimensions in millimeters versus age in years. For each age group, the mean and 95% prediction interval for normal values are depicted. (Reprinted from Gardin et al., J Clin Ultrasound 1979; 7:439–447. Copyright 1979 John Wiley & Sons, Inc., with permission.)

among the six age groups, we could not ascribe the increased wall thickness or mass observed in our subjects to a change in basal arterial blood pressure with aging.

Krovetz reviewed a number of published reports of measurements of aortic valve annulus size made at necropsy (8). When aortic annulus size was corrected for body surface area, progressive increases with age were noted in both men and women over 20 years of age. We noted similar increases in aortic root dimensions as measured by echocardiography. The progressive increase in left atrial dimension with increasing age noted in our normal adult subjects was noted by Roberts and Perloff at necropsy (7). It is important to take this age-related change into account when using echocardiographic measurements of left atrial dimension to make quantitative statements about the effects of various disease states (e.g., hypertension or valvular or coronary disease).

Various investigators have reported functional changes with age in the mitral valve echocardiogram consistent with our findings of decreased E-F slope (9). Factors postulated to explain this decrease in the rate of early diastolic closure

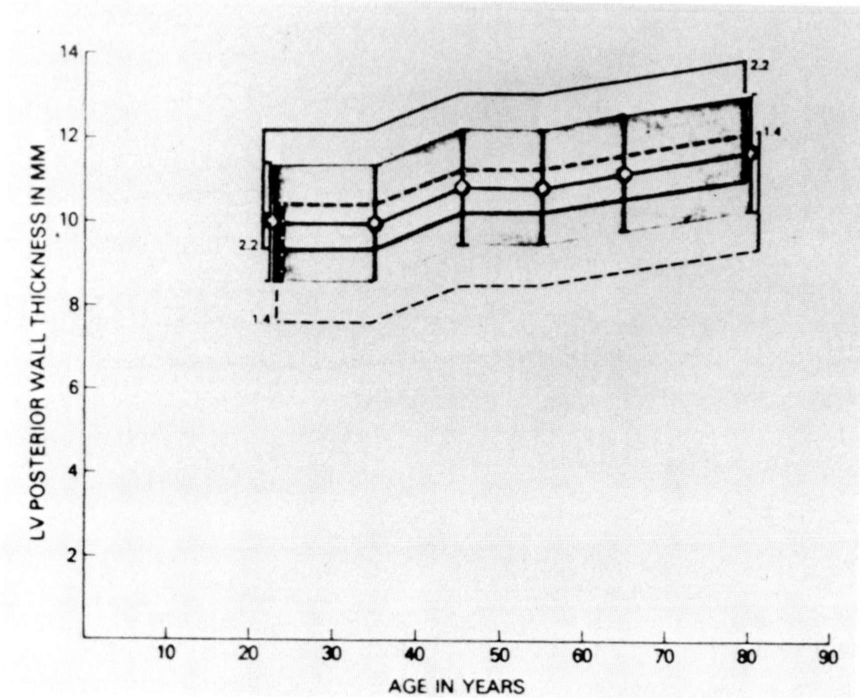


**Figure 8** Left ventricular posterior wall thickness in late diastole in millimeters versus age in years. For each age group, the mean and 95% prediction interval for normal values are depicted. (Reprinted from Gardin et al., J Clin Ultrasound 1979; 7:439–447. Copyright 1979 John Wiley & Sons, Inc., with permission.)

of the anterior mitral valve leaflet have included sclerosis of the mitral leaflets and/or decreased compliance of the left ventricle (9).

In our studies, left ventricular ejection fraction and percentage fractional shortening did not change appreciably as age increased from 20 to 97 years. These findings are consistent with several previous studies (10,11), including one in which left ventricular function was assessed with radionuclide cineangiography (10). If the left ventricular internal dimension at end diastole is mildly reduced in older subjects while ejection fraction and heart rate are unchanged, stroke volume and cardiac output are expected to diminish slightly with advancing age. Data indicating that this is so have been reported using a dye-dilution technique (12,13).

Our findings relating changes in echocardiographic parameters to increasing age are generally in agreement with findings reported by Gerstenblith et al. (14). The major difference is that we found a slight but significant decrease in left ventricular systolic and diastolic internal dimensions with increasing age, whereas Gerstenblith and associates found no change. Furthermore, women

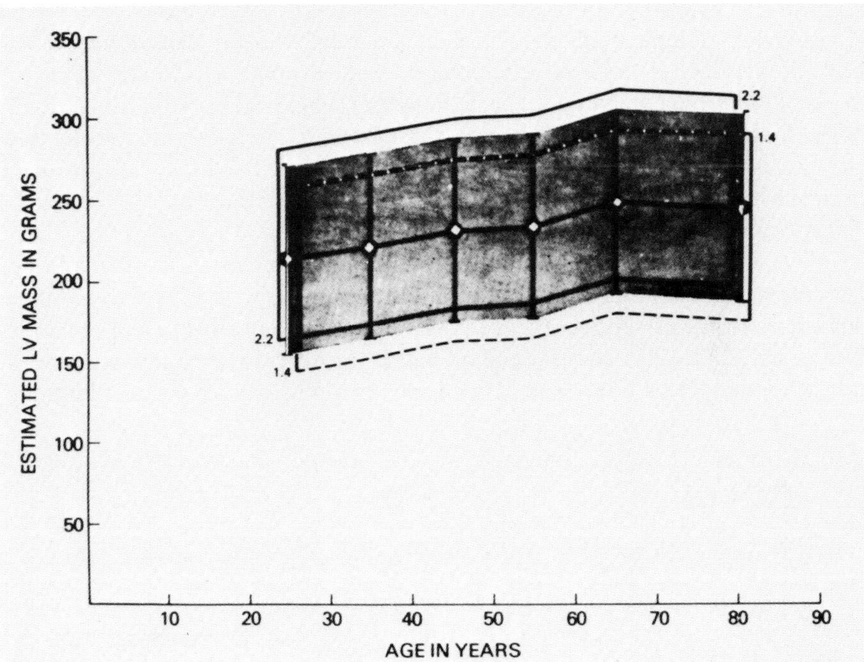


**Figure 9** Estimated left ventricular mass in grams versus age in years. The mean and 95% prediction interval are depicted for each age group. (Reprinted from Gardin et al., Hypertension, 1987, with permission; Ref. 6.)

were not included in their study population, nor did they report measurements of left atrial dimension or left ventricular mass.

Although it is highly likely that these echocardiographic changes reported in the different age groups are related to the aging process, one cannot be certain that this explanation is correct until these changes are documented during serial studies in the same patient. Nonetheless, this analysis makes it clear that it is important to use normal echocardiographic values corrected for both age and body surface area (or another measure of body size) when evaluating adult patients suspected of having heart disease.

## RELATIONSHIP OF AGE TO LEFT VENTRICULAR SYSTOLIC PERFORMANCE AS MEASURED BY DOPPLER AORTIC FLOW VELOCITY PARAMETERS

Doppler flow velocity measurements in the aorta have been shown to be useful in differentiating normal subjects from those with left ventricular dysfunction

(15,16). For example, patients with dilated cardiomyopathy demonstrate aortic peak flow velocity, flow velocity integral, and average acceleration that are markedly reduced compared to those in normal subjects (Fig. 10) (15). Furthermore, in patients with congestive heart failure undergoing vasodilator therapy, changes in Doppler aortic peak flow velocity and flow velocity integral have been shown to be useful in estimating changes in systemic vascular resistance and stroke volume, respectively (16).

We evaluated the relationship between age and Doppler aortic flow velocity measurements in 97 adults (45 men and 52 women, aged 21–78 years) without clinical evidence of cardiac disease (18). No subject had a history of hypertension or cardiovascular disease, and all had a normal cardiac examination, electrocardiogram, chest x-ray, and M-mode and two-dimensional echocardiogram.

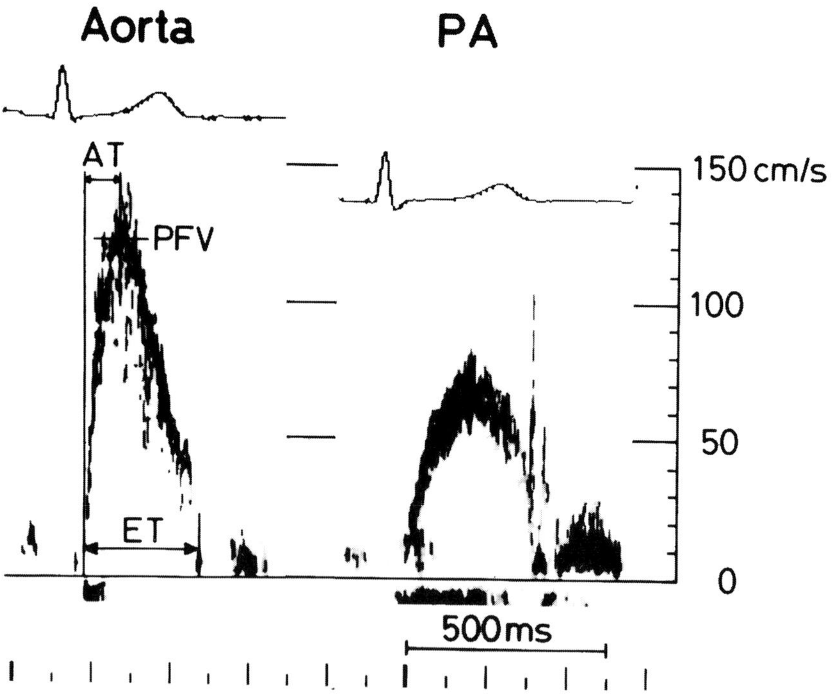


**Figure 10** Doppler aortic and pulmonary flow velocity recording from a normal subject. Measurements made included peak flow velocity (PFV) in cm/s; ejection time (ET) in ms; acceleration time (AT), in ms; and average acceleration in cm/s$^2$ (calculated by dividing PFV by AT). In addition, the aortic flow velocity integral, or area under the flow velocity curve in cm, was estimated. (See text for details.) (Reprinted from Gardin et al., Am Heart J 1984, with permission, Ref. 17.)

Figure 10 demonstrates an aortic flow velocity recording from a normal subject (17,18). Peak flow velocity was measured in centimeters per second at the midpoint of the darkest area of the spectrum at the time of maximum flow velocity. Ejection time (ET) was measured in milliseconds from the onset of the systolic flow velocity curve to the time the curve crossed the zero-flow line at end systole. Aortic flow velocity integral (centimeters), which represents the area under the flow velocity curve, was estimated by the following formula: Flow velocity integral = 0.5 × peak flow velocity × ET (16). Acceleration time in milliseconds was measured from the onset of ejection to the midpoint of the tracing at the time of peak flow velocity. Average acceleration was calculated by dividing the peak flow velocity by the acceleration time and was expressed in centimeters per second per second.

Multiple linear regression analysis revealed that age was significantly correlated with aortic peak flow velocity, average acceleration, and flow velocity integral (all $p < 0.001$) (18). Figure 11 depicts the relationship between aortic peak flow velocity and age. The two parameters were related by the following

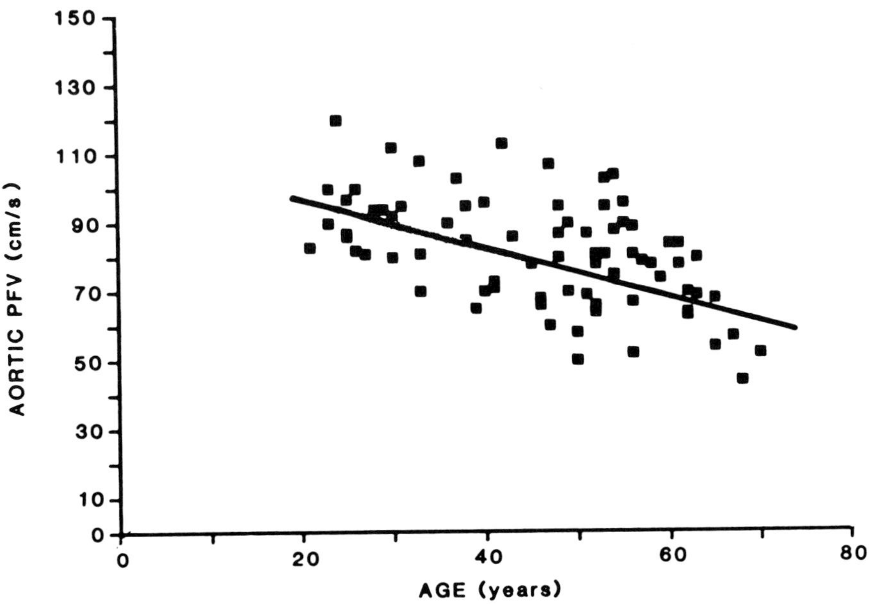


**Figure 11** Relationship between aortic peak flow velocity (cm/s) and age (years) in 80 subjects. The solid line represents the line of regression. Note the negative slope of the relationship between the two parameters ($r = -0.54$). Aortic PFV is significantly lower in the 60–70-year age group than in the 21–30 year age group ($p < 0.001$). (Reprinted from Gardin et al., Am Heart J 1987, with permission, Ref. 18.)

regression equation: Aortic peak flow velocity $= -0.6(\text{age}) + 110$ ($r = -0.54$, $p = 0.001$). Aortic peak flow velocity was significantly lower in the 61–70 year age decade (mean ± standard deviation, SD, = 65 ± 12 cm/s) than in the 21–30 year age decade (mean ± SD = 93 ± 11 cm/s) (18). The correlation of aortic peak flow velocity with age remained significant ($p < 0.001$) after division of peak flow velocity by the square root of the R-R interval.

Figure 12 depicts the relationship between aortic flow velocity integral and age. Note the significantly lower ($p < 0.001$) aortic flow velocity integral in the 61–70-year age decade (mean ± SD = 9.5 ± 2.3 cm) compared with the 21–30-year age decade (13.8 ± 2.1 cm). Aortic flow velocity integral and age are related by the following regression equation: Aortic flow velocity integral $= -0.09(\text{age}) + 16.5$ ($r = -0.44$, $p < 0.001$) (18). This correlation with age remained significant ($p < 0.01$) after correction of aortic flow velocity integral for the square root of the R-R interval.

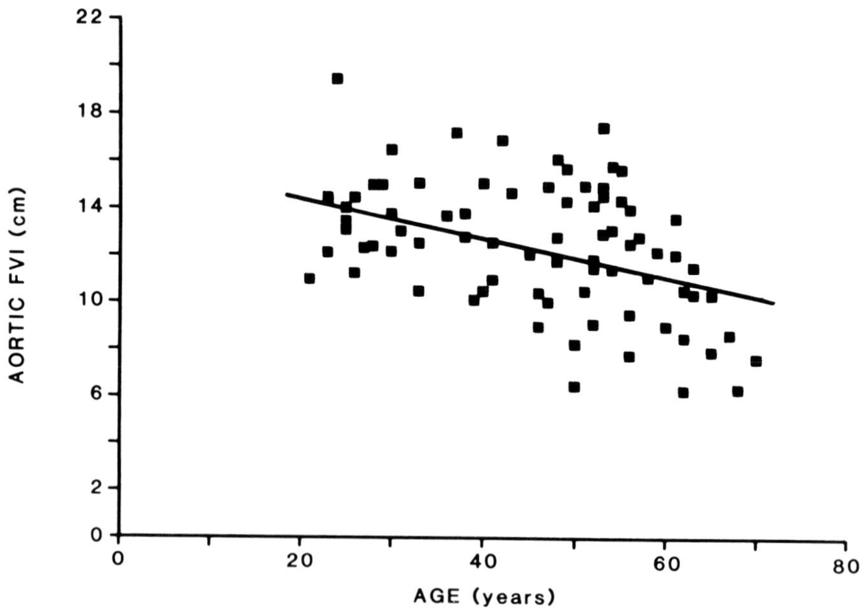


**Figure 12** Relationship between aortic flow velocity integral (cm) and age (years). Note the significantly lower flow velocity integral in the 61–70-year age group than in the 21–30 year age group ($p < 0.001$). (Reprinted from Gardin et al., Am Heart J 1987, with permission, Ref. 18.)

Figure 13 displays the relationship between aortic average acceleration and age. Note the significantly lower ($p < 0.005$) average acceleration in the 61–70-year age decade (mean ± SD = 695 ± 254 cm/s$^2$) compared to the 21–30-year age decade (939 ± 157 cm/s$^2$). Average acceleration in the aorta and age were related by the following regression equation: Aortic average acceleration = −6.55(age) + 1109 ($r = -0.42$, $p < 0.001$) (18). Correlation between aortic average acceleration and age remained significant ($r = -0.29$, $p < 0.02$) after dividing average acceleration by the square root of the R-R interval.

There was no significant relationship ($p > 0.05$) between aortic acceleration time and age. Furthermore, there was no significant relationship between ejection time and age. However, ejection time divided by the square root of the R-R interval increased significantly ($p < 0.001$) with increasing age (18).

The decrease in aortic peak flow velocity and flow velocity integral noted with increasing age are probably due, at least in part, to the increases in aortic

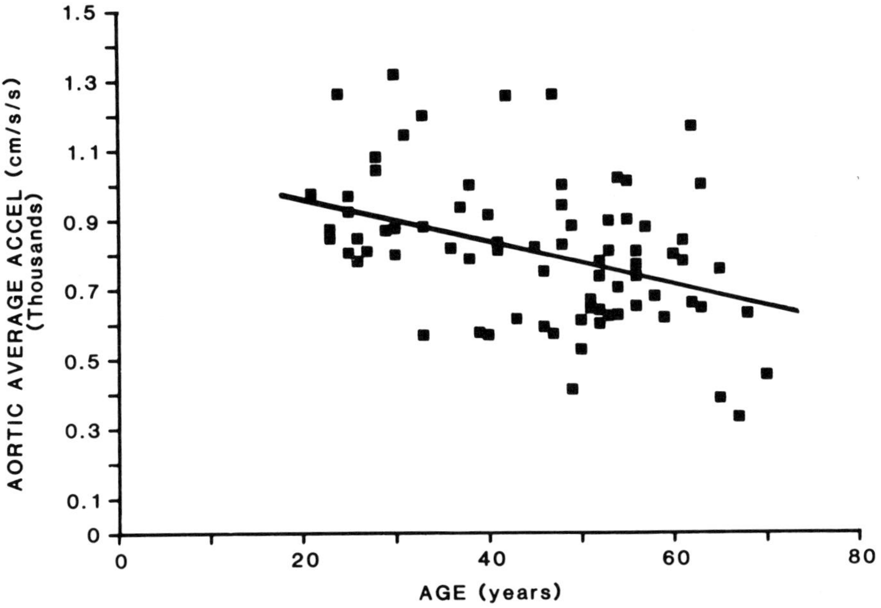


**Figure 13** Relationship between aortic average acceleration (cm/s$^2$) and age. Note the significantly lower average acceleration in the 61–70 year age decade compared to the 21–30 year age group ($p < 0.005$). (Reprinted from Gardin et al., Am Heart J 1987, with permission, Ref. 18.)

root diameter noted with aging (3,5,8,14). It was previously shown that resting stroke volume (3,5) and cardiac output (19) do not change significantly with aging. Since Doppler stroke volume can be estimated by multiplying the aortic flow velocity integral by the aortic root area, it follows that a decrease in flow velocity integral must be accompanied by an increase in aortic root area (and diameter) to maintain a constant stroke volume. Furthermore, since aortic flow velocity integral is approximately equal to ½ peak flow velocity × ejection time (16) and since we did not find any change in aortic ejection time with aging in this study, it follows that aortic peak flow velocity is expected to decrease with aging.

There were no significant differences in Doppler aortic flow velocity measurements between men and women of the same age. Furthermore, there was no significant relationship between body surface area or blood pressure and any of the aortic flow velocity parameters in this group of normal subjects (18).

## RELATIONSHIP OF AGE TO LEFT VENTRICULAR SYSTOLIC PERFORMANCE WITH UPRIGHT EXERCISE AS MEASURED BY DOPPLER AORTIC FLOW VELOCITY RECORDING DURING TREADMILL TESTING

To evaluate the effect of upright exercise on aortic peak flow velocity and acceleration, 60 normal subjects, aged 15–74 years, were evaluated by continuous wave Doppler during treadmill stress testing using the Bruce protocol (20). Subjects were divided into three age groups, each with 20 subjects: group I, 21 ± 4 years of age (mean ± standard deviation); group II, 36 ± 5 years; and group III, 58 ± 7 years. Periodic measurements of heart rate, blood pressure, and Doppler blood flow velocity and acceleration were made before, during, and after exercise. Continuous wave Doppler measurements were recorded from the suprasternal notch. The relationship between Doppler aortic measurements and age, gender, heart rate, and blood pressure responses during exercise were evaluated.

Age alone was significantly related (inversely) to immediate postexercise Doppler aortic peak blood flow velocity (group I, 1.1 ± 0.2; group II, 1.0 ± 0.2; and group III, 0.8 ± 0.2 m/s, respectively; $p < 0.01$) and peak acceleration (group I, 55 ± 15; group II, 46 ± 11; and group III, 36 ± 9 $m/s^2$; $p < 0.05$; Figs. 14 and 15). Gender, heart rate, and blood pressure changes during exercise, as well as exercise preconditioning, had no significant effect on these aortic flow characteristics.

These findings suggest that age is an important factor influencing aortic peak blood flow velocity and acceleration with exercise, as well as at rest. These changes in peak velocity and acceleration with exercise may reflect, in part, changes in exercise left ventricular function with age. Earlier studies (21–23)

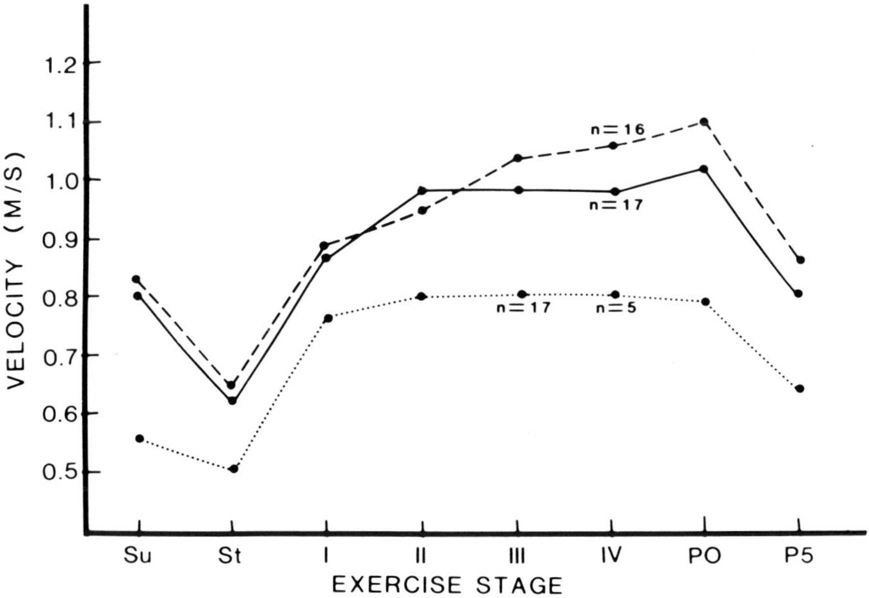


**Figure 14** Doppler peak aortic blood flow velocity measurements before, during, and immediately after exercise. Su = supine, St = standing, PO = immediate postexercise, P5 = 5 min after exercise. Data are shown as the mean for 20 subjects in each of the three groups, except as noted by *n* value in exercise stages III and IV. (Reprinted from Lazarus et al., Am J Cardiol 1988, with permission, Ref. 20.)

showed close correlations between these flow parameters and muscle contractility. However, alterations in aortic configuration, size, and compliance, as well as in impedance (afterload), probably affect these Doppler parameters to an important degree. Importantly, these age-dependent changes must be kept in mind when using Doppler-determined peak velocity and acceleration in evaluating left ventricular performance.

## RELATIONSHIP OF AGE TO LEFT VENTRICULAR DIASTOLIC FUNCTION AT REST AS EVALUATED BY DOPPLER TRANSMITRAL FLOW VELOCITY MEASUREMENTS

Although left ventricular systolic function is generally maintained with aging in healthy subjects (19), alterations in diastolic function are known to occur with "normal" aging (see Chap. 1) (24,25). We evaluated the relationship between age and pulsed Doppler transmitral flow velocity measurements in 66 adult men

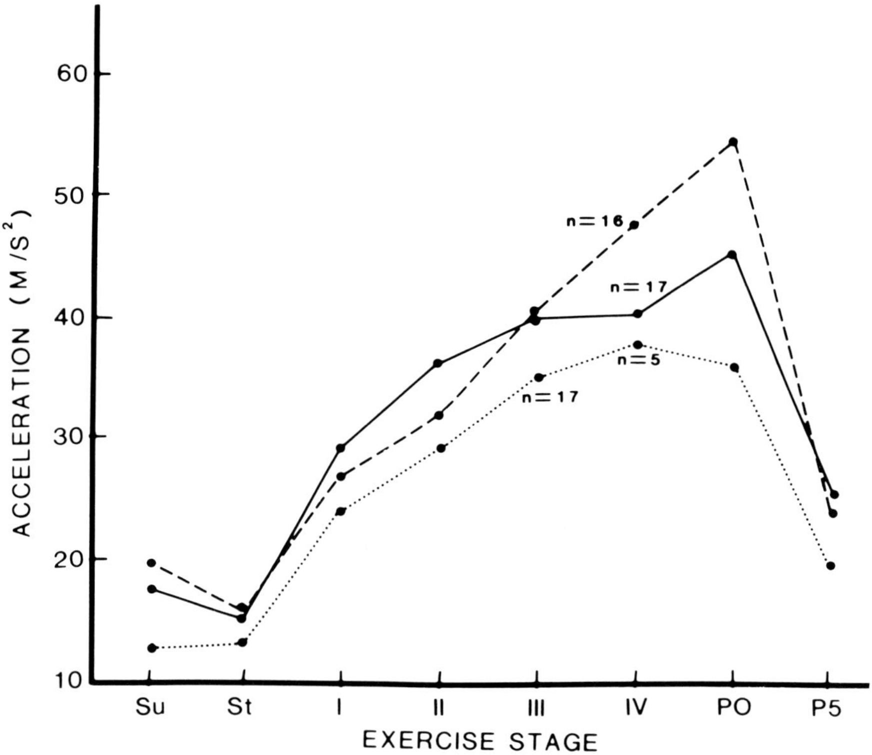


**Figure 15** Doppler peak acceleration measurements before, during, and immediately after exercise. Abbreviations and data display are as in Figure 14. (Reprinted from Lazarus et al., Am J Cardiol 1988, with permission, Ref. 20.)

and women aged 21–78 years without a history of hypertension or cardiovascular disease (25). Measurements of early and late diastolic transmitral peak flow (filling) velocities, flow times and flow velocity integrals, and early diastolic flow acceleration and deceleration were made at the level of the mitral leaflet tips. As shown in Figure 16, transmitral peak flow velocities in centimeters per second were measured in early and late diastole (i.e., at the time of atrial systole) at the midpoint of the darkest portion of the spectrum at the time of peak flow velocity.

Differences in Doppler transmitral flow velocity patterns between 30-year-old and 63-year-old normal adults are depicted in Figure 17 (25). Mitral peak flow velocity in early diastole (PFVE) was significantly lower ($p < 0.01$) in the 61–70-year age decade (45 ± 10 cm/s) than in the 21–30-year age decade (66 ± 11 cm/s; Fig. 18). Mitral peak flow velocity in late diastole (PFVA) was

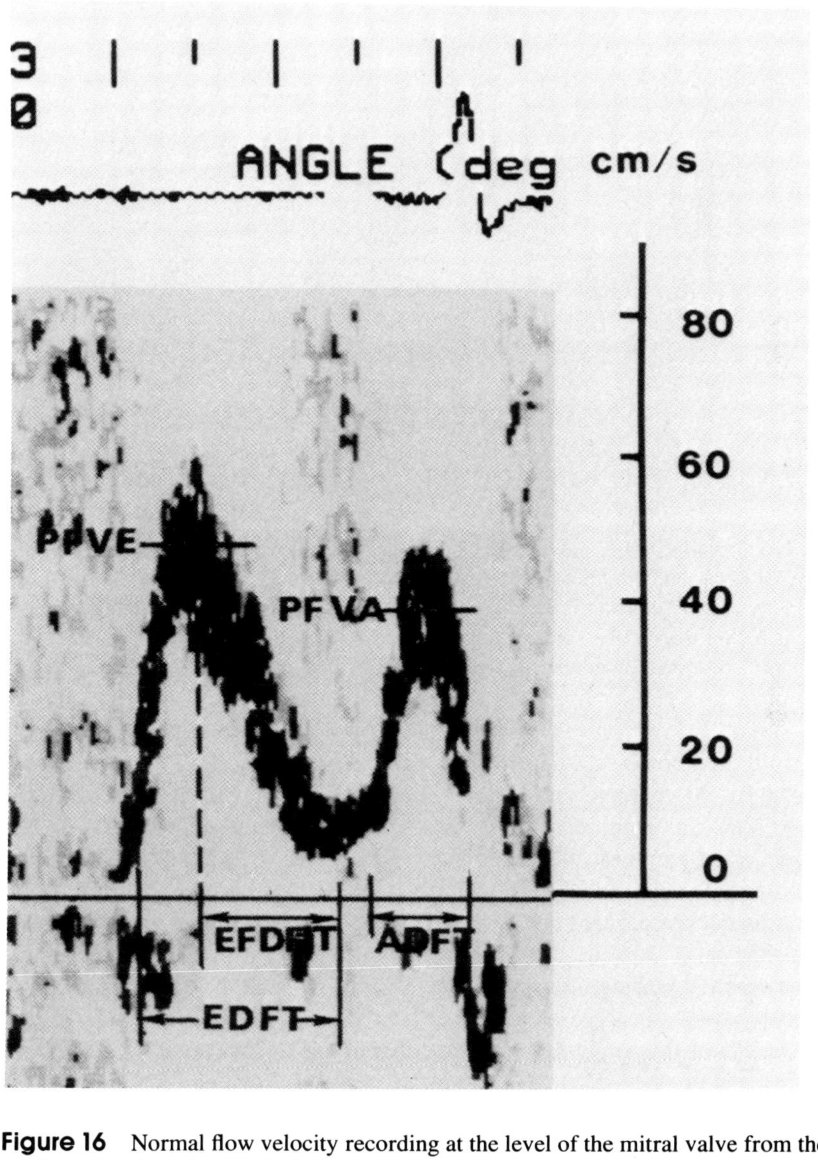


**Figure 16** Normal flow velocity recording at the level of the mitral valve from the apical four-chamber view depicting the method for making Doppler measurements. Mitral peak flow velocity in early diastole (PFVE) and in late diastole (PFVA) were measured (cm/s) at the midpoint of the darkest portion of the spectrum at the time of the maximal flow velocity in early and late diastole, respectively. Early diastolic flow time (EDFT), late diastolic flow time (ADFT), and early diastolic deceleration time (EFDFT) were measured as noted. (Reprinted from Gardin et al. Am J Noninvas Cardiol 1987, with permission.)

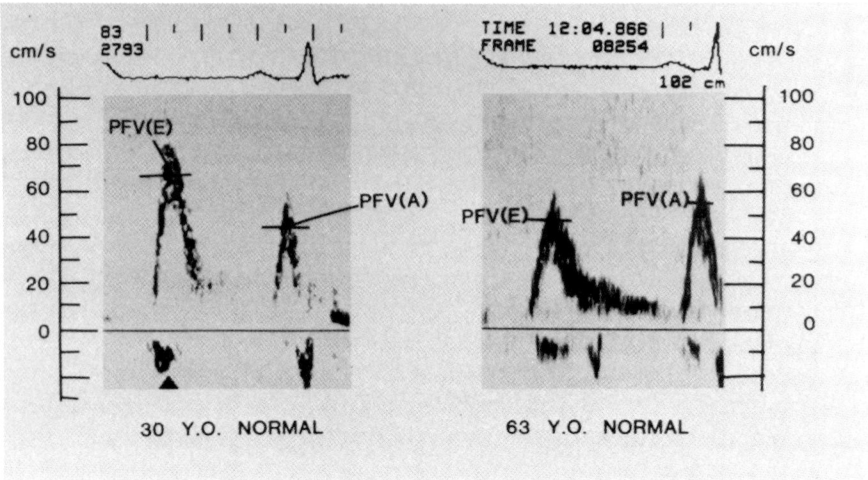


**Figure 17** Doppler mitral valve flow velocity recordings from a younger normal subject, age 30 (left), and from an older normal subject, age 63 (right). Note that the peak flow velocity at early diastole in the older subject is lower and the late diastolic peak flow velocity is higher than in the younger normal subject. (Reprinted from Gardin et al., Am J Noninvas Cardiol 1987, with permission, Ref. 25.)

significantly higher ($p < 0.05$) in the 61–70-year age decade (55 ± 11 cm/s) than in the 21–30-year age group (41 ± 7 cm/s; Fig. 19). Mitral A/E ratio (i.e., PFVA/PFVE) was significantly higher ($p < 0.01$) in the oldest (1.2 ± 0.3) compared to the youngest (0.6 ± 0.1) age group (Fig. 20). Early diastolic flow time increased with age ($r = 0.36$, $p < 0.001$), whereas early diastolic deceleration decreased with age ($r = -0.59$, $p < 0.001$). The combination of a diminished early diastolic peak flow velocity divided by a prolonged deceleration time resulted in a significant ($p < 0.001$) decrease in the rate of early diastolic deceleration with increasing age.

The results of this study demonstrated that aging is associated with progressive decreases in early diastolic transmitral peak flow velocity and early diastolic deceleration and progressive increases in late diastolic transmitral peak flow velocity and the ratio of late to early diastolic peak flow velocity. These findings are similar to those reported by Miyatake and associates (24).

Evidence that the decrease in early diastolic transmitral peak flow velocity is related to impaired early diastolic left ventricular filling has been provided by a number of workers. Dabestani et al. (26) showed in 10 patients who underwent both Doppler mitral flow velocity recording and videodensitometric analysis of left ventricular filling from digital subtraction left ventriculograms that the per-

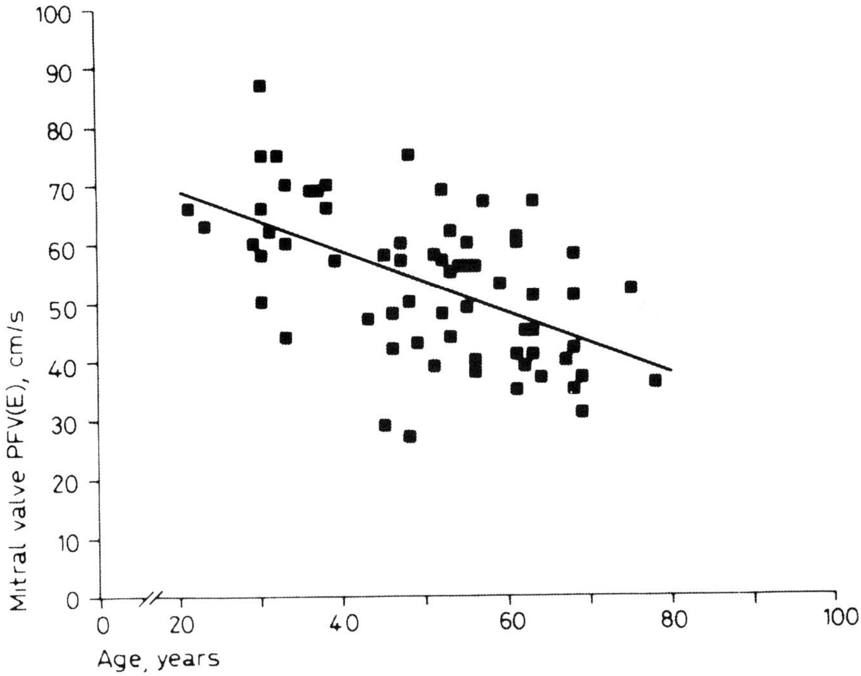


**Figure 18** Data for mitral peak flow velocity in early diastole, PFV(E) (cm/s) is displayed on the vertical axis versus age in years on the horizontal axis ($n = 66$). Note the negative slope of the regression equation mitral, PFVE = −0.52(age) + 79. The correlation coefficient $r = -0.55$. (Reprinted from Gardin et al., Am J Noninvas Cardiol 1987, with permission, Ref. 25.)

centage of total filling completed by middiastole was directly related to the early diastolic peak flow velocity measured by Doppler. These findings suggest that Doppler measurements of peak flow velocity in early diastole are related to the rate of ventricular filling. Rokey et al. (27) also reported a significant correlation between early diastolic transmitral peak flow velocity and angiographic peak filling rate ($r = 0.64$). They noted even better correlations between Doppler echocardiographic and angiographic peak filling rates ($r = 0.87$).

Miyatake et al. (24) postulated that the increase in *late* diastolic peak transmitral flow velocity with aging reflects an augmentation of ventricular filling by atrial contraction that compensates for decreased early diastolic ventricular filling. Our study demonstrated not only age-related increases in late diastolic peak flow *velocity,* but also in late diastolic flow *time* and flow velocity *integral* (25). These findings are further evidence for an age-related increase in the contribution of atrial systole to ventricular filling.

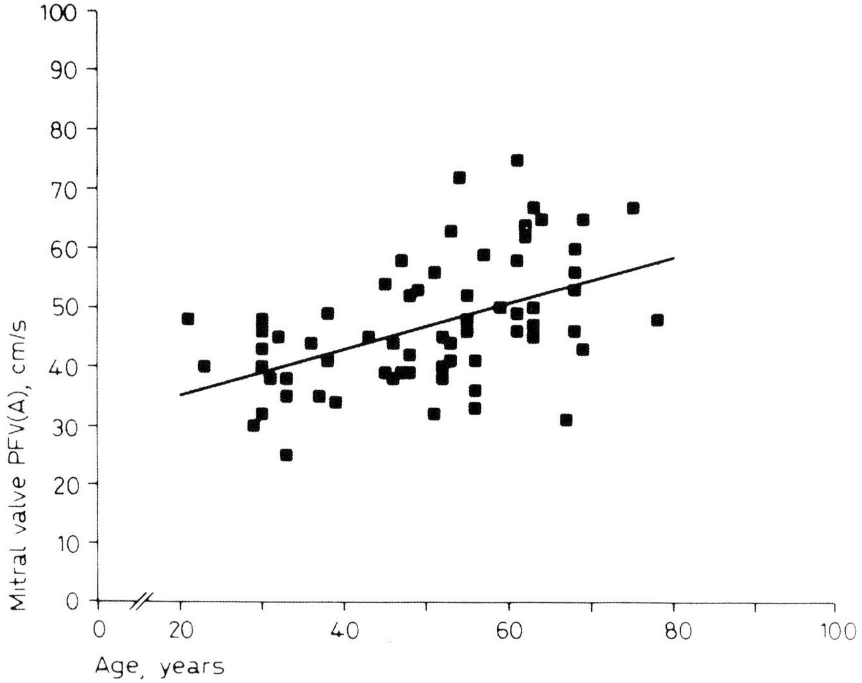


**Figure 19** Data for mitral peak flow velocity in late diastole, PFV(A) (cm/s) is displayed versus age in years ($n = 66$). Note the positive slope of the relationship, mitral PFVA = 0.39(age) + 27. (Reprinted from Gardin et al., Am J Noninvas Cardiol 1987, with permission, Ref. 25.)

## EPIDEMIOLOGICAL STUDIES IN THE ELDERLY

The Framingham study has shown by M-mode echocardiography that (1) left ventricular hypertrophy is a powerful, independent predictor for mortality and morbidity from coronary heart disease, and (2) increased left atrial dimension is associated with an increased risk of stroke (28–30). However, no previous population-based study has evaluated specifically in the elderly the risk factor correlates and predictive value for coronary heart disease and stroke of two-dimensional and Doppler, as well as M-mode, echocardiography.

The Cardiovascular Health Study is a multiyear prospective epidemiological study of 5201 men and women older than 65 years recruited from four U.S. field centers: Davis, California, Hagerstown, Maryland, Winston-Salem, North Carolina, and Pittsburgh, Pennsylvania. The main objectives of incorporating echocardiography were to determine whether echocardiographic measurements,

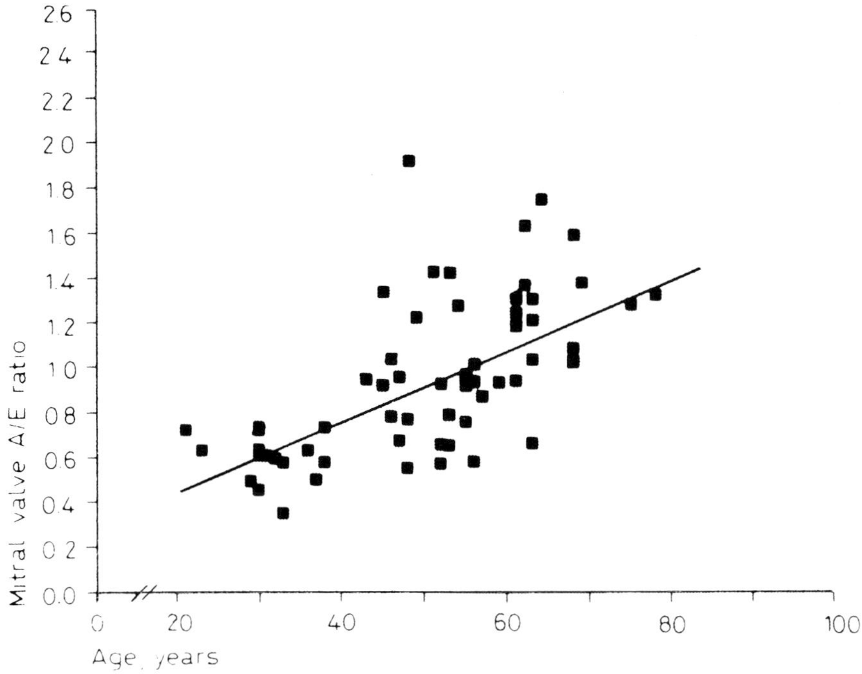


**Figure 20** Data for mitral A/E ratio is depicted versus age in years. Note the positive slope of the relationship, mitral A/E ratio = 0.016 (age) + 0.13. (Reprinted from Gardin et al., Am J Noninvas Cardiol 1987, with permission, Ref. 25.)

or changes in these measurements, are (1) correlated with traditional risk factors for coronary heart disease and stroke and (2) independent predictors of morbidity and mortality from coronary heart disease and stroke.

Echocardiographic measurements obtained include those related to global and segmental left ventricular systolic and diastolic structure and function and left atrial and aortic root dimension. For each subject, a baseline echocardiogram was recorded on super-VHS tape using a standard protocol and equipment. All studies were sent to a reading center (University of California, Irvine), where images were digitized and measurements made using customized computer algorithms. Calculated data and images were stored on optical disks to facilitate retrieval and future comparisons in longitudinal studies. Quality control measures included standardized training of echocardiography technicians and readers, technician observation by a trained echocardiographer, periodic blind duplicate readings with reader review sessions, phantom studies, and quality control audits (32). A second echocardiogram is scheduled in year 7, with the goal of determining whether changes in cardiac anatomy or function over a 5-year period are predictors of morbidity or mortality from coronary heart disease and stroke.

A number of initial cross-sectional associations with baseline echocardiographic data have been described in the Cardiovascular Health Study. Left ventricular mass was found to be significantly higher in men than women, even after multivariate adjustments, and modestly increased with aging (33). Of interest, 3.9% of men and 2.1% of women with no clinical heart disease had LV segmental wall motion abnormalities, suggesting silent disease (33). Borderline and definite isolated systolic hypertension were positively associated with LV mass ($p < 0.001$) and with increases in transmitral atrial peak flow velocity and the ration of atrial-to-early diastolic peak flow velocity (34). Longitudinal follow-up studies should provide fascinating insights related to possible preclinical predictors of incident cardiovascular disease and stroke, as well as associated morbidity and mortality.

In summary, echocardiographic imaging and Doppler flow recording have provided convincing evidence of structural and functional cardiac changes related to aging. These noninvasive ultrasound techniques have provided important insights into the cardiovascular epidemiology of aging, as well as the clinical evaluation of elderly patients with suspected cardiovascular disease.

## ACKNOWLEDGMENT

The author acknowledges the expert assistance of Marcia Johannsen in the preparation of this manuscript.

## REFERENCES

1. Feigenbaum H. Echocardiography, 4th ed. Philadelphia: Lea & Febiger, 1986:1–126.
2. Talano JV, Gardin JM. Textbook of Two-Dimensional Echocardiography. New York: Grune & Stratton, 1983:1–64, 325–355.
3. Gardin JM, Henry WL, Savage DD, Ware JH, Burn C, Borer JS. Echocardiographic measurements in normal subjects: Evaluation of an adult population without clinically apparent heart disease. J Clin Ultrasound 1979; 7:439–447.
4. Pombo JE, Troy BL, Russell RD Jr. Left ventricular volumes and ejection fraction by echocardiography. Circulation 1971; 43:480–490.
5. Henry WL, Gardin JM, Ware JH. Echocardiographic measurements in normal subjects from infancy to old age. Circulation 1980; 62:1054–1061.
6. Gardin JM, Savage DD, Ware JH, Henry WL. Effect of age, sex and body surface area on echocardiographic left ventricular wall mass in normal subjects. Hypertension 1987; 9:II36–II39.

7. Roberts WC, Perloff JK. Mitral valve disease. A clinicopathologic survey of the conditions causing the mitral valve to function abnormally. Ann Intern Med 1972; 77:939–975.
8. Krovetz J. Age-related changes in size of the aortic valve annulus in man. Am Heart J 1975; 90:569–574.
9. Derman U. Changes of the mitral echocardiogram with aging and the influence of atherosclerotic risk factors. Atherosclerosis 1972; 15:349.
10. Borer JS, Bacharach SL, Green MV, et al. Evaluation of clinical utility of real-time computer-based radionuclide cineangiography. In: Proceedings of the IEEE Computer Society, Rotterdam, 1977.
11. Strandell T. Heart rate, arterial lactate concentration and oxygen uptake during exercise in old men compared with young men. Acta Physiol Scand 1964; 60:197–216.
12. Brandfonbrener M, Landowne M, Shock NW. Changes in cardiac output with age. Circulation 1955; 12:557–566.
13. Granath A, Strandell T. Relationships between cardiac output, stroke volume and intracardiac pressures at rest and during exercise in supine position and some anthropometric data in healthy old men. Acta Med Scand 1964; 176:447–466.
14. Gerstenblith G, Frederiksen J, Yin FCP, et al. Echocardiographic assessment of a normal adult aging population. Circulation 1977; 56:273–278.
15. Gardin JM, Iseri LT, Elkayam U, Tobis J, Childs W, Burns CS, Henry WL. Evaluation of dilated cardiomyopathy by pulsed Doppler echocardiography. Am Heart J 1983; 106:1057–1065.
16. Elkayam U, Gardin JM, Berkley R, Hughes C, Henry WL. The use of Doppler flow velocity measurements to assess the hemodynamic response to vasodilators in patients with heart failure. Circulation 1983; 67:377–383.
17. Gardin JM, Burn CS, Childs WJ, Henry WL. Evaluation of blood flow velocity in the ascending aorta and main pulmonary artery of normal subjects by Doppler echocardiography. Am Heart J 1984; 107:310–319.
18. Gardin JM, Davidson DM, Rohan MK, Butman S, Knoll M, Garcia R, Dubria S, Gardin SK, Henry WL. Relationship between age, body size, gender and blood pressure and Doppler flow measurements in the aorta and pulmonary artery. Am Heart J 1987; 113:101–109.
19. Rodeheffer RJ, Gerstenblith G, Becker LC, Fleg JL, Weisfeldt ML, Lakatta EG. Exercise cardiac output is maintained with advancing age in healthy human subjects: Cardiac dilation and increased stroke volume compensate for a diminished heart rate. Circulation 1984; 69:203–213.
20. Lazarus M, Dang TY, Gardin JM, Allfie A, Henry WL. Evaluation of age, gender, heart rate and blood pressure changes and exercise conditioning on Doppler measured aortic blood flow acceleration and velocity during upright treadmill testing. Am J Cardiol 1988; 62:439–443.
21. Rushmer RF. Initial ventricular impulse. A potential key to cardiac evaluation. Circulation 1964; 29:268–283.
22. Noble M, Tenchard D, Guz A. Left ventricular ejection in conscious dogs. I. Mea-

surement and significance of the maximum acceleration of blood from the left ventricle. Circ Res 1966; 19:139–147.
23. Jewitt D, Gabe I, Millis C, Maurer B, Thomas M, Shillingford J. Aortic velocity and acceleration measurements in the assessment of coronary heart disease. Eur J Cardiol 1974; 1:299–305.
24. Miyatake K, Okamoto M, Kinishita N, et al. Augmentation of atrial contribution to left ventricular inflow in aging as assessed by intracardiac Doppler flowmetry. Am J Cardiol 1984; 53:586–589.
25. Gardin JM, Rohan MK, Davidson DM, Dabestani A, Sklansky M, Garcia R, Knoll ML, White DB, Gardin SK, Henry WL. Doppler transmitral flow velocity parameters: Relationship between age, body surface area, blood pressure and gender in normal subjects. Am J Noninvas Cardiol 1987; 1:3–10.
26. Dabestani A, Johnston WD, Tobis JM, et al. Relation between Doppler transmitral diastolic flow and left ventricular filling (abstr). J Am Coll Cardiol 1984; 3:612.
27. Rokey R, Kuo LK, Zoghbi WA, et al. Determination of parameters of left ventricular diastolic filling with pulsed Doppler echocardiography: Comparison with cineangiography. Circulation 1985; 71:543–550.
28. Levy D, Garrison RJ, Savage DD, Kannel WB, Castelli WP. Prognostic implications of echocardiographically determined left ventricular mass in the Framingham Heart Study. N Engl J Med 1990; 322:1561–1566.
29. Levy D, Garrison RJ, Savage DD, Kannel WB, Castelli WP. Left ventricular mass and incidence of coronary heart disease in an elderly cohort: The Framingham Heart Study. Ann Intern Med 1989; 110:101–107.
30. Benjamin E, Levy D, Plehn J, Belanger A, D'Agostino R, Wolf P. Left atrial size: An independent risk factor for stroke (abstr). Circulation 1989; 80(Suppl II):615.
31. Fried L, Borhani N, Enright P, Furberg C, Gardin J, Kronmal R, Kuller L, Manolio T, Mittelmark M, Newman A, O'Leary D, Psaty B, Rautaharju P, Tracy R, Weiler P, for the CHS Collaborative Research Group. Cardiovascular Health Study: Design and rationale. Ann Epidemiol 1991; 1:263–276.
32. Gardin JM, Wong ND, Bommer W, Klopfenstein HS, Smith VE, Tabatznik B, Siscovick D, Lobodzinski S, Anton-Culver H, Manolio TA. Echocardiographic design of a multicenter investigation of free-living elderly subjects: The Cardiovascular Health Study. J Am Soc Echocardiogr 1992; 5:63–72.
33. Gardin JM, Siscovick D, Anton-Culver, H, Smith V-E, Klopfenstein S, Bommer W, Fried LP, O'Leary D, Manolio TA. Age and gender relations of left ventricular mass and wall motion in elderly subjects with no clinical heart disease: The Cardiovascular Health Study (CHS). (Abstract) Circulation 1992; 84(4):I.-672.
34. Psaty BM, Furbert CD, Kuller LH, Borhani NO, Rautaharju PM, O'Leary DH, Bild DE, Robbins J, Fried LP, Reid C. Isolated systolic hypertension and subclinical cardiovascular disease in the elderly. Initial findings from the Cardiovascular Health Study. JAMA 1992; 268:1287–1291.

# 5

# Epidemiology of Coronary Heart Disease in the Elderly

**Pantel S. Vokonas**
*Boston University School of Medicine and*
*Veterans Affairs Medical Center, Boston, Massachusetts*

**William B. Kannel**
*Boston University School of Medicine, Boston, Massachusetts*

## INTRODUCTION

Coronary heart disease (CHD) is the central component of a broad spectrum of disease conditions affecting the heart and circulation, collectively termed cardiovascular disease, that progress dramatically as age advances. Although CHD in all its clinical manifestations contributes significantly to disability and death throughout life, its toll is clearly heaviest in the elderly (1–3).

A common observation made by clinical practitioners is that increasingly larger numbers of older persons are admitted to coronary care units with acute cardiac events and receive a full array of medical interventions, including treatment with thrombolytic drugs and beta-adrenergic blockers (4–6). Older patients are also routinely subjected to invasive cardiac studies and undergo revascularization procedures, such as percutaneous transluminal coronary angioplasty and coronary artery bypass grafting (7,8). In many outpatient settings, older patients represent the largest segment of the active clinic population under medical surveillance. Not only is CHD quite prevalent in this population, but older patients often inquire about health measures that may help prevent CHD, stroke, and other cardiovascular conditions. They also often voice concerns regarding the necessity of certain therapies for the treatment of hypertension or diabetes mellitus initiated by their physicians. Despite the already widespread application of such clinical interventions, and to a lesser extent corresponding preventive approaches, in older persons, there is a substantial paucity of information regarding the efficacy of many such measures, especially in the elderly (9–11). In this context, a thorough evaluation of the role of risk factors for CHD in older persons and the potential benefits of their amelioration would represent an important contribution to our understanding and ultimately our clinical and preventive management of this disease in a large segment of the U.S. and world population.

Considerations regarding the character of CHD and the role of risk factors for its development in older persons, which may appear straightforward, are in actuality quite complex because, of necessity, they involve interactions of the multiple and overlapping domains of aging, disease, and risk factors (12) (Fig. 1).

In this representation, aging represents the constellation of processes occurring over time in the adult organism resulting in characteristic alterations of structure and function of body tissues and organs, including the heart and blood vessels (12). CHD represents "disease" in this context with underlying anatomical and pathophysiological features ultimately manifested as clinical symptoms and complications. Risk factors, in turn, index an array of atherogenic personal traits as well as life-style characteristics, including diet and exercise, that are associated with the development of CHD (13).

Separate perspectives for each interaction among these three domains will therefore constitute the framework for further discussion. First, we will examine the relation of CHD occurrence to advancing age and the character of CHD in older persons. Next, we will examine how established risk factors for CHD change with advancing age and their prevalence in the elderly. Finally, we will examine associations between specific risk factors and CHD in the elderly and comment on available information regarding the efficacy of treating such factors.

Each of these perspectives is systematically examined in 30-year follow-up data from the Framingham Study, focusing on findings in subjects aged 65–94

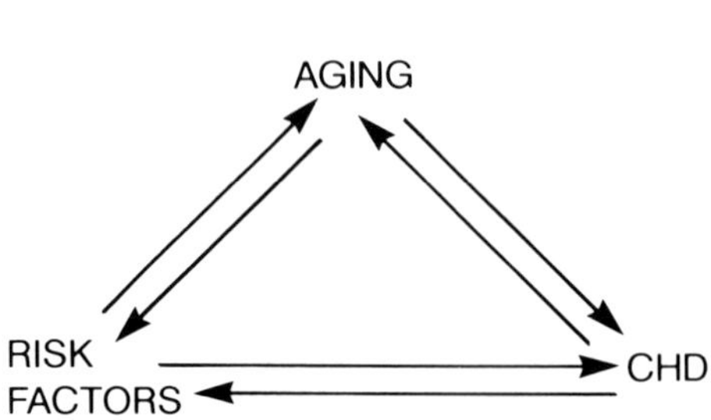


**Figure 1** Conceptualized model of interactions between aging, coronary heart disease (CHD), and risk factors for CHD in older persons. (Modified from Ref. 12.)

years. Details of the examination and laboratory procedures, response rates, and the criteria for disease outcomes in the Framingham Study have been previously described (14,15).

## CHD IN THE ELDERLY

A fundamental observation of cardiovascular disease epidemiology is the distinct age-related rise in the incidence of nearly all manifestations of heart and circulatory disease across the life span. In addition to CHD, such cardiovascular disease conditions include stroke, peripheral arterial disease, and congestive heart failure. The increase in incidence of CHD with advancing age is clearly the most striking (Fig. 2) and illustrates the most important element of the first perspective, i.e., the relationship between aging and CHD. Although calculated incidence rates in men and women at far-advanced age are based on relatively small numbers of CHD events, such rates clearly follow trends established ear-

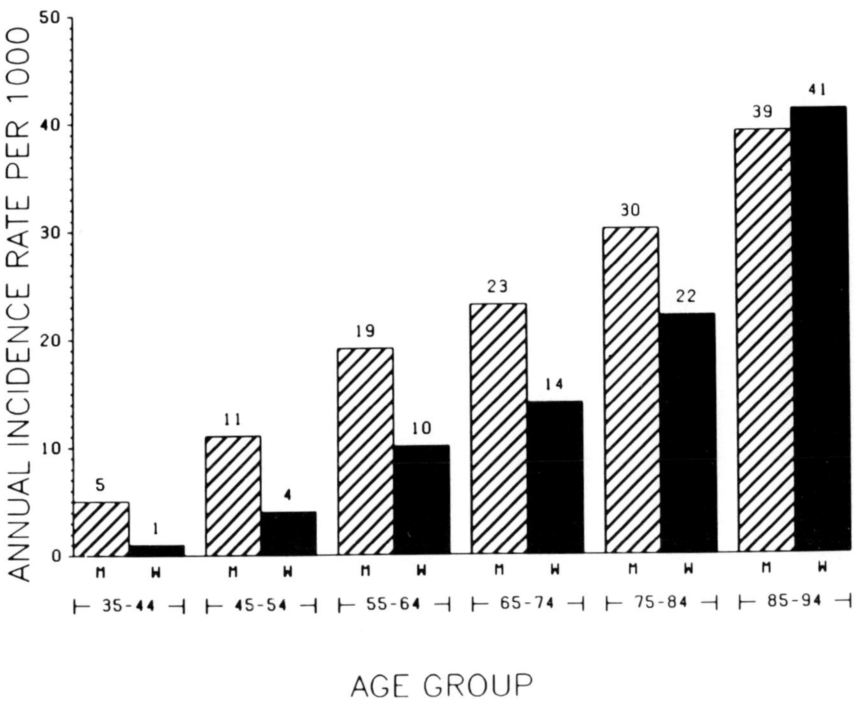


**Figure 2** Age trends in total CHD incidence for men and women, Framingham Study, 30-year follow-up.

lier in life. Also, whereas incidence rates in men increase linearly with age, those in women tend to increase more steeply at advanced age approximating an exponential function.

Similar trends of increasing incidence of disease events with age as noted in Figure 2 are observed in Framingham Study data for both men and women up to age 84 for nearly every major clinical manifestation of CHD, including angina pectoris, myocardial infarction, sudden death, and death due to CHD (15).

Another important observation regarding the relationship of CHD and advancing age is the progressive attenuation of male predominance of disease. This is illustrated in Figure 3, which shows the marked decline in male-to-female ratio of incidence rates for CHD with the relationship crossing the line of identity at far-advanced age.

The character of CHD according to specified clinical manifestations for older men and women in the Framingham cohort is presented in Table 1. Data indicate the proportion of total coronary events represented by a specific manifestation. Symptomatic categories are not mutually exclusive, and percentages exceed 100% because a given subject may have more than one clinical manifes-

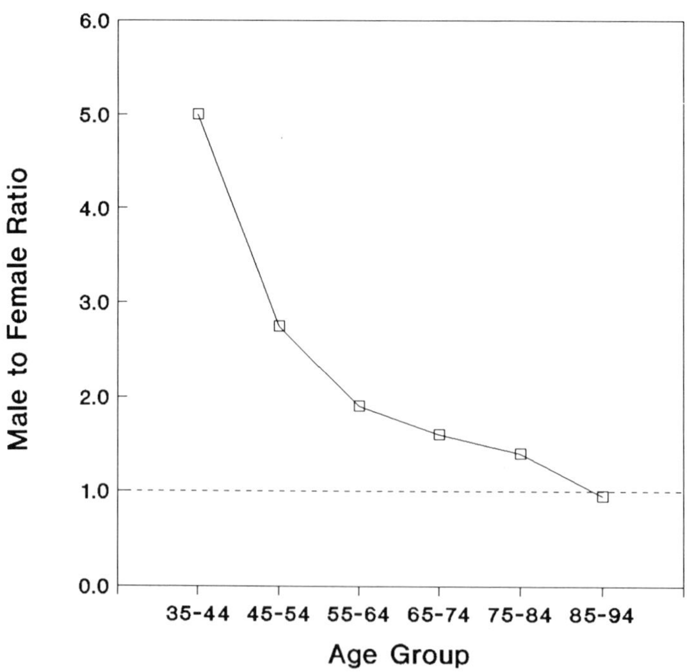


**Figure 3** Age-related change in male-to-female ratios for total CHD incidence, Framingham Study, 30-year follow-up.

**Table 1** Specified Clinical Manifestations of CHD: Men and Women; Aged 65–94, Framingham Study, 30-Year Follow-up

| Manifestation | Men | Women |
|---|---|---|
| Myocardial infarction | 135/244 (55%) | 108/269 (40%) |
| Angina pectoris | 73/244 (30%) | 123/269 (45%) |
| Coronary insufficiency | 16/244 (07%) | 21/269 (08%) |
| Sudden death | 37/244 (15%) | 31/269 (12%) |

tation at the time of initial presentation within a biennial period. Myocardial infarction is the most common initial manifestation for CHD in older men, whereas angina pectoris appears to be the most common presenting feature in older women. Angina pectoris in older women frequently occurs as an isolated clinical entity. Angina pectoris in older men, however, is more often associated with acute myocardial infarction, either preceding or following the acute event. Coronary insufficiency is the traditional term for unstable angina pectoris referring to the clinical situation of either prolonged chest pain or a progressive increase in the frequency and/or intensity of ischemic chest pain. This manifestation occurs at similar frequencies in older men and women. Sudden death, as an initial manifestation of CHD, occurs somewhat more frequently in older men than women.

Another characteristic of CHD in the elderly is the tendency for a larger proportion of myocardial infarction events to be clinically unrecognized (Table 2). The diagnosis of myocardial infarction in such instances is based on the occurrence of unequivocal electrocardiographic changes consistent with infarction between biennial examinations, where neither the subject nor his/her physician has suspected the diagnosis (16). Symptoms associated with such events are

**Table 2** Proportion of Unrecognized Myocardial Infarctions by Age and Sex, Framingham Study, 30-Year Follow-up

| Age (years) | Men | Women |
|---|---|---|
| 30–44 | 29% | — |
| 45–54 | 18% | 41% |
| 55–64 | 25% | 31% |
| 65–74 | 25% | 35% |
| 75–84 | 42% | 36% |
| 85–95 | 33% | 46% |
| Average | 28% | 35% |

usually attributed to musculoskeletal chest discomfort, upper gastrointestinal tract upset, gallbladder disease or other conditions. Approximately one-half of such infarctions are completely silent. Unrecognized events represent a larger proportion of all infarctions in women, particularly older women.

## CHANGES IN CHD RISK FACTORS WITH ADVANCING AGE

Nearly all the established CHD risk factors change with advancing age. These include changes in blood pressure, serum lipids, cigarette smoking, glucose metabolism, body weight, and other factors. Several age-related trends in risk factors and their prevalence in older persons are described below. This constitutes the second perspective of the discussion, i.e., the interaction between aging and risk factors.

The most well-characterized change in an established CHD risk factor with age is elevation of blood pressure. In longitudinal data from the Framingham Study, systolic blood pressure is observed to rise nearly linearly with advancing age in both men and women (Fig. 4). Diastolic blood pressure, in contrast, tends to rise throughout middle age in both sexes and actually declines at advanced age. Diastolic blood pressures in women, however, usually remain 5–10 mm Hg lower than those in men throughout the life span (1).

The consistent increase in systolic blood pressure is due to progressive vascular stiffening attributable, in turn, to alterations of the physicochemical properties of media of the arterial wall, including overall thickening and changes in the nature and content of collagen, elastin, and possibly other structural proteins that occur with advancing age (17). This process is dissimilar to that of atherosclerosis, which underlies the preponderance of cardiovascular disease observed in older people. Although previous investigators have argued that age-related stiffening of arterial walls represent the primary risk factor and not elevated blood pressure per se, which in this context is considered a secondary sign of vascular rigidity, subsequent analyses from the Framingham Study have shown that systolic blood pressure remains an independent contributor to risk for cardiovascular disease events including stroke and CHD, even when arterial rigidity as determined by pulse pressure recordings is taken into account (18).

Although progressive elevation of systolic blood pressure with advancing age is consistently observed in nearly every Western-industrialized population studied, it does not appear to represent a universal feature of the aging process. Data from a number of isolated primitive populations suggest that this relationship is markedly blunted (19). Possibilities accounting for differences in age-related change in blood pressure between populations likely include genetic factors as well as dietary influences, especially the higher intake of salt in industrialized nations (20).

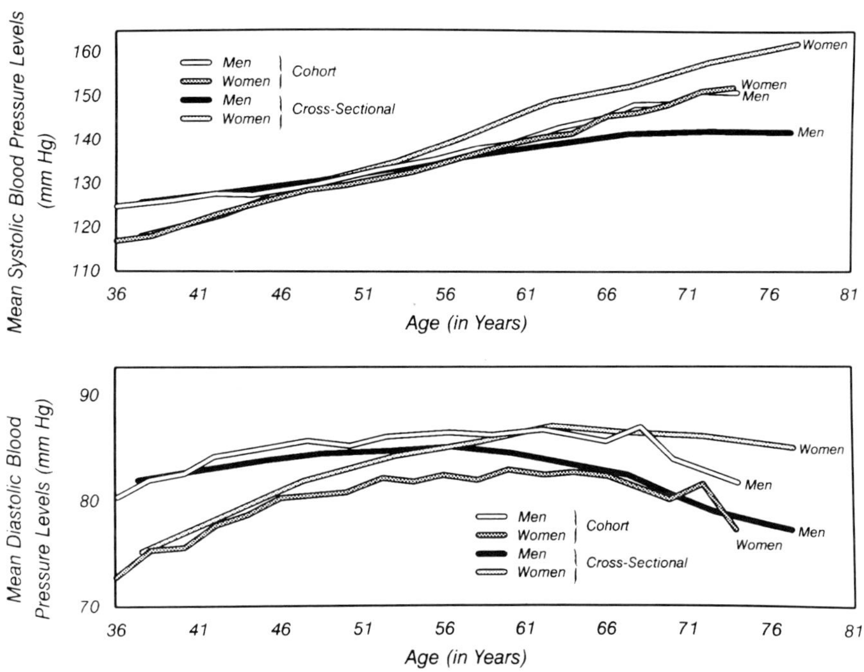


**Figure 4** Average age trends in systolic and diastolic blood pressure levels for men and women based on cross-sectional and longitudinal (cohort) data, Framingham Study, biennial exams 3–10. (Modified from Ref. 1.)

Despite its ubiquity, however, progressive elevation of systolic blood pressure with advancing age should not be construed as an innocuous concomitant of the aging process since it clearly confers increased risk for stroke, CHD, and other cardiovascular disease events in both elderly men and women (21). Elevated diastolic blood pressure also occurs commonly in the elderly and remains an important risk factor for cardiovascular disease, particularly in older men.

As a consequence of the progressive age-related increase, primarily in systolic blood pressure, approximately 40–50% of men and women in a typical Westernized population such as Framingham meet one or more of the established criteria for hypertension after the age of 65. For persons categorized as being hypertensive, isolated systolic hypertension (defined as systolic blood pressure > 160 mm Hg with diastolic blood pressure ≤ 95 mm Hg) accounts for nearly two-thirds of the total prevalence of hypertension in both older men and women (22). Combined hypertension characterized by abnormal elevations of both systolic and diastolic blood pressures accounts for less than one-third of the total prevalence. Isolated diastolic hypertension is considerably less prevalent in older men and women, accounting for less than 15% of the prevalence.

Blood lipids, including total serum cholesterol, also vary with age across the life span and trends appear to be different in women than in men. Figure 5 shows longitudinal trends in average levels of serum cholesterol in the Framingham Study as a function of age. Note that levels in men tend to peak in early middle age and then slowly decline with advancing age. Levels in women peak later in middle age and remain relatively high until advanced age before a decline occurs. The practical implication of this trend is the relatively high prevalence of hypercholesterolemia likely to be encountered in comparable populations of older women.

Corresponding age trends for specific lipoprotein-cholesterol subfractions in the Framingham Study are illustrated in Figure 6. Trends for low-density-lipoprotein cholesterol (LDL), in general, are similar to those for total serum cholesterol. Mean levels of high-density-lipoprotein cholesterol (HDL) are consistently higher in women than in men across the age span but tend to decline slightly after menopause. Trends in men remain essentially unchanged throughout life. Mean values of very-low-density lipoproteins (VLDL) tend to be higher in men than women, but trends in both tend to rise throughout middle age and then remain relatively stable thereafter. Presumably, these trends reflect fluctuations in body weight occurring at corresponding ages in the sexes.

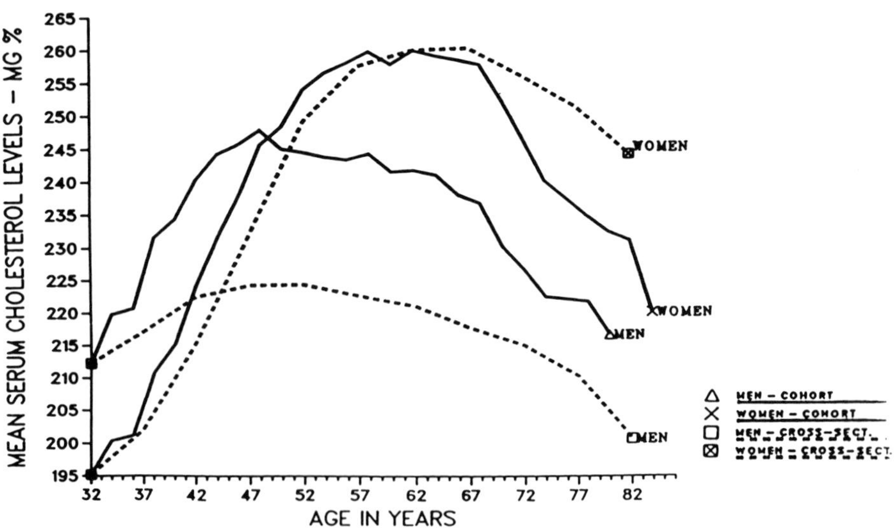


**Figure 5** Average age trends in serum cholesterol levels in cross-sectional and longitudinal (cohort) data, Framingham Study, biennial exams 1–16.

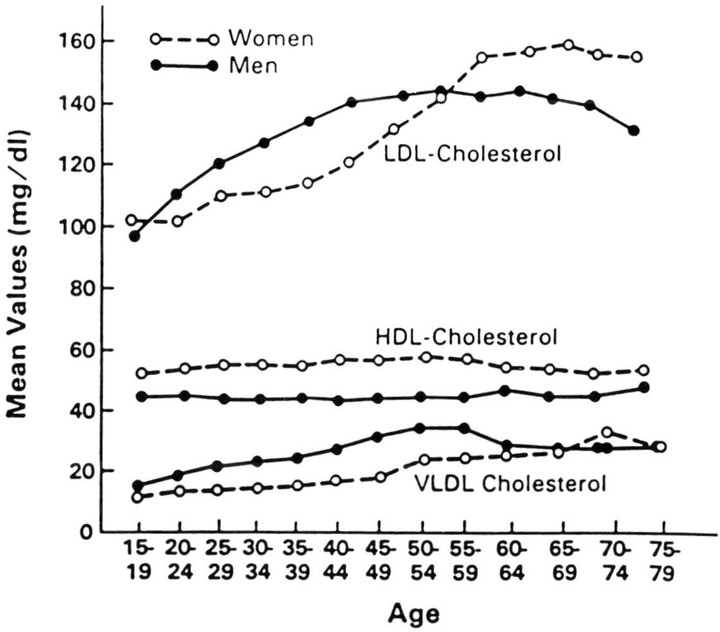


**Figure 6** Average age trends in lipoprotein cholesterol subfractions, Framingham Study (2). (Reproduced by permission.)

The percentage prevalence of a number of cardiovascular risk factors in older subjects of the Framingham Study is presented in Table 3. Data are arrayed for each decade of age from 65 to 94 years and separately for men and women.

As would be expected from age trends observed earlier, hypercholesterolemia appears to be quite prevalent in older women. Glucose metabolism becomes progressively impaired with advancing age, resulting in increasing prevalence of glucose intolerance in both older men and women (23). Body weight tends to decrease at far-advanced age. Weight loss, however, represents a reduction primarily in lean body mass, i.e., muscle and bone tissue, rather than adipose tissue. The result is an alteration of body composition in older persons with higher proportional adiposity per unit of weight (24). Despite the tendency for lower body weights at advanced age, obesity appears to be well represented in both older men and women in this analysis. The prevalence of cigarette smoking appears to decrease with advancing age. This can be attributed not only to higher mortality rates in smokers, but also to discontinuation of smoking because of health problems or concerns in older persons. The preva-

**Table 3** Percentage Prevalence of Cardiovascular Risk Factors in the Elderly: Framingham Study, Exam 16

| Age (years) | Definite hypertension | | Hypercholesterolemia | | Glucose intolerance | | Obesity | | Cigarette smoking | | ECG-LVH | |
|---|---|---|---|---|---|---|---|---|---|---|---|---|
| | Men | Women | Men | Women | Men | Women | Men | Women | Men | Women | Men | Women |
| 65–74 | 42.1 | 48.9 | 16.6 | 39.7 | 29.5 | 17.5 | 52.2 | 47.8 | 21.9 | 23.0 | 5.5 | 4.2 |
| 75–84 | 45.5 | 61.1 | 9.7 | 36.3 | 30.9 | 26.0 | 35.4 | 39.3 | 13.9 | 8.5 | 6.0 | 7.8 |
| 85–94 | 20.7 | 64.8 | 9.4 | 18.4 | 33.3 | 29.0 | 7.7 | 30.0 | 9.4 | 3.2 | 10.4 | 13.0 |

Definite hypertension: BP > 160/95 mm Hg; hypercholesterolemia: serum cholesterol > 250 mg/dl; glucose intolerance: blood glucose > 120 mg/dl, glycosuria, or diabetes mellitus; obesity: relative weight > 120%; cigarette smoking: any (Exam 15); ECG-LVH: evidence of left ventricular hypertrophy on electrocardiogram.

lence of left ventricular hypertrophy as determined by the electrocardiogram (ECG-LVH) increases with advancing age in both older men and women.

From the foregoing analysis, it is clear that the majority of established risk factors for CHD in middle-aged persons are prevalent in the elderly. What remains is the task of marshalling evidence to determine whether such risk factors continue to remain operative in the development of CHD in older persons. This constitutes the third and final perspective of interactions alluded to earlier, i.e., associations between specific risk factors and CHD in older persons, which will be reviewed next.

## ASSOCIATIONS BETWEEN SPECIFIC RISK FACTORS AND CHD IN THE ELDERLY

Associations for a number of specific risk factors and CHD are summarized in Table 4. Putative risk factors are listed in the first column. Standardized, age-adjusted (bivariate) logistic regression coefficients are categorized for younger and older subjects of the Framingham cohort and also arrayed separately for men and women. Regression coefficients are derived using a logistic regression model to mathematically relate the level of a risk factor or its categorical value to the development of CHD events. The magnitude of the coefficient and also the level of statistical significance reflect the strength of the association between the specific risk factor and CHD for the age group and sex under consideration.

A cursory inspection of the results indicates that the majority of significant associations between risk factors and CHD apparent in younger men and women

**Table 4** Impact of Risk Factors on Incidence of Coronary Heart Disease, Framingham Study, 30-Year Follow-up

| | Bivariate standardized regression coefficients (age-adjusted) | | | |
|---|---|---|---|---|
| | Ages 35–64 | | Ages 65–94 | |
| Risk factors | Men | Women | Men | Women |
| Systolic pressure | 0.338*** | 0.418*** | 0.401*** | 0.286*** |
| Diastolic pressure | 0.321*** | 0.363*** | 0.296*** | 0.082 |
| Serum cholesterol | 0.322*** | 0.307*** | 0.121 | 0.213*** |
| Cigarettes | 0.259*** | 0.095 | −0.017 | −0.034 |
| Blood glucose | 0.043 | 0.206*** | 0.166*** | 0.209*** |
| Vital capacity | −0.112* | −0.331*** | −0.127 | 0.253*** |
| Relative weight | 0.190*** | 0.264*** | 0.177** | 0.124* |

Significant at $*p < 0.05$, $**p < 0.01$, $***p < 0.001$.

remain significant in older age groups, but not consistently in both sexes. Systolic blood pressure, for example, demonstrates strong risk associations for CHD in younger men and women and maintains strong associations in both older men and women. The risk association for diastolic blood pressure, in contrast, appears to lose significance in older women. Total serum cholesterol demonstrates strong risk associations for CHD in younger men and women; however, the strength of this risk association clearly weakens in older men but remains significant in older women. Cigarette smoking modeled using this methodology fails to show significant risk associations in either older men or women. Blood glucose levels, as well as other parameters reflecting impaired glucose metabolism, including glucose intolerance and diabetes mellitus, show strong risk associations for CHD, in both older men and women. Vital capacity demonstrates strong negative risk associations, particularly in older women. Of interest, significant risk associations between CHD and body weight expressed as Metropolitan Relative Weight are maintained in both older men and women. A number of these risk associations will be discussed in detail below.

Similar data for associations between specific risk factors and CHD incidence can be derived using an alternative regression methodology, the Cox proportional hazards model (25).

## Blood Pressure

Risk associations between CHD and blood pressure in men are shown in Figure 7. CHD incidence, expressed as age-adjusted annual rate of CHD events per 1000, appears on the ordinate. Systolic and diastolic blood pressures appear on the abscissas of the left and right panels, respectively. Two risk relations are illustrated in each panel, one for younger men aged 35–64 and another for older men aged 65–94. Note that CHD risk for systolic and diastolic blood pressure rises with increasing pressure in both age groups and that the risk is even more striking in older than in younger men. These trends are interpreted as marked increases in relative risk indicating that progressively higher levels of blood pressure confer additional risk for CHD. Although these trends do not establish causality, they emphasize an important role for blood pressure in the extended sequence of pathophysiological events that result in manifest CHD. Note that risk relations in older men are configured well above those of younger men, indicating substantially higher incidence rates for CHD at similar blood pressures. This is interpreted as an increase in absolute risk for CHD in older men, suggesting a substantially higher burden of disease at all levels of the blood pressure in older than in younger men, even at normal or low blood pressures. Thus, for older men, both systolic and diastolic blood pressures confer substantial risk of similar magnitude in terms of either absolute or relative risk.

Risk relations for systolic and diastolic blood pressures in women are shown in Figure 8. Although overall incidence rates for CHD in women are lower than

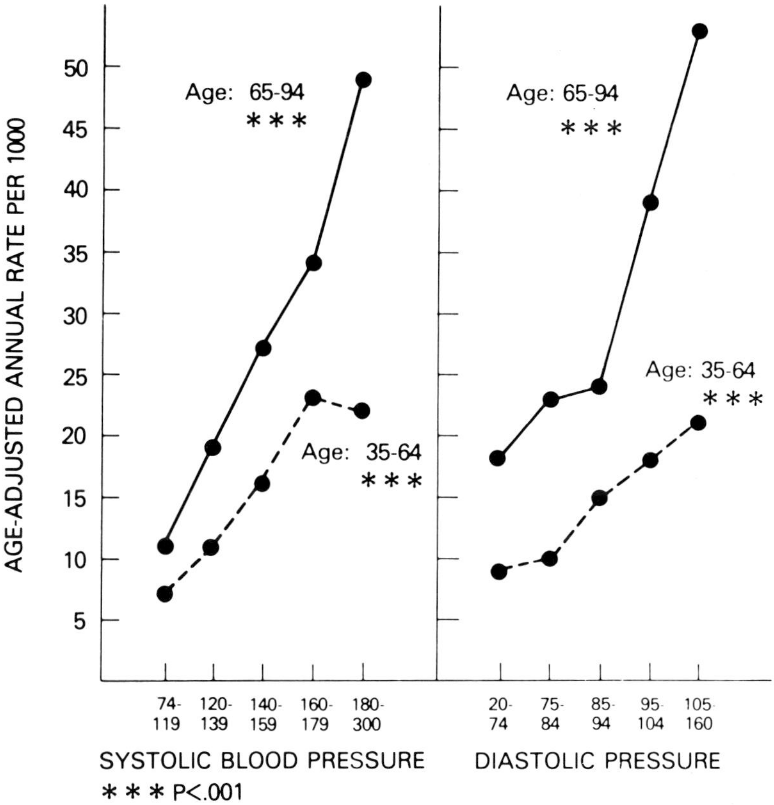


**Figure 7** Risk of CHD by systolic and diastolic blood pressure according to specified age groups in men, Framingham Study, 30-year follow-up.

rates at corresponding blood pressures in men, some of the risk relations previously described in men also pertain to women. Risk appears to rise with increasing blood pressure in both age groups, i.e., increased relative risk, and incidence rates at the same level of blood pressure are higher in older than in younger women, i.e., increased absolute risk. Although there is a minor deviation from the nearly linear trend for the relation between systolic blood pressure and CHD incidence in older women, the relation maintains strong statistical significance. In contrast, the deviation in the relation corresponding to the fourth level of diastolic blood pressure (95–104 mm Hg) yields a statistically insignificant result using the logistic regression model, despite an apparent upper curvilinear trend. Although the discontinuity in the curve remains unexplained, these findings suggest a more consistent and reliable role for systolic blood pressure as a predictor for CHD in the elderly.

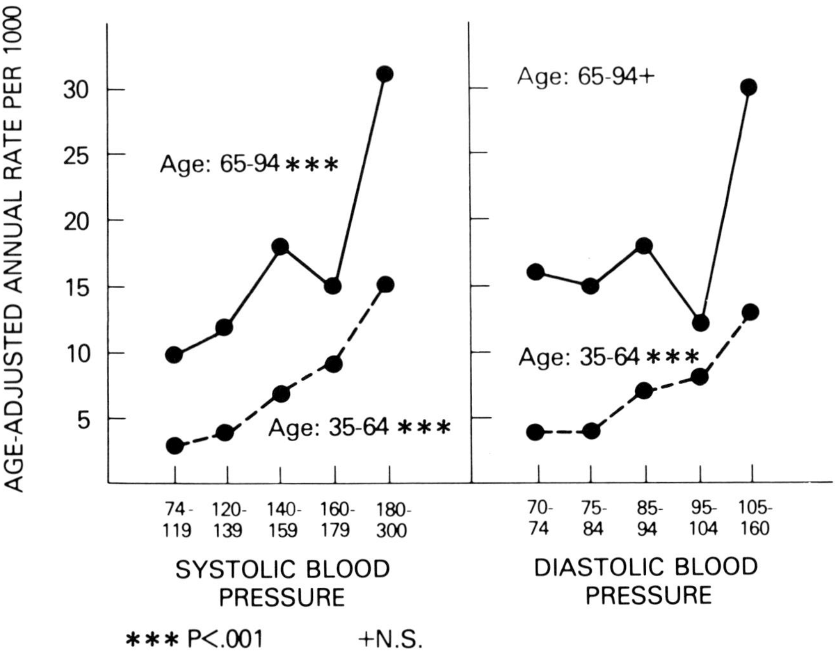


**Figure 8** Risk of CHD by systolic and diastolic blood pressure according to specified age groups in women, Framingham Study, 30-year follow-up.

In the next part of the analysis, CHD risk is evaluated on the basis of age, sex, and specified categories of hypertension. In general, risk gradients for CHD that are similar in direction and magnitude to those suggested earlier are observed when individuals are classified according to hypertensive status instead of absolute levels of blood pressure (Table 5). For all age and sex groups considered, the overall risk of CHD is two to three times higher in subjects with definite hypertension than in normotensives, while risk is intermediate for those with mild hypertension. Absolute risk is two to three times higher in older subjects, in both men and women, and risk is nearly always higher in men than in women, irrespective of age. Similar patterns of risk attributable to hypertension have been observed specifically for cerebrovascular events, congestive heart failure, and peripheral vascular disease (21). When considered alone, isolated systolic hypertension also confers substantial risk for CHD and other cardiovascular disease outcomes (18).

Previous data from randomized clinical trials have established a strong case for the efficacy of treating combined elevations of systolic and diastolic blood pressure in older hypertensives (26–31), although considerable uncertainty

**Table 5** Risk of CHD by Hypertensive Status According to Age and Sex, Framingham Study, 30-Year Follow-up

| | Average annual age-adjusted rate per 1000, coronary heart disease | | | |
|---|---|---|---|---|
| | 35–64*** years | | 65–94*** years | |
| Hypertensive status | Men | Women | Men | Women |
| Normal (< 140/90 mm Hg) | 8 | 3 | 14 | 11 |
| Mild (140–160/90–95 mm Hg) | 15 | 7 | 28 | 16 |
| Definite (> 160/95 mm Hg) | 21 | 10 | 41 | 22 |

***All trends significant at $p < 0.001$.

remained regarding the treatment of isolated systolic hypertension. The recent report of the Systolic Hypertension in the Elderly Program (SHEP) has dispelled much of this uncertainty (32). This study documented impressive reductions in total numbers of fatal and nonfatal strokes in the active treatment group compared to the placebo group. Statistically significant reductions in nonfatal myocardial infarctions plus coronary death, as well as combined CHD and total cardiovascular disease outcomes, were also noted in the group on active treatment. In addition, there was a favorable trend for mortality in the group on active treatment that failed to achieve statistical significance. There appeared to be little or no evidence in this study that lowering of either systolic or diastolic blood pressure resulted in an increased risk of CHD events or mortality, particularly at the lower end of the distribution for blood pressure, the so-called J-shaped curve (33–35).

Two other recent clinical trials of drug therapy for hypertension in the elderly that included patients with isolated systolic hypertension also showed beneficial effects (36,37). In addition to substantial reductions in cerebrovascular events and congestive heart failure, the majority of such studies performed in older persons to date have consistently demonstrated either beneficial trends or significant reductions in CHD events and mortality. Such findings appear to be considerably less prominent in clinical trials experiences derived from predominantly middle-aged hypertensives (31,38).

Details regarding clinical evaluation and treatment of the elderly hypertensive patient appear elsewhere (Chap. 7).

## Blood Lipids

The relationships between CHD incidence and total serum cholesterol in the Framingham Study are shown in Figure 9. Separate trends are plotted in

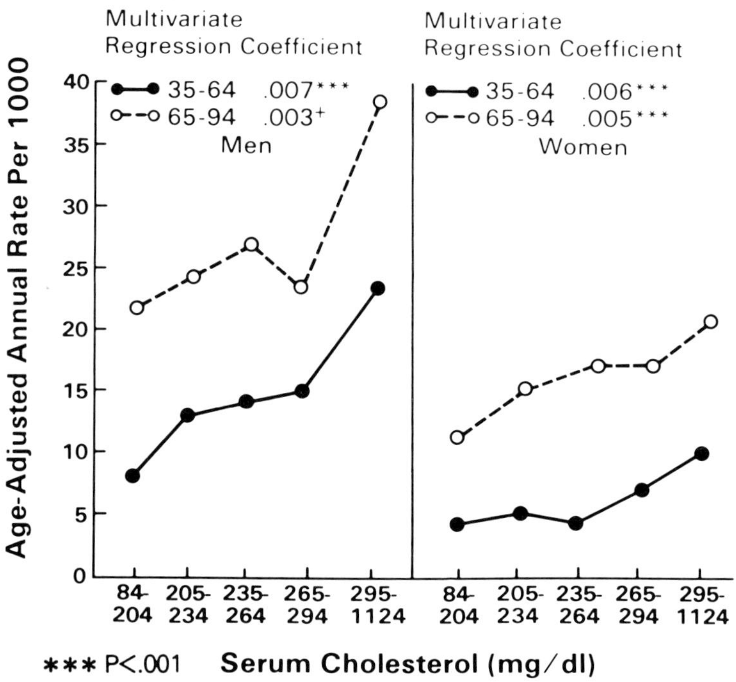


**Figure 9** Risk of CHD by serum cholesterol according to specified age groups in men and women, Framingham Study, 30-year follow-up.

younger and older subjects for men and women, respectively. Note that absolute risk is substantially increased in older as compared to younger men. Note also that relative risk clearly rises over the entire distribution of total serum cholesterol in younger as well as older men. The break in continuity of the risk relation at the fourth level of distribution in older men, however, yields results that narrowly miss statistical significance in both bivariate (age-adjusted) and multivariate estimates using the logistic regression model, whereas the association remains strongly predictive in younger men. Although incidence rates for CHD at corresponding levels of cholesterol are lower in women than in men, the same overall pattern pertains, i.e., an increase in both absolute and relative risk. In this instance, however, statistical significance is maintained in both younger and older women.

The finding that total serum cholesterol loses strength as a risk factor for CHD, particularly in older men of the Framingham cohort, has resulted in serious misinterpretation by some authors who have used this information to argue that serum lipids do not represent important risk factors for CHD in the elderly and thus justify neither detection nor treatment (39,40). This view is both extreme and unreasonable, since several other studies have clearly validated the role of total serum cholesterol as a predictor of CHD events in older men (41–50) and also older women (41,42,44,48,51). Recent data from the Honolulu Heart Study, in particular, provide the strongest support for serum cholesterol as a potent predictor of CHD in older men (45,52). In this prospective study, risk associations were based on CHD events occurring during a follow-up period of 12 years based on total serum cholesterol levels determined at the beginning of the period. An analysis using a comparable statistical approach but based on data from the Framingham Study is shown in Table 6. Risk of CHD events after age 65, in this instance, is based on average levels of serum cholesterol for the 12-year period prior to age 65. Note that trends in risk associations for serum cholesterol are statistically significant for both older men and women.

Despite these findings, however, a recent meta-analysis encompassing data from 22 U.S. and international cohort studies concluded that serum cholesterol did indeed lose strength as a risk predictor for CHD in older men and also in older women (53), a finding consistent with original observations made in data from the Framingham Study.

Focusing on serum cholesterol as the sole measure of risk for CHD attributable to serum lipids should now be considered obsolete based on our current understanding of lipoprotein subfractions and the availability of standardized laboratory methods to measure them in clinical practice. Substitution of either LDL or HDL cholesterol in the regression model fully restores statistical predictability for the risk relation between serum lipids and CHD (54,55). HDL cholesterol, in particular, has emerged as an important lipid moiety that adds substantial precision in assessing coronary risk at limited additional cost. Con-

**Table 6** Risk of Coronary Heart Disease After Age 65 Based on Serum Cholesterol in Middle Age,[a] Framingham Study, 30-Year Follow-up

| | 10-year rate per 1000[b] | |
|---|---|---|
| Cholesterol (mg/dl) | Men** | Women*** |
| <200 | 158 | 49 |
| 200–239 | 214 | 86 |
| 240–279 | 225 | 122 |
| 280+ | 321 | 160 |

[a] Average level during the 12 years prior to age 65.
[b] Kaplan-Meier age-adjusted rates.
Trends significant at $^{**}p < 0.01$, $^{***}p < 0.001$.

struction of a serum cholesterol/HDL ratio provides a highly accurate characterization of CHD risk in older men and women in the Framingham Study, as illustrated in Figure 10. Indeed, data from Framingham as well as other studies confirm the overall reliability of the cholesterol/HDL ratio in assessing CHD risk in younger and older persons and in men as well as women (44,55,56,57). The rationale for this approach is that the ratio reliably captures the effect of a dynamic equilibrium of lipid transport into and out of body tissues possibly including the intima of blood vessels.

Several studies have suggested that serum triglycerides may be important predictors for CHD in either older men or older women, but not consistently in both sexes (44,45,56,58). Despite these observations, the present consensus holds that elevated levels of serum triglycerides represent a risk marker for obesity, glucose intolerance, and low HDL levels, all of which confer risk for CHD and, to the extent possible, deserve preventive attention.

Systematic information from clinical trials regarding the efficacy and safety of treating lipid abnormalities in the elderly, despite their prevalence in this population, is not yet available. A strong case for the widespread application of drug therapy to lower LDL, and/or to elevate HDL, to reduce risk of CHD in older persons is not warranted at present. Management of hypercholesterolemia for now should consist of a highly individualized approach beginning with appropriate dietary measures and weight control before initiation of a trial of

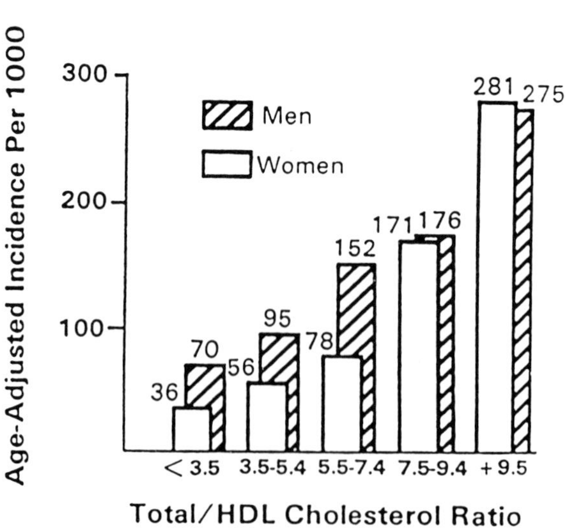


**Figure 10** Risk of CHD by total/HDL cholesterol ratios among men and women aged 50–90 years, Framingham Study, 26-year follow-up.

specific drug therapy, preferably at lower doses, to achieve a carefully monitored lipid-lowering effect (59).

Details regarding the treatment of dyslipidemias in elderly patients appear elsewhere (Chap. 8).

## Cigarette Smoking

Cigarette smoking fails to demonstrate strong risk associations for total CHD events in either older men or older women using the logistic regression methodology indicated in Table 4. Significant risk associations, however, are discerned between cigarette smoking and death due to CHD (15). One explanation for this phenomenon is that smoking may be more closely related to lethal events than to outcomes comprised of combinations of morbid and lethal events. Another explanation is that the cross-sectional pooling approach used in the analysis may classify long-term smokers who have discontinued cigarettes for relatively brief periods as nonsmokers, in effect diluting the strength of the association between the risk factor and the outcome (60). Because of these difficulties, the most reliable approach in assessing risk associations between cigarette smoking and cardiovascular morbidity or mortality is to model these events prospectively for defined categories of smoking behaviors (e.g., current smoker, former smoker, and never smoker) and for longer time intervals. Such approaches yield strong risk associations between cigarette smoking and a broad array of cardiovascular outcomes, including CHD, stroke, and peripheral arterial disease, even in older men and women. These observations have been documented using data from Framingham as well as other studies (44,61–66).

Reducing the risk of cardiovascular disease is not the only reason to encourage discontinuation of smoking in older persons. Cigarettes contribute to the development of chronic bronchitis and obstructive lung disease as well as lung cancer and other malignancies. These conditions also exact a heavy toll in terms of disability and death in the elderly. Thus, the clinician can make a compelling case that it is never too late to stop smoking and extend appropriate advice and encouragement to assist patients in their effort to discontinue cigarette smoking.

## Glucose Tolerance

Impaired glucose metabolism is not only highly prevalent in the elderly, but also confers substantial risk for CHD as well as other cardiovascular events in both older men and women. Various measures of glucose tolerance are employed and nearly all demonstrate significant risk associations with CHD in the Framingham Study (15). These measures include blood glucose levels (Table 4), glycosuria, and the composite risk categories designated as glucose intolerance and diabetes mellitus. Although diabetes mellitus confers enhanced risk for both younger and older men, overall risk increases dramatically for both younger and older women (Table 7). Similar patterns of risk are noted for coronary and cardiovascular mortality (15,67). Diabetes also emerges as an important risk factor in the development of congestive heart failure, particularly in older women with insulin-dependent diabetes mellitus (68). Presumably, the microvascular disease that is unique to diabetes, as well as other mechanisms, serve to produce progressive damage to heart muscle, ultimately resulting in compromised ventricular function and heart failure.

There is little evidence that control of hyperglycemia, by either oral hypoglycemic agents or insulin, effectively forestalls either the development or complications of cardiovascular disease (67,69–71). Present evidence, therefore, suggests that there is more to be gained in reducing risk by correcting associated cardiovascular risk factors in persons with diabetes than by attention confined to early detection and control of hyperglycemia.

## Left Ventricular Hypertrophy

ECG-LVH is a strong risk factor for CHD in older men and women (Fig. 11). Marked increases in CHD incidence are noted for voltage criteria for LVH alone with additional risk conferred by definite LVH, which, in addition to voltage criteria, includes repolarization (ST and T wave) abnormalities consistent with LVH. These electrocardiographic findings presumably reflect abnormalities of myocardial structure and function related to early compromise of underlying coronary circulation that antedates the development of clinical manifestations of CHD (72,73).

In this context, left ventricular hypertrophy (LV mass) as determined by cardiac echocardiography has emerged as an extremely potent independent predictor of CHD as well as other cardiovascular disease events especially in older persons (74–77).

**Table 7** Risk of CHD in Diabetic Subjects by Age and Sex, Framingham Study, 30-Year Follow-up

| | Age-adjusted annual incidence per 1000 | | Age-adjusted risk ratio[a] | |
|---|---|---|---|---|
| | 35–64 years | 65–94 years | 35–64 years | 65–94 years |
| Men | 20 | 34 | 1.7** | 1.4* |
| Women | 19 | 32 | 3.8*** | 2.1*** |

[a] Diabetic versus nondiabetic.
Significant at $*p < 0.05$, $**p < 0.01$, $***p < 0.001$.

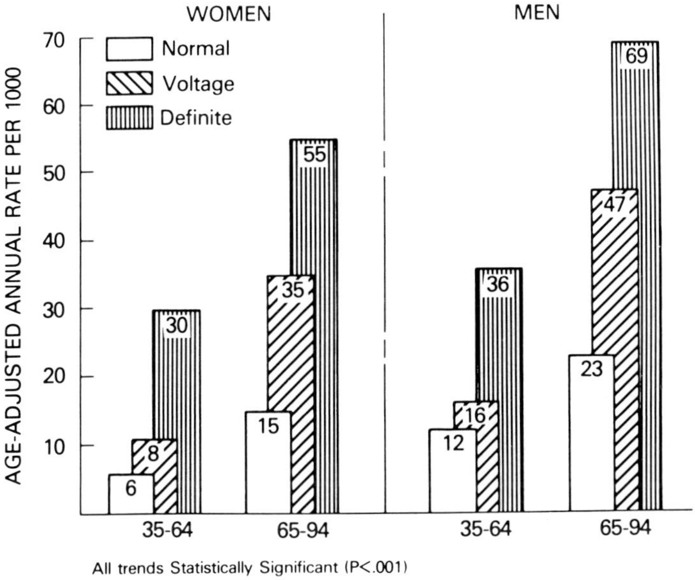


**Figure 11** Risk of CHD according to ECG-LVH status, Framingham Study, 30-year follow-up.

## Body Weight

The association between body weight and risk for CHD in older subjects of the Framingham Study is illustrated in Figure 12. Note that while CHD risk rises more strikingly with increasing body weight in older men, trends in older women clearly indicate enhanced risk at higher body weights. Progressive increases in body weight occurring earlier in life correlate closely with changes in the levels of several risk factors considered to be more directly related to pathogenesis of atherosclerosis (78,79). These include increases in blood pressure, serum cholesterol and triglycerides, and blood glucose with a reduction in HDL cholesterol. These findings serve to emphasize the need to incorporate measures ultimately designed to either control or, if necessary, gradually reduce body weight as part of risk management even in older persons. When coupled with appropriate dietary measures, weight control would be particularly useful in the initial management of elderly patients with hypertension, dyslipidemia, and diabetes or combinations of these conditions.

## Vital Capacity

Vital capacity is a simple, sensitive clinical technique for assessing compromise of pulmonary or cardiac function, or both, in individuals of all ages. In contrast

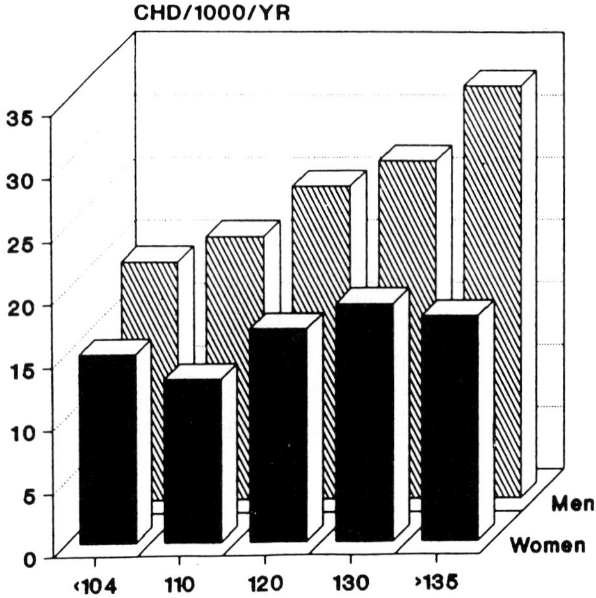


**Figure 12** Risk of CHD according to body weight in men and women, aged 65–94 years, Framingham Study, 30-year follow-up.

to inconsistent risk associations with CHD found in younger subjects, vital capacity is an important risk factor in the elderly, particularly with respect to risk for major coronary events (2,15). Vital capacity normally declines with advancing age, an effect that is strongly exacerbated by cigarette smoking and obesity (80,81). Diminished vital capacity in older people is also correlated with loss of muscular strength as assessed by hand grip, presumably reflecting overall neuromuscular debility (82). Low vital capacity remains a strong predictor of cardiovascular mortality, as well as mortality from all causes. Measurement of this parameter, therefore, should be considered as part of the standard risk assessment of all older patients.

## Heart Rate

Recent data from the Framingham Study demonstrate that resting heart rate confers additional risk for CHD in both younger and older men, although no similar risk association is observed in either younger or older women (2,15). An explanation for this finding is not readily apparent. Heart rate in men may be a more sensitive indicator of underlying cardiac dysfunction than in women, or the net impact of sympathetic nervous system influences in precipitating CHD events may be greater in men. High heart rates may also reflect physical deconditioning.

## Physical Activity

Accumulating evidence now suggests that lifetime vigorous physical activity may forestall CHD in the elderly (83–85). Previously reported data from Framingham indicated that overall mortality, including coronary mortality, was inversely related to level of physical activity in men (86,87). A benefit for exercise in older men was also suggested; however, the levels of exercise involved were quite modest. Although regular physical activity in the elderly is desirable and should be strongly encouraged, it would be unwise to place undue emphasis on this approach alone in attempting to reduce the risk for CHD.

## Prevalent CHD

An important predictor of CHD events at all ages is the presence of antecedent CHD. It is therefore of interest that several of the risk factors associated with the initial development of CHD in the elderly not only continue to have strong correlations with prevalent disease, but also maintain predictive associations for new CHD events in older persons with preexisting disease (42,44,47,88–90). Serum lipids, cigarette smoking, and diabetes appear to be more prominent in this context than hypertension. Blood pressure may fall substantially following myocardial infarction, especially extensive anterior myocardial infarction, which carries a poorer prognosis, thereby confounding the relation between hypertension and CHD morbidity and mortality (91). Blood pressure, however, reemerges as a significant predictor of recurrent CHD events in long-term survivors of myocardial infarction (92).

These findings emphasize the critical role of controlling risk factors in older persons with established CHD.

## Other Risk Factors

Several hematological or hemostatic factors have been described as risk variables in the Framingham Study. Hematocrit appeared to contribute to CHD in younger men and women in this analysis, but not in older persons (15). White blood cell count, which was strongly correlated with the number of cigarettes smoked per day, hematocrit, and vital capacity, was also associated with enhanced risk for CHD and other cardiovascular end-points in older men, both smokers and nonsmokers, but only in women who smoked (93). These data were consistent with reports from other studies (94–96). Plasma fibrinogen showed strong risk associations for CHD and other cardiovascular disease outcomes in men, including older men (97), similar to findings from other studies

(98,99). Significant risk associations, however, were not apparent in older women.

An extensive array of psychosocial, occupational, dietary, and other factors have been described as putative risk parameters for CHD in the Framingham Study (13,100); however, only limited information is available regarding specific associations of these factors with CHD in older persons. Although family history of CHD is strongly related to early development of CHD (before age 60) in both men and women in the Framingham Study, predictive associations also remained significant for the late onset of CHD (101).

## CHD RISK PROFILES IN THE ELDERLY

Although associations between a specific risk factor and CHD can be considered in isolation as a single relation, in many instances combinations of several risk factors may constitute the observed risk profile, especially in older persons. In such instances, risk of CHD can be reliably estimated by synthesizing a number of risk factors into a composite score, based on a multiple logistic function (102). Risk factors are assessed by standard clinical procedures (smoking history, blood pressure, and electrocardiogram) and by routine laboratory studies (total serum cholesterol, HDL cholesterol, and blood glucose). This type of composite index permits detection of individuals at relatively high risk, either on the basis of marked elevation of a single factor or because of marginal abnormalities of several risk factors.

This multivariate risk scenario is illustrated in Figure 13, which characterizes the risk of CHD at two predefined levels of serum cholesterol and then consid-

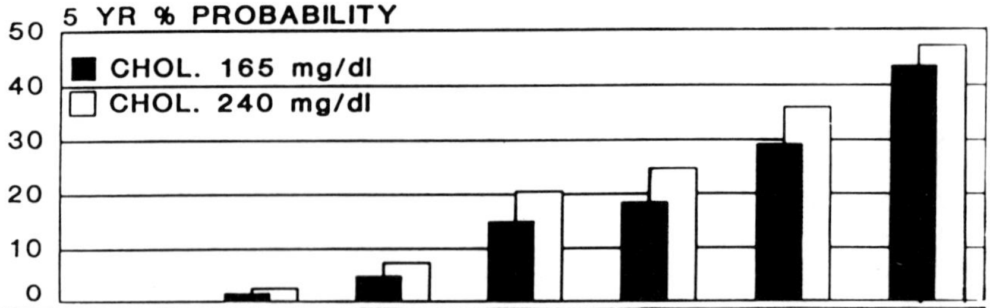


| | | | | | | |
|---|---|---|---|---|---|---|
| SYSTOLIC BP | 100 | 180 | 180 | 180 | 180 | 180 |
| HDL-CHOL. | 65 | 65 | 35 | 35 | 35 | 35 |
| CIG'S | - | - | - | + | + | + |
| GLUC. INTOL. | - | - | - | - | + | + |
| ECG-LVH | - | - | - | - | - | + |

**Figure 13** Risk of CHD of two levels of serum cholesterol according to specified levels or categories of other risk factors for 70-year-old women in the Framingham Study.

ers changes in the levels or values of other risk factors toward worsening risk, as indicated in the table at the bottom of the figure. Note that risk increases progressively with the additional impact of other risk factors for both categories of serum cholesterol, even in instances where a factor such as cigarette smoking has a relatively weak risk association with CHD when considered alone.

When taken together, the major risk factors, including age, explain only a limited proportion of the variance of CHD incidence in younger as well as older persons (102). It is likely that other major risk attributes exist among both the young and the elderly, but are yet to be identified. It must be emphasized, however, that the factors that have already been delineated do identify high-risk subgroups of the elderly population that should be targeted for preventive management.

## PERSPECTIVES FOR PRIMARY PREVENTION OF CHD IN THE ELDERLY

An important principle of prevention is the concept that measures limiting the effect of known risk factors should be initiated as early in life as possible to minimize the subsequent development of disease in both the young and the elderly. It is unreasonable to conclude, however, that modifications of risk factors initiated at advanced age are likely to be ineffective in reducing the toll of related disease in older persons. A simple but important observation in this context is that the incidence of CHD in the elderly varies widely within distributions of continuous risk factors such as blood pressure or serum cholesterol. Incidence also appears to differ markedly for values of categorical variables such as the presence or absence of left ventricular hypertrophy. In addition, data presented earlier indicate that the incidence of CHD, as well as other cardiovascular disease events, is not only substantially higher in populations of older persons, but also continues to rise with advancing age across the life span. Because incidence is usually higher in older persons, the beneficial effect of a given intervention such as treatment of hypertension or hypercholesterolemia, as assessed by reduction in relative risk, may be similar to or lower than that observed in younger persons (2,31,59,103). In many such instances, however, the same effect measured as a difference in absolute risk, reflecting reduction in numerical toll of disease outcomes, actually remains higher in the elderly. A corollary of this effect is that a smaller number of older as compared to younger people must be treated to yield the same benefit in terms of numbers of disease events prevented.

These considerations are more relevant today than ever before. Recently, a marked and progressive decline in mortality due to coronary and cardiovascular disease has occurred in the United States (Fig. 14) and several other industrialized nations (104,105). Age-specific trends indicate decreasing mortality due to

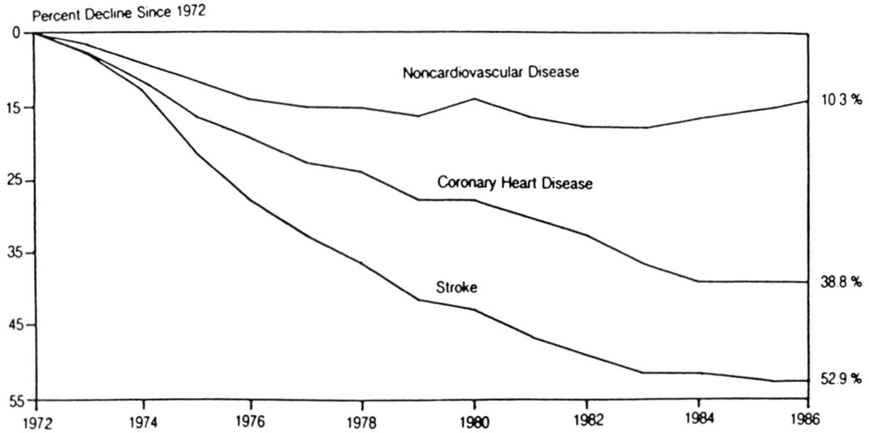


**Figure 14** Trends in mortality for cardiovascular disease (CVD) and non-CVD causes of death. Decline in age-adjusted death rates in the United States, 1972–1986. (From the National Center for Health Statistics.)

CHD and cardiovascular disease, both in the elderly and in younger adults of both sexes. Similar trends in cardiovascular mortality have been identified in the Framingham population (106). At the same time, the prevalence of several coronary risk factors, such as untreated hypertension, elevated serum cholesterol levels, and cigarette smoking, has diminished in the population at large, including the elderly, while impressive improvements have occurred in the diagnosis and treatment of CHD. Although the available information supports the contention that both these potentially beneficial effects have contributed to the observed decline in mortality from CHD, the present consensus gives greater weight to the success of widespread primary preventive strategies, resulting in lowered levels of major risk factors that contribute to disease, rather than to improved diagnosis and treatment of established disease (107).

In this context, hypertension clearly emerges as the dominant, potentially remediable, risk factor for both CHD and cerebrovascular disease morbidity and mortality in the elderly. Hypertension is highly prevalent in the aged, easily detected, and can be corrected by the careful application of appropriate measures, including drug therapy. As mentioned earlier, direct evidence from clinical trials has already established the efficacy of antihypertensive measures in reducing the frequency of stroke and CHD events in elderly hypertensives. Available information also makes a compelling case for discontinuation of cigarette smoking at all ages including the elderly. Information is needed, however, regarding the feasibility and effectiveness of nonpharmacological approaches such as diet and weight reduction in treating older persons with hypertension and lipid abnormalities, both as initial therapy and as adjuncts to specific drug therapy. Also, as a matter of critical importance, the efficacy and safety of drug therapy for the treatment of lipid abnormalities in the elderly should be established in large, well-designed clinical trials. Lack of such information severely limits our confidence in extending what may be a potentially beneficial preventive measure to greater numbers of older persons.

The emphasis of this approach is not a quest for immortality, but for maintenance of a worthwhile quality of life for the aged. In many instances, the sequelae of myocardial infarction or stroke destroy the functional capabilities and independence of elderly persons, ultimately making them dependent on others for their care and support. Thus, appropriate preventive measures that forestall cardiovascular disease in the elderly could well enhance the quality, if not the duration, of the remaining years of life.

## REFERENCES

1. Kannel WB, Gordon T. Evaluation of cardiovascular risk in the elderly: The Framingham Study. *Bull NY Acad Med* 1978; 54:573–591.
2. Kannel WB, Vokonas PS. Primary risk factors for coronary heart disease in the elderly: The Framingham Study. In: Wenger NK, Furberg CD, Pitt E, eds. Coronary Heart Disease in the Elderly. New York: Elsevier, 1986:60–92.
3. Kannel WB, Vokonas PS. Demographics of prevalence, incidence and management of coronary heart disease in the elderly and in women. *Ann Epidemiol* 1992; 2:5–14.
4. Rich M. Acute myocardial infarction in the elderly. *Cardiology* 1990; 7:79–90.
5. Forman DE, Bernal JLG, Wei JY, Management of acute myocardial infarction in the very elderly. *Am J Med* 1992; 93:315–326.
6. Wenger NK. Cardiovascular disease in the elderly. *Curr Probl Cardiol* 1992; 10:615–690.
7. Bedotto JB, Rutherford BP, McConahay DR, Johnson WL, Giorgi LV, Shimshak TM, O'Keefe JH, Ligon RW, Hartzler GO. Results of multivessel percutaneous transluminal coronary angioplasty in persons aged 65 years and older. *Am J Cardiol* 1991; 67:1051–1055.
8. Gersh BJ, Kronmal RA, Schaff HV, Frye RL, Ryan TJ, Mock MB, Myers WO, Athearn MW, Gosselin AJ, Kaiser GC, Bourassa MG, Killip T III, and the Participants in the Coronary Artery Surgery Study: Comparison of coronary artery bypass surgery and medical therapy in patients 65 years of age or older. A nonrandomized study from the Coronary Artery Surgery Study (CASS) registry. *N Engl J Med* 1985; 313:217–224.
9. Wenger NK, Furberg CD, Pitt E. Coronary heart disease in the elderly: Review of current knowledge and research recommendations. In: Wenger NK, Furberg CD, Pitt E, eds. Coronary Heart Disease in the Elderly. New York: Elsevier, 1986:1–7.
10. Kannel WB, Doyle JT, Shepard RJ, Stamler J, Vokonas PS. Prevention of car-

diovascular disease in the elderly. 18th Bethesda Conference: Cardiovascular disease in the elderly. *J Am Coll Cardiol* 1987; 19(Suppl A):25A–28A.
11. Gurwitz JH, Col NF, Avorn J. The exclusion of the elderly and women from clinical trials in acute myocardial infarction. *JAMA* 1992; 268:1417–1422.
12. Lakatta EG. Cardiovascular function in later life. *Cardiovasc Med* 1985; 10:37–40.
13. Kannel WB, Sytkowski PA. Atherosclerosis risk factors. *Pharmacol Ther* 1987; 32:207–235.
14. Dawber TR. The Framingham Study: The Epidemiology of Atherosclerotic Disease. Cambridge: Harvard University Press, 1980.
15. Cupples LA, D'Agostino RB. Section 34. Some risk factors related to the annual incidence of cardiovascular disease and death using pooled repeated biennial measurements: Framingham Heart Study, 30-year follow-up. In: Kannel WB, Wolf PA, Garrison RJ, eds. The Framingham Study: An Epidemiological Investigation of Cardiovascular Disease. Bethesda, MD: National Heart, Lung, and Blood Institute publication No. (NIH) 87-2703, 1987.
16. Kannel WB, Abbott RD. Incidence and prognosis of unrecognized myocardial infarction: An update from the Framingham Study. *N Engl J Med* 1984; 11:1144–1147.
17. Learoyd BM, Taylor MG. Alterations with age in the viscoelastic properties of human arterial walls. *Circ Res* 1966; 18:278–292.
18. Kannel WB, Wolf PA, McGee DL, Dawber TR, McNamara P, Castelli WP. Systolic blood pressure, arterial rigidity, and risk of stroke: The Framingham Study. *JAMA* 1981; 245:1225–1229.
19. Maddocks I. Possible absence of essential hypertension in two complete Pacific Island populations. *Lancet* 1976; 2:327–331.
20. Avolio AP, Deng FQ, Li WG, Luo YF, Huang ZD, Xing LF, O'Rourke MF. Effects of aging on arterial distensibility in populations with high and low prevalence of hypertension: Comparison between urban and rural communities in China. *Circulation* 1985; 71:202–210.
21. Vokonas PS, Kannel WB, Cupples LA. Epidemiology and risk of hypertension in the elderly: The Framingham Study. *J Hypertens* 1988; 8(Suppl I):53–59.
22. Wilking SV, Belanger AJ, Kannel WB, D'Agostino RB, Steel K. Determinants of isolated systolic hypertension. *JAMA* 1988; 260:3451–3455.
23. DeFronzo RA. Glucose intolerance and aging. *Diabetes Care* 1981; 4:493–501.
24. Borkan GA, Norris AH. Fat redistribution and the changing body dimensions of the adult male. *Hum Biol* 1977; 49:495–514.
25. Harris T, Cook EF, Kannel WB, Goldman L. Proportional hazards analysis of risk factors for coronary heart disease in individuals 65 or older. The Framingham Heart Study. *J Am Geriatr Soc* 1988; 36:1023–1028.
26. Veterans Administration Cooperative Study Group on Antihypertensive Agents, Effects of treatment on morbidity in hypertension. III. Influence of age, diastolic pressure and prior cardiovascular disease: further analysis of side effects. *Circulation* 1972; 45:991–1004.
27. Hypertension Detection and Follow-up Program Cooperative Group. Five year

findings of the Hypertension Detection and Follow-up Program. II. Mortality by race-sex and age. *JAMA* 1979; 242:2572–2577.
28. Management Committee. Treatment of mild hypertension in the elderly: A study initiated and administered by the National Heart Foundation of Australia. *Med J Aust* 1981; 2:398–402.
29. Amery A, Birkenhager W, Brixko P, Clement D, Bulpitt C, Deruyttere M, deSchaepdryver A, Dollery C, Fagard R, Forette F, Forte J, Hamdy R, Henry JF, Joossens JV, Leonetti G, Lund-Johansen P, O'Malley K, Petrie J, Strasser T, Tuomilehto J, Williams B. Mortality and morbidity results from the European Working Party on High Blood Pressure in the Elderly Trial. *Lancet* 1985; 1:1349–1354.
30. Coope J, Warrender T. Randomized trial of treatment of hypertension in the elderly patients in primary health care. *Br Med J* 1986; 293:1145–1151.
31. Applegate WB. Hypertension in elderly patients. *Ann Intern Med* 1989; 110:901–915.
32. SHEP Cooperative Research Group. Prevention of stroke by antihypertensive drug treatment in older persons with isolated systolic hypertension: Final results of the Systolic Hypertension in the Elderly Program (SHEP). *JAMA* 1991; 265:3255–3264.
33. Cruickshank JM, Thorp JM, Zacharias FJ. Benefits and potential harm of lowering high blood pressure. *Lancet* 1987; 1:581–584.
34. Berglund G, Samuelsson O. Lowering blood pressure and the J-shaped curve. *Lancet* 1987; 1:1154–1155.
35. Amery A, Birkenhager W, Bulpitt C, et al. Efficacy of antihypertensive drug treatment according to age, sex, blood pressure, and previous cardiovascular disease in patients over the age of 60. *Lancet* 1986; 1:589–592.
36. Dahlof B, Lindholm LH, Hausson K, Schersten B, Ekbom T, Wester PO. Morbidity and mortality in the Swedish Trial in Old Patients with Hypertension (STOP-Hypertension). *Lancet* 1991; 338:1281–1285.
37. MRC Working Party. Medical Research Council trial of treatment of hypertension in older adults: Principal results. *Br Med J* 1992; 304:405–412.
38. Strandgaard S, Haunso S. Why does anti-hypertensive treatment prevent stroke but not myocardial infarction? *Lancet* 1987; 2:658–661.
39. Garber AM, Littenberg B, Sox HC Jr, Gluck ME, Wagner JL, Duffy BM. Costs and Effectiveness of Cholesterol Screening in the Elderly. Washington, DC: Health Program, Office of Technology Assessment, Congress of the United States; April, 1989. GPO publication no. 052-003-01151-4.
40. Beaglehole R. Coronary heart disease and elderly people: No mass treatment for risk factors yet (editorial). *Br J Med* 1991; 303:69–70.
41. Barret-Connor E, Suarex L, Khaw KT, Criqui MH, Wingrad DL. Ischemic heart disease factors after age 50. *J Chronic Dis* 1984; 37:903–908.
42. Aronow WS, Starling L, Etienne F, D'Alba, Edwards M, Lee NH, Parungno RF. Risk factors for coronary artery disease in persons older than 62 years in a long-term health care facility. *Am J Cardiol* 1986; 57:518–520.
43. Stamler J, Wentworth D, Neaton JD, for the MRFIT Research Group. Is the rela-

tionship between serum cholesterol and risk of premature death from coronary heart disease continuous and graded? Findings in 356, 222 primary screenees of the Multiple Risk Factor Intervention Trial (MRFIT). *JAMA* 1986; 256:2835–2838.

44. Aronow WS, Herzig AH, Etienne F, D'Alba P, Ronquillo J. 41-month follow-up of risk factors correlated with new coronary events in 708 elderly patients. *J Am Geriatr Soc* 1989; 37:501–506.
45. Benfante R, Reed D. Is elevated serum cholesterol level a factor for coronary heart disease in the elderly? *JAMA* 1990; 263:393–396.
46. Rubin SM, Sidney S, Black DM, Browner WJ, Hulley SB, Cummings JR. High blood cholesterol in elderly men and the excess risk for coronary heart disease. *Ann Intern Med* 1990; 113:916–920.
47. Pikkanen J, Linn S, Heiss G, Suchindran CM, Leon A, Rifkin BM, Tyroler HA. Ten-year mortality from cardiovascular disease in relation to cholesterol level among men with and without preexisting cardiovascular disease. *N Engl J Med* 1990; 322:1700–1707.
48. Rossouw JE, Bangdiwala S, Gordon DJ, Bush TL, Rifkind BM. Plasma lipids as predictors of CHD in older men and women: The LRC Follow-up Study (abstract). *Circulation* 1990; 82(Suppl III):III–346.
49. Shipley MH, Pocock SJ, Marmot MG. Does plasma cholesterol concentration predict mortality from coronary heart disease in elderly people? *Br Med J* 1991; 303:89–92.
50. Sorkin JD, Andres R, Muller DC, Baldwin HL, Fleg JL. Cholesterol as a risk factor for coronary heart disease in elderly men. The Baltimore Longitudinal Study of Aging. *Ann Epidemiol* 1992; 2:59–67.
51. Keil JE, Sutherland SE, Knapp RG, Gazes PC. Serum cholesterol—Risk factor for coronary heart disease mortality in younger and older blacks and whites. The Charleston Heart Study, 1960–1988. *Ann Epidemiol* 1992; 2:93–99.
52. Reed D, Benfante R. Lipid and lipoprotein predictors of coronary heart disease in elderly men in the Honolulu Heart Program. *Ann Epidemiol* 1992; 2:29–34.
53. Manolio TA, Pearson TA, Wenger NK, Barret-Connor E, Payne GH, Harlan WR. Cholesterol and heart disease in older persons and women: Review of an NHLBI Workshop. *Ann Epidemiol* 1992; 2:161–176.
54. Gordon T, Castelli WP, Hjortland MC, Kannel WB, Dawber TR. Predicting coronary heart disease in middle-aged and older persons. The Framingham Study. *JAMA* 1977; 238:497–499.
55. Castelli WP, Wilson PWF, Levy D, Anderson K. Cardiovascular risk factors in the elderly. *Am J Cardiol* 1989; 63:12H–19H.
56. Castelli WP, Anderson K, Wilson PWF, Levy D. Lipids and risk of coronary heart disease. The Framingham Study. *Ann Epidemiol* 1992; 2:23–28.
57. Hong MK, Romm PA, Reagan K, Green CE, Rackley CE. Total cholesterol/HDL ratio is the best predictor of anatomic coronary artery disease among elderly patients (abstract). *J Am Coll Cardiol* 1991; 17:151A.
58. Welin L, Eriksson H, Larsson B, Ohlon LO, Svardsudd K, Tibblin G, Wilhelmsen L. Triglycerides, a major coronary risk factor in elderly men: A study of men born in 1913. *Eur Heart J* 1991; 6:700–704.

59. Denke MA, Grundy SM. Hypercholesterolemia in elderly persons: Resolving the treatment dilemma. *Ann Intern Med* 1990; 112:780–792.
60. Cupples LA, D'Agostino RB, Anderson K, Kannel WB. Comparison of baseline and repeated measure covariate techniques in the Framingham Heart Study. *Stat Med* 1988; 7:205–218.
61. Wolf PA, D'Agostino RB, Kannel WB, Bonita R, Belanger AJ. Cigarette smoking as a risk factor for stroke: The Framingham Study. *JAMA* 1988; 259:1025–1029.
62. Kannel WB, Higgins M. Smoking and hypertension as predictors of cardiovascular risk in population studies. *J Hypertens* 1990; 8(Suppl 5):S3–S8.
63. Jajich CL, Ostfeld AM, Freeman DH Jr. Smoking and coronary heart disease mortality in the elderly. *JAMA* 1984; 252:2831–2834.
64. Hermanson B, Omenn GS, Kronmal RA, Gersh BJ. Participants in the Coronary Artery Surgery Study, Beneficial six-year outcome of smoking cessation in older men and women with coronary artery disease: Results from the CASS registry. *N Engl J Med* 1988; 319:1365–1369.
65. Benfante R, Reed D, Frank J. Does smoking have an independent effect on coronary heart disease incidence in the elderly? *Am J Public Health* 1991; 81:897–899.
66. LaCroix AZ, Lang J, Scherr P, Wallace RB, Cornoni-Huntley J, Berkman L, Curb JD, Evans D, Hennekens CH. Smoking and mortality among older men and women in three communities. *N Engl J Med* 1991; 324:1619–1625.
67. Kannel WB, McGee DL. Diabetes and cardiovascular disease: The Framingham Study. *JAMA* 1979; 241:2035–2038.
68. Kannel WB, Hjortland M, Castelli WB. Role of diabetes in congestive heart failure: The Framingham Study. *Ann Intern Med* 1970; 72:813–822.
69. Assman G, Shulte H. Diabetes mellitus and hypertension in the elderly: Concomitant hyperlipidemia and coronary heart disease risk. *Am J Cardiol* 1989; 63:33H–37H.
70. Wilson PWF, Cupples L, Kannel WB. Is hyperglycemia associated with cardiovascular disease? The Framingham Study. *Am Heart J* 1991; 121:586–590.
71. Mykannen L, Laakso M, Penttila I, Pyorala K. Asymptomatic hyperglycermia and cardiovascular risk factors in the elderly. *Atherosclerosis* 1991; 88:153–161.
72. Kannel WB, Dannenberg AL, Levy D. Population implications of electrocardiographic left ventricular hypertrophy. *Am J Cardiol* 1987; 60:851–931.
73. Aronow WS. Left ventricular hypertrophy. *J Am Geriatr Soc* 1992; 40:71–80.
74. Casale PN, Devereux RB, Milner M, Zullo G, Harshfield GA, Pickering TG, Laragh JH. Value of echocardiographic measurement of left ventricular mass in predicting cardiovascular morbid events in hypertensive men. *Ann Intern Med* 1986; 105:173–178.
75. Aronow WS, Koenigsberg M, Schwartz KS. Usefulness of echocardiographic left ventricular hypertrophy in predicting new coronary events and atherothrombotic brain infarction in patients over 62 years of age. *Am J Cardiol* 1988; 61:1130–1132.
76. Levy D, Garrison RJ, Savage DD, Kannel WB, Castelli WP. Left ventricular mass and incidence of coronary disease in an elderly cohort. The Framingham Heart Study. *Ann Intern Med* 1989; 110:101–107.

77. Aronow WS, Ahn C, Kronzon I, Koenigsberg M. Congestive heart failure, coronary events, and atherothrombotic brain infarction in elderly blacks and whites with systemic hypertension and with and without echocardiographic and electrocardiographic evidence of left ventricular hypertrophy. *Am J Cardiol* 1991; 67:295–299.
78. Ashley FW, Kannel WB. Relation of weight change to changes in atherogenic traits: The Framingham Study. *J Chronic Dis* 1974; 27:103–114.
79. Borkan GA, Sparrow D, Wisnieski C, Vokonas PS. Body weight and coronary risk: Patterns of risk factor change associated with long-term weight change. The Normative Aging Study. *Am J Epidemiol* 1986; 124(3):410–419.
80. Ashley F, Kannel WB, Sorlie P, Masson R. Pulmonary function: Relation to aging, cigarette habit and mortality: The Framingham Study. *Ann Intern Med* 1975; 82:739–745.
81. Sparrow D, Weiss ST. Pulmonary system. In: Rowe JW, Besdine R, eds. Geriatric Medicine. Boston: Little Brown, 1988:266–275.
82. Kannel WB, Hubert H, Lew EA. Vital capacity as a predictor of cardiovascular disease: The Framingham Study. *Am Heart J* 1983; 34:1022–1033.
83. Paffenbarger RS, Hyde RT, Wing AL, Hsieh CC. Physical activity, all-cause mortality, and longevity of college alumni. *N Engl J Med* 1986; 314:605–613.
84. Ekeland LG, Haskell WL, Johnson JL, Whaley FS, Criqui MH, Sheps DS. Physical fitness as a predictor of cardiovascular mortality in asymptomatic North American men. The Lipid Research Clinics Mortality Follow-up Study. *N Engl J Med* 1988; 319:1379–1384.
85. Donahue RP, Abbott RD, Reed DM, Yano K. Physical activity and coronary heart disease in middle-aged and elderly men: The Honolulu Heart Program. *Am J Public Health* 1988; 78:683–685.
86. Kannel WB, Sorlie P. Some health benefits of physical activity. The Framingham Study. *Arch Intern Med* 1979; 139:857–861.
87. Kannel WB, Belanger AJ, D'Agostino RB, Israel I. Physical activity and physical demand on the job and risk of cardiovascular disease and death: The Framingham Study. *Am Heart J* 1986; 112:820–825.
88. Wong ND, Wilson PWF, Kannel WB. Serum cholesterol as a prognostic factor after myocardial infarction: The Framingham Study. *Ann Intern Med* 1991; 115:687–693.
89. Simons LA, Friedlander Y, McCallum J, Simons J, Powell I, Heller R, Berry G. The Dubbo Study of health of elderly: Correlates of coronary heart disease at study entry. *J Am Geriatr Soc* 1991; 39:584–590.
90. Applegate WB, Hughes JP, Vander-Zwaag R. Case-control study of coronary heart disease risk factors in the elderly. *J Clin Epidemiol* 1991; 44:409–415.
91. Kannel WB, Sorlie PD, Castelli WP, McGee DL. Blood pressure and survival after myocardial infarction. The Framingham Study. *Am J Cardiol* 1980; 45:326–330.
92. Wong ND, Cupples LA, Ostfeld AM, Levy D, Kannel WB. Risk factors for long-term coronary prognosis after initial myocardial infarction. The Framingham Study. *Am J Epidemiol* 1989; 130:469–480.

93. Kannel WB, Anderson K, Wilson PWF. White blood cell count and cardiovascular disease. *JAMA* 1992; 267:1253–1256.
94. Friedman GD, Klatsky AL, Siegelaub AB. The leukocyte count as a predictor of myocardial infarction. *N Engl J Med* 1974; 290:1275–1278.
95. Zalokar JB, Richards JL, Claude JR. Leukocyte count, smoking and myocardial infarction. *N Engl J Med* 1981; 394:465–468.
96. de Labry LO, Campion EW, Glynn RJ, Vokonas PS. White blood cell count as a long term predictor of mortality: Results over 18 years from the Normative Aging Study. *J Clin Epidemiol* 1990; 43:153–157.
97. Kannel WB, Wolf PA, Castelli WP, D'Agostino RB. Fibrinogen and risk of cardiovascular disease. The Framingham Study. *JAMA* 1987; 258:1183–1186.
98. Korsan-Bengtsen K, Wilhelmsen L, Tibblin G. Blood coagulation and fibrinolysis in a random sample of 788 men 54 years old. II. Relations of the variables to "risk factors" for myocardial infarction. *Thromb Diathes Haemorrh* 1972; 28:99–108.
99. Wilhelmsen L, Swardsudd K, Korsan-Bengsten K, Larsson B, Welin L. Fibrogen as a risk factor for stroke and myocardial infarction. *N Engl J Med* 1984; 311:501–505.
100. Kannel WB, Eaker ED. Psychosocial and other features of coronary heart disease: Insights from the Framingham Study. *Am Heart J* 1986; 112:1066–1073.
101. Schildkraut JM, Myers RH, Cupples LA, Kiely DK, Kannel WB. Coronary risk associated with age and sex of parental heart disease in the Framingham Study. *Am J Cardiol* 1989; 64:555–559.
102. Gordon T, Kannel WB. Multiple risk functions for predicting heart disease: The concept, accuracy and application. *Am Heart J* 1982; 103:1031–1039.
103. Malenka DJ, Baron JA. Cholesterol and coronary heart disease. The importance of patient-specific attributable risk. *Arch Intern Med* 1988; 148:2247–2252.
104. Kannel WB, Thom TJ. Implications of the recent decline in cardiovascular mortality. *Cardiovasc Med* 1979; 4:983–997.
105. Walker WJ. Changing U.S. life style and declining vascular mortality—A retrospective. *N Engl J Med* 1983; 308:649–651.
106. Sytkowski PA, Kannel WB, D'Agostino RB. Changes in risk factors and the decline in mortality from cardiovascular disease. The Framingham Heart Study. *N Engl J Med* 1990; 322:1635–1641.
107. Goldman L, Cook EF. The decline in ischemic heart disease mortality rates: An analysis of medical interventions and changes in lifestyles. *Ann Intern Med* 1984; 101:825–836.

# 6

# Cerebrovascular Disease in the Elderly

**Philip A. Wolf**
*Boston University School of Medicine, Boston, Massachusetts*

## INTRODUCTION

The toll in death and disability from cardiovascular disease increases steadily with age; above the age of 65 years, it accounts for nearly half of all deaths. Much of this morbidity and mortality is attributable to stroke, which accounts for almost 20% of all cardiovascular disease deaths in the elderly. Although cerebrovascular disease is the third leading cause of death in the United States, stroke is far more likely to produce disability than death. In fact, stroke is the leading cause of neurological disability leading to institutionalization in the elderly. The American Heart Association estimated that in 1988, 500,000 Americans sustained a stroke and 150,300 of them died of stroke (1). Many of the estimated 2,930,000 stroke survivors required chronic care. In addition, death statistics underestimate the stroke survivors and their families, whose lives are irrevocably altered by this neurological catastrophe. To the functionally independent elderly person, stroke represents a condition worse than death itself, robbing the individual of function and independence and serving as a signal of the end of useful life.

Although medical and surgical therapies for impending or recent-onset stroke should be pursued, it is likely that *prevention* holds the key to reducing cerebrovascular disease. Prevention will be facilitated by a more complete understanding of modifiable host and environmental factors that predispose to stroke. During recent years, these risk factors have been identified and their impact assessed, chiefly through prospective epidemiological study. Furthermore, it has been demonstrated that modification of key risk factors, notably control of hypertension, can substantially reduce stroke occurrence. This review of the epidemiology of stroke in the elderly patient will rely heavily on data collected in the Framingham Study and on evidence garnered from clinical trials that demonstrate the efficacy of risk factor modification in reducing stroke incidence or severity.

Risk factor assessment in an epidemiological study such as Framingham provides special advantages for study of stroke in the elderly since data are collected systematically, often years prior to the appearance of clinical disease. Prospective longitudinal study thereby provides the least distorted picture of the impact of risk factors on the development of cerebrovascular disease.

Stroke is chiefly a disease of the elderly, and a discussion of risk factors for stroke generally is pertinent to stroke in the geriatric age group. However, some factors that may predispose to premature stroke—congenital cardiac lesions, antiphospholipid antibody syndrome, most blood coagulation abnormalities, pregnancy, oral contraceptives, migraine, and arteriovenous malformations—are less important in persons over age 60 years.

## INCIDENCE OF STROKE

### Stroke Incidence According to Age and Gender

Stroke incidence rates depend on the age distribution of the source population, whether recurrent as well as initial strokes are counted, and on completeness of case ascertainment. The occurrence of cardiovascular disease, including stroke and transient ischemic attack (TIA), has been under study in the general population sample at Framingham, Massachusetts, since 1950. The Framingham cohort of 5070 men and women, aged 30–62, who were free of cardiovascular disease at entry into the study, has been followed for 36 years. On each biennial examination, subjects were specifically and systematically queried about the sudden occurrence of speech difficulty, muscular weakness, numbness or tingling, visual defect, or other neurological symptoms, including dizziness and double vision. Subjects with these symptoms of TIA or stroke were evaluated by the study neurologists for the past 20 years to clarify the details and to determine whether minimal criteria for these end-points were met. These clinic and in-hospital assessments have documented the circumstances surrounding the event, served to differentiate stroke and TIA from other neurological diseases, and facilitated classification according to stroke type (particularly during the years prior to computerized tomography (CT) scan availability). It has been possible to determine whether the stroke mechanism was infarct or hemorrhage and whether the bleeding was subarachnoid from a ruptured berry aneurysm (or, rarely, arteriovenous malformation) or intraparenchymatous. Furthermore, the neurological assessments have helped to distinguish cerebral infarction due to large vessel atherothrombosis from lacunar infarction and from stroke secondary to embolism from the heart.

After 36 years of follow-up in the Framingham Study, stroke or isolated TIA occurred in 693 persons; 318 in men and 375 in women. It is informative to compare the incidence, by age and sex, of atherothrombotic brain infarction (ABI) with the coronary circulation analog, myocardial infarction (MI) (Fig. 1). While both increase with age, approximately doubling in successive decades, there are clear differences. Below age 65, MI has a striking male predominance, with a male:female ratio of 4 to 1. Incidence of MI in women lags 20 years behind that of men: the rate of MI in women aged 65–74 years approximates that of men aged 45–54 years. While ABI incidence is approximately 30% higher in men, the ratio is relatively constant across the adult age span, with no striking male predominance at younger ages.

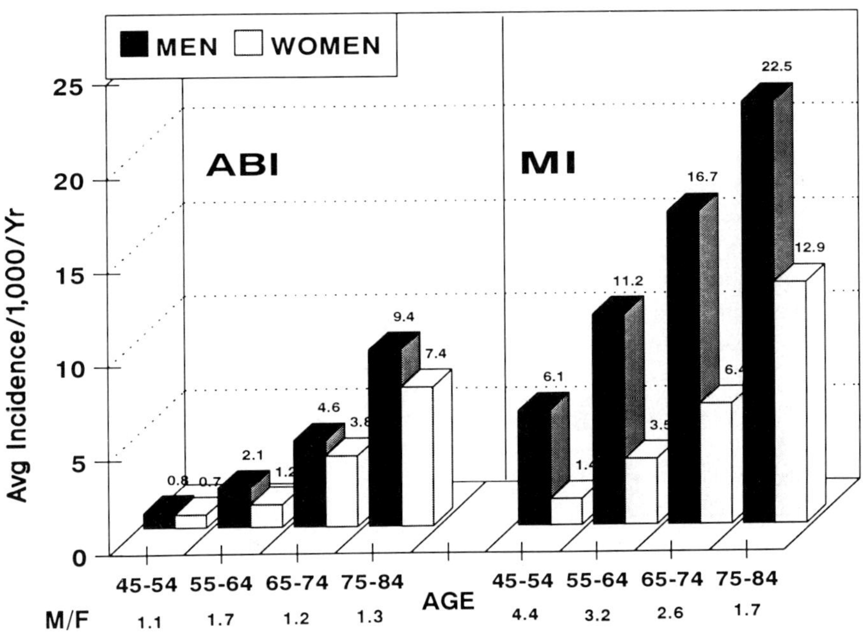


**Figure 1** Incidence of ABI and MI, 36-year follow-up, the Framingham Study.

## Frequency of Stroke by Type

Little substantive difference occurred in the distribution of specific stroke types in persons aged 35–64 years and in the elderly, 65–94 years of age (Table 1). In the older age group, there was more stroke due to cerebral embolism (CE) and somewhat less from subarachnoid hemorrhage (SAH). Overall, however, the relative frequency of stroke by type is approximately the same in younger and older adults and in men and women. In the elderly, aged 65–94 years, atherothrombotic brain infarction (ABI), which includes infarction resulting from large vessel atherothrombosis, lacunar infarction, and infarct of undetermined cause, was the most frequent manifestation and comprised approximately 50% of all strokes regardless of age. Since isolated TIAs are also a manifestation of occlusive arterial disease, this category may be combined with ABI to represent stroke events resulting from atherothrombosis. Together they account for approximately two-thirds of all symptomatic cerebrovascular disease. Intracranial hemorrhage was the mechanism in only 12% of strokes; hemorrhage was intraparenchymatous as often as subarachnoid in men; in younger women the hemorrhage was more than twice as frequently subarachnoid (from a ruptured berry aneurysm) as intraparenchymatous.

Amyloid or congophilic angiopathy is likely to be responsible for a portion of intracerebral hemorrhages, particularly above age 70. Incidence of both types, hypertensive intracerebral hemorrhage and intraparenchymatous bleeding from amyloid angiopathy, increases with age, and distinguishing between them is difficult. Characteristics such as advanced age, absence of a history of hypertension, presence of Alzheimer's disease, a lobar location of the hemorrhage, and other features such as multiple hemorrhages in different sites occurring simultaneously or serially are thought to be characteristic of amyloid angiopathy. However, because of these nosological difficulties, no epidemiological study of the incidence of relative frequency of hemorrhage due to amyloid angiopathy has been made. A diagnostic "gold standard" will be needed to substantiate this diagnosis before convincing epidemiological assessment of the importance of this mechanism of hemorrhage can be made.

# RISK FACTORS FOR STROKE

## Atherogenic Host Factors

Atherosclerotic involvement of the intima of arteries supplying the brain leads to compromise of the arterial lumen with resulting stroke due to atherothrombosis. Since cerebral infarction from atherothrombosis is the mechanism of stroke in two-thirds of cases, an understanding of predisposing factors may provide clues leading to the prevention of stroke. Since the pathological processes underlying stroke from atherothrombotic cerebrovascular disease differ from

**Table 1** Distribution of Stroke Types—36-Year Follow-up

| | Men | | | | Women | | | |
|---|---|---|---|---|---|---|---|---|
| | Age group 35–64 No. cases | Percent of all strokes | Age group 65–94 No. cases | Percent of all strokes | Age group 35–64 No. cases | Percent of all strokes | Age group 65–94 No. cases | Percent of all strokes |
| Atherothrombotic brain infarction | 52 | 43.3% | 89 | 44.9% | 42 | 44.2% | 122 | 43.6% |
| Cerebral embolus | 17 | 14.2% | 42 | 21.2% | 16 | 16.8% | 70 | 25.0% |
| Intracerebral hemorrhage | 7 | 5.8% | 11 | 5.6% | 3 | 3.2% | 14 | 5.0% |
| Subarachnoid hemorrhage | 10 | 8.3% | 9 | 4.5% | 11 | 11.6% | 16 | 5.7% |
| Transient ischemic attack only | 32 | 26.7% | 42 | 21.2% | 17 | 17.9% | 56 | 20.0% |
| Stroke from other causes | 2 | 1.7% | 5 | 2.5% | 6 | 6.3% | 2 | 0.7% |
| Total | 120 | 100.0% | 198 | 100.0% | 95 | 100.0% | 280 | 100.0% |

those predisposing to subarachnoid and intracerebral hemorrhage and to cerebral embolus, it seems reasonable to relate risk factor levels specifically to specific stroke types. Since brain infarction secondary to atherothrombosis (ABI) is the most frequent stroke subtype, and may be considered the cerebral analog of MI, greatest emphasis will be given to ABI.

### *Hypertension*

Hypertension is the dominant precursor of stroke. For atherothrombotic brain infarction, incidence of stroke was approximately 3 times greater in persons with definite hypertension (>160/95 mm Hg) and 50% higher in borderline hypertensives than in normotensives (<140/90 mm Hg) (Fig. 2). This was true in both sexes and in all age categories including 75–84 years. There was no support for the belief that women tolerate hypertension better than men or that hypertension is unimportant or has fewer dire consequences in the elderly.

The relative impact of the major risk factors may be inferred from the size of their multivariate regression coefficients (Table 2). These coefficients, stan-

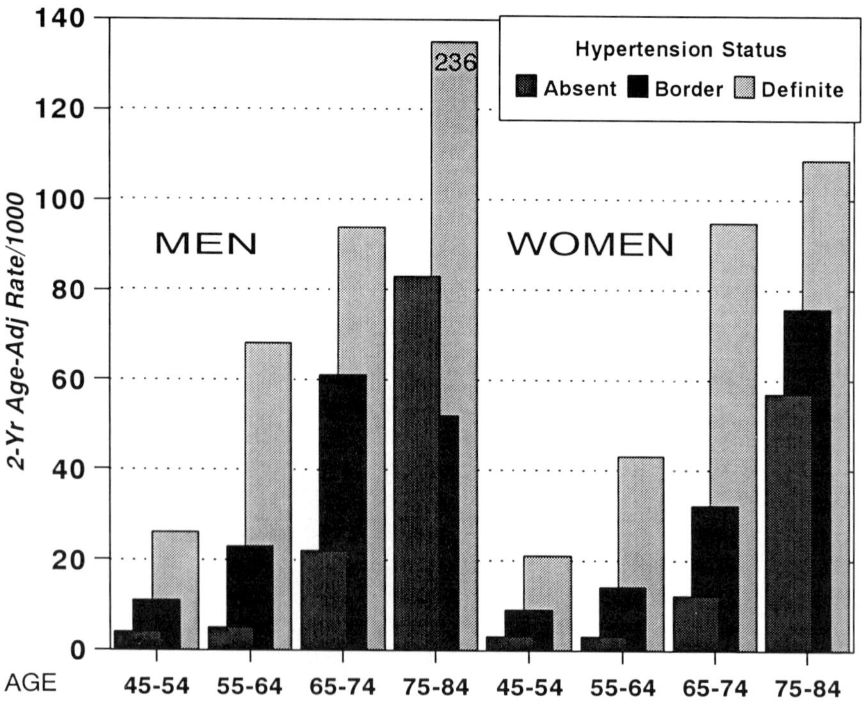


**Figure 2** Incidence of ABI and hypertensive status, 36-year follow-up, the Framingham Study.

**Table 2** Risk Factors for ABI: Standardized Multivariate Regression Coefficients*, Men and Women, Aged 35–64 and 65–94 Years, 36-Year Follow-up, The Framingham Study

| | Standardized multivariate regression coefficients | | | |
|---|---|---|---|---|
| | Men | | Women | |
| Risk factor | 35–64 | 65–94 | 35–64 | 65–94 |
| Hypertension | .761[a] | .426[a] | .814[a] | .477[a] |
| Systolic BP | .613[a] | .395[a] | .629[a] | .396[a] |
| Diastolic BP | .642[a] | .228[b] | .615[a] | .369[a] |
| LVH by ECG | .113 | .192[c] | .130[b] | .228[a] |
| Cigarettes | .468[a] | .197[b] | .090 | .274[a] |
| Total Chol. | −.060 | −.114 | .096 | −.097 |
| Glucose Intol. | .108 | 0.115 | .054 | .156[b] |
| Rel. Weight | .266[b] | .009 | .157 | .195[b] |
| Hematocrit | .324[b] | .105 | .051 | −.098 |

*Multivariate contains systolic blood pressure, LVH by ECG, cigarette smoking, glucose intolerance, total serum cholesterol, and the other appropriate variable.

[a] $p < 0.001$

[b] $p < 0.05$

[c] $p < 0.01$

dardized for the varied units and scales, take into account the contribution made by the other risk factors to incidence of ABI. The bigger the coefficient, the greater is its impact on ABI incidence. Those risk factors with statistically significant coefficients made an *independent* contribution to risk even after age and other pertinent risk factors had been accounted for. For hypertension, in both younger and older age categories, the standardized multivariate regression coefficient was large, denoting a powerful and independent contribution of definite hypertension to ABI.

Most of the numerous trials assessing the impact of blood pressure control since 1970 have dealt with diastolic hypertension in persons below age 70 years. A recently completed trial, the Swedish Trial of Old Patients with Hypertension (STOP-Hypertension) (2), has clearly demonstrated the efficacy and safety of blood pressure control in persons above the age of 70 and will be discussed below.

*Systolic Versus Diastolic Pressure Level.* While incidence of cerebrovascular disease is increased in hypertensives, it is apparent that incidence of stroke generally and ABI specifically is related to the level of the blood pressure. Certain insights into the relative impact of systolic and diastolic components of blood pressure may be attained by cross-classifying rates by each pressure level and examining stroke incidence rates in each category (Fig. 3). At all levels of diastolic blood pressure, incidence of stroke increases directly as level of systolic pressure increases, including persons with diastolic hypertension (>95 mm Hg). However, in persons with systolic hypertension (those with a systolic pressure of 160 mm Hg or greater), incidence of stroke does not increase with increasing levels of diastolic pressure. These data tend to discredit the contention that the diastolic is of greater importance than the systolic component. Although most studies of the efficacy of hypertension control in stroke prevention have classified subjects by the diastolic level, evidence for the ascendancy of diastolic blood pressure over systolic is lacking.

*Isolated Systolic Hypertension.* With the disproportionate rise in systolic pressure that occurs with advancing age, isolated systolic hypertension becomes highly prevalent; above age 75, 18% of men and 30% of women have this condition (Fig. 4). Although common, it is far from innocuous. Not only is systolic blood pressure as powerful a predictor of brain infarction as the diastolic component, but isolated elevations of systolic pressure are also important. Among

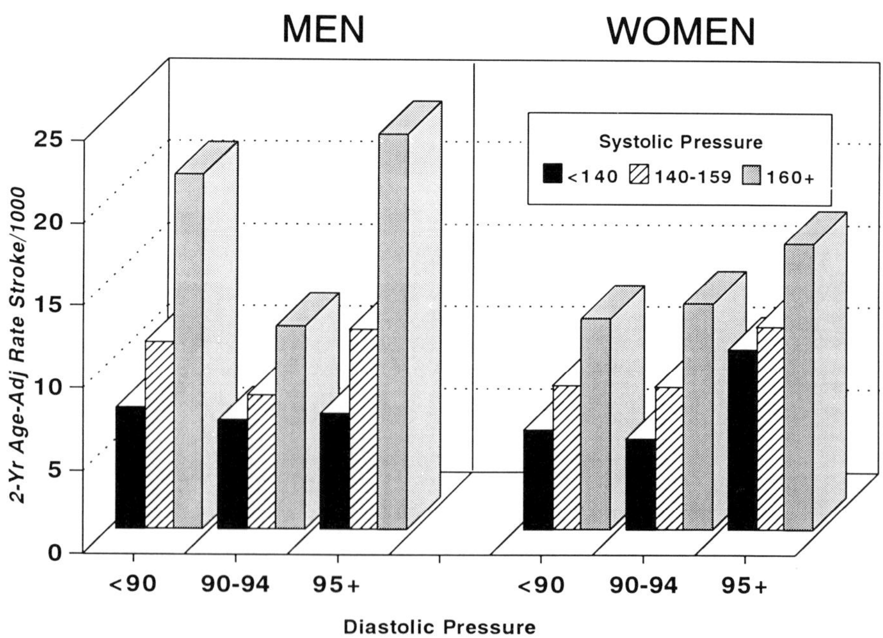


**Figure 3** Level of systolic and diastolic blood pressure (mm Hg), 36-year follow-up, the Framingham Study. Ages 35–84 years.

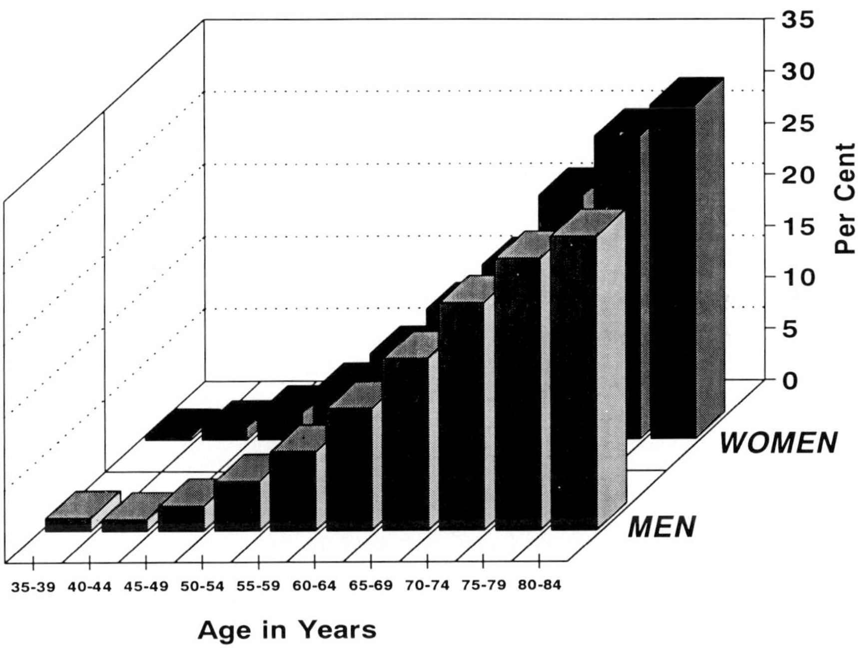


**Figure 4** Prevalence of isolated systolic hypertension, 36-year follow-up, the Framingham Study.

those with isolated systolic hypertension, in both age groups of elderly subjects in the Framingham Study, those 65–74 years and those 75–84 years, there is at least a two-fold increased risk of stroke in men and 1.5-fold increased risk in women (Table 3). Since isolated systolic hypertension was a consequence of reduced elasticity of the great arteries, it had been suggested the arterial rigidity

**Table 3** Incidence of Stroke with ISH, 36-Year Follow-up, The Framingham Study. (Average annual incidence of stroke per 1000 persons.)

| Age at biennial exam | | NO ISH | ISH | Risk ratio |
|---|---|---|---|---|
| 65–74 | Men | 8.7 | 17.0 | 2.0 |
| | Women | 7.3 | 12.6 | 1.7 |
| 75–84 | Men | 17.4 | 37.6 | 2.2 |
| | Women | 15.1 | 20.4 | 1.4 |

rather than the systolic blood pressure was responsible for the increased stroke rate. If so, reduction of the systolic pressure would have no impact on stroke incidence. However, data from Framingham demonstrated increased risk of stroke with isolated systolic hypertension even after arterial rigidity was taken into account. Furthermore, incidence of stroke rose as systolic pressure increased.

It had also been suggested the isolated systolic elevations would be resistant to antihypertensive medications and that treatment with attendant reduced cerebral perfusion might even increase the incidence of stroke. It was felt the use of medications to treat elevated systolic pressures in the elderly would be poorly tolerated, leading to syncope or dizziness with increased falls and fractures, or to confusion and altered mental status. After a successful pilot study, a randomized clinical trial of treatment of isolated systolic hypertension in persons aged 60 years and older was conducted. The Systolic Hypertension in the Elderly Program (SHEP) has recently been completed, and the findings have refuted virtually all of these notions, as will be discussed further below (3).

### *Heart Disease and Impaired Cardiac Function*

Although hypertension is the preeminent risk factor for stroke of all types, at all blood pressure levels persons with evidence of impaired cardiac function, occult or overt, have a significant increase in incidence of stroke. The major cardiac contributors to stroke include prior coronary heart disease (CHD), cardiac failure, electrocardiographic abnormalities (particularly left ventricular hypertrophy), and atrial fibrillation.

*Coronary Heart Disease.* The age-adjusted incidence of stroke was increased severalfold in the presence of these cardiovascular abnormalities (Fig. 5) (4–6). In Framingham, persons with any of the manifestations of CHD, including uncomplicated angina pectoris and clinically silent as well as overt MI, had a significantly increased incidence of stroke. Overall, age-adjusted incidence of stroke was more than doubled in the presence of CHD. Similarly, cardiac failure (CHF) increased stroke incidence more than fourfold.

*Left Ventricular Hypertrophy by Electrocardiogram.* Definite left ventricular hypertrophy by electrocardiogram (LVH by ECG), increases in prevalence with age and blood pressure. LVH by ECG is a powerful contributor to stroke incidence generally and to brain infarction incidence specifically. Incidence of stroke was increased more than fourfold in persons with this ECG pattern. This excess risk persisted even after the influence of other atherogenic precursors, including blood pressure and age, was taken into account (Table 3). A powerful relationship between left ventricular mass, a more precise echocardiographic determination of an enlarged left ventricular wall, and cardiovascular disease including stroke has been demonstrated.

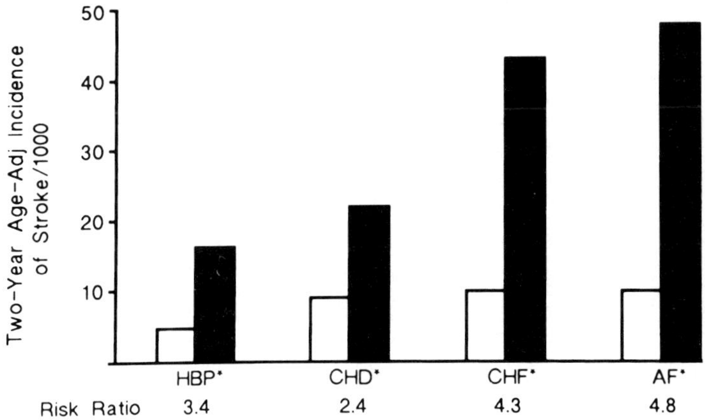


**Figure 5** Two-year age-adjusted incidence of stroke according to presence (filled bars) and absence (open bars) of cardiovascular condition. HBP, hypertension; CHD, coronary heart disease; CHF, cardiac failure; AF, atrial fibrillation. *$p < 0.001$ different from unity. (From Wolf PA, Abbott RD, Kannel WB. *Stroke* 1991; 22:983–988.)

*Atrial Fibrillation.* It is now clear that risk of stroke is increased approximately five-fold in the presence of atrial fibrillation (AF). Incidence is even higher, 18-fold, when AF is associated with rheumatic heart disease and mitral stenosis. AF is the most prevalent cardiac arrhythmia in the elderly (5,6). In the Framingham Study, incidence of nonvalvular AF more than doubled in successive decades, rising from 0.2 per 1000 at ages 30–39 to 39.0 per 1000 at ages 80–89 years. It is also highly prevalent, particularly among those affected by stroke; overall, prevalence of nonvalvular AF among stroke patients was 15%. However, prevalence was not uniform and increased dramatically with age. Nonvalvular AF was particularly important in the elderly since the proportion of strokes occurring in persons with this arrhythmia increased steadily with age, rising from 6.5% for ages 50–59 years to 30.7% for ages 80–89 years (Table 4). Thus, nearly one-third of all stroke events in the 80–89-year age group occurred in persons with nonvalvular AF and in nearly one-fifth (18.8%) of all initial stroke events in persons aged 70–79 years. The stroke was not a consequence of the often associated CHD or cardiac failure since relative risk of stroke rose with age for AF while relative risk of stroke attributable to cardiac failure, CHD, and hypertension declined with age (Table 4).

In addition to clinically evident stroke, a number of case-control studies have disclosed persons with nonvalvular AF had a higher prevalence with silent infarcts, as well as a greater number of silent lesions, than did controls in regular rhythm.

**Table 4** Attributable Risk of Stroke for Hypertension, Coronary Heart Disease, Cardiac Failure, and Atrial Fibrillation by Age

| Cardiovascular condition | Age group: 50–59 yr (92 stroke events) | 60–69 yr (213 stroke events) | 70–79 yr (192 stroke events) | 80–89 yr (75 stroke events) |
|---|---|---|---|---|
| Hypertension | | | | |
| Attributable risk (%) | 48.8 | 53.2 | 48.6 | 33.4 |
| Events occurring with condition (%) | 72.8 | 80.3 | 83.9 | 84.0 |
| Coronary heart disease | | | | |
| Attributable risk (%) | 11.1 | 12.4 | 12.6 | 0.0 |
| Events occurring with condition (%) | 25.0 | 32.9 | 38.0 | 28.0 |
| Cardiac failure | | | | |
| Attributable risk (%) | 2.3 | 3.1 | 5.6 | 6.0 |
| Events occurring with condition (%) | 9.8 | 11.7 | 18.2 | 18.7 |
| Atrial fibrillation | | | | |
| Attributable risk (%)* | 1.5 | 2.8 | 9.9 | 23.5 |
| Events occurring with condition (%) | 6.5 | 8.5 | 18.8 | 30.7 |

*Significant increase with age ($p < 0.01$).

Although most persons with nonrheumatic atrial fibrillation do not sustain a stroke, 35% do over the course of their lifetime. Despite the concern about hemorrhage, particularly intracerebral hemorrhage, in elderly persons on long-term warfarin anticoagulation, this complication occurred infrequently (<0.5% per year) in five recently completed clinical trials that strongly support the use of low-intensity warfarin anticoagulation therapy (7,8). Attempts to identify a subset of persons at particularly high risk of stroke have not been successful. However, since "low-intensity" anticoagulation with warfarin, with prolongation of the prothrombin time 1.2–1.5 times control, has significantly reduced stroke incidence, this is the preferred method of stroke prevention today.

### *Blood Lipids*

Total serum cholesterol is significantly and independently related to the development of CHD in men and women, although the impact seems to diminish with advancing age, particularly in men. However, there is a clear direct relationship between MI and total and LDL cholesterol, and an inverse impact of HDL cholesterol can be seen in older persons. When these lipid fractions are expressed as the total cholesterol/HDL cholesterol ratio, the relationship to CHD is quite strong (Fig. 6). The association between total serum cholesterol,

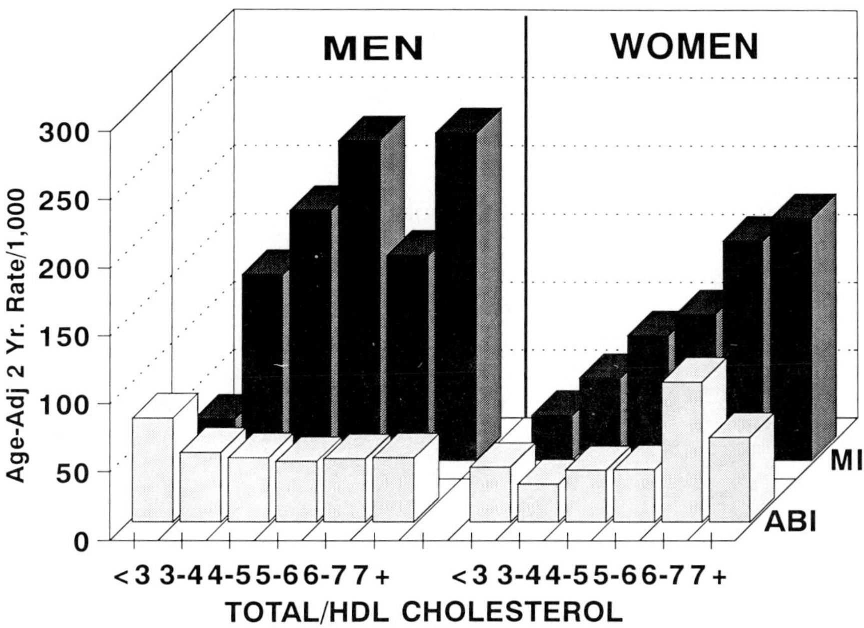


**Figure 6** Total/HDL cholesterol and incidence of ABI and MI, exams 10–12, the Framingham Study. Men—ABI p = .919; MI p = .0001; Women—ABI p = .020; MI p = .0000;

or the lipoprotein cholesterol fractions, and the occurrence of stroke or brain infarction is far less clear or consistent. Although a number of case-control studies have found a modest increase in risk of ischemic stroke, Framingham data have not.

Recently, a relationship between high levels of total serum cholesterol and ischemic stroke and low levels of serum cholesterol and intracerebral hemorrhage (9,10) was found after 6-year death certificate follow-up of predominantly white men in the United States. These data from the 350,977 Multiple Risk Factor Intervention Trial (MRFIT) screenees, based on a single measure of total serum cholesterol at entry and death certificate diagnosis of stroke, are nonetheless persuasive (11).

However, since CHD is an important disease state that predisposes to stroke, it seems reasonable to try to modify blood lipid levels to reduce MI incidence and thereby prevent cardiovascular disease generally.

### *Diabetes*

Clinical observations, including surveys of diabetic patients, and prospective studies have disclosed an increased susceptibility to atherosclerosis including stroke. In the United States in 1976–1980, prior stroke was 2.5–4 times more common in diabetics than in nondiabetics (12). In the Framingham Study, intermittent claudication was more than four times more prevalent in diabetics (13). The coronary and cerebral circulations were also affected. In a population-based cohort in Rancho Bernardo, California, the relative risk of stroke was 1.8 in men and 2.2 in women even after adjusting for the impact of other pertinent risk factors (14).

### *Obesity*

Obese persons have higher blood pressures and higher blood glucose levels (as well as higher levels of serum lipids), which could be expected to increase stroke incidence on that account alone. However, when these other relevant risk factors are taken into account, no residual independent increase in risk from overweight persists. Obviously, obesity exerts an adverse influence on health status by promoting higher blood pressures, blood sugar, and lipids and through other mechanisms. The pattern of obesity is important, and abdominal deposition of fat is more strongly associated with stroke and hypertensive disease (15).

### *Fibrinogen*

Serum fibrinogen has been implicated in stroke and in atherogenesis (16). In addition, levels of fibrinogen and hematocrit have substantial effects on blood viscosity and cerebral blood flow. In a prospective study in Sweden, fibrinogen was found to be a potent risk factor for stroke in a sample of 54-year-old men followed for 13 years (17).

### *Race*

Stroke is a greater public health problem for blacks than whites in the United States. Compared with whites, blacks have death rates from stroke that are 1.5-fold greater in men and 2.3-fold higher in women; overall, age-adjusted mortality was 1.98 times that of whites (18).

Japanese have been known to have high incidence and death rates from stroke. Although intracerebral hemorrhage is far more frequent among Japanese than Caucasian Americans, autopsy studies have shown infarction to be the most frequent mechanism of stroke. In contrast to whites, Japanese, like U.S. blacks, have a predominance of intracranial small vessel disease (19).

### *Family History of Stroke*

Although family history of atherosclerotic disease, including stroke, is commonly perceived to be an important marker of increased risk, evidence for this notion has been lacking. Recently, in a Swedish cohort born in 1913, stroke incidence was significantly increased in men whose mothers had died from stroke (20). This family history of fatal maternal stroke was independent of other significant risk factors, including hypertension, abdominal pattern of obesity, and fibrinogen level.

## Environmental Factors

### *Cigarette Smoking*

Several large-scale prospective studies, including the Framingham Study, have linked cigarette smoking to stroke (21,22). Even after other cardiovascular risk factors, such as systolic blood pressure level, total serum cholesterol, LVH by ECG, obesity, and glucose intolerance, were taken into account, stroke incidence was 40% higher in men and 60% higher in women smokers. There was also a significant relationship between cigarette smoking and ABI. Incidence of stroke increased with number of cigarettes smoked daily, and the impact of smoking did not wane with advancing age. After smoking cessation, stroke incidence fell substantially within 2 years of quitting cigarettes. Within 5 years of quitting, risk of stroke had fallen to the level of a nonsmoker. There was no evidence of any less benefit of smoking cessation in the elderly. These data suggest cigarette smoking acts by precipitating stroke in susceptibles rather than by promoting atherosclerosis and that it is never too late in life to quite.

In a cohort of female nurses, risk of stroke in light smokers, $<15$ cigarettes per day, was more than twice that of nonsmokers (23). Heavy smokers, $>25$ cigarettes per day, had nearly a fourfold increased stroke risk compared with nonsmokers. This significantly increased stroke risk persisted after other risk factors, including alcohol consumption, oral contraceptive and postmenopausal estrogen use, and other standard risk factors, were taken into account.

Of considerable interest, relative risk of subarachnoid hemorrhage also showed a dose-response relationship from fourfold in light smokers to 9.8-fold in heavy smokers. The association between cigarette smoking and subarachnoid hemorrhage from aneurysm was found in men as well as women, in Framingham, Massachusetts (24), New Zealand (25), and recently in King County, Washington (26), in case-control analyses. A similar relationship between cigarette smoking and stroke was seen in Hawaiian Japanese men after 10 years of follow-up in the Honolulu Heart Study, where cigarette smoking made a significant independent contribution to cerebral infarction and intracranial hemorrhage risk (27).

### *Alcohol Consumption*

The impact of alcohol consumption on stroke risk, like its influence on CHD, is related to the amount of alcohol consumed (28). Nondrinkers and heavy users have high stroke and coronary disease rates, while light or moderate alcohol consumers have lower rates of these diseases. The protective effect of moderate drinking and CHD incidence may relate to the increased HDL cholesterol level promoted by alcohol, while heavy imbibers have more hypertension and higher triglyceride levels. The adverse impact of both total abstinence and heavy alcohol consumption seems to be true for ischemic stroke; heavy drinking is related to hemorrhagic stroke, both intraparenchymatous and subarachnoid hemorrhage (29,30). Some of this effect is probably mediated through higher blood pressures in heavy imbibers and the frequent association between heavy drinking and cigarette smoking. Both lead to hemoconcentration, increased blood hematocrit, and viscosity, and rebound thrombocytosis during abstinence has been observed. Acute alcohol intoxication may provoke cardiac rhythm disturbances, notably AF (31), as a precipitant of acute infarction in young people and in subarachnoid hemorrhage.

### *Physical Activity*

Leisure-time and work-associated vigorous physical activity has also been linked to reduced CHD incidence; longshoremen had lower rates of MI (32). There was no corresponding decreased stroke incidence. The more physically active of 17,000 former Harvard University students experienced half the risk of fatal CHD and one-third the mortality rate of their least active fellow alumni (33). No such data exist demonstrating a reduction in stroke occurrence from vigorous habitual leisure-time physical activity. However, moderate exercise should be encouraged because it exerts a beneficial influence on risk factors for atherosclerotic disease by promoting weight reduction, lowering blood pressure, reducing the pulse rate, raising the HDL cholesterol and lowering the LDL cholesterol, improving glucose intolerance, and promoting a healthy lifestyle.

## Signs of Compromised Cerebral Circulation

There are two clinical indicators of a compromised cerebral circulation: asymptomatic carotid bruit and transient ischemic attack.

### *Asymptomatic Carotid Bruits*

In the Framingham Study, carotid bruit in the neck was associated with a doubling of the incidence of subsequent stroke. The stroke was not directly related to the carotid artery with the bruit; the site and type of stroke were appropriate to carotid artery stenosis in only 19% of persons. Incidence of myocardial infarction was also doubled in persons with bruit, and mortality was also increased, 1.7-fold in men and 1.9-fold in women, with 79% of the deaths being due to cardiovascular disease. Furthermore, not all the strokes were cerebral infarction due to carotid stenosis. Ruptured aneurysm, posterior circulation atherosclerosis, emboli from the heart, and lacunar infarction were stroke mechanisms in nearly half the cases. Thus, carotid bruit served only as a sign of atherosclerosis, rather than indicating specific propensity to internal carotid artery territory infarction. In keeping with this predisposition, incidence of myocardial infarction was also increased twofold in those with asymptomatic carotid bruit.

### *Transient Ischemic Attacks*

For secondary prevention generally and to prevent stroke secondary to extracranial internal carotid artery stenosis specifically, attempts have been made to educate physicians and the general population about TIAs. TIAs are reversible focal neurological deficits persisting for less than 24 h; duration is usually minutes rather than hours. Based on retrospective data from clinical series of stroke patients, TIAs were believed to be frequent harbingers of brain infarction. Risk of stroke is clearly increased following TIA, perhaps by as much as 10-fold in the first days or weeks following the TIA.

Although the indications for carotid endarterectomy have been debated for more than 3 decades, and the annual number of procedures grew rapidly to nearly 100,000 in the United States in 1986, guidelines based on firm data have become available only in the past year. In persons with recent TIAs that are referable to an cervical internal carotid artery stenosis of >70%, surgery was clearly superior to best medical therapy in preventing stroke (34). Several important qualifiers must be noted. These findings do not apply to *symptomatic* persons with carotid stenosis of 30-69% or to asymptomatic persons or to those with <30% stenosis.

In addition, estimates indicate that only 10–20% of all strokes are actually preceded by TIAs. It is also estimated that atherothrombotic disease of the surgically accessible carotid artery accounts for less than 15% of strokes.

In the Framingham Study, 12% of cerebral infarcts were preceded by a TIA. The average annual incidence of TIAs was similar in men and women and increased with age. Subjects reported nonspecific, non-TIA neurological symptoms nearly four times as frequently as bona fide TIAs. Stroke developed in about 40% of the persons with TIA; half occurred within 3 months of the TIA onset and two-thirds within 6 months. In most cases, fewer than four attacks occurred prior to completed stroke.

## SECULAR TRENDS IN INCIDENCE AND MORTALITY

Over the past 25 years there has been a decline in stroke death rates of more than 50% in the United States. Similar improvement in stroke mortality has occurred in most industrialized nations. The acceleration of a 1% annual decline from 1915 to 1965 to 5% per year since 1968 strongly supports a role of modifiable environmental factors in stroke mortality. Stroke death rates have declined concurrent with declining death rates of total and cardiovascular disease. The accelerated decline in stroke mortality has been linked to an appreciation of the importance of hypertension as the major risk factor for stroke, hemorrhage, or infarction and the finding in clinical trials that hypertension control will reduce stroke incidence and death by 42% (35,36) (Fig. 7).

Stroke death rates have declined either as a result of decreased incidence or from improved survival. Evidence supporting the role of declining *incidence* of stroke has come from a number of populations, including the community-based study of Rochester, Minnesota, where stroke incidence declined coincident with improved hypertension detection and control (37). In other populations, evidence of decline in stroke case-fatality rates but no change in incidence, has been found (38). The introduction of CT of the brain in the mid-1970s has substantially improved diagnostic sensitivity and facilitated identification of many milder strokes with minimal neurological symptoms and signs. Identifying these less severe neurological events as stroke may increase the apparent incidence while apparent stroke severity declines. The widespread availability of imaging studies, CT scan and magnetic resonance imaging of the brain has introduced a diagnostic test for stroke that has made analysis of secular trends difficult (39).

## PREVENTIVE IMPLICATIONS

Since 1970 when stroke and other hypertensive outcomes were reduced by drug treatment of severely hypertensive patients, a large number of clinical trials have consistently demonstrated that stroke can be prevented in severe, moderate, and, recently, mild hypertensives (35–40).

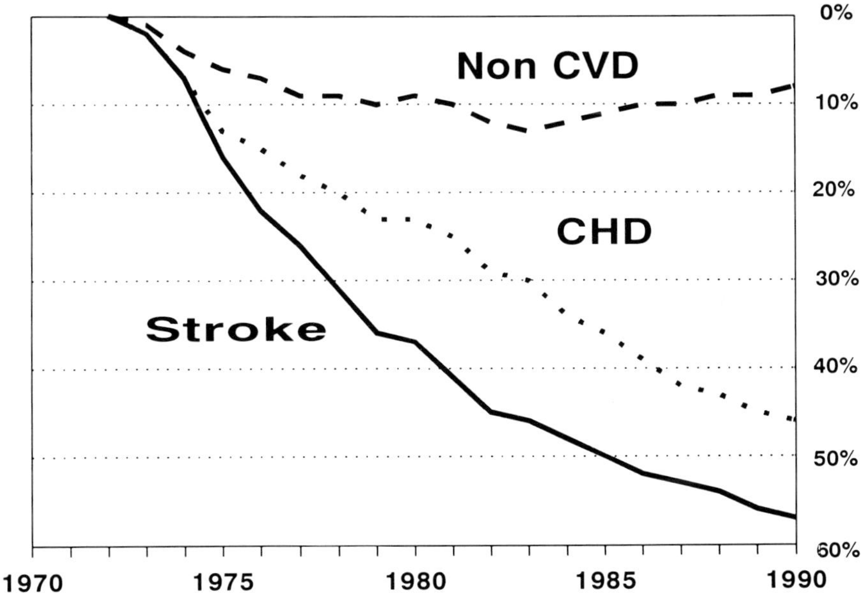


**Figure 7** Decline in mortality 1972 to 1990.

## Antihypertensive Treatment in the Elderly

While it was clear that treatment and control of hypertension prevented stroke in middle-aged persons with diastolic hypertension, there was no consensus on the safety or efficacy of hypertension control in the elderly. The European Working Party on Hypertension in the Elderly (EWPHE) study (41) and the STOP-Hypertension study (2) determined that antihypertensive medication was well tolerated and was effective in the elderly, i.e., persons aged 60–85 years (41). In the STOP-Hypertension study, 1627 patients with diastolic hypertension (mean blood pressure 195/102 mm Hg) were randomized and followed for 25 months. Compared with placebo, active treatment significantly reduced total stroke events by 47% and deaths by 43%; treatment benefit was discernible up to age 84 years.

Emphasis has been placed on the diastolic component in virtually all treatment trials although stroke risk is clearly related to systolic pressure levels (Table 2). In the elderly, where isolated elevation of the systolic pressure is common, reduction of systolic pressure was thought to be difficult to achieve, hazardous in terms of side effects, and unwarranted on the basis of available data. The SHEP examined this question in a clinical trial (3). They randomized

4736 persons, above age 60, who had systolic levels above 160 mm Hg and diastolic pressures below 90 mm Hg and followed them for 4.5 years on average. Good blood pressure control was achieved, approximately half with chlorthalidone alone, and medication was well tolerated with no excess of significant side effects in this elderly group. Treatment was associated with significant reduction in stroke (36%), as well as MI and coronary death (27%). Death from all causes was reduced 13%. These findings have great importance since two-thirds of all individuals with hypertension between the ages of 65 and 89 years have isolated systolic hypertension. The bulk of strokes occur in this age group. Since increased blood pressure is the most powerful risk factor for stroke, and since the benefits of treatment occur so promptly, control of increased blood pressure, systolic as well as diastolic levels, is the cornerstone of stroke prevention.

Acceleration in the decline in the incidence and mortality from cerebrovascular disease in recent years is a clear indication that stroke is not an inevitable consequence of aging or genetic constitution. Decrease in stroke mortality has occurred at all ages, including the eighth and ninth decades of life, providing evidence that control of hypertension and changes in environmental factors can reduce stroke occurrence.

## ACKNOWLEDGMENT

This work was supported in part by Grants 2-RO1-NS-17950-11 (National Institute of Neurological Disorders and Stroke), 1-RO1-AG-08122-04 (National Institute on Aging), and Contract NIH-N01-HC-38038 (National Heart, Lung, and Blood Institute).

## REFERENCES

1. 1992 Heart and Stroke Facts. American Heart Association, Dallas TX: 1992.
2. Dahlof B, Lindholm LH, Hansson L, Schersten B, Ekbom T, Wester P-O. Morbidity and mortality in the Swedish Trial in Old Patients with Hypertension (STOP-Hypertension). *Lancet* 1991; 338:1281–1285.
3. SHEP Cooperative Research Group. Prevention of stroke by antihypertensive drug treatment in older persons with isolated systolic hypertension: Final results of the Systolic Hypertension in the Elderly Program (SHEP). *JAMA* 1991; 265:3255–3264.
4. Kannel WB, Wolf PA, Verter J. Manifestations of coronary disease predisposing to stroke: The Framingham Study. *JAMA* 1983; 250:2942–2946.
5. Wolf PA, Abbott RD, Kannel WB. Atrial fibrillation: A major contributor to stroke in the elderly: The Framingham Study. *Arch Intern Med* 1987; 147:1561–1564.

6. Wolf PA, Abbott RD, Kannel WB. Atrial fibrillation, an independent risk factor for stroke: The Framingham Study. *Stroke* 1991; 22:983–988.
7. Albers GW, Sherman DG, Gress DR, Paulseth JE, Petersen P. Stroke prevention in nonvalvular atrial fibrillation: A review of prospective randomized trials. *Ann Neurol* 1991; 30:511–518.
8. Singer DE. Randomized trials of warfarin for atrial fibrillation. *N Engl J Med* 1992; 327:1451–1452.
9. Tanaka H, Ueda Y, Hayashi M, Date C, Baba T, Yamashita H, Shoji H, Tanaka Y, Owada K, Detels R. Risk factors for cerebral hemorrhage and cerebral infarction in a Japanese rural community. *Stroke* 1982; 13:62–73.
10. Yano K, Reed DM, MacLean CJ. Serum cholesterol and hemorrhagic stroke in the Honolulu Heart Program. *Stroke* 1989; 20:1460–1465.
11. Iso H, Jacobs DR, Wentworth D, Neaton JD, Cohen JD. Serum cholesterol levels and six-year mortality from stroke in 350,977 men screened for the multiple risk factor intervention trial. *N Engl J Med* 1989; 320:904–910.
12. Kuller LH, Dorman JS, Wolf PA. Cerebrovascular disease and diabetes. In: Diabetes in America, Diabetes Data Compiled for 1984. National Diabetes Data Group, Department of Health and Human Services. NIH Publication No. 85-1468, August 1985; XVIII:1–18.
13. Kannel WB, McGee DL. Diabetes and cardiovascular disease, the Framingham Study. *JAMA* 1979; 241:2035–2038.
14. Barrett-Connor E, Khaw K. Diabetes mellitus, an independent risk factor for stroke. *Am J Epidemiol* 1988; 128:116–123.
15. Folsom AR, Prineas RJ, Kaye SA, Munger RG. Incidence of hypertension and stroke in relation to body fat distribution and other risk factors in older women. *Stroke* 1990; 21:701–706.
16. Kannel WB, Wolf PA, Castelli WP, D'Agostino RB. Fibrinogen and risk of cardiovascular disease: The Framingham Study. *JAMA* 1987; 258:1183–1186.
17. Wilhelmsen L, Svardsudd K, Korban-Bengsten K, Larsson B, Welin L, Tibblin G. Fibrinogen as a risk factor for stroke and myocardial infarction. *N Engl J Med* 1984; 311:501–505.
18. Otten MW, Teutsch SM, Williamson DF, Marks JS. The effect of known risk factors on the excess mortality of black adults in the United States. *JAMA* 1990; 263:845–850.
19. Reed DM. The paradox of high risk of stroke in populations with low risk of coronary heart disease. *Am J Epidemiol* 1990; 131:579–588.
20. Welin I, Svardsudd K, Wilhelmsen L, Larsson B, Tibblin G. Analysis of risk factors for stroke in a cohort of men born in 1913. *N Engl J Med* 1987; 317:521–526.
21. Wolf PA, D'Agostino RB, Kannel WB, Bonita R, Belanger AJ. Cigarette smoking as a risk factor for stroke. *JAMA* 1988; 259:1025–1029.
22. Shinton R, Beevers G. Meta-analysis of relation between cigarette smoking and stroke. *Br Med J* 1989; 298:789–794.
23. Colditz GA, Bonita R, Stampfer MJ, Willett WC, Rosner B, Speizer FE, Hennekens CH. Cigarette smoking and risk of stroke in middle-aged women. *N Engl J Med* 1988; 318:937–941.

24. Sacco RL, Wolf PA, Bharucha NE, Meeks SL, Kannel WB, Charette J, McNamara PM, Palmer EP, D'Agostino RB. Subarachnoid and intracerebral hemorrhage: Natural history, prognosis, and precursive factors in the Framingham Study. *Neurology* 1984; 34:847–854.
25. Bonita R. Cigarette smoking, hypertension and the risk of subarachnoid hemorrhage: A population-based case-control study. *Stroke* 1986; 17:831–835.
26. Longstreth WT, Koepsell TD, Yerby MS, van Belle G. Risk factors for subarachnoid hemorrhage. *Stroke* 1985; 16:377–385.
27. Abbott RD, Yin Yin MA, Reed DM, Yano K. Risk of stroke in male cigarette smokers. *N Engl J Med* 1986; 315:717–720.
28. Gorelick BP. The status of alcohol as a risk factor for stroke. *Stroke* 1989; 12:1607–1610.
29. Stampfer MJ, Colditz GA, Willett WC, Speizer FE, Hennekens CH. A prospective study of moderate alcohol consumption and the risk of coronary disease and stroke in women. *N Engl J Med* 1988; 319:267–273.
30. Donahue RP, Abbott RD, Reed DM, Yano K. Alcohol and hemorrhagic stroke: The Honolulu Heart Program. *JAMA* 1986; 255:2311–2314.
31. Ettinger PO, Wu CF, DeLaCruz C Jr, Weisse AB, Ahmed SS, Regan TJ. Arrhythmias and the "holiday heart": Alcohol-associated cardiac rhythm disorders. *Am Heart J* 1985; 95:55.
32. Paffenbarger RS, Laughlin ME, Gina AS, et al. Work activity of longshoremen as related to death from coronary heart disease and stroke. *N Engl J Med* 1970; 282:1109–1114.
33. Paffenberger RS, Wing AL, Hyde RT. Physical activity as an index of heart attack risk in college alumni. *Am J Epidemiol* 1978; 108:161–175.
34. North American Symptomatic Carotid Endarterectomy Trial, methods, patient characteristic, and progress (NASCET), Steering Committee. *Stroke* 1991; 22:711–720.
35. MacMahon S, Peto R, Cutler J, et al. Blood pressure, stroke and coronary heart disease. Part I. Effects of prolonged differences in blood pressure—Evidence from nine prospective observational studies corrected for regression dilution bias. *Lancet* 1990; 335:765–774.
36. Collins R, Peto R, MacMahon S, et al. Blood pressure, stroke and coronary heart disease. Part II. Effects of short-term reductions in blood pressure—An overview of the unconfounded randomised drug trials in an epidemiological context. *Lancet* 1990; 335:827–838.
37. Garraway WM, Whisnant JP. The changing pattern of hypertension and the declining incidence of stroke. *JAMA* 1987; 258:214–217.
38. Howard G, Toole JF, Becker C, Lefkowitz DS, Truscott BL, Rose L, Evans GW. Changes in survival following stroke in five North Carolina counties observed during two different periods. *Stroke* 1989; 20:345–350.
39. Broderick JP, Phillips SJ, Whisnant JP, O'Fallon WM, Bergstralh EJ. Incidence rates of stroke in the eighties: The end of the decline in stroke? *Stroke* 1989; 20:577–582.
40. Cooper R, Sempos C, Hsieh S-C, Kovar MG. Slowdown in the decline of stroke mortality in the United States, 1978–1986. *Stroke* 1990; 21:1274–1279.

41. Amery A, Birkenhager W, Brixko P, et al. Mortality and morbidity results from the European Working Party on High Blood Pressure in the Elderly Trial. *Lancet* 1985; 1:1349–1354.
42. Wilking SVP, Belanger A, Kannel WB, D'Agostino RB, Steel K. Determinants of isolated systolic hypertension. *JAMA* 1988; 260:3451–3455.

# 7

# Hypertension in the Elderly

**Deanna G. Cheung and Michael A. Weber**
*University of California, Irvine, and*
*Veterans Affairs Medical Center, Long Beach, California*

## INTRODUCTION

The increased prevalence and associated morbidity of hypertension in the elderly population establish an urgent need to understand and treat this precursor of disabling disease. Ironically, high blood pressure in the aged, perhaps because it occurs so often, has generally been disregarded as an important medical condition. Because blood pressure tends to increase with increasing age, clinicians have been reluctant to diagnose hypertension in patients whose blood pressures have been apparently normal at younger ages. It has been assumed that hypertension in older persons is simply a manifestation of an irreversible arteriosclerotic process that is not amenable to therapy (1). Furthermore, the tendency to define hypertension on the basis of diastolic blood pressure has contributed to the neglect of this condition in the elderly, in whom increased blood pressure tends to be predominantly of the systolic type. Although there has been a gradual change in physician attitudes and practices over the last two decades (2), a recent survey of physician practices in New Jersey indicated that only 26% of clinicians routinely considered using drugs to treat isolated systolic hypertension for all persons aged 60 and older (3). People in this age group belong to the most rapidly increasing group in the United States, accounting for 12% of the population (4) and the consumption of at least one-third of all U.S. health care dollars (5,6). This represents approximately 31 million people over age 65, of whom 3 million are over age 85 (7). Prevention of disability and premature mortality in this group could result in a significant reduction in human suffering as well as in economic costs. The relationship between hypertension and cardiovascular disease, which is the major cause of morbidity and mortality in this group, emphasizes the importance of an effective approach to this problem in clinical practice.

## EPIDEMIOLOGY

Both systolic and diastolic blood pressure increase with advancing age, especially during the first 50–60 years of life (Fig. 1). This increase averages 5–10 mm Hg per year for systolic blood pressure and 5–6 mm Hg for diastolic blood pressure in the United States (8). At older ages there is a tendency for blood pressure to reach a plateau or even decrease, especially in men (9). Diastolic blood pressure tends to stabilize at a younger age than systolic pressure (10). This, combined with the fact that the increase in systolic pressure is greater than that in diastolic pressure, results in a characteristic rise in pulse pressure with increasing age. Both the increases in systolic and diastolic blood pressure and the increase in pulse pressure are of clinical significance (11–17). These trends may be a characteristic of westernized or acculturated societies, for in isolated primitive populations in South America and the South Pacific no such association between increasing blood pressure with advancing age has been observed (18,19). Interestingly, the tendency for blood pressure to increase with increasing age may be accentuated in populations characterized by economic or educational deprivation (20).

Because cardiovascular risk associated with hypertension increases continuously with increasing blood pressure, the definition of hypertension is arbitrarily reached by consensus about the level of blood pressure at which the benefits of treatment exceed the risks of nontreatment. The Joint National Committee on Detection, Evaluation and Treatment of High Blood Pressure has defined this level as a systolic blood pressure of 140 mm Hg or a diastolic blood pressure of 90 mm Hg (21), but the Working Group on Hypertension in the Elderly considers systolic blood pressures between 140 and 159 mm Hg to be borderline (22). In most elderly patients, hypertension is diagnosed by a systolic blood pressure of 160 mm Hg or more. Diastolic blood pressure may be elevated as well (combined systolic–diastolic hypertension) or may be normal (isolated systolic hypertension). A useful classification is given in Table 1. Using these criteria, the prevalence of hypertension in an ambulatory population was found by the 1976–1980 National Health and Nutrition Examination Survey to be 64% in men and women between the ages of 65 and 74 (23). Table 2 illustrates the prevalence of hypertension in the elderly population utilizing two alternative criteria for diagnosis.

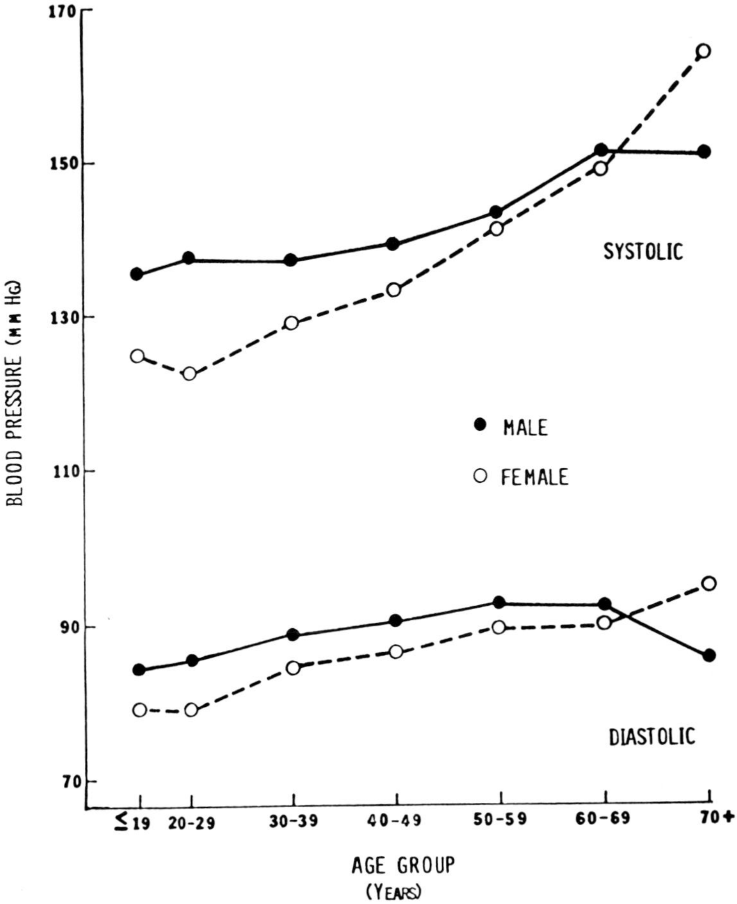


**Figure 1** Systolic and diastolic blood pressures in 1972 men and 2032 women attending a free screening clinic (23).

**Table 1** Classification of Hypertension in the Aged

| Classification | Systolic BP[a] (mm Hg) | Diastolic BP (mm Hg) | Pulse BP |
|---|---|---|---|
| Isolated systolic | >160 | <90 | Elevated |
| Predominant systolic | > 2 × (diastolic BP − 15) | >90 | Elevated |
| Combined systolic-diastolic | >160 | >90 | Unchanged |
| Borderline | 140–159 | <90 | Unchanged |

[a] Blood pressure.

**Table 2** Prevalence of Hypertension in Persons Aged 65–74 According to Different Criteria

| | Blood pressure, systolic/diastolic (%) | |
|---|---|---|
| | 165/95 mm Hg | 140/90 mm Hg |
| Black women | 73 | 83 |
| Black men | 43 | 67 |
| White women | 48 | 66 |
| White men | 38 | 59 |

These and other data (24) indicate that this problem occurs more frequently in women than in men and more often in blacks than in whites. Even when the more conservative criterion is used (165/95 mm Hg), the overall prevalence is 45%. The distribution of the different types of hypertension among men and women aged 65–89 is depicted in Figure 2 (25). The prevalence of isolated systolic hypertension (ISH) is about 7% at age 60–69 and increases with age to 25% by age 90 years (26–29). Because the fastest growing part of the population comprises persons older than 80 years, the importance of isolated systolic hypertension is expected to increase in the next decades, so that the projected number of persons with this diagnosis is nearly 8 million in the year 2025 (30).

The importance of hypertension as a risk factor for cardiovascular disease in elderly persons is well established. In the Framingham Study Kannel et al. (31) found a three- to fourfold increase in the risk of cardiovascular disease in hyper-

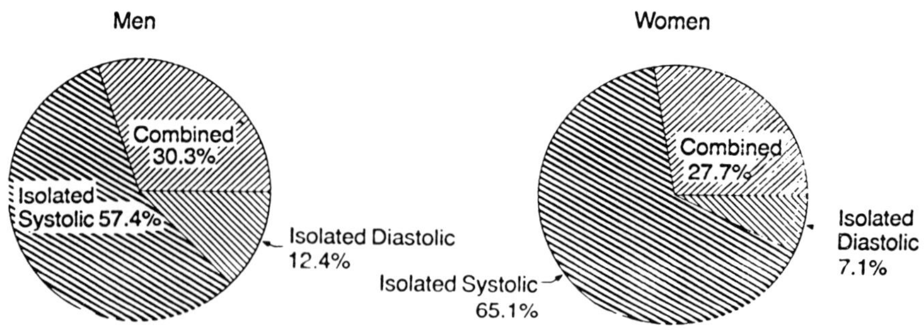


**Figure 2** Distribution of hypertensive diagnoses in elderly patients aged 65–89 years in the Framingham Heart Study. Systolic hypertension refers to systolic blood pressure ≥ 160 mm Hg; diastolic hypertension, diastolic blood pressure ≥ 95 mm Hg; combined hypertension, systolic blood pressure ≥ 160 mm Hg and diastolic blood pressure ≥ 95 mm Hg (25).

tensive patients aged 65–74 (Table 3). Diastolic blood pressure increased the risk of cardiovascular events in men from 24.2 to 42.9 and 55.6 per 1000 population (18 year follow-up) for blood pressures 90–109 and ⩾ 110 mm Hg, respectively. Comparable increases were also observed in women (11). Although the risk from hypertension was related to both systolic and diastolic components, with advancing age the systolic blood pressure had a greater influence on the risk of stroke, left ventricular hypertrophy, and congestive heart failure than did diastolic pressure (31). Thus, it was also shown that isolated systolic hypertension resulted in a twofold increase in the risk of death from all causes, including a twofold increase in the risk of death from cardiovascular disease in men and a fivefold increase in women (31).

Even borderline hypertension increased the cardiovascular mortality by a factor of 4 in men and a factor of 2 in women aged 65–74, in comparison with normotensive persons of the same age (11). Data from the Framingham Study demonstrate that both the absolute cardiovascular risk and the rise in cardiovascular risk related to systolic blood pressure levels increase with age (Fig. 3). Thus, elderly persons are not only more likely to have systolic hypertension than younger persons but also appear to be more sensitive to the adverse effects associated with it. Whether this represents progression of an underlying process manifesting itself in a more advanced stage with greater age or whether the aging process itself predisposes target organs to hypertensive damage is not known. It is possible that both processes contribute to this observed sensitivity. Other observers have also documented increases in the likelihood of major cardiovascular events in older age groups, even in the range of 80–100 years (32). Likewise, the Pooling Project Research Group found that first coronary events correlated closely with prior diastolic or systolic blood pressure at any age, including the elderly (33), whereas in the Chicago Stroke Study it was found that cerebrovascular accidents occurred at least twice as often in elderly subjects with hypertension than in those with normal blood pressure (34).

**Table 3** 20 Year Risk of Cardiovascular Disease in Relation to Hypertensive Status in the Elderly (Aged 65–74) in the Framingham Study (Incidence per 1000 Population)

| Hypertensive status[a] | Men | Women |
|---|---|---|
| Normal | 17.1 | 8.6 |
| Borderline | 32.7 | 22.5 |
| Hypertension | 51.0 | 35.6 |

[a] Normal pressure < 140/90 mm Hg; borderline pressure 140–159/90–95 mm Hg; hypertension pressure > 160/95 mm Hg (11).

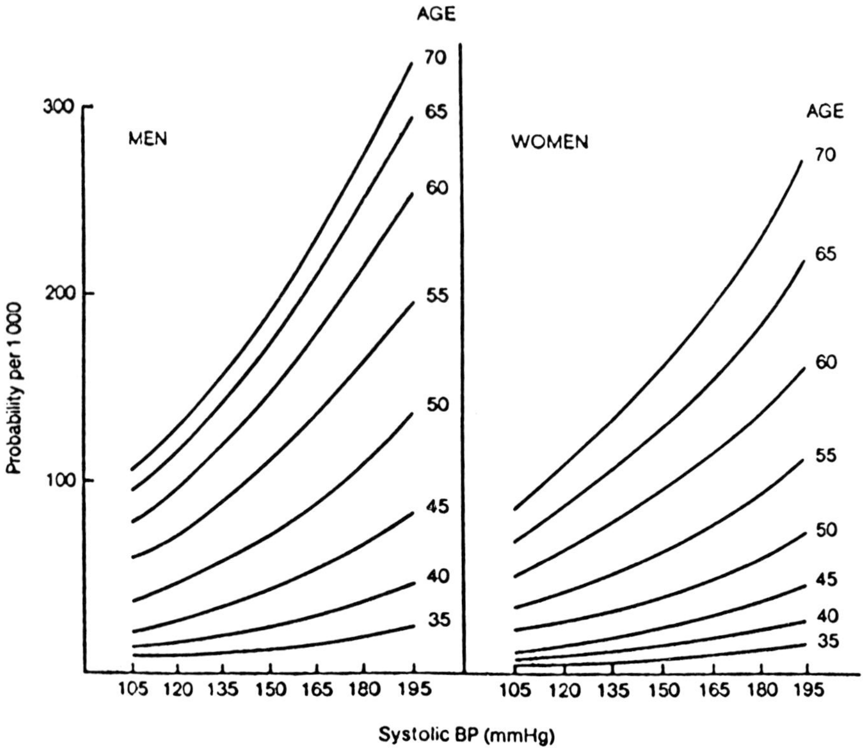


**Figure 3** Relationship between systolic blood pressure and 8 year probability of cardiovascular disease at different ages (31).

A high prevalence of systolic hypertension is characteristic of the elderly population and increases steadily with age. Because systolic hypertension in the elderly may be linked to advanced arteriosclerotic changes, it has been argued that the apparent complications of this form of hypertension may instead simply reflect underlying vascular disease (35). However, Kannel et al. (31) have argued that systolic hypertension leads to cardiovascular disease independently of any associated arteriosclerosis. If cardiovascular disease resulting from systolic hypertension were due to underlying vascular disease alone, atheromatous cardiovascular complications, such as coronary disease and peripheral vascular disease, should predominate; instead, strokes and congestive heart failure, which are more likely to reflect the direct effects of hypertension, occur at least as frequently.

The predominance of systolic hypertension in determining cardiovascular risk in this age group has been inadequately appreciated, especially since so many earlier reports emphasized the importance of diastolic blood pressure. Most studies in hypertension continue to use diastolic blood pressure as the basis for classifying patients and for including or excluding them from participation. This is one of the reasons that elderly hypertensive patients, whose systolic hypertension is often associated with normal or only minimally increased diastolic pressures, rarely participate in major hypertension investigations. It has been thought that systolic hypertension in the elderly may simply be a later stage of what had once been a diastolic-dominated hypertension at a younger age. When patients with a known history of diastolic hypertension are excluded from the analysis of hypertension, however, systolic hypertension can still be demonstrated to account for the excess risk of cardiovascular events (36). Thus, hypertension in older persons is usually a de novo condition arising for the first time in the later years of life, and it differs clinically and mechanistically from hypertension in the young (37,38).

Isolated systolic hypertension has been associated with cardiovascular risk in both prospective epidemiological studies and life insurance actuarial data (39–42). The increase in mortality in men and women aged 60–69 with ISH is approximately twofold (39,43), and the risk of stroke is increased by a factor of 3 (43). Similar dramatic increases in the incidence of nonfatal cardiovascular events, such as stroke, myocardial infarction, intermittent claudication, and congestive heart failure, have been observed (31).

Other risk factors, such as elevated low-density lipoprotein (LDL)- or reduced high-density lipoprotein-cholesterol levels, smoking, diabetes mellitus, and electrocardiographic evidence of left ventricular hypertrophy, are also associated with an increased risk of atherosclerotic disease in the elderly (11), but the importance of other risk factors appears to decrease with advancing age, making hypertension (especially systolic) the dominant risk factor in this age group. In a detailed analysis of risk factors found in patients presenting with myocardial infarctions, it was found that elderly patients (aged 65 and older) were less likely than younger patients to have a history of smoking or obesity or a family history of coronary disease (44). Only the presence of hypertension and diabetes mellitus was comparable in the two groups. An increased association between hypertension and diabetes mellitus in the aged has been observed (32) and cannot be explained by the relation between these conditions and obesity, suggesting some more basic link between them. In another study of elderly patients, performed in France, both myocardial infarction and cerebrovascular accidents were strongly linked to the presence of hypertension but not to other risk factors, including age itself.

## PATHOPHYSIOLOGY

The cause of hypertension in the elderly, as with essential hypertension in younger persons, is not known. Hypertension in the aged has characteristics that differ from those in younger patients in several respects, but most obviously in the dominance of the systolic blood pressure. Although the basic etiology of systolic hypertension is not clear, a number of mechanisms appear to contribute to this form of hypertension and are listed in Table 4.

Arteriosclerotic changes in the large arterial circulation are believed to play a significant role in the genesis of systolic hypertension in the aged. The aorta and its major branches, often referred to as the Windkessel vessels, normally play a major role in dampening the pulsatile nature of blood flow from the left ventricle, allowing blood to be distributed to vital organs and peripheral tissues in a more continuous manner. The elastic or distensible properties of the aorta and other major vessels play a critical role in this function, allowing them to store potential energy from the systolic thrust of the left ventricle for subsequent release during diastole, resulting in the maintenance of the required mean perfusion pressure throughout the cardiac cycle (45). About half the pressure attenuation and half the stroke volume are stored in the thoracic aorta during systole and released during diastole (46–48). Loss of compliance in these vessels is associated with two principal characteristics: an increase in systolic blood pressure related to the diversion of the entire contractile force along the axis of the blood vessels rather than partly into the walls, and a relative decrease in diastolic blood pressure related to the loss of elastic tension, which no longer accumulates during systole to provide force during diastole. Substitution of the descending thoracic aorta by a rigid tube, imitating this mechanistic abnormality in a canine model, has been shown to produce these anticipated changes in the pattern of blood pressure. Furthermore, cardiac index and ejection fraction were also decreased in this model, a finding that is also characteristic of systolic hypertension in the aged (49).

**Table 4** Pathophysiological Mechanisms in the Development of Systolic Hypertension of the Aged

1. Changes in compliance of large arterial circulation: loss of Windkessel properties
2. Decreased baroreceptor sensitivity (secondary to local atheromatous changes)
3. Increased responsiveness to sympathetic nervous system stimuli
4. Altered renal and sodium metabolism
5. Altered renin-angiotensin-aldosterone relationships

The aging process in the cardiovascular system is characterized by an increase in aortic wall thickness and a decrease in aortic elasticity. These changes are partially caused by the fracturing and uncoiling of the elastic fibers and the deposition of calcium and collagenous matrix within vessel walls (50,51). Human aortic tissue obtained at postmortem examinations has been found to exhibit age-related differences in pressure-volume relations. The fluid volume required to achieve comparable pressure increases in tissues from older persons was found to be one-third as much as was required in tissues from younger persons (less than 25 years old) (52). Messerli et al. found that both central and total blood volume were significantly lower in elderly hypertensive patients than in younger patients with comparable mean arterial pressures (53). Thus, for the same amount of volume, greater pressures developed in older, less compliant aortas. Aortic elongation and tortuosity are associated with concomitant increases in diameter and volume during aging, resulting in a linear increase in vascular stiffness and pulsed wave velocity between the ages of 20 and 60 years (48,54,55).

Measurable decreases in arterial compliance that correlate negatively and significantly with systolic blood pressure have been observed in patients with systolic hypertension (56). The existence of normal left ventricular function in these patients indicates that the reduction in large-vessel compliance is a major factor in sustaining systolic hypertension. It is possible that the loss in elasticity of arterial vessels may be a result of hypertension rather than its cause. However, studies in a rat model have indicated that both mechanisms exist (20). Thus, whereas hypertension per se can lead to increased collagen deposition in the vascular media, the presence of increased collagen in arterial walls itself may stimulate an increase in blood pressure. It is now well established that smooth muscle cells in the arterial media, which normally are responsible for the elastic properties of the vessel, can actually produce connective tissue components, such as collagen, and may thereby contribute to the genesis of arteriosclerotic changes (56).

Sequelae of these vascular changes include elevation in peripheral vascular resistance and an increase in left ventricular work, with resultant left ventricular hypertrophy (50,51,57). Left ventricular ejection time increases, and a reduction in stroke volume leads to decreased cardiac output (58). In response to exercise, the rise in left ventricular end-diastolic pressure is exaggerated, and both maximal oxygen consumption and maximal heart rate are decreased (57). Corresponding findings have been observed in elderly hypertensive patients in a study that compared hemodynamics, echocardiographic measurements, intravascular volumes, and hormonal levels of elderly subjects with a group of younger subjects matched for arterial blood pressure, race, and body build (53). In this study elderly hypertensive patients were found to have lower heart rates, lower stroke volumes, lower cardiac outputs, lower left ventricular ejection rates, and higher total peripheral resistance and left ventricular mass than younger patients with comparable mean arterial blood pressures.

A further mechanism by which senescent changes in vascular tissue may contribute to hypertension is linked to alterations in baroreceptor sensitivity, which has been shown to be decreased in the elderly (59,60). Atherosclerotic changes in the region of the carotid sinus may alter baroreceptor sensitivity, allowing the maintenance of higher blood pressure levels on a chronic basis. Baroreceptor sensitivity in older hypertensive patients with atherosclerotic disease has been shown to be considerably less than that in younger hypertensives (61). However, the role of this mechanism in sustaining hypertension chronically is still speculative. In canine models, an acute increase in blood pressure, together with a tendency for greater blood pressure lability, has been associated with baroreceptor destruction, but sustained resting hypertension was not observed (62). Diminished baroreceptor sensitivity may explain the variability in blood pressure seen during continuous monitoring in the elderly (63–65) and is probably the cause of the impairment of postural reflexes that predisposes elderly patients to orthostatic hypotension regardless of treatment status (66).

Changes in the activity of the various components of the sympathetic nervous system may also influence blood pressure characteristics of the aged. $\alpha$-Adrenergic responsiveness remains unchanged (67), but the $\beta$-adrenergic responsiveness of vascular smooth muscle clearly declines with age (68,69). In particular, elderly hypertensive patients have slower heart rates at rest and after exercise, have lower plasma renin activity values, require a greater amount of isoproterenol to increase the heart rate by a standard increment, and have lesser vasodilation measured by forearm blood flow after administration of isoproterenol than normotensive persons or younger patients with hypertension (70,71). Reduced drug sensitivity to propranolol in elderly patients compared with younger subjects despite higher drug plasma levels is another manifestation of this decrease in $\beta$-adrenergic responsiveness (71). It has also been found that there is decreased $\beta$-adrenoreceptor binding capacity in lymphocyte preparations in older persons, although other studies have indicated that the decrease in $\beta$-adrenergic-mediated activity occurs distal to the receptor (70,72). Consistent with these possibilities, cyclic adenosine monophosphate production, a marker of intracellular $\beta$-adrenergic activity, tends to decrease with advancing age (73).

The increased vascular resistance characteristic of the hypertensive state in the elderly may relate to diminished $\beta$-adrenergic vasodilation together with unchanged and unopposed $\alpha$-adrenergic vasoconstriction (67). Thus, an age-related shift in the balance between $\beta$-adrenergic vasodilation and $\alpha$-adrenergic vasoconstriction in favor of vasoconstriction may underlie the observed increases in peripheral vascular resistance and blood pressure. In support of this, Palmer et al. (74) showed that the pressor response to a standardized sympathetic stress (cold pressor test) increases with advancing age. It is also possible that the increased variability of blood pressure observed in the aged may reflect the absence of the buffering effect of $\beta$-adrenoreceptors on blood pressure responses to sympathetic activity. Although there may be some degree of imbalance between $\alpha$- and $\beta$-adrenergic activity in older persons, there is limited evidence for an overall increase in sympathetic activity. It has been shown that plasma epinephrine levels, which may reflect sympathetic activity more closely than norepinephrine itself, tend to be higher in older persons (70) and that there is a tendency for plasma norepinephrine concentrations to be somewhat higher in older hypertensive patients than in younger patients (49,53). Both increased systolic blood pressure and aortic rigidity (ratio of pulse pressure to stroke volume) have been linked with plasma norepinephrine levels (75). In support of these findings, Buhler et al. (70) observed that the peripheral $\alpha$-adrenergic blocking agent prazosin is more effective than the direct-acting vasodilatory agent sodium nitroprusside in producing forearm vasodilation in elderly hypertensive patients. This evidence tends to strengthen the possibility that the increased total peripheral resistance that characterizes hypertension of the elderly may be at least as much dependent on $\alpha$-adrenergic-mediated mechanisms as on intrinsic structural changes.

There is little evidence for a direct role of the renin-angiotensin system in the pathogenesis of hypertension in the elderly. Plasma renin activity declines with age and tends to be low in both normotensive and hypertensive elderly persons, making it unlikely that a direct vasoconstrictor effect of the renin-angiotensin system is involved in maintaining blood pressure. The renin response to sodium depletion (76), diuretic administration (77), and upright posture (78) declines with age as well. Low renin levels and diminished renin response may be related to the generalized decrease in $\beta$-adrenergic activity that governs renin release (79). Alternatively, hyaline degeneration in the afferent arterioles of the kidney in the elderly may make the juxtaglomerular apparatus less responsive to normal stimuli (80). Reductions in renal mass and renal blood flow may also be contributory (81), especially since renin suppression is greater in elderly hypertensive patients than in normotensive subjects (82). An additional possibility is that renin release is suppressed by virtue of sodium expansion (83). It has been shown that elderly patients with low renin hypertension respond better to diuretic therapy than those whose renin values are normal. However, renin activity remains low in the elderly, even on a fixed sodium diet or after diuretic therapy (82,84). Furthermore, the low blood volumes observed in elderly hypertensive patients (53,80) are not consistent with this mechanism.

Plasma aldosterone does not appear to decrease in elderly hypertensive patients (85,86). Morimoto et al. (87) showed that a heterogeneous relation exists between renin and aldosterone in older persons; although approximately two-thirds of these patients have a normal renin-aldosterone relation, the remaining patients appear to exhibit a heightened aldosterone response to angiotensin II. In another study it was observed that plasma renin activity in hypertensive patients with low renin (chiefly older subjects) was relatively insensitive to changes in sodium balance, but that the sensitivity of aldosterone to relatively small changes in renin (i.e., angiotensin II) appeared to be heightened (38). Aldosterone levels were closely similar in almost 1000 hypertensive patients subdivided into high-, medium-, and low-renin categories, despite marked disparities in renin values (Table 5) (37). It could be concluded that the low-renin subgroup contains at least a portion of patients in whom aldosterone production is exceptionally responsive to the renin-angiotensin system. It has not been possible, however, to determine whether the relatively high aldosterone production results in an increased mineralocorticoid (sodium-retaining) activity that contributes to the hypertensive state. It is also possible that aldosterone may have blood pressure-raising effects that are independent of its intrarenal mineralocorticoid actions (88), but there is no evidence that such a mechanism plays a part in sustaining clinical hypertension.

Evidence exists to support the possibility that sodium retention may contribute to hypertension in older persons. Both excessive sodium intake (50,89) and a decrease in the ability of the kidney to excrete sodium (90,91) may play a role in sustaining hypertension. Although total-body sodium has been shown to be increased in various forms of secondary hypertension, the findings in essential hypertension have not been as clear. However, sodium status in essential hypertension may be age dependent. Young hypertensive individuals (less than 35 years old) tend to have lower exchangeable sodium values than normal controls; older hypertensive patients tend to have increased exchangeable sodium values (92). The correlation between total-body sodium or exchangeable sodium and blood pressure observed in hypertensive patients does not exist in normotensive persons.

Salt sensitivity in the elderly may also be related to reduced production of natriuretic substances in response to a high salt intake. Elderly hypertensive

**Table 5** Characteristics of Hypertensive Patients Classified into High ($n$ = 105), Medium ($n$ = 592), and Low ($n$ = 259) Renin Subgroups

| | High | Medium | Low |
|---|---|---|---|
| Age, years | 40.2 ± 13.3 | 48.5 ± 13.3 | 55.5 ± 10.3 |
| Plasma renin activity, ng/ml/h | 7.1 ± 4.6 | 2.7 ± 2.4 | 1.0 ± 0.8 |
| Aldosterone excretion rate, μg per 24 h | 13.1 ± 7.6 | 11.9 ± 8.9 | 11.0 ± 6.9 |

patients have been found to have decreased renal excretion of the vasodilatory prostaglandin $E_2$ (50). Sodium-potassium ATPase activity in myocardial cells and erythrocytes decreases with age (93–95), which may result in an accumulation of intracellular sodium. This decrease in membrane sodium transport activity probably contributes to calcium-dependent smooth muscle contraction, resulting in increased smooth muscle tone, peripheral vascular resistance, and peripheral vascular responsiveness to circulating vasoconstrictor factors and reflex neural stimuli (95,96). There is no clear explanation of why sodium retention characterizes hypertension in older patients; presumably, the pressure-natriuresis relations that govern the regulation of sodium excretion by blood pressure have been reset in this group.

## DIAGNOSIS AND CLINICAL EVALUATION

Because elderly patients may be particularly susceptible to adverse drug effects (96), accurate determination of the blood pressure is crucial to making treatment decisions. There has been some concern that conventional methods for measuring blood pressure using the standard brachial artery cuff may not provide accurate blood pressure measurements. Arteriosclerotic changes in the artery may prevent normal compression, resulting in falsely elevated blood pressure readings (97) (pseudohypertension). Berliner et al. (98) found that cuff blood pressure measurements were approximately 7 mm Hg higher than direct intraarterial measurements, but he also noted that the discrepancy between the two methods decreased in patients older than 70 years. The correlation between the two methods is reported to be very good (99,100), however, and a more recent comparison between them found no greater discrepancy in elderly than in young subjects (99). Despite the possible discrepancies, direct blood pressure measurements based on full 24 h monitoring appear to be very close to blood pressures at rest measured with the standard technique. The actual prevalence of pseudohypertension is not known, but it is believed to be an uncommon condition. The conventional cuff measurement is adequate for most elderly hypertensives; pseudohypertension should be considered in elderly patients with no evidence of hypertension-related end-organ damage despite very high blood pressure. Other suggestive signs of pseudohypertension include palpably incompressible peripheral arteries, inadequate response to pharmacological therapy despite the appearance of hypotensive side effects, and vascular calcification on roentgenograms of the arm (101). The finding of a palpable pulseless brachial or radial artery when the blood pressure cuff is inflated above the systolic pressure (Osler's maneuver) may be helpful, but direct intraarterial blood pressure measurement is required to make the diagnosis.

Special considerations in measuring blood pressure in the elderly include the increase in systolic blood pressure variability with age (65) and an increasing prevalence of postural hypotension (66). Adequate cuff inflation should be ensured to avoid falsely low blood pressure readings related to an auscultatory gap, which may be more prevalent in elderly patients. Baseline blood pressure should be determined by the average of three readings on at least three occasions using a cuff of an appropriate size (22,102). A significant number of patients being treated for hypertension may have been classified as normotensive if an adequate number of initial measurements were taken (103). The importance of repeated blood pressure measurements cannot be underestimated. A misdiagnosis of hypertension is much more likely to be related to an inadequate number of blood pressure determinations than to pseudohypertension. In addition to measurements in the sitting position, standing blood pressure should be determined in patients both before and during therapy (22). The likelihood of clinically important postural hypotension may be as low as 4% in ambulatory patients aged 50–99 years old (104), but the frequency of orthostatic hypotension increases with age and in the presence of neurological and metabolic disorders (105). Furthermore, antihypertensive therapy may be associated with the development or exacerbation of this disorder.

Clinical evaluation should be directed toward assessing end-organ damage, detecting causes of secondary hypertension, and determining the presence of associated disorders that could influence therapeutic decisions or are associated with additional cardiovascular risk. Recommendations for the initial evaluation do not differ substantially from those given for younger hypertensive patients (106). Left ventricular hypertrophy, which is associated with a higher risk of cardiovascular complications (107), is more common in elderly hypertensive individuals. Detection of this entity by electrocardiography may indicate the need for more intensive therapy with agents that have been associated with regression of left ventricular hypertrophy (108,109). The baseline evaluation should include a thorough history and physical examination, an electrocardiogram, a hemogram, urinalysis, and a blood chemistry profile, including serum creatinine, plasma glucose, electrolytes, serum uric acid, and a fasting lipid profile.

The likelihood of secondary hypertension is low in elderly hypertensive patients in the absence of suggestive symptoms or signs, the sudden onset of increased diastolic pressure greater than 105 mm Hg, poor response to rational pharmacological intervention, accelerated hypertension, or spontaneous hypokalemia in the absence of diuretic therapy (22). Renal artery stenosis is the most frequent cause of reversible hypertension in this population (110). Although bilateral renal artery stenosis may be more common and difficult to repair surgically, medical control of the blood pressure can often be achieved. A rise in serum creatinine in response to the use of an angiotensin converting enzyme inhibitor is suggestive of this disorder. Surgical revascularization should be considered in patients with renovascular disease, declining renal function, and hypertension resistant to medical therapy (110,111). Both surgical revascularization and balloon angioplasty can be well tolerated by elderly patients and may be associated with a lower incidence of renal deterioration (112). Even with improvement, however, many patients still need some antihypertensive treatment after such interventions.

The prevalence of concomitant diseases that may influence the therapeutic approach is higher in elderly patients than in their younger counterparts. Cognitive impairment may adversely affect medication compliance. Certain conditions, such as obstructive lung disease, diabetes mellitus, and sinoatrial node dysfunction, may limit antihypertensive drug choices. A subgroup of elderly hypertensives with heart failure has been found who have hypertensive hypertrophic cardiomyopathy characterized by severe concentric cardiac hypertrophy, a small left ventricular cavity, excessive systolic emptying, and impaired diastolic function (113). This disorder may be associated with a paradoxical increase in blood pressure during treatment with vasodilators, which reduce the load on the heart; the diagnosis is usually made by echocardiography in elderly hypertensive women presenting with pulmonary congestion, angina, or syncope.

The likelihood of adverse antihypertensive drug effects is increased by both the presence of additional diagnoses and the drugs used to treat them. In the Multiple Risk Factor Intervention Trial (MRFIT) (114), a higher risk of death in patients with nonspecific abnormalities on the baseline electrocardiograms was found to be associated with sudden death in patients treated with high doses of diuretics, presumably due to hypokalemia and fatal arrhythmia. A strong correlation between the number of drugs prescribed for patients and adverse drug reactions has been observed (115). Early identification of factors that may predispose patients to adverse events can reduce the number of complications related to treatment.

Systolic hypertension predominates as the major cardiovascular risk factor in elderly patients, but other contributory risk factors should be identified and treated in elderly hypertensives. Almost 60% of adults aged 60–74 years may have serum LDL-cholesterol levels requiring treatment (116). The strength of the association between serum cholesterol and cardiovascular risk declines with age (117), but the total attributable risk does not (118,119). The incidence of diabetes mellitus increases with age to a level of 18% in the 64- to 74-year-old class (120) and is even more prevalent among the hypertensive elderly. Impairment of glucose tolerance in this group may be associated with the development of overt diabetes in response to treatment with thiazide diuretics.

## TREATMENT

The benefits of treating hypertension in the elderly population are no longer in dispute. A number of randomized clinical trials have demonstrated reductions in cardiovascular morbidity and mortality associated with treatment of both diastolic and isolated systolic hypertension. In the High Blood Pressure Detection and Follow-up Program, elderly patients aged 60–69 years experienced a 45% decrease in the incidence of fatal and nonfatal stroke associated with antihypertensive therapy of diastolic blood pressures greater than 90 mm Hg (121). In the Australian National Blood Pressure Study, treatment of diastolic blood pressures in the range 95–109 mm Hg resulted in a 39% reduction in fatal and nonfatal trial end points in patients aged 60–69 years (122). The European Working Party on High Blood Pressure in the Elderly focused exclusively on elderly patients over age 60 with diastolic blood pressures of 90–109 mm Hg and/or systolic blood pressures of 160–239 mm Hg. They observed a 38% statistically significant reduction in total cardiovascular mortality in actively treated patients compared with those who received placebo. This included a 60% reduction in fatal myocardial infarctions. A 43% decrease in cerebrovascular deaths was not statistically significant. It was concluded that treatment of hypertension in this group of hypertensive patients resulted in 29 fewer cardiovascular events and 14 fewer cardiovascular deaths per 1000 patient-years of treatment (123). Isolated systolic hypertension was addressed by the Systolic Hypertension in the Elderly Program (SHEP), in which patients older than 60 years of age with systolic blood pressure ranging from 160 to 219 mm Hg and diastolic blood pressure less than 90 mm Hg were randomized to active treatment with chlorthalidone and/or atenolol or placebo (124). A 36% reduction in fatal and nonfatal stroke rate was observed in actively treated patients (Fig. 4) and was associated with a decrease in systolic blood pressure, from an average of 170 mm Hg at baseline to 143 mm Hg during treatment. Reductions in coronary artery disease incidence and deaths, left ventricular failure, and total mortality were also associated with active treatment (Table 6).

Based on these data, treatment can be recommended for elderly hypertensive patients who have diastolic blood pressures greater than 90 mm Hg or systolic blood pressures greater than 160 mm Hg. Therapy should also be considered for patients with multiple risk factors and borderline systolic hypertension (systolic blood pressure 140–159 mm Hg). The goal of treatment should be the reduction in diastolic blood pressure to below 90 mm Hg or by at least 10 mm Hg and the reduction in systolic blood pressure to below 160 mm Hg while maintaining a diastolic pressure of 70 mm Hg or above (22). A reduction in systolic blood pressure to less than 140 mm Hg may result in additional benefit without excess risk (125); in the SHEP trial, systolic blood pressures averaging 143 mm Hg during treatment were well tolerated and were associated with an average reduction in diastolic blood pressure from 77 to 68 mm Hg. This should not be done at the expense of adverse effects or unnecessary complexity of treatment, however. In addition, autoregulatory mechanisms are sluggish in elderly patients,

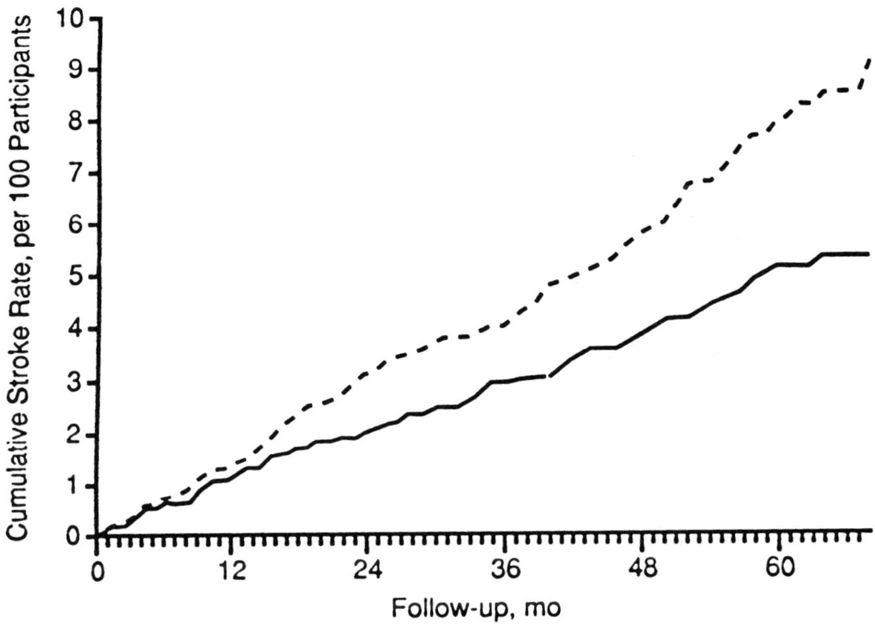


**Figure 4** Cumulative rate of fatal and nonfatal stroke per 100 participants in the active treatment (solid line) and placebo (broken line) groups during the Systolic Hypertension in the Elderly Program (16).

**Table 6** Morbidity and Mortality in the Systolic Hypertension in the Elderly Trial

| Event | Active treatment group ($n$ = 2365) | Placebo group ($n$ = 2371) | Relative risk |
|---|---|---|---|
| Nonfatal stroke | 96 | 149 | 0.63 |
| TIA | 62 | 82 | 0.75 |
| Fatal stroke | 10 | 14 | 0.71 |
| Nonfatal MI | 50 | 74 | 0.67 |
| Nonfatal CHD[a] | 99 | 143 | 0.62 |
| Fatal MI | 15 | 26 | 0.57 |
| Cardiac deaths[b] | 59 | 73 | 0.80 |
| LV failure | 48 | 102 | 0.46 |
| Total CVD | 289 | 414 | 0.68 |
| All cause deaths | 213 | 242 | 0.87 |

TIA = transient ischemic attack; MI = myocardial infarction; CHD = coronary heart disease; LV = left ventricle; CVD = cardiovascular disease.

[a] Nonfatal CHD includes nonfatal MI, coronary artery bypass graft, and angioplasty.

[b] Cardiac deaths include fatal MI, sudden death (< 1 h), and rapid death (1–24 h).

*Source Data*: from Reference 124.

and goal blood pressures should be achieved slowly over periods of months rather than days or weeks.

Nonpharmacological therapy should be the initial approach to therapy in elderly patients with mild to moderate hypertension. Recommended measures include weight loss, sodium restriction, decreased alcohol intake, and regular aerobic exercise (126,127). Because elderly patients may already have marginal diets, it is important to ensure the adequacy of any prescribed restricted diet. Although most studies of the efficacies of these measures have been restricted to younger patients (128,129), it is reasonable to adopt this approach in this group of patients, who may be particularly susceptible to adverse drug effects. If nonpharmacological therapy fails to reduce blood pressure to acceptable levels, pharmacological intervention will be necessary. It is generally desirable to continue nonpharmacological measures during drug therapy because of their beneficial effect on cardiovascular risk and to reduce the amount of medication required to achieve blood pressure control.

The use of drugs of all types in the aged is more difficult than in younger patients, because the aging process is associated with altered pharmacokinetics and drug responses. Both hepatic metabolism and renal clearance of pharmacological agents tend to be decreased in the elderly. Furthermore, low blood volume, reduced baroreflex sensitivity, and postprandial reduction in blood pressure may frequently be present in elderly persons and may increase their responsiveness to antihypertensive drugs (130). A wide experience with the use of antihypertensive and cardiovascular drugs in the elderly has indicated that a comparatively high incidence of symptomatic side effects can be anticipated (131–133). The use of small doses and slow titration may minimize such effects and should underlie the management of these patients at every step.

In most instances, adverse effects of drugs in the elderly are not unique to this age group but simply reflect a more exaggerated form of problems that may be seen in younger persons. Thus, drugs that tend to cause drowsiness, sedation, or orthostatic symptoms may do so with marked severity in older patients (132). This can be due to decreased drug metabolism, resulting in a relative drug overdose, as well as to increased sensitivity to such adverse effects. Diuretic agents, if given in full or large doses, may produce serious adverse effects. Older patients often have difficulty in protecting their serum sodium concentrations during diuretic treatment, and a number of instances of hyponatremia, some of which result in fatal outcomes, have been reported (134). Thus, even though there is a possibility that hypertension in the elderly subject may at times be linked to excessive sodium retention (92), it is also true that older patients often have difficulty in conserving sodium (135) and thus may be vulnerable to hyponatremia during diuretic treatment. Hypokalemia also appears to occur frequently in the aged, even when diuretics are administered in comparatively low doses. Because diuretic-induced hypokalemia has been linked to the genesis of potentially hazardous cardiac dysrhythmias, there may be particular concern in older patients, in whom underlying arteriosclerotic heart disease is often present. Even in the absence of treatment, elderly subjects experience a significantly greater frequency of ventricular ectopic beats than younger subjects (136). Additionally, elderly patients with renal impairment may be at greater risk for the development of hyperosmolar nonketotic diabetic coma during therapy with thiazide diuretics (137).

Physicians are sometimes concerned about the effects of the decreased blood flow to certain organs produced by a reduction in blood pressure. For example, it is well established that renal function tends to be decreased during various forms of antihypertensive therapy, and it is commonplace for serum indicators, such as blood urea nitrogen or creatinine concentration, to increase. This should not be a major concern, however, for it has generally been observed that cessation of treatment (or even persistence with long-term treatment) allows renal function to return to its baseline value, indicating that no intrinsic alteration in the kidney has taken place.

A more difficult problem may arise with blood supply to the central nervous system. Not much information is available on treatment-induced changes; in one study in which diuretics were used to treat systolic hypertension, cerebrovascular resistance tended to decrease, but there were variable changes in gray matter flow (138). In general, cerebral autoregulation is active over a wide range of blood pressures, but in the elderly there may be a diminution in the ability of the cerebral circulation to vasodilate adequately at lower blood pressure levels. This shift of autoregulation to a higher range in the elderly means that symptoms of cerebral ischemia may occur at blood pressures higher than would occur in younger subjects. It is likely that this inability to vasodilate rapidly or fully is due to atheromatous changes in the small arterial circulation. Potentially, stepwise decreases in blood pressure could actually result in an improvement in cerebral blood flow without bringing about untoward symptoms. Most studies have not shown significant adverse effects on either renal or cerebral perfusion to be associated with the judicious use of antihypertensive medications (139–141).

The association of antihypertensive therapy with undesirable changes in blood lipids is well established (142). However, only a transient adverse effect on serum lipids was observed in the European Working Party on High Blood Pressure in the Elderly study and in the SHEP pilot study (143,144). Whether this was due to age-related metabolic differences or the lower doses of diuretics used in these studies is not known. Although a lipid-related increase in cardiovascular risk may play a role in counteracting some of the benefits of antihypertensive therapy, the clinical significance of this effect is not clear. Certainly, the lipid profile of elderly hypertensive patients should be monitored during therapy and appropriate treatment prescribed based on individual risk assessment. In some cases selection of antihypertensive agents not associated with adverse effects on lipids ($\alpha$-blockers, sympatholytics, angiotensin converting enzyme inhibitors, and calcium antagonists) may be necessary.

Although differing mechanisms appear to be involved in sustaining hypertension in the aged, the three principal factors appear to be a tendency to sodium expansion, enhanced sympathetic nervous system responsiveness, and a decrease in compliance of the large arterial circulation. In addition, the cardiovascular system of elderly patients may be less sensitive to both $\beta$-adrenergic stimulation and $\beta$-blockade (145,146). The best approach to the pharmacological treatment of hypertension in this age group is therefore to select agents that counter each or all of these mechanisms. It might be predicted on this basis that diuretics, vasodilators, and calcium channel blockers will prove to be most effective, but all classes of antihypertensive agents currently available have been successfully used in treating hypertension in elderly patients.

Diuretics have provided the basis for treatment in all major trials of antihypertensive therapy in the elderly. In view of the cardiovascular benefits demonstrated in these studies, it is probably most reasonable to start therapy with diuretic agents, as suggested in the standard stepped-care approach for the treatment of hypertension (21). The effectiveness of this class of agents in reducing blood pressure in the aged is well established (123,147,148). To minimize the possibility of adverse biochemical effects, relatively low doses, equivalent to 12.5–25 mg per day of hydrochlorothiazide, should be used. The routine use of a thiazide-triamterene combination may reduce the likelihood of hypokalemia. Unless the patient has renal insufficiency or diabetes mellitus, thiazide diuretics are preferred to loop diuretics because they are at least as effective and need to be given only once daily. Low cost is often cited as an advantage of these agents. A 60–70% response rate can be expected, with blood pressure reductions averaging about 25/10 mm Hg. Despite their efficacy, however, the diuretics appear to be associated with more frequent metabolic abnormalities and symptomatic complaints than alternative agents (149). More frequent biochemical monitoring to detect the hypokalemia and hypomagnesemia associated with therapy may be required (150,151). In consideration of the concerns raised by the MRFIT study discussed earlier, it seems advisable to avoid diuretics in elderly men with significant baseline abnormalities.

If a diuretic is not effective or well tolerated, the use of alternative or additional drugs is indicated. Sympatholytic drugs are a useful class of agents in this population. They do not cause significant changes in cardiac output, heart rate, renal blood flow, or glomerular filtration rate (131,154,163). The combination of clonidine with a low-dose diuretic has been used with good results in treating systolic hypertension (152,153). Systolic blood pressure was decreased by at least 20 mm Hg in most patients in response to therapy with 0.1 mg clonidine combined with 15 mg chlorthalidone in a single daily dose. A few patients required this combination to be administered twice daily. An advantage of this regimen was the simplicity of administration combined with relatively few adverse effects. Guanabenz, earlier alone or in combination with a diuretic, is another effective form of therapy in older patients (154). Similarly, good results have been reported with the sympatholytic agent methyldopa. Concerns that treatment with centrally acting adrenergic inhibitors may be associated with detrimental effects on quality of life (155) have been cited as a reason for avoiding this class of agents in elderly patients, who may experience excessive sedation (156). However, the use of low doses and vigilance in maintaining a high level of sensitivity to drug-induced symptoms can allow physicians to take advantage of this useful class of agents in those patients who are able to tolerate them. Side effects may be minimized by administering clonidine as a single small nighttime dose or by utilizing a once weekly transdermal clonidine preparation (157).

The $\alpha$-blockers, including prazosin and terazosin, produce clear antihypertensive effects in this age group and appear to have an acceptable adverse event profile (158). The half-life of terazosin, which is the longer lived of the two agents, may be increased in elderly patients; the half-life of prazosin is unaffected by age. Because these agents may be associated with postural hypotension, they should be avoided in patients who have a significant postural change in blood pressure at baseline (systolic pressure drop greater than 15 mm Hg). Few adverse metabolic effects and no central nervous system symptoms are associated with these agents. Labetalol is a combined $\alpha_1$- and $\beta$-blocking agent that is effective alone or in combination with a diuretic (159). Peak plasma concentrations and the half-life of this agent are both increased in elderly patients. Labetalol has been used successfully in treating isolated systolic hypertension, with a low incidence of side effects and adverse orthostatic changes (160). Whole-day blood pressure monitoring data suggest that labetalol may be more effective than enalapril in reducing ambulatory blood pressure and heart rate throughout the day (161). Hypotension during therapy with $\alpha$-blocking agents may be more frequent in the presence of volume depletion, diuretic therapy, and concomitant use of other antihypertensive medications. Patients should be cautioned to maintain adequate fluid intake during warm weather or activities that may result in increased fluid losses. By starting with small doses and administering the first dose after each change in dose at bedtime while supine, the likelihood of first-dose hypotension can be minimized.

The value of $\beta$-blockers in treating elderly hypertensive patients requiring therapy in addition to or in place of diuretic agents is not clear. $\beta$-Blockers reduce cardiac output and heart rate and increase peripheral resistance. Although many clinicians have found these agents to work satisfactorily in their elderly patients, it has been reported that they are less effective in older patients than in the young (162). However, the use of low doses (25–50 mg per day) of atenolol in the SHEP trial was associated with substantial reductions in both blood pressure and cardiovascular risk. The success of this trial suggests that β-blockers can have a role in treating elderly patients, but it is not known to what degree cardioprotective effects and possible adverse effects on serum lipids and glucose disposition contributed toward improvement or worsening of the outcomes. When β-blockers are used for treating hypertension in elderly patients, it should be remembered that their metabolism is often slower than in younger patients, and it follows that plasma concentrations tend to be higher. Thus, unless low doses are used, it can be anticipated that the incidence of adverse effects during β-blocking treatment may be relatively high in older hypertensive patients. Fatigue and exercise intolerance sometimes associated with these agents may significantly reduce functional capacity in this group of patients, many of whom may be only marginally functional to begin with. As in younger patients, β-blocking treatment should be avoided in patients with concomitant bronchoconstrictive disease, allergic rhinitis, peripheral vascular disease, diabetes mellitus, left ventricular dysfunction, atrioventricular conduction abnormalities, bradycardia, and depression. Conversely, β-blockade is a good choice in patients with migraine headaches, senile tremor, certain arrhythmias, and coronary heart disease, especially after nonfatal myocardial infarction.

The vasodilatory agent hydralazine has also been shown to be effective in elderly hypertensive patients. It can be used as a third step in patients not responding well to a diuretic-sympatholytic combination, or it can be administered directly with a diuretic. In younger patients this is not possible because the stimulatory effects of hydralazine on the sympathetic nervous system normally demand that a β-blocker or sympatholytic agent be given concurrently to prevent tachycardia. In older patients, however, this stimulatory effect is often minimal or absent, thereby allowing hydralazine to be given in a simple combination with a diuretic. Minoxidil, a more potent vasodilator, is more likely to cause tachycardia, fluid retention, and greater cardiac work. Similarly, the marked postural hypotension associated with guanethidine limits its use in elderly patients.

Newer classes of antihypertensive drugs can also play an important role in the treatment of the elderly. The calcium channel blockers are clearly effective in these patients (163,164). They are at least as efficacious as diuretics and perhaps are better tolerated (149). Postural hypotension, sedation, depression, and biochemical abnormalities are generally not associated with these agents. A higher percentage of older hypertensives respond to calcium channel blockers than to β-adrenergic blockers (165). These drugs act as peripheral vasodilators; negative inotropic and chronotropic effects may be associated with verapamil and diltiazem. Because these two agents affect atrioventricular and sinus node function, a combination of these with β-blockers may be associated with some degree of heart block (166). This effect may be uncommon in clinical practice, but such combinations should be used with caution. Nifedipine has been frequently used to effect rapid blood pressure reduction in patients with severe range hypertension. Because cerebral blood flow in the elderly may be particularly sensitive to sudden large decreases in blood pressure, this approach is indicated only rarely. On the other hand, slow-release formulations of nifedipine may be well tolerated. Dizziness, tachycardia, edema, and headache may be associated with calcium channel blockade; constipation has been particularly associated with verapamil.

Although low serum renin values characteristic of elderly hypertensives might suggest that angiotensin converting enzyme (ACE) inhibitors should be among the less effective antihypertensive agents for this group, elderly patients appear to respond well to therapy with both captopril and enalapril (167). It is known that ACE inhibitors may lower blood pressure in patients with low serum renin values, possibly because of effects on kinins and prostaglandins (108). Total peripheral resistance is reduced without reflex stimulation of heart rate and cardiac output. These agents appear to be particularly effective in elderly patients when combined with diuretic therapy (168). When used with diuretic agents, an additional advantage may result from a tendency of these agents to raise serum potassium levels, decreasing the likelihood of clinically significant hypokalemia. Side effects are infrequent. Furthermore, ACE inhibitors may be useful in managing coexisting congestive heart failure. Care should be taken to avoid using these agents in patients with bilateral renal artery stenosis, who may develop severe azotemia. Because of the possibility of hyperkalemia, ACE inhibitors should be used carefully in patients with renal impairment or who are taking potassium-retaining diuretics, potassium salts, or nonsteroidal anti-inflammatory drugs.

The presence of left ventricular hypertrophy is an important issue in elderly hypertensives. This condition often heralds a poor prognosis, presumably because it is associated with increased possibilities of serious arrhythmias, ischemic heart disease, and ventricular dysfunction. It has not been established that the pharmacological regression of left ventricular hypertrophy can decrease the likelihood of these complications, but there has been a growing interest in antihypertensive drugs that can decrease echocardiographically measured left ventricular muscle mass in such patients. The sympatholytic agents, the ACE inhibitors, and the calcium channel blockers (169) appear most effective in this regard. Both centrally acting sympatholytic inhibitors, such as methyldopa and clonidine, and peripheral $\alpha$-blockers significantly decrease left ventricular muscle mass and wall thickness in patients with enlarged hearts (170,171). The ACE inhibitors and calcium channel blockers likewise produce regression of hypertrophy and preserve left ventricular function (109,172).

## SUMMARY

Hypertension is a highly prevalent condition among the elderly and is associated with a substantial risk of cardiovascular morbidity and mortality. Hypertension in the elderly is a distinct entity from hypertension in younger persons and is characterized by the predominance of systolic blood pressure elevation. There is convincing evidence that reduction in elevated blood pressure, using pharmacological measures when necessary, decreases the risk of cardiovascular death and disability in the aged. This holds true for diastolic hypertension, systolic–diastolic hypertension, and isolated systolic hypertension. Antihypertensive therapy should be individualized and should take into consideration concurrent medical conditions, social situations that may affect compliance, and individual responses to therapy. The greater likelihood of adverse effects in this population may be related to alterations in metabolism, changes in cardiovascular sensitivity, and the increased prevalence of concomitant medical diagnoses associated with aging. The goal of therapy should be the reduction of cardiovascular risk while maintaining an acceptable quality of life and a high degree of functional capacity.

## REFERENCES

1. Master AM, Lasser RP. Blood pressure elevation in the elderly. In: Brest AN, Moyer JH, eds. Hypertension: Recent Advances—Second Hahneman Symposium on Hypertensive Disease. Philadelphia: Lea and Febiger, 1961:23–24.
2. Breckenridge MB, Kostis JB. Isolated systolic hypertension in the elderly: results of a statewide survey of clinical practice in New Jersey. *Am J Med* 1989; 86:370–375.
3. Curb JD, Borhani NO, Entwisle G, et al. Isolated systolic hypertension in 14 communities. *Am J Epidemiol* 1985; 121:362–370.
4. Torrey BB, Kinsella K, Tacuber CM. An aging world international population report. Series P-95, No. 78. U.S. Bureau of the Census, September 1987.
5. Wenger NK, Marcus FI, O'Rourke RA. Cardiovascular disease in the elderly. *J Am Coll Cardiol* 1987; 10:80a–87a.
6. U.S. Senate Special Committee on Aging. Aging America: Trends and Projections. Publication PL3377-584. U.S. Government Printing Office, 1984.
7. Wetrogran S. Projections of the Population of States by Age, Sex, and Race: 1989 to 2010. Current Population Reports, Population Estimates and Projections, Series P-25, No. 1053, January 1990.
8. Miller HW. National Center of Health Statistics. Plan and Operation of the National Health and Nutrition Examination Survey. United States 1971–1973 Vital and Health Statistics, Series 1, Nos. 10a and 10b. U.S. Dept. of Health, Education and Welfare Publication No. 73-1310. Washington, DC: U.S. Government Printing Office 1973:46.

9. Master AM, Lasser RP, Jaffe HL. Blood pressure in white people over 65 years of age. *Ann Intern Med* 1958; 48:284–290.
10. Kannel WB. In: Caird FE, Dall JLC, Kennedy RD, eds. Cardiology in Old Age. New York: Plenum Press, 1976:160.
11. Kannel WB, Gordon T. Evaluation of cardiovascular risk factors in the elderly: the Framingham study. *Bull NY Acad Med* 1978; 54:573–591.
12. Abernathy J, Borhani NO, Hawkins CM, et al. Systolic blood pressure as an independent predictor of mortality in the Hypertension Detection and Follow-up Program. *Am J Prev Med* 1986; 2:123–132.
13. Amery A, Birkenhager W, Brixko P, et al. Mortality and morbidity results from the European Working Party on High Blood Pressure in the elderly trial. *Lancet* 1985; 1:1349–1354.
14. MacMahon S, Peto R, Cutler J, et al. Blood pressure, stroke, and coronary heart disease. Part 1. Prolonged differences in blood pressure: prospective observational studies corrected for the regression dilution bias. *Lancet* 1990; 335:765–774.
15. Staessen J, Bulpitt C, Clement D, et al. Relation between mortality and treated blood pressure in elderly patients with hypertension: report of the European Working Party on High Blood Pressure in the Elderly. *Br Med J* 1989; 298:1552–1556.
16. SHEP Cooperative Research Group. Prevention of stroke by antihypertensive drug treatment in older persons with isolated systolic hypertension. *JAMA* 1991; 265:3255–3264.
17. Sleight P. Blood pressure, hearts, and U-shaped curves. *Lancet* 1988; 1:235.
18. Lowenstein WF. Blood pressure in relation to age and sex in the tropics and subtropics. *Lancet* 1961; 1:389–393.
19. Maddocks I. Possible absence of essential hypertension in two complete Pacific island populations. *Lancet* 1961; 2:396–399.
20. Weber MA, Neutel JM, Cheung DG. Hypertension in the aged: a pathophysiologic bias for treatment. *Am J Cardiol* 1989; 63:25H–32H.
21. Joint National Committee on the Detection, Evaluation and Treatment of High Blood Pressure. The 1988 Report of the Joint National Committee on the Detection, Evaluation, and Treatment of High Blood Pressure. *Arch Intern Med* 1988; 148:1023–1038.
22. Working Group on Hypertension in the Elderly. Statement on hypertension in the elderly. *JAMA* 1986; 256:70–74.
23. Subcommittee of Definition and Prevalence of the 1985 Joint National Committee. Hypertension prevalence and the status of awareness, treatment, and control in the United States: final report. *Hypertension* 1985; 7:457–468.
24. Wing S, Aubert RE, Hansen JP. Isolated systolic hypertension in Evans County. I. Prevalence and screening considerations. *J Chron Dis* 1982; 35:735–742.
25. Wilking SVB, Belanger A, Kannel WB, D'Agostino RB, Steel K. Determinants of isolated systolic hypertension. *JAMA* 1988; 260:3451–3455.
26. Vogt TM, Ireland CC, Black D, Camel G, Hughes G. Recruitment of elderly

volunteers for a multicenter clinical trial: the SHEP Pilot Study. *Controlled Clin Trials* 1986; 7:118–133.

27. Rowland M, Roberts J. Blood pressure level and hypertension in persons 6 to 74 years. United States, 1976–80. Advance Data in Vital and Health Statistics. DHHS Publication No. (PHS) 82-1250, 1982.
28. Curb JD, Borhani NO, Schnaper H, et al. Detection and treatment of hypertension in older individuals. *Am J Epidemiol* 1985; 121:371–376.
29. Wing S, Aubert RE, Hansen JP, Hames CG, Slome C, Tyroler HA. Isolated systolic hypertension in Evans county. I. Prevalence and screening considerations. *J Chron Dis* 1982; 35:735–742.
30. Borhani NO, Applegate WB, Cutler JA, et al. Part 1. Rationale and design. *Hypertension* 1991; 17(Suppl. 3):II2–II15.
31. Kannel WB, Dawber TR, McGee DL. Perspectives on systolic hypertension. The Framingham Study. *Circulation* 1979; 61:1179–1182.
32. Barrett-Connor E, Criqui MH, Klauber MR. Diabetes and hypertension in a community of older adults. *Am J Epidemiol* 1981; 113:276–284.
33. Georas MC, Haverback BJ. The aging gastrointestinal tract. *Am J Surg* 1969; 117:881–892.
34. Norris AH, Lundy T, Shock NW. Trends in elected indices of body composition in men between the ages of 30 and 80 years. *Ann NY Acad Sci* 1963; 110:623–639.
35. Brest AN, Haddad M. Should systolic hypertension be treated? In: Corday E, ed. Controversies in Cardiology. Philadelphia: F. A. Davis, 1978:217–220.
36. Kannel WB, Dawber TR. Hypertension as an ingredient of a cardiovascular risk profile. *Br J Hosp Med* 1974; 2:508–516.
37. Drayer JIM, Weber MA, Laragh JH. Renin subgroups in essential hypertension. *Clin Exp Hypertens* 1982; [A]4:1817–1834.
38. Drayer JIM, Weber MA, Sealey JE, Laragh JH. Low and high renin essential hypertension: a comparison of clinical and biochemical characteristics. *Am J Med Sci* 1981; 281:135–142.
39. Society of Actuaries. Build and Blood Pressure Study. Vol. 1, 1959.
40. Kannel WB, Dawber TR, Sorlie P. Components of blood pressure and risk of atherothrombotic brain infarction. *Stroke* 1976; 7:327–331.
41. Colandrea MA, Friedman GD, Nichaman MZ, Lynd CN. Systolic hypertension in the elderly: an epidemiologic assessment. *Circulation* 1970; 41:239–245.
42. Garland C, Barrett-Conner E, Suarez L, Criqui MH. Isolated systolic hypertension and mortality after age 60 years: a prospective population-based study. *Am J Epidemiol* 1983; 118:365–376.
43. Shekelle R, Ostfeld A, Klawans H. Hypertension and risk of stroke in an elderly population. *Stroke* 1974; 5:71–75.
44. Stebbins PT, Taylor GJ, Gibson RS. Risk factors and myocardial infarction in the elderly. *Circulation* 1981; 62(Suppl. III):220–228.
45. Hallock P, Benson IC. Studies on the elastic properties of human isolated aorta. *J Clin Invest* 1937; 16:595–602.
46. Bader H. Dependence of wall stress in the human thoracic aorta on age and pressure. *Circ Res* 1967; 20:354–361.

47. Gerstenblith G, Lakatta EG, Weisfeldt ML. Age changes in myocardial function and exercise response. *Prog Cardiovasc Dis* 1976; 19:1–21.
48. Yin FCP. The aging vasculature and its effects on the heart. In: Weisfeldt ML, ed. The Aging Heart. New York: Raven Press, 1980:137–213.
49. Messerli FH, Glade LB, Dreslinski GR. Hypertension in the elderly: haemodynamic, fluid volume and endocrine findings. *Clin Sci* 1981; 61:393s–394s.
50. Sowers JR, Zawada ER. Hypertension in the aged. In: Zawada EJ, Sica DA, eds. Geriatric Nephrology and Urology. Littleton, MA: PSG Publication Co., 1985:265–281.
51. Gifford RW. Isolated systolic hypertension in the elderly. *JAMA* 1982; 247:781–785.
52. Hallock P, Benson IC. Studies of the elastic properties of human isolated aorta. *J Clin Invest* 1937; 16:595–600.
53. Messerli FH, Sundgaard-Riise K, Ventura HO, Dunn FG, Glade LB, Frohlich ED. Essential hypertension in the elderly: haemodynamics, intravascular volume, plasma renin activity, and circulating catecholamine levels. *Lancet* 1983; 2:983–985.
54. Gozna ER, Marble AE, Shaw A, Holland JG. Age-related changes in the mechanics of the aorta and pulmonary artery of man. *J Appl Physiol* 1974; 36:407–411.
55. Lakatta EG. Alterations in the cardiovascular system that occur in advanced age. *Fed Proc* 1979; 38:163–167.
56. Ross R. The smooth muscle cell. II. Growth of smooth muscle in culture and formation of elastic fibers. *J Cell Biol* 1971; 50:172–178.
57. Granath A, Jonsson B, Strandell T. Circulation in healthy old men, studied by right heart catheterization of rest and during exercise in supine and sitting position. *Acta Med Scand* 1964; 176:425–446.
58. Lund-Johansen P. Hemodynamics in essential hypertension at rest and during exercise—a 20-year follow-up study. *Ann Clin Res* 1988; 20(Suppl. 28):31–8.
59. Shimada K, Kitazumi T, Sadakane N, Ogura H, Ozawa T. Age-related changes of baroreflex function, plasma norepinephrine, and blood pressure. *Hypertension* 1985; 7:113–117.
60. Gribbin B, Pickering LTG, Sleight P, Petro R. Effect of age and high blood pressure on baroreflex sensitivity in man. *Circ Res* 1971; 29:424.
61. Vlachakis ND, Mendlowitz M, Degusman DD. Diminished baroreceptor sensitivity in elderly hypertensives. Possible role of atherosclerosis. *Atherosclerosis* 1976; 24:243–248.
62. Cowley AW, Liard JF, Guyton AC. Role of the baroreceptor reflex in daily control of arterial blood pressure and other variables in dogs. *Circ Res* 1973; 32:564–570.
63. Drayer JIM, Weber MA, DeYoung JL, Wyle FA. Circadian blood pressure patterns in ambulatory hypertensive patients. Effect of age. *Am J Med* 1982; 73:493–499.
64. DeGaudemaris R, Mallion JM, Battistella P, et al. Ambulatory blood pressure and variability by age and sex in 200 normotensive subjects: reference population values. *J Hypertens* 1987; Suppl. 5:S429–S430.
65. Zachariah PK, Sheps SG, Bailey KR, Wiltgen CM, Moore AG. Age-related

characteristics of ambulatory blood pressure load and mean blood pressure in normotensive subjects. *JAMA* 1991; 265:1414–1417.
66. Caird FI, Andrews GR, Kennedy RD. Effects of posture on blood pressure in the elderly. *Br Heart J* 1973; 35:527–530.
67. Abrass IB. Catecholamine levels and vascular responsiveness in aging. In: Horan MJ, Steinberg GM, Dunbar JB, Hadley EC, eds. Blood Pressure Regulation and Aging, an NIH Symposium. New York: Biomedical Information Corporation, 1986:123–130.
68. Fleisch JH, Maling HM, Brodie BB. Beta-receptor activity in aorta: variations with age and species. *Circ Res* 1970; 26:151–162.
69. Fleisch JH, Hooker CS. The relationship between age and relaxation of vascular smooth muscle in the rabbit and rat. *Circ Res* 1976; 38:243–249.
70. Buhler FR, Kiowski W, Landmann R, et al. Changing role of beta- and alpha-adrenoreceptor-mediated cardiovascular responses in the transition from high-cardiac output into a high-peripheral resistance phase in essential hypertension. In: JH Laragh, F Buhler, D Selden, eds. Frontiers in Hypertension Research. New York: Springer-Verlag, 1982:316–326.
71. Vestal RE, Wood AJJ, Shand DG. Reduced β-adrenoreceptor sensitivity in the elderly. *Clin Pharmacol Ther* 1979; 26:186–191.
72. Doyle V, O'Malley K, Kelly JG. Human lymphocyte beta-adrenoreceptor density in relation to age and hypertension. *J Cardiovasc Pharmacol* 1982; 4:738–740.
73. Lowder SC, Hamet P, Liddle GW. Contrasting effects of hypoglycemia on plasma renin activity and cyclic adenosine 3′,5′-mono-phosphate (cyclic AMP) in low renin and normal renin essential hypertension. *Circ Res* 1976; 38:105–108.
74. Palmer GJ, Ziegler MG, Lake CR. Response of norepinephrine and blood pressure to stress increases with age. *J Gerontol* 1978; 33:482–487.
75. Alicandri CL, Agabiti-Rosei E, Fariello R. Aortic rigidity and plasma catecholamines in essential hypertensive patients. *Clin Exp Hypertens* 1982; 4:1073–1083.
76. Noth RH, Lassman MN, Tan SY, Fernandez-Crug A Jr, Mulrow PJ. Age and the renin-aldosterone system. *Arch Intern Med* 1977; 137:1414–1417.
77. Luft FC, Grim CE, Fineberg N, Weinberger MC. Effects of volume expansion and contraction in normotensive whites, blacks, and subjects of different ages. *Circulation* 1979; 59:643–650.
78. Stern N, Tuck ML. Homeostatic fragility in the elderly. *Geriatr Cardiol* 1986; 4:201–211.
79. Osborne JL, DiBona FG, Thames MD. Beta-1 receptor mediation of renin secretion elicited by low frequency renal nerve stimulation. *J Pharmacol Exp Ther* 1981; 216:265–270.
80. Gavrus I, Gavrus H, Chobanian AV, Tifft JC, Melby JC, Jick H. Hypertension and age: clinical and biochemical correlates. *Clin Exp Hypertens* 1982; 4:1097–1106.
81. Sowers JR. Hypertension in the elderly. *Am J Med* 1987; 82(Suppl. 1B):1–8.
82. Tuck ML, Williams GH, Cain JP. Relation of age, diastolic pressure and known duration of hypertension to pressure of low renin essential hypertension. *Am J Cardiol* 1973; 32:632–637.

83. Laragh JH. Vasoconstriction-volume analysis for understanding and treating hypertension. The use of renin and aldosterone profiles. *Am J Med* 1973; 55:201–274.
84. Crane MG, Harris JJ. Effect of aging on renin activity and aldosterone excretion. *J Lab Clin Med* 1976; 87:949–959.
85. Nowarcynski W, Genest J, Kuchel O, et al. Age- and posture-related changes in plasma protein binding and metabolism of aldosterone in essential and secondary hypertension. *J Lab Clin Med* 1977; 90:475–490.
86. Hegstag R, Brown RD, Jaing N. Aging and aldosterone. *Am J Med* 1983; 74:442–448.
87. Morimoto S, Uchida K, Miyamoto M. Plasma aldosterone response to angiotensin II in sodium-restricted elderly subjects with essential hypertension. *J Am Geriatr Soc* 1981; 29:302–307.
88. Weber MA, Purdy RE. Catecholamine mediated pressor effects of aldosterone on vascular smooth muscle. *Life Sci* 1982; 30:2009–2017.
89. Meneely GR, Batterbee HD. High sodium, low potassium, environment and hypertension. *Am J Cardiol* 1976; 38:768–785.
90. Guyton AC, Colemen TG, Cowley AW. Arterial pressure regulation: overriding dominance of the kidneys in long term regulation and in hypertension. *Am J Med* 1972; 52:584–594.
91. Luft FC, Grim CE, Fineberg N. Effects of volume expansion and contraction in normotensive whites, blacks and subjects of different ages. *Circulation* 1979; 59:643–650.
92. Beretta-Piccoli C, Davies DL, Boddy K. Relation of arterial pressure with body sodium, body potassium and plasma potassium in essential hypertension. *Clin Sci* 1982; 63:257–270.
93. Kroening BH, Weintraub M. Age-associated differences in guinea pig myocardial $Na^+$, $K^+$ ATPase activity and ouabain inhibition and in $Mg^{2+}$ ATPase activity. *Pharmacology* 1980; 21:193–197.
94. Gamberg SR, Duthie EH. Effect of age on red cell membrane sodium-potassium dependent adenoside triphosphatase ($Na^+$-$K^+$ ATPase) activity in healthy men. *J Gerontol* 1983; 38:23–28.
95. Sowers JR, Monhanty PK, Thames MD. Age related forearm vascular resistance and neurohumoral responses to unloading of cardiopulmonary baroreceptors in hypertensives (abstract). *Clin Res* 1986; May:2–5.
96. Nolan L, O'Malley K. Prescribing for the elderly. Part I. Sensitivity of the elderly to adverse drug reactions. *J Am Geriatr Soc* 1988; 36:142–149.
97. Kierman PJ, Isaacs JB. Use of drugs by the elderly. *J R Soc Med* 1981; 74:196–200.
98. Berliner K, Fujry H, Lee DH. Blood pressure measurement in obese persons. Comparison of intra-arterial and auscultatory measurements. *Am J Cardiol* 1961; 8:10.
99. O'Callaghan WG, Fitzgerald DJ, O'Malley K, O'Brien E. Accuracy of indirect blood pressure measurement in the elderly. *Br Med J* 1983; 286:1545–1546.
100. Vardan S, Mookherjee S, Warner R, et al. Systolic hypertension. Direct and indirect BP measurements. *Arch Intern Med* 1983; 143:935–938.

101. Messerli FH, Ventura HO, Amodes C. Osler's maneuver and pseudohypertension. *N Engl J Med* 1985; 312:1548–1551.
102. Joint National Committee on Detection, Evaluation and Treatment of High Blood Pressure. Report of the Joint National Committee on Detection, Evaluation, and Treatment of High Blood Pressure. Bethesda: National Heart, Lung, and Blood Institute, NIH Publication No. 84-1088, 1984.
103. Furberg CD, Black DM. The systolic hypertension in the elderly pilot program: methodological issues. *Eur Heart J* 1988; 9:223–227.
104. Myers MG, Kearns PM, Kennedy DS, Fisher RH. Postural hypotension and diuretic therapy in the elderly. *Can Med Assoc J* 1978; 119:581–585.
105. Caird FI, Andrews GR, Kennedy RD. Effect of posture on blood pressure in the elderly. *Br Heart J* 1973; 35:527–530.
106. Muller FB, Laragh JH. Clinical evaluation and differential diagnosis of the individual hypertensive patient. In: JH Laragh and BM Brenner, eds. Hypertension. New York: Raven Press, 1990, 1385–1396.
107. Kannel WB, Gordon T, Castelli WB, Margolis JR. Electrocardiographic left ventricular hypertrophy and risk or coronary heart disease: the Framingham Study. *Ann Intern Med* 1970; 72:813–822.
108. Dzau VJ. Evolution of the clinical management of hypertension: emerging role of "specific" vasodilators as initial therapy. *Am J Med* 1987; 82:36–43.
109. Schulman SP, Weiss JL, Becker LC, et al. The effects of antihypertensive therapy on left ventricular mass in elderly patients. *N Engl J Med* 1990; 322:1350–1356.
110. Novick AC, Ziegelbaum M, Vidt DG, Gifford RW Jr, Pohl MA, Goormastic M. Trends in surgical revascularization for renal artery disease: ten years' experience. *JAMA* 1987; 257:498–501.
111. Pickering TG, Herman L, Devereux DB, et al. Recurrent pulmonary ocedema in hypertension due to bilateral renal artery stenosis: treatment by angioplasty or surgical revascularization. *Lancet* 1988; 2:551–552.
112. Olin JW, Vidt DG, Gifford RW Jr, Novick AC. Renovascular disease in the elderly: an analysis of 50 patients. *J Am Coll Cardiol* 1985; 2:1232–1238.
113. Topal EJ, Traill TA, Fortuin JN. Hypertensive hypertrophic cardiomyopathy of the elderly. *N Engl J Med* 1985; 312:277–283.
114. Kuller LH, Hulley SB, Cohen JD, et al. Unexpected effects of treating hypertension in men with electrocardiographic abnormalities: a critical review. *Circulation* 1986; 73:114–123.
115. Nolan L, O'Malley K. Prescribing for the elderly. Part II. Prescribing patterns: differences due to age. *J Am Geriatr Soc* 1988; 36:245–254.
116. Sempos C, Fulwood R, Haines C, et al. The prevalence of high blood cholesterol levels among adults in the United States. *JAMA* 1989; 262:45–52.
117. Pooling Project Research Group. Relationship of blood pressure, serum cholesterol, smoking habit, relative weight, and ECG abnormalities to incidence of major coronary events: final report of the Pooling Project. *J Chron Dis* 1978; 31:201–306.
118. Benfante R, Reed D. Is elevated serum cholesterol level a risk factor for coronary heart disease in the elderly? *JAMA* 1990; 263:393–396.

119. Harris T, Cook EF, Kannel WB, Goldman L. Proportional hazards analysis of risk factors for coronary heart disease in individuals aged 65 or older. The Framingham Heart Study. *J Am Geriatr Soc* 1988; 36:1023–1028.
120. Harris MI. Epidemiologic characteristics of impaired glucose tolerance in the United States population. In: Bab S, Gould MK, Zimmet P, eds. Diabetes Mellitus. Recent Knowledge on Etiology, Complications and Treatment. Orlando, FL: Academic Press, 1984:105–109.
121. Hypertension Detection and Follow-up Program Cooperative Group. Five-year findings of the Hypertension Detection and Follow-up Program. II. Mortality by race, sex and age. *JAMA* 1979; 242:2572–2577.
122. National Heart Foundation of Australia. Treatment of mild hypertension in the elderly: report by the management committee. *Med J Aust* 1981; 2:398–402.
123. Amery A, Birkenhager W, Bixko P, et al. Mortality and morbidity results from the European Working Party on High Blood Pressure in the Elderly Trial. *Lancet* 1985; 1:1329–1354.
124. Final results of the Systolic Hypertension in the Elderly Program (SHEP). Prevention of stroke by antihypertensive drug treatment in older persons with isolated systolic hypertension. SHEP Cooperative Research Group. *JAMA* 1991; 265:3255–3264.
125. Fletcher AE, Bulpitt CJ. How far should blood pressure be lowered? *N Engl J Med* 1992; 326:251–254.
126. Kaplan NM. Non-drug treatment of hypertension. *Ann Intern Med* 1985; 102:359–373.
127. Subcommittee on Nonpharmacological Therapy of the 1984 Joint National Committee on Detection, Evaluation, and Treatment of High Blood Pressure. Nonpharmacological approaches to the control of high blood pressure: final report. *Hypertension* 1986; 8:444–467.
128. Langford HG, Blanfox D, Oberman A, et al. Dietary therapy slows the return of hypertension after stopping prolonger medication. *JAMA* 1985; 253:657–664.
129. Stamler R, Stamler J, Grimm R, et al. Nutritional therapy for high blood pressure. *JAMA* 1987; 257:1484–1491.
130. Lipsitz LA, Nyquist RP Jr, Wei JY, et al. Postprandial reduction in blood pressure in the elderly. *N Engl J Med* 1983; 309:81–83.
131. Hurwitz N. Predisposing factors in adverse reactions to drugs. *Br Med J* 1969; 1:536–539.
132. Jackson G, Pierscianowski TA, Mahon W. Inappropriate antihypertensive therapy in the elderly. *Lancet* 1976; 2:1317–1318.
133. Montamat SC, Cusack BJ, Vestal RE. Management of drug therapy in the elderly. *N Engl J Med* 1989; 321:303–308.
134. Ashraf N, Locksley R, Arieff AI. Thiazide-induced hyponatremia associated with death or neurologic damage in outpatients. *Am J Med* 1981; 70:1163–1168.
135. Kampmann JP, Molhom-Hansen JE. Renal excretion of drugs. In: Crooks J, Stevenson IH, eds. Drugs and the Elderly. Baltimore: University Park Press, 1979:77–87.
136. Hinkle LE, Carver ST, Argyros DC. The prognostic significance of ventricular

premature contractions in healthy people and in people with coronary heart disease. *Acta Cardiol* 1974; 18:5.
137. Sowers JR. The impact of diuretics on potassium and glucose. *J Cardiovasc Pharmacol* 1984; 6:5477–5482.
138. Traub YM, Shapiro AP, Dujovny M. Cerebral blood flow changes with diuretic therapy in elderly subjects with systolic hypertension. *Clin Exp Hypertens* 1982; 4:1193–1201.
139. Strandgaard S. Cerebral blood flow and antihypertensive drugs in the elderly. *Acta Med Scand* 1983; 676:103–109.
140. Ram CV, Meese R, Kaplan NM, et al. Antihypertensive therapy of the elderly: effects on blood pressure and cerebral blood flow. *Am J Med* 1987; 82(1A):53–57.
141. Bertel O, Marx BE, Conen D. Effects of antihypertensive treatment on cerebral perfusion. *Am J Med* 1987; 82(3B):29–36.
142. Wilking SVB, Belaner A, Kannel WB, et al. Determinants of isolated systolic hypertension. *JAMA* 1988; 260(23):3451–3455.
143. Hulley SB, Furberg CD, Gurland B, et al. Systolic hypertension in the elderly program: antihypertensive efficacy of chlorthalidone. *Am J Cardiol* 1985; 56:913–920.
144. Amery A, Birkenhager W, Bulpitt C. Influence of antihypertensive therapy on serum cholesterol in elderly hypertensive patients. *Acta Cardiol* 1982; 37:235–244.
145. Vestal RE, Wood AJJ, Schand DG. Reduced beta-adrenoceptor sensitivity in the elderly. *Clin Pharmacol Ther* 1979; 26:181–186.
146. Vestal RE, Wood AJJ, Branch RA, et al. Effects of age and cigarette smoking on propranolol disposition. *Clin Pharmacol Ther* 1979; 26:8–15.
147. Meyers MG. Hydrocholorothiazide with or without amiloride for hypertension in the elderly. *Arch Intern Med* 1987; 147:1026–1030.
148. Freis ED. Age and antihypertensive drugs (hydrochlorothiazide, bendromethiazide, nadolol and captopril). *Am J Cardiol* 1988; 61:117–121.
149. Byyny RL, LoVerde M, Mitchell W. Treatment of hypertension in the elderly with a new calcium channel blocking drug, nitrendipine. *Am J Med* 1989; 86:49–55.
150. Onyer J, Weber M, DeYoung J, Wyle FA. Circadian blood pressure patterns in ambulatory hypertensive patients. *Am J Med* 1982; 73:493–499.
151. Sowers JR. Managing geriatric hypertension: a brief overview. *Geriatrics* 1985; 40:63–66.
152. Thananopavarn C, Golub MS, Sambhi MP. Clonidine in the elderly hypertensive: monotherapy and therapy with a diuretic. *Chest* 1983; 83:410–411.
153. Weber MA, Drayer JIM, Gray DR. Combined diuretic and sympatholytic therapy in elderly patients with predominant systolic hypertension. *Chest* 1983; 83:S416–S418.
154. Weber MA, Drayer JIM. Treatment of hypertension in the elderly. *South Med J* 1986; 79:323–326.
155. Crogg SH, Levine S, Testa MA, et al. The effects of antihypertensive therapy on the quality of life. *N Engl J Med* 1986; 314:1657–1664.
156. Messerli FH, Deslinski GR, Husseri FE, et al. Anti-adrenergic therapy: special

aspects of hypertension in the elderly. *Hypertension* 1981; 3(Suppl. 2):II226–II229.

157. Burris JF. Transdermal clonidine compared to sustained-release verapamil in elderly hypertensive persons. *Choices Cardiol* 1991; 5(Suppl. 2):25–30.
158. Cheung DG, Hoffman CA, Weber MA, Ricci ST. Mild hypertension in the elderly: a comparison of prazosin and enalapril. *Am J Med* 1989; 86(Suppl. 1B):87–90.
159. Eisalo A, Virta P. Treatment of hypertension in the elderly with labetalol. *Acta Med Scand* 1984; 665S:129–133.
160. Giles TD, Weber MA, Bartels DW, Silberman HM, Gilderman LP, Burris JF. Treatment of isolated systolic hypertension with labetalol in the elderly. *Arch Intern Med* 1990; 150:974–976.
161. Applegate WB, Borhani N, DeQuattro V, et al. Comparison of labetalol versus enalapril as monotherapy in elderly patients with hypertension: results of 24-hour ambulatory blood pressure monitoring. *Am J Med* 1991; 90:198–205.
162. Buhler FR, Burkhart F, Lutold BE, Kung M. Antihypertensive beta blocking action as related to renin and age: a pharmacologic tool to identify mechanisms in essential hypertension. *Am J Cardiol* 1975; 36:653–669.
163. Fritschka E, Distler A, Gotzen R, Thiede HM, Philipp T. Crossover comparison of nitrendipine with propranolol in patients with essential hypertension. *J Cardiovasc Pharmacol* 1984; 6(Suppl. 7):S1100–S1104.
164. Kiowski W, Buhler FR, Fadayomi MO. Age, race, blood pressure and renin: predictors for antihypertensive treatment with calcium antagonists. *Am J Cardiol* 1985; 56:81H–85H.
165. Buhler FR. Age and cardiovascular response adaptation. Determinants of an antihypertensive concept primarily based on beta-blockers and calcium entry blockers. *Hypertension* 1983; 5(Suppl. 3):III94–III100.
166. Evans MG, Olanoff LS, Hurwitz G, Cowart TD, Conradi EC. Use of nifedipine as an adjunct to current antihypertensive. *Arch Intern Med* 1984; 144:985–987.
167. Veterans Administration Cooperative Study Group on Antihypertensive Agents. Low-dose captopril for the treatment of mild to moderate hypertension. *Hypertension* 1983; Suppl. 5:III136–144.
168. Cheung DG, Gasster JL, Weber MA. Assessing duration of antihypertensive effects with whole-day blood pressure monitoring. *Arch Intern Med* 1989; 149:2021–2025.
169. Pedrinelli R, Fouad FM, Tarazi RC, Bravo EL, Textor SC. Nitrendipine, a calcium-entry blocker. Renal and humoral effects in human arterial hypertension. *Arch Intern Med* 1986; 146:62–65.
170. Weber MA, Drayer JIM, Baird WM. Echocardiographic evaluation of left ventricular hypertrophy. *J Cardiovasc Pharmacol* 1986; 8(Suppl. 3):S61–S68.
171. Leenen FHH, Smith DL, Farkas RM, Reeves RA, Marquez-Julio A. Vasodilators and regression of left ventricular hypertrophy: hydralazine versus prazosin in hypertensive humans. *Am J Med* 1987; 82:969–978.
172. Ventura HO, Frohlich ED, Messerli FH, Kobrin I, Kardon MB. Cardiovascular effects and regional blood flow distribution associated with angiotensin converting enzyme inhibition (captopril) in essential hypertension. *Am J Cardiol* 1985; 55:1023–1026.

# 8

# Hyperlipidemia in the Elderly

**Donald B. Hunninghake**
*University of Minnesota Hospital and Clinic, Minneapolis, Minnesota*

## INTRODUCTION

The major cause of death in older persons is atherosclerotic vascular disease (1). Men and women over 65 years of age have a higher prevalence of elevated serum cholesterol levels than younger groups (2,3). Although the evidence is more limited in older individuals than in middle-aged individuals, total and low-density lipoprotein cholesterol (LDL-C) appear to predict risk for developing coronary heart disease (CHD) (4). Thus it appears that lowering total and LDL-C levels in older individuals should be considered. However, there are some major unanswered questions regarding the benefits of cholesterol lowering in this age group. What is the reduction in risk, the effect on quality of life, the cost, and who should be treated? The National Cholesterol Education Program (NCEP) Expert Panel on the Detection and Management of High Blood Cholesterol in Adults presented an approach to the management of patients with high serum cholesterol levels, but it did not define management for patients greater than 60 years of age in any detail (5). The management of older patients is especially challenging because if a large segment of the older population receives active treatment for high blood cholesterol levels, this would significantly increase the total health care cost for the entire nation and for a segment of the population with limited incomes. On the other hand, if reduction of blood cholesterol levels significantly reduces the risk of CHD, the cost of medical therapy may be justified. In this chapter the term "older patient" refers to individuals $\geqslant$ 65 years. The focus is on summarizing the available information and approaches to management.

## LIPIDS AND LIPOPROTEINS

Cholesterol, cholesterol esters, and triglycerides are lipids that are insoluble in water. To circulate in the aqueous environment of blood, these lipids are complexed with phospholipids and protein in particles called lipoproteins. The protein components are called apoproteins, which serve the function of solubilization of fats in the blood, and they also regulate the uptake and metabolism of lipids by cells. The lipoproteins are frequently broken down into six classes based upon size, density, and composition (Table 1). Generally, only three lipoproteins—very low density lipoproteins (VLDL), LDL, and high-density lipoproteins (HDL)—are found in the serum of fasting individuals. LDL, HDL, and triglycerides are the primary clinical measures used to assess risk and to determine the need for and the type of therapeutic intervention.

### Low-Density Lipoprotein

LDL is the major cholesterol-containing lipoprotein. It is considered the major atherogenic lipoprotein and is the primary target of therapeutic interventions (5,6). It may be increased because of environmental reasons, including increased dietary saturated fat and cholesterol and obesity (7). It may also be increased in a variety of genetic disorders involving LDL receptor defects, such as familial hypercholesterolemia) and familial combined hyperlipidemia (overproduction of apoprotein $B_{100}$, apo-$B_{100}$-containing lipoproteins), and defective apo-$B_{100}$ (defective binding to LDL receptors) (8). There are also many secon-

**Table 1** Lipoprotein Classes and Composition

| Lipoprotein | Density (water = 1.000) | Composition (w %) Cholesterol | Triglycerides | Protein | Major apoprotein |
|---|---|---|---|---|---|
| Chylomicron | 0.940 | 5 | 85–90 | 1–2 | $B_{48}$, E, $C_{II}$ |
| VLDL | 0.940–1.006 | 20 | 60–70 | 5–10 | $B_{100}$, E, $C_{II}$ |
| Chylomicron remnant | 1.006–1.019 | 30 | 30 | 15–20 | $B_{48}$, E |
| VLDL remnant (IDL) | 1.006–1.019 | 30 | 30 | 15–20 | $B_{100}$, E |
| LDL | 1.019–1.063 | 50–60 | 4–8 | 20 | $B_{100}$ |
| HDL | 1.063–1.210 | 15–20 | 2–7 | 45–55 | $A_I$, $A_{II}$ |

HDL = high-density lipoprotein; IDL = low-density lipoprotein; VLDL = very-low-density lipoprotein.

dary causes, including hypothyroidism, nephrotic syndrome, renal failure, biliary cirrhosis, and drug administration, including thiazide diuretics, immunosuppressant drugs, and anabolic steroids (9).

## High-Density Lipoprotein

HDL seems to exert a protective effect on the development of atherosclerosis and is synthesized in both the liver and the intestine (10,11). One mechanism proposed for its protective effect is reverse cholesterol transport, the removal of cholesterol from cells to be delivered directly to the liver or indirectly via transfer of other lipoproteins for catabolism (12). It may also promote cholesterol efflux from macrophages or prevent oxidation and aggregation of LDL in the arterial wall. Unfortunately, no current tests directly measure the function of HDL. Low HDL levels may be genetically determined or related to nutritional and life-style habits: obesity, cigarette smoking, and lack of exercise. Certain drugs, such as $\beta$-adrenergic blocking agents, anabolic steroids, and progestational agents, also lower HDL levels. There is also a strong inverse relationship between HDL and triglyceride levels.

## VLDL (Triglycerides)

VLDL is a triglyceride-rich lipoprotein synthesized and secreted by the liver. Triglycerides are removed from VLDL by the action of lipoprotein lipase with the formation of more cholesterol-enriched lipoproteins (IDL), which can then either be taken up and catabolized by the LDL receptors on hepatocytes or converted to LDL. A number of genetic disorders are associated with hypertriglyceridemia, including familial hypertriglyceridemia, familial combined hyperlipidemia, and familial dysbetaliproproteinemia (type III) (13). Hypertriglyceridemia is closely associated with obesity and heavy ethanol intake. Estrogens, $\beta$-blockers, diabetes mellitus, and renal failure are also common causes. Plasma triglyceride levels are associated with the development of CHD, but they have not been documented as independent predictors of risk (14,15).

## Other Lipoprotein Risk Factors

A number of other components of the lipoprotein system are under investigation as predictors of CHD risk (16,17). The HDL subfractions ($HDL_2$ and $HDL_3$) are occasionally measured, with $HDL_2$ generally more predictive of risk than either the total or $HDL_3$. Small LDL particles, remnants of chylomicrons, and VLDL and IDL may also be predictors of risk (18,19). All these parameters are difficult and expensive to measure. There are no standardized measures, and their current application is limited to research. Apoproteins $A_1$ and B are frequently measured, but there is no standardized assay. There is one apo-$B_{100}$ in each atherogenic particle (VLDL, IDL, and LDL), so this test is an indirect measure of the number of atherogenic particles. Apo-$A_I$ is occasionally a better predictor of risk than total HDL. Lipoprotein(a) appears to be an independent risk factor for CHD, but it may be less important in the older population (20,21). There is also considerable interest in oxidized or modified LDL particles (22). At present, there is no need to measure any of these parameters routinely.

## RELATIONSHIP OF LIPIDS AND LIPOPROTEINS TO CARDIOVASCULAR DISEASE RISK

CHD is a major cause of death for middle-aged as well as older individuals of both sexes (Table 2) (23). Although the risk of developing CHD is considerably higher for middle-aged men than middle-aged women, the difference in risk gradually narrows, with only a small difference after age 75 for the two sexes (23). Of the 500,000 plus deaths due to CHD each year in the United States, the total number is approximately equal for the two sexes; women simply die at an older age (1,24). Thus the potential role of lipid and lipoprotein abnormalities in the development of CHD in the older age group is of considerable interest. The basic pathophysiological processes leading to atherosclerosis appear to be similar at all age groups (25), suggesting that it may be reasonable to extrapolate the principles of detection and intervention of lipid disorders to the older age groups.

Unfortunately, the majority of the studies that define the relative contribution of individual lipid and lipoprotein abnormalities to the risk of developing CHD and epidemiological studies have been done primarily in middle-aged men (26). Similarly, intervention studies that have demonstrated the benefit of lipid and lipoprotein alteration have been done primarily in middle-aged men (27,28). Recent studies have also shown that aggressive lipid intervention may slow the rate of progression or even cause regression of coronary atherosclerosis (29,30). In addition to CHD, other atherosclerotic cardiovascular diseases, including stroke, abdominal aneurysm, and various manifestations of peripheral arterial vascular disease, are a significant concern in the older population. There

**Table 2** Heart Disease Death Rates per 100,000, 1989

| | 65–74 Years | 75–84 Years | ≥85 Years |
|---|---|---|---|
| Total deaths | 2730 | 6321 | 15,594 |
| All heart disease | 984 | 2543 | 7,098 |
| Ischemic heart disease | 677 | 1738 | 4,617 |
| Other cardiovascular disease | 155 | 554 | 1,707 |

*Source*: Adapted from Ref. 23.

is minimal information on the significance of lipid and lipoprotein abnormalities in the development of these disease processes in the elderly (19,31). Thus, we are left with making decisions regarding the management of lipid disorders in the elderly by extrapolation of data in middle-aged men rather than good, scientific data in this specific age group.

A number of studies have investigated the relationship of total serum cholesterol to the development of CHD in older persons. Most studies have utilized CHD death as the principal end point. The most comprehensive evaluation of this problem was presented at a recent National Heart, Lung, and Blood Institute (NHLBI) workshop. The most recent follow-up data from 25 populations in 22 U.S. and international cohort studies were analyzed. Crude, relative, and absolute risk of fatal CHD were determined for individual studies and pooled across studies to determine a pooled estimate of risk. The duration of follow-up varied from 3 to 28 years. Risk was compared for those less than 65 years to those greater than 65 years. This aggregate analysis included approximately 475,000 men < 65 years and 24,000 men ⩾ 65 years. There were approximately 75,000 women < 65 years and 15,000 women ⩾ 65 years. There were a large number of men < 65 years, which was heavily influenced by the inclusion of the Multiple Risk Factor Intervention Trial, which has been extensively used to form the basis of U.S. policy. Total cholesterol values were available for most participants; LDL-C, HDL-C, and triglyceride levels were done for a more limited subfraction of the population. It should also be noted that these lipid determinations were frequently made many years before the eventual documentation of presence or absence of CHD and do not reflect the predictive value of recently determined lipids. The results of this extensive meta analysis are included in Table 3. It should be emphasized that the data in Table 3 refer to

**Table 3** Relative Risk of Fatal CHD from Pooled Data

| | Men | | Women | |
|---|---|---|---|---|
| | <65 | ≥65 | <65 | ≥65 |
| Cholesterol | 1.73 | 1.32 | 2.44 | 1.12 |
| LDL-cholesterol | 1.51 | 1.51 | 3.27 | 1.13[a] |
| HDL-cholesterol | 2.31 | 1.09[a] | 2.13 | 1.75 |
| Triglycerides | 1.16 | 1.24 | 1.98 | 1.39 |

Cholesterol = ⩾6.2 mM (240 mg/dl) versus <5.17 mM (200 mg/dl); LDL-cholesterol = ⩾4.14 mM (160 mg/dl) versus <3.62 mM (140 mg/dl); HDL-cholesterol = <1.20 mM (50 mg/dl) versus ⩾1.55 mM (60 mg/dl); triglycerides = ⩾1.47 mM (130 mg/dl) versus <1.13 mM (100 mg/dl).

[a] Not statistically significant.

*Source*: Adapted from Manolio TA, et al. *Ann Epidemiol* 1992; 2:18.

relative risk. Thus the relative risk for total LDL and HDL-C was higher for the middle-aged individuals than for the older individuals. It should be noted that the differences between the cut points for high and low values were quite small, especially for HDL-C and triglycerides.

There is very little information on the importance of the age at which lipids are measured as predictors of risk. For example, if a person is currently 75 years of age, do the cholesterol measurement done at age 55 and the current measurement have the same predictability? In the Honolulu Heart Program, cholesterol measurements at ages 52–59 had essentially the same predictability as cholesterol measurements made at age 65–74 (32). In contrast, data from the Whitehall Study suggested that cholesterol measurements made earlier in life were more predictive for developing disease at any given age than those made later in life (33).

The data presented in Table 3 on relative risk do not appear to be very dramatic. However, one must also consider absolute or excess risk. Absolute risk is relative risk times the expected frequency in the population. Thus a small increase in relative risk could markedly increase the frequency of disease in an older population with a high frequency of disease. The excess risk or absolute difference in disease rates is a better guide to the potential value of treating high blood cholesterol than the relative risk. This is illustrated in Table 4, where the relative risk associated with high blood cholesterol levels was similar between ages 60 and 79 years. However, the excess risk of CHD death due to high blood cholesterol levels was five times higher in the 75–79 year age group compared to the 60–64 year age group (34).

There is considerable epidemiological evidence that lipid management in the elderly would be beneficial. However, one would also like to have data from intervention trials that document the benefit of treatment in this age group, but definitive studies are lacking. The Stockholm Ischemic Heart Disease Study showed a decrease in both ischemic heart disease and total mortality in a small number of patients > 60 years of age when treated with a combination of clofibrate and niacin, but the numbers are small (35). At one time, the feeling was that if atherosclerosis were present, treatment was no longer beneficial. A variety of secondary prevention trials and regression studies have now demonstrated that the atherosclerotic process can be retarded or even reversed (29,30). Thus the severity of atherosclerotic disease in older patients should not be considered a contraindication for initiating therapy.

The pilot study for the Cholesterol Reduction in Seniors Program, which was funded by the National Heart, Lung, and Blood Institute, has been successfully completed, but the definitive study to document the benefits of lowering total and LDL-C levels in patients over 65 years has not been initiated. Gordon and Rifkind (37) calculated the theoretical benefit of cholesterol lowering in older individuals (Table 5), but documentation of benefit is still required in a major

**Table 4** Relative Risk and Excess Risk for Mortality from Coronary Heart Disease in 2746 White Men by 5-Year Age Intervals

| Age at entry (years) | Deaths due to coronary heart disease[a] cholesterol quartile | | | | Relative risk[b] | Excess risk[c] |
|---|---|---|---|---|---|---|
| | QI | QII | QIII | QIV | | |
| 60–64 | 5.3 | 5.2 | 6.5 | 7.8 | 1.4 (0.9–2.2) | 2.2 (−1.2 to 5.5) |
| 65–69 | 9.3 | 7.5 | 9.8 | 14.1 | 1.6 (1.0–2.5) | 5.2 (−0.3 to 10.8) |
| 70–74 | 12.3 | 9.0 | 13.6 | 19.6 | 1.7 (1.0–2.8) | 11.3 (−6.6 to 29.2) |
| 75–79 | 8.6 | 7.2 | 9.1 | 12.6 | 1.5 (1.2–2.0) | 4.3 (1.3–7.2) |

[a] Deaths per 1000 persons-years.
[b] Comparing mortality from coronary heart disease in men in the highest quartile of serum cholesterol with mortality in men in the three lower quartiles.
[c] Difference between mortality from coronary heart disease in the highest quartile of serum cholesterol and mortality in the three lower quartiles. QI is lowest quartile and QIV is the highest.
*Source*: Adapted from Rubin SM, et al. *Ann Intern Med* 1990; 113:916–920.

**Table 5** Potential Benefit of Reducing Cholesterol from 185 to 200 mg/dl

| Age group (years) | Decrease in CHD risk (%) | "Preventable" CHD deaths[a] | | "Preventable" CHD cases[b] | |
|---|---|---|---|---|---|
| | | Men | Women | Men | Women |
| 35–44 | 77.4 | 1.8 | 0.7 | 11.8 | 3.2 |
| 45–54 | 61.8 | 6.3 | 0.9 | 23.4 | 6.0 |
| 55–64 | 46.3 | 8.7 | 1.8 | 26.0 | 10.2 |
| 65–74 | 33.1 | 9.5 | 3.8 | 20.4 | 10.6 |
| 75–84 | 22.9 | 12.7 | 6.5 | 20.4 | 12.3 |

[a] Per 1000 patients per year. Estimated by applying calculated age-specific percentage decrease in CHD risk to age- and sex-specific CHD mortality rates in the Framingham Heart Study (1).

[b] Per 1000 patients per year, estimated as above. Totals include cases of myocardial infarction, coronary insufficiency, and agina pectoris in subjects without prior CHD manifestations, and all CHD deaths.

*Source*: Adapted from Gordon DJ, Rifkind BM. *Am J Cardiol* 1989; 63:48H–52H.

clinical trial. Their projections suggest that cholesterol lowering should be beneficial in older patients.

## NONLIPID RISK FACTORS

Other risk factors for developing coronary heart disease, such as cigarette smoking, hypertension, diabetes mellitus, and obesity, are associated with an increased risk of CHD in older patients (38–42). The frequency of these risk factors, with the exception of smoking, increases with increasing age. Obesity also contributes to the development of hypertension, hyperlipidemia, and diabetes mellitus. These risk factors also increase the likelihood of developing cerebrovascular and peripheral vascular disease (19,31). The benefits of smoking cessation are especially important in older patients (43), as are those related to management of hypertension, diabetes mellitus, and obesity. The recently completed Systolic Hypertension in the Elderly Program, which used chlorthalidone plus a $\beta$-adrenergic antagonist, if needed, for the treatment of isolated hypertension, demonstrated a significant reduction in cardiovascular events (44). There was a reduction in total and cardiovascular mortality and stroke. A 25% reduction in CHD events was also observed, which is greater than that observed in other studies, primarily in younger age groups. This study increases the expectation that lipid-lowering therapy may also reduce the risk of CHD, and possibly other CVD diseases, in older patients.

Since the benefits of lipid lowering have not been clearly established in this age group, it is very important to assess the projected quality of life, life expectancy, and benefits and risks of lipid-lowering therapy. Patients who have significant concomitant illnesses, such as congestive heart failure, stroke, dementia, chronic lung disease, or other debilitating diseases, such as severe arthritis, may not gain much in terms of either quality of life or life expectancy. A decrease in total mortality has not been documented for primary prevention but has been observed in secondary intervention trials (45,46). The benefits of cholesterol lowering in studies of middle-aged men were demonstrated within 2 years and were apparent after 5 years of treatment in the older patients in the Stockholm Ischemic Heart Disease Study (27–30,35). Thus, the benefit expected in older persons would be primarily a decrease in cardiac events, possibly cardiovascular, rather than an increase in life expectancy.

## APPROACH TO PATIENT MANAGEMENT

The preceding discussion emphasized that a definitive benefit of cholesterol lowering has not been documented in individuals who are 65 years and older. Thus, a highly individualized approach to the management of each patient is indicated. The need for screening and medical management requires an evaluation of physiological, psychological, sociological, and medical factors in each patient. Clinicians interpret these data differently and adopt their own approaches. The general approach that I have followed for primary prevention is to adhere to the guidelines proposed by the Adult Treatment Panel of NCEP if the patient is 75 years or younger. The conservative approach of individualized assessment of older patients for screening and medical management that is proposed in this chapter is shared by the majority (5,47), but others have criticized the approach as too costly if benefit has not been conclusively demonstrated (48). This is contingent upon the patient not having severe concomitant disease, that medical therapy does not pose a major impediment to their interpretation of quality of life, which includes financial considerations, and their desire to implement dietary and/or drug treatment. Occasional patients who are more than 75 years of age may be considered for medical management. There are fewer restrictions for dietary therapy than for drug therapy. Older patients are frequently interested in whether lipid reduction will reduce their risk of developing a stroke. The available information is even more limited for cerebrovascular disease than for CHD.

If the patient has CHD or other cardiovascular disease, the patient is treated irrespective of current age. Again, this is done only if there are no severe functional or quality of life restrictions or significant concomitant disease that would severely limit life expectancy. Patients with clinical evidence of arterial vascular disease would be expected to benefit more from treatment than those who are being treated for primary prevention. The majority of patients with evident CHD are older than 65 years. A paradox currently exists in the United States in that we aggressively utilize interventional strategies, such as coronary artery bypass graft surgery and angioplasty, in progressively older populations, but yet we are reluctant to manage the risk factors for the development of CHD in this age group.

## SCREENING AND DIAGNOSIS

The current recommendation of NCEP is that a total cholesterol be obtained on all adult patients 20 years and over (5). If one adhered to the current NCEP guidelines, some type of medical intervention would be required in 24 million individuals age 60 years or older (49). Thus screening efforts should be limited to individuals in whom one is willing at least to proceed to dietary intervention, if needed.

The current NCEP recommendations for initial classification and recommended follow-up are contained in Table 6. For this population, several changes are recommended. One is that all patients should have an HDL-C measurement. This is especially true for women who frequently have a high total cholesterol

**Table 6** Initial Classification and Recommended Follow-up Proposed by National Cholesterol Education Program

| Cholesterol reading | Classification |
|---|---|
| <200 mg/dl (<5.2 mM) | Desirable |
| 200–239 mg/dl (5.2–6.2 mM) | Borderline |
| ⩾240 mg/dl (⩾6.2 mM) | High |
| **Cholesterol reading** | **Recommended follow-up** |
| Total cholesterol < 200 mg/dl | Repeat within 5 years |
| Total cholesterol 200–239 mg/dl | Dietary information and recheck annually |
| • Without definite coronary heart disease or two other risk factors, one of which can be male sex | |
| • With definite coronary heart disease or two other risk factors, one of which can be male sex | Lipoprotein analysis; further action based on LDL cholesterol level |
| Total cholesterol ⩾ 240 mg/dl | Lipoprotein analysis; further action based on LDL cholesterol level |

Suggested modification for older patients

1. All patients should minimally have a total and HDL-C measurement (can be nonfasting).
2. All patients with CHD or symptomatic peripheral artery disease (PAD) should have a lipoprotein analysis.
3. Risk factors are defined as
   All older individuals
   Cigarette smoking
   Hypertension
   HDL-C ⩽ 35 mg/dl, confirmed by repeat measurement.
   Diabetes mellitus

because of an increase in HDL-C, especially if they are receiving estrogen replacement. Also, patients who have CHD or symptomatic peripheral vascular disease should immediately have a lipoprotein analysis. This is because both groups have a very high risk of having a myocardial infarction within the next few years (6,46,50). More than 35–50% of patients with symptoms of intermittent claudication will die within 5 years, primarily of CHD, if risk factor intervention is not employed (50). Lipoprotein analysis is defined as follows, with the Friedewald formula used for calculation of LDL-C when the triglyceride levels are $\leqslant$400 mg/dl (51):

$$\text{LDL-cholesterol} = \text{total} - \text{HDL-cholesterol} - \frac{\text{triglycerides}}{5}$$

LDL-cholesterol is still the major target for treatment in the NCEP guidelines (5). The current recommendations of NCEP are listed in Table 7. Low HDL-C levels are treated as a major risk factor and are secondary targets for treatment if they are low. Life-style modification and selection of LDL-C-lowering drugs that also increase HDL-C levels are recommended (discussed later). Triglyceride levels should be maintained below 500 mg/dl to reduce the risk of pancreatitis, and triglyceride levels $\geqslant$ 250 mg/dl after diet and life-style may be considered for drug therapy in patients with CHD or who have a high risk for developing CHD.50. The recommendations for management of HDL and trigly-

**Table 7** Classification and Treatment Decisions Based on LDL-Cholesterol Level Proposed by National Cholesterol Education Program

| | | |
|---|---|---|
| LDL-cholesterol reading | Classification | |
| < 130 mg/dl (< 3.4 mM) | Desirable | |
| 130–159 mg/dl (3.4–4.1 mM) | Borderline | |
| ≥ 160 mg/dl (≥ 4.1 mM) | High | |
| Dietary treatment | Initiation level | Minimum goal |
| Without coronary heart disease or two other risk factors | ≥ 160 mg/dl | < 160 mg/dl |
| With coronary heart disease or two other risk factors[a] | ≥ 130 mg/dl | < 130 mg/dl |
| Drug treatment | Initiation level | Minimum goal |
| Without coronary heart disease or two other risk factors | ≥ 190 mg/dl (≥ 4.9 mM) | < 160 mg/dl |
| With coronary heart disease or two other risk factors[a] | ≥ 160 mg/dl | < 130 mg/dl |

[a] Patients with coronary heart disease or symptomatic peripheral vascular disease. Many lipid specialists believe that dietary intervention should be implemented if the LDL-C levels are ≥ 100 mg/dl and that drug therapy should be initiated if the LDL-C is ≥ 130 mg/dl, with a minimum target level of < 100 mg/dl. These proposed modifications to the current guidelines may be too aggressive for many older patients.

cerides were reviewed in an NHLBI-sponsored consensus conference held on February 26 and 27, 1992, and no major changes were recommended in the original guidelines (52).

It is important to do an appropriate history and physical examination and perform laboratory tests to rule out secondary causes of hyperlipidemia. Diabetes mellitus and hypothyroidism are important considerations in this age group. Since hypothyroidism is frequently not clinically evident, routine measurement of thyroid stimulating hormone is recommended. Other secondary causes include chronic renal disease, liver disease, and various drugs. Secondary causes of hyperlipidemia should be corrected, if possible, to avoid the need for lipid intervention.

Rapid cholesterol determinations are now common in both physicians' offices and screening centers. Three widely used office analyzers—Abbot-Vision, Boehringer-Mannheim Reflotron, and Kodak Ektachem DT60 Analyzer—meet the National Cholesterol Education Program guidelines for accuracy and precision (53). There are many potential sources of inaccuracy, however, including the possibility of significant mistakes made by test operators. Field trials of cholesterol screening outside physicians' offices have demonstrated considerable error. If office testing is done, it is important to validate measurements by comparing the results of split specimens that are also analyzed by a certified laboratory guidelines for quality control, reagents, and other factors that influence measurement accuracy and precision (54–58). In general, cholesterol readings are more reliable than measures of triglycerides and HDL.

There are two major sources of variations in cholesterol measurements, assuming that appropriate collection methods are used and that diet is stable. The standard deviation for repeated measurements in an individual patient with average cholesterol values is 18 mg/dl. Therefore, 65% of the determinations are within $\pm 18$ mg/dl and 95% are within $\pm 36$ mg/dl of the mean value of multiple determinations. Variations can also be attributed to differing standards among laboratories. Current standards for laboratory certification require cholesterol measurements to be within 5% of the true value but will be reduced to 3% in the future. Thus 95% of the values for a patient with a true mean blood cholesterol measurement would be between 216 and 264 mg/dl. Measurement variability is an important consideration not only for initial classification, but also for follow-up during therapy.

## DIETARY THERAPY

The initial approach is always dietary and life-style modification. In the majority of older patients this should be the only type of medical management required. There is marked variation in the ability of older patients to make dietary modifications. On the one extreme are individuals who are quite active, mentally alert, living with a spouse, and sharing meals and who have diverse culinary interests. These individuals can be treated in a manner similar to that for much younger patients. In contrast, other individuals may be borderline or inadequate in intake of various nutrients. This is especially true for total calories, protein, calcium, iron, zinc, and certain vitamins (58). Patients may then also be at risk of poor nutrition because of depression, isolation, or concomitant disease. Some individuals may also have had a lifetime of certain dietary habits, and it will be very difficult for them to make changes and to introduce new foods. Many older patients have a tendency to consume the same diet with little variation because of cost, ease of preparation, or personal preference.

The current dietary recommendations of NCEP are the step 1 and step 2 diets (5). These diets are defined in Table 8. In most older patients the step 1 diet is adequate. For the smaller segment of this population who may be considered for the step 2 diet, this should be done under the supervision of a dietitian. The cost may be higher, but it is essential that the nutritional adequacy of the diet be maintained.

Most of the dietary elevation of LDL-C is due to increased dietary intake of saturated fatty acids and cholesterol and caloric intake greater than is required to maintain ideal body weight (7,59). Saturated fatty acids are primarily derived from high-fat dairy products, including whole milk, ice cream, cheese, cream, and butter; meat products, including beef, pork, lamb, and poultry skin; and tropical oils, such as coconut and palm oil. The intake of tropical oils is low in the United States, but these oils are found in many prepackaged foods used for snacks and desserts. Dietary cholesterol is primarily derived from egg yolks, organ meats, such as liver, and from meat products.

**Table 8** Dietary Therapy for High Blood Cholesterol Level

| | Recommended intake | |
|---|---|---|
| Nutrient | Step 1 diet | Step 2 diet |
| Total fatty acids | Less than 30% of total calories | Less than 30% of total calories |
| Saturated | Less than 10% of total calories | Less than 7% of total calories |
| Polyunsaturated | Up to 10% of total calories | Up to 10% of total calories |
| Monounsaturated | 10–15% of total calories | 10–15% of total calories |
| Carbohydrates | 50–60% of total calories | 50–60% of total calories |
| Protein | 10–20% of total calories | 10–20% of total calories |
| Cholesterol | Less than 300 mg/day | Less than 200 mg/day |
| Total calories | Achieve and maintain desirable weight | Achieve and maintain desirable weight |

Obesity is a major contributor not only to hyperlipidemia but also to other risk factors for CHD, including hypertension and diabetes mellitus (60–62). If a successful weight reduction program can be implemented, weight loss can significantly reduce the overall risk of CHD. Weight loss, especially if it is associated with increased exercise levels, also tends to increase HDL-C levels and lower triglyceride levels in addition to lowering LDL-C levels.

Dramatic changes in diet should not be made in older patients. Lean cuts of beef and pork, poultry, and fish can be substituted for fatty meats. Lean cuts of beef and pork have a cholesterol content similar to that of poultry and most seafood (63). The saturated fat content of fish is lower, but there is no significant difference in blood cholesterol levels between patients consuming lean beef or poultry and fish. A gradual change from high-fat to lower fat dairy products should be recommended. One should not eliminate dairy products because they are a necessary source of calcium, especially in older women, who are at increased risk of osteoporosis. If a patient is unable to reduce the fat content of dairy products, then the benefits of reducing saturated fat must be carefully weighed against the need for calcium supplementation.

Low-fat, high-carbohydrate diets may increase glucose intolerance in older patients (64). If total fat and calories are reduced by a decrease in saturated fat, it is best to substitute monounsaturated fats (olive and canola oil) if calorie balance must be maintained. Monounsaturated fatty acids do not lower HDL-C levels (65). Polyunsaturated fats of the $n - 6$ type are found in vegetable oils and should not exceed 10% of total calories. Although no adverse effects have been proven in humans, they can decrease HDL-C levels and suppress the immune system in animals (65,66). Older patients have depressed immune systems and are at increased risk for developing cancer. Fish is a good source of the $n - 3$ polyunsaturated fatty acids, which theoretically could reduce the risk of thrombus formation (67).

The diets of older patients should also have increased fiber intake. A variety of disorders, such as diverticulosis, diverticulitis, constipation, and cancer, can be benefited by dietary fiber. Additionally, soluble fibers, such as psyllium, oat bran, and pectins, may also produce some small additional cholesterol lowering (69,70).

There is limited evidence of the benefit of cholesterol-lowering diets in older patients. Dayton et al. studied the effect of a high polyunsaturated fat–low saturated fat diet in 846 men ranging in age from 50 to 89 years who were residing in a domiciliary (68). There was a 23% reduction in total cholesterol levels in the experimental group compared to a 10% reduction in the control group. The overall results of the study suggested a reduction in mortality from CHD and cerebral infarction in patients with pretreatment cholesterol levels above 233 mg/dl over an 8 year period of follow-up. The beneficial effects appeared to be equal for both the younger and older age groups. These results are not conclusive, but the data from this trial suggest that dietary treatment of hypercholesterolemia reduces the risk for cardiovascular events. Confirmation studies are desirable.

## DRUG THERAPY

Drug therapy should be considered for patients who can reasonably expect some long-term benefit since conclusive evidence of a reduction in risk for CHD has not been shown in this age group. This decision is based upon clinical expectation. The decision to initiate drug therapy should be made jointly by the patient and physician. The patient should understand that evidence of benefit from therapy has not been established, and the costs and side effects of drug therapy should be explained. Older patients may be more susceptible to the side effects of drugs because of decreased hepatic metabolism or renal excretion or presence of concomitant disease. The recommendations of NCEP for initiating drug therapy and the suggested target goals are listed in Table 7. The dose of drug should not be pushed to the point of toxicity or severe side effects simply to achieve the suggested target goal. Careful selection of candidates for drug therapy is also required because of the large number of older patients who are potentially candidates for drug therapy. The distribution of LDL-C levels for selected age groups in the U.S. population are indicated in Table 9.

## SPECIFIC DRUGS

### Bile Acid Sequestrants

The two major drugs in this category are cholestyramine and colestipol (71–73). These drugs are primarily used to lower low-density lipoprotein cholesterol, and they also produce a slight increase in high-density lipoprotein cholesterol and either have no effect or modestly elevate triglycerides. These drugs are primarily used in patients who have elevated LDL-C levels and triglycerides less than 200–250 mg/dl. The reductions in LDL-C are dose dependent, as are the side effects. The side effects are primarily gastrointestinal in nature, both upper and lower. Constipation is frequent and is one of the major reasons for poor acceptance in older patients.

Equivalent doses of cholestyramine and colestipol are 4 and 5 g, respectively. These medications are available in both individual packets as well as bulk containers. The usual amount of LDL-C lowering with two packets or scoops of these medications is about 15 and 25% for four packets or scoops per day. Patients who have lower LDL-C levels at baseline tend to have greater percentage reductions than those who have very high LDL-C levels. The sequestrants

**Table 9** Calculated Levels of Fasting (12 h or more) Serum LDL-Cholesterol for Persons Aged 20–74 Years by Sex and Age

| Sex and age (years) | Mean | Percentile 10th | 25th | 50th | 75th | 90th |
|---|---|---|---|---|---|---|
| Male | | | | | | |
| 20–74 | 140 | 92 | 113 | 136 | 164 | 181 |
| 35–44 | 145 | 96 | 116 | 138 | 176 | 203 |
| 45–54 | 150 | 103 | 119 | 146 | 171 | 195 |
| 55–64 | 148 | 101 | 118 | 147 | 171 | 206 |
| 65–74 | 149 | 105 | 120 | 144 | 174 | 199 |
| Female | | | | | | |
| 20–74 | 141 | 91 | 110 | 136 | 164 | 199 |
| 34–44 | 129 | 90 | 107 | 126 | 150 | 171 |
| 45–54 | 157 | 104 | 125 | 156 | 184 | 213 |
| 55–64 | 159 | 113 | 129 | 150 | 188 | 219 |
| 65–74 | 162 | 109 | 135 | 158 | 186 | 226 |

Means and selected percentiles in the United States, 1976–1980.

are generally administered either once or twice daily. If administered once daily, they should be administered within an hour of the evening meal.

The sequestrants produce modest increases in HDL-C in the range of 3–5%. The triglyceride levels may not be altered or may increase by 10% in patients with triglyceride levels below 200 mg/dl. There may be a much more marked increase in triglyceride and cholesterol levels in patients who are treated with these drugs if the triglyceride levels are greater than 500 mg/dl or in patients who have type III hypercholesterolemia. These two conditions are absolute contraindications to single-drug therapy. Generally, the sequestrants are not used in patients who have triglyceride levels above 200 mg/dl as single-drug therapy.

The sequestrants interfere with the normal enterohepatic recirculation of bile acids. They produce a marked increase in the fecal excretion of bile acids. There is an associated increased rate of conversion of cholesterol to bile acids in the liver, resulting in decreased hepatic cholesterol levels. This decrease in hepatic cholesterol levels stimulates the production of LDL receptors, with an increase in the uptake of LDL by the liver and increased catabolism of LDL.

The adverse effects of the sequestrants are primarily related to gastrointestinal complaints. Upper gastrointestinal complaints include belching, bloating, gas, abdominal pain, and nausea. The other major complaint is constipation, which frequently limits the use of this class of drugs, especially in this age group. The degree of constipation can be lessened by increased fluid intake and especially by increased consumption of fiber in the diet or use of fiber supplements. The use of soluble fiber, such as psyllium and oat bran, may also slightly increase the degree of cholesterol lowering that is achieved (68,69). Many patients also dislike the gritty consistency of the medication, which must be ingested.

These medications may also decrease the absorption of other drugs that are administered simultaneously. Although the general recommendation is that all drugs be administered either 1 h before or 4 h after the use of sequestrants, significant decreases in absorption have only been documented for the β-blockers, cardiac glycosides, coumarin anticoagulants, diuretics, and exogenously administered thyroid hormone (74). They also decrease the bioavailability of HMG coenzyme A (CoA)-reductase inhibitors, and if both drugs are used, it is probably best to administer the resin with the evening meal and the HMG CoA-reductase inhibitors at bedtime. There is a suggestion that the risk of cholelithiasis may be slightly greater with these drugs.

These drugs have been shown to reduce the risk of coronary disease in the Lipid Research Clinics–Coronary Primary Prevention Trial and when used in combination with other drugs in regression studies (27,29,30). These drugs are primarily used in patients with elevated LDL-C levels and relatively normal triglycerides. Smaller doses are frequently tolerated, especially if administered in association with a high-fiber diet or fiber supplements.

## Nicotinic Acid

Nicotinic acid or niacin has lipid-altering properties, but nicotinamide does not (73,75,76). Since these drugs are available in "over-the-counter" status, it is important to distinguish between the various preparations. Nicotinic acid lowers total and LDL-C and triglycerides and also increases HDL-C levels. It also favorably affects all other lipoprotein measures associated with increased risk for coronary heart disease, such as lowering Lp(a) and apolipoprotein B levels. It has been shown to reduce the risk of CHD, and long-term follow-up in the Coronary Drug Project was associated with decreased mortality. The drug has multiple side effects and thus is poorly tolerated in many patients. A major advantage is the relatively low cost, being the cheapest of all current hypolipidemic agents. Its over-the-counter status, however, precludes coverage by most third-party payers.

The dose-response effect of nicotinic acid has not been carefully defined in clinical trials. The available information suggests that lower doses ($\leqslant$1.5 g) per day are more effective in increasing HDL-C levels and in lowering triglycerides. Higher doses are generally required to lower LDL-C levels significantly. Increases in HDL-C levels ranging from 15 to 35% have been noted, and triglyceride reductions in the range of 20–50% are usually observed. The majority of these effects can be obtained with daily doses of 1.5 g or less. These doses generally reduce LDL-C by 10–15%, and 25–30% reductions are only noted when daily doses or 3 g or more is used.

Administration of nicotinic acid is associated with many side effects. Flushing, sense of warmth, pruritus, and other symptoms of venodilation are noted in essentially all patients when this drug is initiated. Many patients rapidly develop tolerance to these symptoms, but others do not. In some patients, the initial symptoms of flushing may be so severe and frightening that the patient may be unwilling to continue the medication. The degree of flushing can be decreased by taking the medication during or after meals or by pretreatment with aspirin or other inhibitors of prostaglandin synthesis. Several sustained-release or slow-release preparations are also available that usually cause significantly less flushing, but the frequency of other adverse effects may be greater. The degree of flushing is also greater in patients who are receiving other vasodilators, especially antihypertensive medication, and there may be a greater tendency for hypotensive symptoms. The drug should also be used cautiously in patients with angina pectoris. Increased frequency of angina has been reported, but it is not clear whether this is related to circulatory effects or increased anxiety.

There are also multiple other side effects, including upper gastrointestinal effects, such as nausea and heartburn, with some increased risk for developing peptic ulcer. Other major forms of toxicity include hyperglycemia, hyperuricemia, and hepatotoxicity. The risk of these complications increases with increasing dose and is generally believed to be significantly elevated if the total daily dose is 3 g or more. However, the older patient is especially vulnerable to these effects. They tend to have much more hyperglycemia, and the decreased renal function predisposes to the development of hyperuricemia and possibly gout, especially in males. The risk of hepatotoxicity appears to be greater with the sustained-release preparations. There are occasional reports of severe hepatic failure, even death, with the use of nicotinic acid. The usual pattern of hepatotoxicity is that of increased transaminase, alkaline phosphatase, and bilirubin. These symptoms can also be associated with other systemic complaints, including malaise, fatigue, and poor appetite. Sudden and dramatic decreases in cholesterol levels can be an indication of hepatotoxicity.

## HMG CoA-Reductase Inhibitors

Currently, three drugs are marketed in this category, including lovastatin, pravastatin, and simvastatin (73,77–81). This class of drugs is the most effective for lowering LDL-C levels. They also produce modest increases in HDL-C and decrease triglyceride levels. They are very easy to administer, and there are relatively few drug-drug interactions. Their use is well accepted by both physicians and patients. In general, they have been tolerated very well by older patients, with few adverse reactions. Lovastatin was marketed in 1987, and thus the long-term experience with these drugs is more limited than with the sequestrants and nicitonic acid. However, they are the most frequently prescribed class of drugs, they have been extensively evaluated in clinical trials, and there is also a large clinical experience. Early studies have shown a reduction in CHD risk, primarily in regression studies, but many clinical trials in both primary and secondary prevention are currently underway to assess the effect on both morbidity and mortality.

Equivalent doses of lovastatin and pravastatin are similar, and simvastatin is approximately twice as potent on a milligram basis. This class of drugs is primarily used to lower LDL-C, and they can be used in all kinds of lipid abnormalities, except those characterized by hypertriglyceridemia without an increase in LDL-C levels. The dose response is not linear. There is a greater percentage of reduction in LDL-C per milligram of drug administered with the smaller doses. Although the effects on HDL-C and triglycerides tend to be somewhat greater with the higher doses, there are only modest differences in these effects between the various doses of drug. Generally, 5–15% increases in HDL-C are noted, and 10–25% reductions in triglycerides are observed. Older patients, especially women, tend to have slightly greater decreases in LDL than younger patients.

The dose response for the various HMG CoA-reductase inhibitors is similar to that reported with lovastatin in the EXCEL Study (Table 10) (78). The dose of simvastatin would be reduced by one-half. If a single dose of drug is administered, it is most effective if given in the evening. Lovastatin is generally administered with the evening meal, pravastatin at bedtime, and simvastatin without regard for meals. At doses equivalent to 20 mg pravastatin or lovastatin, there is a slightly greater decrease in LDL-C if given twice daily compared to once daily.

The major adverse effects associated with administration of HMG CoA-reductase inhibitors are increases in transaminase levels and myopathy (defined as an elevated creatine kinase and myalgia). The frequency of transaminase elevations $\geqslant$ three times the upper limit of normal at daily doses equivalent to 20 mg lovastatin is generally the same as in a placebo group. With higher doses the frequency of these transaminase elevations ranges from 1 to 2%. The transaminase elevations are rapidly reversible with discontinuance of the drug or reduction in dosage. There is a sense that the frequency of transaminase elevations is greater in heavy consumers of alcohol and potentially other hepatotoxic drugs. Although there are no reported definitive trials, there is a general sense that elevated transaminase levels occur less frequently in older individuals, probably because of their decreased alcohol consumption.

**Table 10** Change from Baseline in Plasma Lipid and Lipoprotein Levels

| | Treatment group | | | | |
|---|---|---|---|---|---|
| | | Lovastatin | | | |
| Variable | Placebo | 20 mg, four times per month | 40 mg, four times per month | 20 mg, twice per day | 40 mg, twice per day |
| LDL-cholesterol | 0.4 (11) | −24.0 (11) | −30.0 (11) | −34.0 (11) | −40.0 (11) |
| HDL-cholesterol | 2.0 (12) | 6.6 (13) | 7.2 (13) | 8.6 (13) | 9.5 (13) |
| Total cholesterol | 0.7 (8) | −17.0 (8) | −22.0 (8) | −24.0 (8) | −29.0 (9) |
| Triglycerides | 3.6 | −10.0 | −14.0 | −16.0 | −19.0 |

*Source*: Adapted from Bradford R, et al. Expanded Clinical Evaluation of Lovastatin (EXCEL) Study results. I. Efficacy in modifying plasma lipoproteins and adverse event profile in 8245 patients with moderate hypercholesterolemia. *Arch Intern Med* 1991; 151:43–49.

The frequency of myopathy in the EXCEL Study was 0.1% at 40 mg lovastatin and about 0.2% for 80 mg per day of drug (78). These patients were not taking any drugs known to predispose to the development of myopathy. The risk of myopathy is increased if patients are taking other drugs, such as cyclosporine, gemfibrozil, niacin, and possibly erythromycin (82). The risk of myopathy also appears to be increased in patients with multiple disease states and is probably increased in any condition that tends to decrease the excretion of the drug. Thus, older patients may be at slightly greater risk for developing myopathy. It is not clear whether there is a difference in the risk for myopathy among the various drugs, but there are fewer case reports to date with pravastatin. A very limited number of patients have developed rhabdomyolysis and have required dialysis. Most of these cases of rhabdomyolysis were seen early in the development in this class of drugs, when the awareness of the need for early diagnosis and discontinuance of the medication was less well appreciated. Myopathy is a clinical diagnosis based upon symptoms of muscle aches, soreness, tenderness, and weakness and confirmed by the presence of markedly elevated creatine kinase levels. Modest degrees of exercise, including walking in some patients, is sufficient to cause a significant increase in creatine kinase levels, and thus the mere presence of elevated creatine kinase levels is not sufficient for the diagnosis. Some patients have nonspecific aches and pains without increased creatine kinase levels, and these patients probably do not have myopathy; however, the symptoms may disappear if the drug is discontinued, and it is difficult to be sure that the symptoms are not subjective rather than truly drug related.

## Gemfibrozil

Gemfibrozil (73,83,84) is primarily effective in lowering triglyceride levels, and it also increases HDL-C levels. The effect on LDL-C levels is quite variable. A 34% reduction in CHD risk was noted in the Helsinki Heart Study. The drug is easy to administer and is generally well tolerated. The major side effects are primarily gastrointestinal in nature. Fibric acid derivatives, such as gemfibrozil, increase the lithogenicity of bile and the risk of cholelithiasis.

Gemfibrozil is generally administered at a fixed dose of 600 mg twice daily. Gemfibrozil and its metabolites are primarily excreted by the kidney, and thus smaller doses may be indicated if serum creatinine or creatinine clearance is reduced. The drug is also highly bound to serum albumin, and low serum albumin levels necessitate a reduction in dose. It can also potentiate the effect of oral anticoagulants, such as warfarin.

Reductions in triglyceride levels in the range of 25–50% are usually observed with increases in HDL-C ranging from 10 to 25%. The greater increases in HDL-C levels are observed in hypertriglyceridemic patients. The reduction in LDL-C is in the range of 10–15% in patients without hypertriglyceridemia. In the presence of hypertriglyceridemia, the LDL-C levels may actually increase.

Gemfibrozil is primarily used to lower triglycerides. However, patients who had an elevation in both LDL-C and triglyceride levels obtained the greatest reduction in CHD risk in the Helsinki Heart Study. Thus, one of the indications for the use of this drug is to reduce the risk of CHD in patients with combined hyperlipidemia. More recent analyses indicate that the greatest reduction in risk occurs in patients who have an LDL-C/HDL-C ratio > 5 and triglyceride levels > 200 mg/dl (85).

## Probucol and Other Antioxidants

There is increasing evidence that modifications of LDL increase its atherogenic potential and uptake into the arterial wall. There is considerable interest in the possibility that agents that inhibit the oxidation of LDL will also decrease atherogenesis. Evidence for a reduction in the severity of atherosclerosis has been demonstrated in animals with the use of the antioxidant probucol (86). A clinical trial evaluating the effect of probucol on the progression of femoral atherosclerosis in humans is expected to be reported in 1993 (87). At present, the use of probucol is not recommended because of the lack of documented evidence of benefit, and there are limited long-term safety data (88). There are also many other antioxidants with suggestive evidence of benefit in humans. These include vitamin C, vitamin E, and $\beta$-carotene (89). Additional studies are also required with these agents to document benefit, appropriate doses, and the combination of antioxidants that should be used.

## SELECTION OF DRUGS

The major types of lipid and lipoprotein disorders that may be seen in older patients being considered for drug therapy are as follows.

### Elevated LDL-C and Triglycerides < 200 mg/dl

The majority of patients being considered for drug therapy fall into this category. The two major classes of drugs to be considered are the bile acid sequestering agents (BAS) and the HMG CoA-reductase inhibitors (HMGRI). The HMGRI are very effective and well tolerated. The BAS are more difficult to administer, but many older patients tolerate two scoops. Although aggressive management of older patients is not recommended, the combination of an HMGRI plus BAS can produce dramatic reductions in LDL-C, with fewer side effects and less cost than high doses of either drug. For example, a dose of an HMGRI equivalent to 20 mg lovastatin and two packets of BAS reduces LDL-C levels by 40% or more. Nicotinic acid can be used, but relatively high doses are frequently required to achieve the desired reduction in LDL-C.

### Elevated LDL-C and Triglycerides Between 200 and 400 mg/dl

Nicotinic acid is the ideal first drug to use in this disorder because it is an inhibitor of lipoprotein synthesis and decreases both LDL-C and triglyceride levels. However, many patients do not tolerate the high doses that are required. An HMGRI is the next drug of choice and effectively lowers LDL-C, but the triglyericde levels may remain elevated. Gemfibrozil lowers triglyceride levels, but the reduction in LDL-C levels is generally only about 5%. Combination therapy with an HMGRI plus either nicotinic acid or gemfibrozil is used in younger patients. These combinations are not recommended in older patients, who are more prone to develop myopathy or rhabdomyolysis.

### Triglycerides > 400 mg/dl

If drug therapy is indicated in this age group, gemfibrozil is usually the drug of first choice because it does not adversely affect blood glucose or uric acid levels. Nicotinic acid is very effective and less costly, but it has more side effects and increases the frequency of hyperglycemia and hyperuricemia or gout in these patients.

## SUMMARY

The benefits of lipid-lowering therapy have not been conclusively documented in older patients. However, the available epidemiological evidence indicates that high blood cholesterol levels are associated with an increased risk of developing CHD. The available data are sufficient to justify an individualized approach to the selection of patients for medical therapy, including both dietary and drug therapy. The utilization of drug therapy should be more conservative than the criteria selected for dietary therapy. Older patients with clinical evidence of CHD should be treated more aggressively than those selected for treatment for primary prevention.

## REFERENCES

1. Lerner DJ, Kannel WB. Patterns of coronary heart disease morbidity and mortality in the sexes: a 26-year follow-up of the Framingham population. *Am Heart J* 1986; 111:383–390.
2. National Center for Health Statistics. Total Serum Cholesterol Levels of Adults 20–74 Years of Age: United States, 1976–80. Hyattsville, MD: U.S. Department of Health and Human Services, Public Health Services, Public Health Service, National Center for Health Statistics; 1986: Vital and Health Statistics. Series II, No. 236, DHHS Publication No. (PHS) 86-1686.
3. Lipid Research Clinics Program Epidemiology Committee. Plasma lipid distributions in selected North American populations: the Lipid Research Clinics Program Prevalence Study. *Circulation* 1979; 60:427–39.
4. Manolio TA, Pearson TA, Wenger NK, Barrett-Connor E, Payne GH, Harlan WR. Cholesterol and heart disease in older person and women: review of an NHLBI workshop. *Ann Epidemiol* 1992; 2:101–176.
5. Expert Panel. Report of the National Cholesterol Education Program Expert Panel on Detection, Evaluation and Treatment of High Blood Cholesterol in Adults. *Arch Intern Med* 1988; 148:36–69.
6. Pekkanen J, Linn S, Heiss G, et al. Ten-year mortality from cardiovascular disease in relation to cholesterol level among men with and without preexisting cardiovascular disease. *N Engl J Med* 1990; 322:1700–1707.
7. Kris-Etherton PM, Krummel D, Russell ME, et al. The effect of diet on plasma lipids, lipoproteins, and coronary heart disease. *J Am Diet Assoc* 1988; 88:1373–1400.
8. Zannis VI, Breslow JL. Genetic mutations affecting human lipoprotein metabolism. *Adv Hum Genet* 1985; 14:125–215.
9. Durrington PN. Secondary hyperlipidemia. *Br Med Bull* 1990; 46:1005–1024.
10. Gordon DJ, Probstfield JL, Garrison RJ, et al. High-density lipoprotein cholesterol and cardiovascular disease: four prospective American studies. *Circulation* 1989; 79:8–15.
11. Livshits G, Weisbort J, Meshulam N, Brunner D. Multivariate analysis of the twenty-year follow-up of the Donolo-Tel Aviv prospective Coronary Artery Disease Study and the usefulness of high density lipoprotein cholesterol percentage. *Am J Cardiol* 1989; 63:676–681.
12. Tall AR. Plasma high density lipoproteins. Metabolism and relationship to atherogenesis. *J Clin Invest* 1989; 63:676–681.

13. Grundy SM, Vega, GL. Hypertriglyceridemia: causes and relation to coronary heart disease. *Semin Trhomb Hemost* 1988; 14:149–164.
14. Austin MA. Plasma triglyceride and coronary heart disease. *Arterioscler Thromb* 1991; 11:2–14.
15. Schaefer EJ, McNamara JR, Genest J, Ordovas JM. Clinical significance of hypertriglyceridemia. *Semin Thromb Hemost* 1988; 14:143–148.
16. Stampfer MJ, Sacks FM, Salvini S, Willett WC, Hennekens CH. A prospective study of cholesterol apolipoproteins, and the risk of myocardial infarction. *N Engl J Med* 1991; 325:373–381.
17. Miller NE. Associations of high-density lipoprotein subclasses and apolipoproteins with ischemic heart disease and coronary atherosclerosis. *Am Heart J* 1987; 113:589–597.
18. Tell GA, Crouse JR, Furberg CD. Relation between blood lipids, lipoproteins, and cerebrovascular atherosclerosis: a review. *Stroke* 1988; 19:423–430.
19. Pomrehn P, Duncan B, Weissfeld L, et al. The association of dyslipoproteinemia with symptoms and signs of peripheral arterial disease. *Circulation* 1986; 73(Suppl.1):100–107.
20. Scann AM. Lipoprotein(a). A genetic risk factor for premature coronary heart disease. *JAMA* 1992; 267:3326–3329.
21. Rhoads GG, Dahlen G, Berg K, Morton NE, Dannenberg AL. Lp(a) lipoprotein as a risk factor for myocardial infarction. *JAMA* 1986; 256:2540–2544.
22. Ylä-Herttuala S, Palinski W, Rosenfeld ME, et al. Evidence for the presence of oxidatively modified low density lipoprotein in atherosclerotic lesions of rabbit and man. *J Clin Invest* 1989; 84:1086–1095.
23. U.S. Dept. of Health and Human Services. Vital Statistics of the United States 1988. Vol. II. Mortality, Part A. Hyattsville, MD, 1991.
24. Pisa Z, Uemura K. Trends of mortality from ischaemic heart disease and other cardiovascular disease in 27 countries, 1968–1977. *World Health Stat Q* 1982; 35:11–47.
25. Ross R. Atherosclerotic coronary heart disease: factors influencing atherogenesis. In: Hurst JW, Schlant RC, eds. The Heart, Arteries and Veins. New York: McGraw-Hill, 1990:877–892.
26. Simons LA. Interrelations of lipids and lipoproteins with coronary artery disease mortality in 19 countries. *Am J Cardiol* 1986; 57:56–106.
27. Lipid Research Clinics Program. The Lipid Research Clinics Coronary Primary Prevention Trials results. I. Reduction in incidence of coronary heart disease. *JAMA* 1984; 251:351-364.
28. Frick M, Elo O, Haapa K, et al. Helsinki Heart Study: primary-prevention trial with gemfibrozil in middle-aged men with dyslipidemia: safety of treatment, changes in risk factors, and incidence of coronary heart disease. *N Engl J Med* 1987; 317:1237–1245.
29. Blankenhorn D, Nessim S, Johnson R, Sanmarco M, Azen SC. Beneficial effects of combined colestipol-niacin therapy on coronary atherosclerosis and coronary venous bypass grafts. *JAMA* 1987; 257:3233–3240.
30. Brown G, Albers J, Fisher L, et al. Regression of coronary artery disease as a

result of intensive lipid-lowering therapy in men with high levels of apolipoprotein B. *N Engl J Med* 1990; 323:1289–1298.
31. Tell GA, Crouse JR, Furberg CD. Relation between blood lipids, lipoproteins, and cerebrovascular atherosclerosis: a review. *Stroke* 1988; 19:423–430.
32. Benfante R, Reed D. Is elevated serum cholesterol level a risk factor coronary heart disease in the elderly? *JAMA* 1990; 263:393–396.
33. Rose G, Shipley M. Plasma cholesterol concentration and death from coronary heart disease: 10 year results of the Whitehall study. *Br Med J* 1986; 293:306–307.
34. Rubin SM, Sidney S, Black DM, Browner WS, Hulley SB, Cummings SR. High blood cholesterol in elderly men and the excess risk for coronary heart disease. *Ann Intern Med* 1990; 113:916–920.
35. Carlson LA, Rosenhamer G. Reduction of mortality in the Stockholm Ischaemic Heart Disease Secondary Prevention Study by combined treatment with clofibrate and nicotinic acid. *Acta Med Scand* 1988; 223:405–418.
36. Canner PL, Berge KG, Wenger NK, et al. Fifteen year mortality in Coronary Drug Project patients: long-term benefit with niacin. *J Am Coll Cardiol* 1986; 8:1245–1255.
37. Gordon DJ, Rifkind BM. Treating high blood cholesterol in the older patient. *Am J Cardiol* 1989; 63:48H–52H.
38. Anderson KM, Castelli WP, Levy D. Cholesterol and mortality. 30 years of follow-up from the Framingham study. *JAMA* 1987; 257:2176–2180.
39. Kannel W, Brand F. Cardiovascular risk factors in the elderly. In: Andrews R, Bierman EL, Hazzard WR, eds. Principles of Geriatric Medicine. New York: McGraw-Hill, 1985.
40. Applegate WB. Hypertension in elderly patients. *Ann Intern Med* 1989; 110:901–905.
41. Castelli WP, Wilson PWF, Levy D, Anderson K. Cardiovascular disease in the elderly. *Am J Cardiol* 1989; 63:12H–19H.
42. Taylor WC, Pass TM, Shepard DS, Komaroff AF. Cholesterol reduction and life expectancy. A model incorporating multiple risk factors. *Ann Intern Med* 1987; 106:605–614.
43. Hermanson B, Omenn GS, Kronmal RA, Gersh BJ. Beneficial six-year outcome of smoking cessation in older men and women from coronary artery disease. Results from the CASS registry. *N Engl J Med* 1988; 319:1365–136.
44. SHEP Cooperative Research Group. Prevention of stroke by antihypertensive drug treatment in older persons with isolated systolic hypertension. Final results of the Systolic Hypertension in the Elderly Program. *JAMA* 1991; 265:3255–3264.
45. Muldoon MF, Manuck SB, Matthews KA. Lowering cholesterol concentrations and mortality: a quantitative review of primary prevention trials. *Br Med J* 1990; 301:309–314.
46. Roussouw JE, Lewis B, Rifkind BM. The value of lowering cholesterol after myocardial infarction. *N Engl J Med* 1990; 323:1112–1119.
47. Demke MA, Grundy SM. Hypercholesterolemia in elderly persons: resolving the treatment dilemma. *Ann Intern Med* 1990; 112:780–792.
48. Garber AM, Littenberg B, Sox HC, Wagner SL, Gluck M. Costs and health conse-

quences of cholesterol screening for asymptomatic older Americans. *Arch Intern Med* 1991; 151:1089–1095.
49. Sempos C, Fulwood R, Haines C, et al. The prevalence of high blood cholesterol levels among adults in the United States. *JAMA* 1989; 262:45–52.
50. Howell MA, Colgan MP, Seeger RW, Ramsey DE, Sumner DS. Relationship of severity of lower limb peripheral vascular disease to mortality and morbidity: a six-year follow-up study. *J Vasc Surg* 1989; 9:691–696.
51. Friedwald WT, Levy RI, Frederickson DS. Estimation of the concentration of LDL-C in plasma without use of preparatory ultracentrifuge. *Clin Chem* 1972; 18:499–502.
52. Consensus Conference. Treatment of hypertriglyceridemia. *JAMA* 1984; 251:1196–1200.
53. Burke JJ II, Fischer PM. A clinicna's guide to the office measurement of cholesterol. *JAMA* 1988; 259:3444.
54. Koch DD, Hassemer DJ, Wiebe JA, et al. Testing cholesterol accuracy—performance of several common laboratory instruments. *JAMA* 1988: 260:252.
55. Kaufman HW, McNamara JR, Anderson KM, et al. How reliably can compact chemistry analyzers measure lipids? *JAMA* 1990; 263:1245.
56. Myers GL, Cooper GR, Winn CL, Smith SJ. Centers for Disease Control–National Heart, Lung and Blood Institute Lipid Standardization Program. An approach to accurate and precise lipid measurements. *Clin Lab Med* 1989; 9:105–135.
57. Laboratory Standardization Panel, National Cholesterol Education Program. Recommendations for improving cholesterol measurement. Bethesda, MD: National Heart, Lung, and Blood Institute, 1990; DHHS Publication No. (NIH) 90-2964.
58. Morley JE, Mooradian AD, Silver AJ, Herber D, Alfin-Slater RB. Nutrition in the elderly. *Ann Intern Med* 1988; 109:890–904.
59. Grundy SM. Cholesterol and coronary heart disease. A new era. *JAMA* 1986; 256:2849–2858.
60. Garrison RJ, Wilson PW, Castelli WP, Feinleib M, Kannel WB, McNamara PM. Obesity and lipoprotein cholesterol in the Framingham offspring study. *Metabolism* 1980; 29:1053–1060.
61. Chiang BN, Perlman LV, Epstein FH. Overweight and hypertension. A review. *Circulation* 1969; 39:403–21.
62. Huges TA, Gwynne JT, Switzer BR, Herbst C, White G. Effects of caloric restriction and weight loss on glycemic control, insulin release and resistance, and atherosclerotic risk in obese patients with type II diabetes mellitus. *Am J Med* 1984; 77:7–17.
63. National Research Council (U.S.). Committee on Technological Options to Improve the Nutritional Attributes of Animal Products. Designing Foods: Animal Product Options in the Marketplace. Washington, DC: National Academy Press, 1988.
64. Garg A, Bonanome A, Grundy SM, Zhang ZJ, Unger RH. Comparison of a high-carbohydrate diet with a high-monounsaturated-fat diet in patients with non-insulin dependent diabetes mellitus. *N Engl J Med* 1988; 319:829–834.

65. Mattson FH, Grundy SM. Comparison of effects of dietary saturated, monounsaturated, and polyunsaturated fatty acids on plasma lipids and lipoproteins in man. *J Lipid Res* 1985; 26:194–202.
66. Bennett M, Uauy R, Grundy SM. Dietary fatty acid effects in T-cell-mediated immunity in mice infected with *Mycoplasma pulmonis* or given carcinogens by injection. *Am J Pathol* 1987; 126:103–113.
67. Knapp HR, Reilley IA, Alessandrini P, Fitgerald GA. In vivo indexes of platelet and vascular function during fish-oil administration in patients with atherosclerosis. *N Engl J Med* 1986; 314:937–942.
68. Bell LP, Hectorne K, Reynolds H, Balm TK, Hunninghake DB. Cholesterol-lowering effects of psyllium hydrophilic mucilloid. *JAMA* 1989; 261:3419–3423.
69. Davidson MH, Dugan LD, Burns JH, Bova J, Story K, Drennan KB. The hypocholesterolemic effects of β-glucan in oatmeal and oat bran. *JAMA* 1991; 265:1833–1839.
70. Dayton S, Pearce ML, Hoshimoto S, Dixon WJ, Tomiyasu U. A controlled trial of a diet high in unsaturated fat in preventing complications of atherosclerosis. *Circulation* 1969; 60(Suppl.2):1–63.
71. Hunninghake DB, Probstfield JL. Drug treatment of hyperlipoproteinemia. In: Rifkind BM, Levy RI, eds. New York: Grune & Stratton, 1977:327–362.
72. Ast M, Frishman WH. Bile acid sequestrants. *J Clin Pharmacol* 1990; 30:99–106.
73. Hunninghake DB. Drug treatment of dyslipoproteinemia. *Endocrinol Metab Clin North Am* 1990; 19:345–360.
74. Hunninghake DB. Resin therapy: adverse effects and their management. In: Fears R, ed. Pharmacological Control of Hyperlipidemia. Barcelona: J. R. Prous, 1986:67–89.
75. Drood JM, Zimetbaum PJ, Frishman WH. Nicotinic acid for the treatment of hyperlipoproteinemia. *J Clin Pharmacol* 1991; 31:641–650.
76. Figge HL, Figge J, Souney PF, Mutnick AH, Sacks F. Nicotinic acid: a review of its clinical use in the treatment of lipid disorders. *Pharmacotherapy* 1988; 8:287–294.
77. Grundy SM. HMG CoA reductase inhibitors for treatment of hypercholesterolemia. *N Engl J Med* 1988; 319:24–33.
78. Bradford R, Shear C, Chremos A, et al. Expanded Clinical Evaluation of Lovastatin (EXCEL) Study results. I. Efficacy in modifying plasma lipoproteins and adverse event profile in 8245 patients with moderate hypercholesterolemia. *Arch Intern Med* 1991; 151:43–49.
79. McTavish D, Sorkin EM. Pravastatin. A review of its pharmacological properties and therapeutic potential in hypercholesterolemia. *Drugs* 1991; 42:65–89.
80. Hunninghake DB, Mellies MJ, Goldberg AC, et al. Efficacy and safety of pravastatin in patients with primary hypercholesterolemia. II. Once-daily versus twice-daily dosing. *Atherosclerosis* 1990; 85:219–227.
81. Todd PA, Goa KL. Simvastatin. A review of its pharmacological properties and therapeutic potential in hypercholesterolemia. *Drugs* 1990; 40:583–607.
82. Tobert JA. Efficacy and long-term adverse effect pattern of lovastatin. *Am J Cardiol* 1988; 62:28J–34J.

83. Frick M, Elo O, Haapa K, et al. Helsinki Heart Study: primary-prevention trial with gemfibrozil in middle-aged men with dyslipidemia; safety of treatment, changes in risk factors, and incidence of coronary heart disease. *N Engl J Med* 1987; 317:1237–1245.
84. Todd P, Ward A. Gemfibrozil: a review of its pharmacodynamic and pharmacokinetic properties, and therapeutic use in dyslipidaemia. *Drugs* 1988; 36:314–339.
85. Manninen V, Tenkanen L, Koskinen P, et al. Joint effects of serum triglyceride and LDL cholesterol and HDL cholesterol concentrations on coronary heart disease risk in the Helsinki Heart Study. *Circulation* 1992; 85:37–45.
86. Kita T, Nagano Y, Yokode M, et al. Prevention of atherosclerotic progression in Watanabe rabbits by probucol. *Am J Cardiol* 1988; 62(Suppl.B):13–19.
87. Walldius G, Carlson LA, Erikson U, et al. Development of femoral atherosclerosis in hypercholesterolemic patients during treatment with cholestyramine and probucol/placebo: Probucod Quantitative Regression Swedish Trial (PQRST): a status report. *Am J Cardiol* 1988; 62(Suppl. B):37–43.
88. Buckley MMT, Goa KL, Price AH, Brogden RN. Probucol. A reappraisal of its pharmacological properties and therapeutic use in hypercholesterolemia. *Drugs* 1989; 37:761–800.
89. Steinberg D, workshop participants. Antioxidants in the prevention of human atherosclerosis. Summary of the proceedings of a National Heart, Lung, and Blood Institute workshop: September 5–6, 1991, Bethesda, MD. *Circulation* 1992; 85:2337–2344.

# 9

# Anticoagulation Therapy in the Elderly

**James L. Sebastian**
*Medical College of Wisconsin, Milwaukee, Wisconsin*

**Donald D. Tresch**
*Medical College of Wisconsin and University of Wisconsin, Milwaukee, Wisconsin*

## INTRODUCTION

The use of long-term anticoagulation has recently increased, especially in elderly patients. There may be several reasons to account for this. First, less intense treatment regimens have recently been shown to be associated with lower rates of serious bleeding complications compared to more traditional treatment regimens that used higher doses of medication (1–4). Second, data from several large-scale, randomized clinical trials have more clearly defined the risks and benefits of anticoagulating elderly patients. For example, in the setting of nonvalvular atrial fibrillation, older patients (mean age > 65) who were treated with warfarin experienced a 60–70% reduction in their risk of stroke (5–8). This risk reduction was achieved with an acceptably low rate of serious bleeding complications, which averaged only 1–2% per year. Based on such evidence, many clinicians now seem to be more willing to treat their patients, particularly their elderly patients, with long-term anticoagulants.

The issue of anticoagulation in the elderly is important to address because of the sheer frequency of thrombotic disorders in this age group. Clinicians caring for such patients would like to know which individuals are at highest risk for the development of thrombotic complications so that preventive and treatment strategies could be targeted at those who would potentially benefit most from anticoagulation. Is it possible to identify specific risk factors in older individuals that predispose them to develop thrombosis? Are the elderly inherently hypercoagulable?

In general, it seems that there are no differences in coagulation factors when individuals aged 50–80 are compared with younger people (9–11). Although there are no major biochemical differences in the hemostatic mechanisms between young and old (12), some data suggest that the fibrinolytic response may be lower in patients who are older than age 65 (13). The high prevalence of thrombotic disorders in the elderly appears to be in large part related to the frequency of underlying conditions that predispose individuals to develop thrombosis. Examples of such predisposing conditions that are prevalent in the elderly include congestive heart failure, malignancy, surgery, and immobility. Since many of these disease states and conditions are clinically apparent, it seems possible to target high-risk patients for preventive treatment with long-term anticoagulation.

In this chapter we (1) summarize the major indications for long-term anticoagulation; (2) discuss some of the risk factors thought to be responsible for the hemorrhagic complications related to the use of heparin and/or sodium warfarin; and (3) review some practical considerations associated with the use of these drugs. We have attempted to focus on the specific risks and benefits of anticoagulating the elderly, but many of our remarks may also be applied to younger age groups.

Because the intensity of anticoagulation is intimately related to issues of safety and efficacy, we begin our discussion with an explanation of how contemporary oral anticoagulant treatment regimens should be monitored and reported.

## RATIONALE FOR USE OF THE INTERNATIONAL NORMALIZED RATIO

Over the past 40 years, the one-stage prothrombin time (PT) test has become the standard method of monitoring the status of patients who are receiving long-term oral anticoagulation. The PT test is easily performed by adding a mixture of calcium and thromboplastin to a sample of the patient's plasma. Although the PT results from a given laboratory are generally quite reproducible, clinicians may become confused when they attempt to equate the results obtained from different laboratories. Some of this confusion relates to the fact that reporting systems vary between laboratories, and PT results may be expressed in terms of seconds, ratios, or percentage activity (14). More importantly, however, there has been a growing recognition that the results obtained from one laboratory may not be directly comparable to the results obtained from a different laboratory if each utilizes a different tissue thromboplastin to measure the PT (15).

Tissue thromboplastins can be obtained from different sources (human brain, rabbit brain, bovine brain, and others) and prepared by different methods. These differences may result in thromboplastins that vary widely in their sensitivities to the reduction of the vitamin K-dependent clotting factors (16). For example, rabbit brain thromboplastins, commonly used in North America, are generally less sensitive than the human brain thromboplastins more commonly used in European and U.K. laboratories (17).

To further complicate matters, one lot or batch of a specific thromboplastin may be more or less responsive to the anticoagulant effects of warfarin than other lots or batches of the same thromboplastin. Thus, batch-to-batch variations in thromboplastin sensitivity may explain some differences in an individual's degree of anticoagulant control when serial PT measured in the same laboratory are compared over time.

It is also not difficult to see how significant problems may have arisen in both the interpretation and generalizability of PT results reported by different laboratories. Previous reports of clinically important differences in the mean dose of warfarin used in various countries may have been due, at least in part, to significant differences in the sensitivity of uncalibrated thromboplastins (17,18).

When prothrombin time results are expressed only as the ratio of the patient's PT to the control PT, the clinical implications of using different thromboplastins to perform the "same" test are profound. Use of low-sensitivity thromboplastins may lead to overanticoagulation and an increased risk of hemorrhage; use of thromboplastins with greater sensitivity may cause underanticoagulation and lead to an increased risk of thromboembolism (19).

To address these inconsistencies, the World Health Organization (WHO) recently recommended that, when the prothrombin time is used as a measure of long-term anticoagulant control, results should be "normalized" by using a system of thromboplastin calibration (20). An international committee has since recommended the adoption of a uniform reporting system in which the PT results are standardized and reported in terms of an international normalized ratio (INR) (21). The INR is equal to the prothrombin time ratio (PTR) raised to the power of the international sensitivity index (ISI); that is,

$$\text{INR} = \text{PTR}^{\text{ISI}}$$

where PTR represents the patient's PT divided by the control PT. The ISI is simply a measure of thromboplastin responsiveness. It is obtained by calibrating a given thromboplastin reagent against a WHO standard thromboplastin, the international reference preparation (IRP), which has been arbitrarily assigned an ISI of 1.0 (22). Thus, when this IRP is the thromboplastin used to perform the prothrombin time test, the INR is numerically equal to the PTR ($\text{INR} = \text{PTR}^1$).

Manchester Comparative Reagent, the thromboplastin used in almost all U.K. hospitals, has an ISI that is close to 1.0, signifying that it is quite sensitive to the reduction of vitamin K-dependent coagulation factors. Thromboplastins commonly used in the United States generally are less sensitive to the reduction of these same coagulation factors and have higher ISI. Poller found that most of the commercial rabbit brain thromboplastins commonly used in North America had ISI that varied between 2.0 and 2.6 (15). More recently, Bussey and colleagues reported that only a small percentage of the laboratories they surveyed were using thromboplastins with ISI in this range (19). The ISI of most thromboplastins used in the United States were found to vary even more widely with a range between 1.8 and 2.8 (19). Only a small proportion of North American thromboplastin reagents had an ISI value as low as 1.4.

By taking into account the potential for such a wide range of thromboplastin sensitivities, calculation of the INR provides an internationally standardized "common denominator" for reporting the intensity of long-term oral anticoagulation. In the discussion that follows we attempt to report the intensity of all oral anticoagulant treatment regimens in terms of the international normalized ratio.

## INTENSITY OF TREATMENT

Recent guidelines from the American College of Chest Physicians (ACCP) simplify the target treatment goals of long-term anticoagulation. In applying these guidelines to clinical practice, physicians need to consider whether individual patients will require "more intense" or "less intense" treatment regimens (17).

*More intense* levels of anticoagulation are recommended for patients with mechanical heart valves and individuals with a history of previous sytemic emboli. For such patients, the desired goal of treatment is to achieve and maintain a prothrombin time ratio in the range of 1.5–2.0 times control using a typical North American (rabbit brain) thromboplastin. This PTR corresponds to an INR of 3.0–4.5 when a thromboplastin with an ISI of 2.4 is used. *Less intense* treatment regimens, which aim for a target PTR of 1.3–1.5 times control using a typical North American (rabbit brain) thromboplastin, are recommended for all other patients who require long-term oral anticoagulation. The PTR for this *less intense* regimen corresponds to an INR of 2.0–3.0 when a thromboplastin with an ISI of 2.4 is used.

## IMPLEMENTATION OF AN INR REPORTING SYSTEM

The conversion from a laboratory system that reports PT results in terms of seconds, ratios, or percentage activity to one that utilizes the INR can be relatively easy to accomplish. Some laboratories already have autoanalyzers that are equipped to provide PT results in terms of the INR. For other laboratories, INR can be easily calculated by laboratory personnel ($INR = PTR^{ISI}$) or determined from simple charts or conversion tables supplied by thromboplastin manufacturers.

Use of a "double-reporting system" during the period of laboratory transition helps clinicians become acquainted with the usefulness and limitations of the INR calibration system (14). Figure 1 provides an example of the revised PT report currently used in the anticoagulation clinic at our Veterans Affairs Medical Center.

## INDICATIONS FOR TREATMENT

In this section we discuss the following indications for treatment with long-term anticoagulants: (1) nonvalvular and lone atrial fibrillation, (2) venous thromboembolic disease, (3) valvular heart disease and prosthetic heart valves, (4) ischemic heart disease, (5) dilated congestive cardiomyopathy, (6) ischemic cerebral vascular disease, and (7) peripheral vascular disease. The following discussion is by no means comprehensive, but it does address many of the thrombotic diseases and conditions that are common in the elderly.

### Nonvalvular Atrial Fibrillation

Atrial fibrillation (AF) is the most common cardiac rhythm disturbance in elderly patients (23). It has been estimated that AF occurs with a frequency of

**Milwaukee Clinical Laboratory Report**

Smith, John Q. 12/18/91 09:28
SSN: 123-45-6789 Sex: M Age: 67 Loc: LAMB

Ordered by: Sebastian, James L MD
Specimen: Plasma COAG 1218 35 12/18/91 08:56

| Test Name | Result | Units | Reference Range |
|---|---|---|---|
| PROTIME | 17.0 H | Sec | 11.4- 12.9 |
| INR | 2.54 | Ratio | |

INR= International Normalized Ratio

| Indication | PT Ratio | INR |
|---|---|---|
| Mechanical heart valves | 1.5-2.0 | 3.0-4.5 |
| Recurrent systemic embolism | 1.5-2.0 | 3.0-4.5 |
| All other indications | 1.3-1.5 | 2.0-3.0 |

**Figure 1** Example of a double-reporting system for prothrombin times and INR.

about 1–2% in the U.S. public over age 60, but the prevalence of AF in the very elderly may be substantially higher (24). For example, Aronow (25) reported a 13% prevalence of AF in 1153 unselected nursing home patients with a mean age of 82 years. The significance of this finding is underscored by the fact that one-third of all patients with AF eventually have a stroke (26) and many of these strokes are permanently disabling or fatal.

To help place the attributable risk of AF in perspective, Wolf and colleagues examined the impact of nonrheumatic atrial fibrillation, hypertension, coronary heart disease (CHD), and congestive heart failure (CHF) on stroke incidence in over 5000 participants in the Framingham Study (27). In persons with either CHD or CHF, atrial fibrillation doubled the risk of stroke in men and trebled the risk of stroke in women. The effects of hypertension, CHD, and CHF on the risk of stroke became progressively weaker with advancing age, but the impact of atrial fibrillation did not decrease significantly. In fact, for persons in the ninth decade, AF was the sole cardiovascular risk factor to exert an independent effect on stroke incidence. In this study, the attributable risk of stroke for atrial fibrillation increased from 1.5% for those aged 50–59 to 23.5% for those aged 80–89. From these data it seems reasonable to conclude that elderly patients are particularly vulnerable to stroke when atrial fibrillation is present.

It has been known for many years that AF is a powerful and independent risk factor for stroke. Why then have so many physicians remained reluctant to anticoagulate elderly patients with AF (28)? Important factors contributing to this apparent treatment inertia may have included the lack of convincing evidence that treatment with anticoagulants makes a difference in modifying stroke risk, coupled with the fear of excessive hemorrhagic side effects in the elderly. Both concerns have now been addressed by the recent publication of four large-scale, randomized, clinical trials that have evaluated the safety and efficacy of long-term anticoagulation in patients with nonvalvular AF (NVAF). These studies include the Atrial Fibrillation-Aspirin-Anticoagulation (AFASAK) Study (5), the Stroke Prevention in Atrial Fibrillation (SPAF) Study (6), the Boston Area Anticoagulation Trial for Atrial Fibrillation (BAATAF) (7), and the Canadian Atrial Fibrillation Anticoagulation (CAFA) Study (8). Table 1 provides a brief overview of the treatment interventions and major results of each of these clinical trials.

## *AFASAK (5)*

The Copenhagen AFASAK trial randomized 1007 outpatients with chronic nonrheumatic atrial fibrillation to one of three treatment regimens that included placebo, 75 mg aspirin daily, or warfarin administered by an open-label design with doses adjusted to maintain the INR between 2.8 and 4.2. Participants in this study, 54% of whom were men, had a median age of 74.2 years with an age range of 38–91 years.

**Table 1** Randomized, Controlled Clinical Trials in Nonvalvular Atrial Fibrillation

| | AFASAK (5) | SPAF (6) | BAATAF (7) | CAFA (8) |
|---|---|---|---|---|
| No. patients in study | 1007 | 1330 | 420 | 378 |
| No. patients on warfarin | 335 | 210 | 212 | 187 |
| Age of patients on warfarin | 72.8[a] | 65 | 68.5 | 68 |
| Target PT ratio | 1.5–2.0 | 1.3–1.8 | 1.2–1.5 | 1.3–1.6 |
| Target INR | 2.8–4.2 | 2.0–3.5 | 1.5–2.7 | 2.0–3.0 |
| ASA dose | 75 mg/day | 325 mg/day | 46% used ASA | |
| Stroke events per 100 person-years (C) | 4.6 | 7.0 | 3.0 | 3.6 |
| Stroke events per 100 person-years (W) | 1.9 | 2.3 | 0.4 | 2.1 |
| Risk reduction, % | 58 | 67 | 86 | 37 |
| Major bleeding events per 100 person-years (C) | 0 | 1.2 | 1.6 | 0.8 |
| Major bleeding events per 100 person-years (W) | 0.4 | 1.2 | 1.0 | 1.7 |
| Minor bleeding events per 100 person-years (C) | 0 | 0.4 | 4.8 | 11.2 |
| Minor bleeding events per 100 person-years (W) | 8.0 | 1.5 | 7.0 | 15.4 |

ASA = aspirin; C = control groups; INR = international normalized ratio; PT = prothrombin time; W = warfarin-treated group.

[a] Median age; all other studies report mean age.

*Source*: Adapted from References 5–8 and 31.

The yearly incidence of thromboembolic complications was 2.0% for patients receiving warfarin compared with 5.5% for patients receiving low-dose aspirin or placebo. Although bleeding complications were detected in 6.6% of the patients on warfarin compared with 0.6% of the aspirin patients and none of the placebo group, only two of the warfarin-induced hemorrhages were classified as serious. These included one fatal intracerebral bleed and one additional bleeding episode that required a blood transfusion in a patient who was too strongly anticoagulated.

## *SPAF (6)*

The SPAF study, a randomized trial performed at 15 clinical centers in the United States, enrolled 1330 inpatients and outpatients with constant (66%) or intermittent (34%) nonrheumatic atrial fibrillation. Study participants (71% male) had a mean age of 67 years and were categorized at entry as either warfarin eligible (group I) or warfarin ineligible (group II). Group assignments were based on preestablished criteria that initially excluded patients over age 75 from receiving warfarin. Partway through the study, the SPAF investigators relaxed this exclusion criteria to allow patients over age 75 to be assigned to the warfarin-eligible group.

Group I patients were randomized to receive either placebo, 325 mg aspirin daily, or warfarin administered by an open-label design with doses adjusted to maintain the INR between 2.0 and 3.5. Group II patients received 325 mg aspirin or placebo in a double-blind fashion.

The yearly incidence of primary events (ischemic stroke or systemic embolism) was 2.3% in patients receiving warfarin compared with 7.4% in the placebo group, a risk reduction of 67%. Surprisingly, the rate of primary events in patients assigned to receive aspirin was 3.6% compared with 6.3% in the placebo group, a risk reduction of 42%. The risk of significant bleeding was 1.5, 1.4, and 1.6% in patients assigned to warfarin, aspirin, and placebo, respectively.

Although the SPAF investigators concluded that both aspirin and warfarin were effective in reducing ischemic stroke and systemic embolism in patients with nonrheumatic atrial fibrillation, the relative benefits of warfarin versus aspirin were not directly assessed by this study. The continuation of this trial (SPAF-II) will directly compare the risks and benefits of these two drugs in patients of all ages followed for a longer period of time (29).

### *BAATAF (7)*

BAATAF was a randomized clinical trial that enrolled 420 patients with nonrheumatic atrial fibrillation (83% sustained and 17% intermittent). Study participants (72% male) had a mean age of 68 years and were randomly assigned to either treatment or control groups. The treatment group received warfarin administered by an open-label design with doses adjusted to maintain the INR between 1.5 and 2.7. The control group was not given warfarin but could choose to take aspirin. Of all the patient-years in the control group, 46% were contributed by patients who stated they were taking aspirin on a regular basis.

Of the BAATAF participants, 48% had no clinical evidence of heart disease other than AF. Most of the study patients had some echocardiographic abnormalities, however, 47% having a left atrial diameter greater than 40 mm and 29% showing evidence of mitral annular calcification.

There were only 2 strokes in the warfarin-treated group (stroke incidence rate of 0.41% per year) compared with 13 strokes in the control group (stroke incidence rate of 2.98% per year). Although mortality was not a primary end point of the original BAATAF study design, the death rate was also markedly lower in the warfarin-treated group (2.25% per year compared with 5.97% per year in the control group). One fatal hemorrhage was noted in each group. More patients receiving warfarin experienced minor hemorrhages (38 patients versus 21 patients in the control group), but the frequency of bleeding events requiring hospitalization or transfusion was approximately equal in both groups.

### *CAFA (8)*

The CAFA study was the latest in this series of randomized clinical trials designed to assess the potential for warfarin to reduce the risk of systemic embolism in patients with nonrheumatic atrial fibrillation. Of the subjects in this Canadian study, 7% had paroxysmal AF; the remainder had chronic AF that was documented to be present for at least 1 month. CAFA study participants (74.6% male, mean age of 68 years) were randomly allocated to receive either placebo or warfarin. Unlike the other trials just noted, warfarin and placebo were administered in a double-blind fashion. In each clinical center, an unblinded supervisor regulated the dose of warfarin for patients on active treatment to maintain the INR between 2.0 and 3.0

The annual rates of primary events (nonlacunar ischemic stroke, noncentral nervous system embolism, and intracranial or fatal hemorrhage) were 3.5% in the warfarin-treated group compared with 5.2% in the placebo-treated group, a risk reduction of 37%. Fatal or major bleeding occurred at annual rates of 2.5% in the warfarin group compared with 0.5% in the placebo group. Minor bleeding occurred in 16% of the patients receiving warfarin versus 9% of the patients receiving placebo.

### *Summary*

Together these four trials enrolled 3135 patients and convincingly demonstrated both the safety and efficacy of long-term oral anticoagulation to decrease the risk of stroke and systemic emboli in patients with nonvalvular atrial fibrillation.

Using an "intention-to-treat" analysis, the combined results of all these studies demonstrate a stroke risk reduction of 63% in patients who were randomized to receive warfarin. A total of only 18 nonhemorrhagic strokes occurred in the 944 patients (1.9%) who were randomized to the active treatment arms of these studies. The results favoring treatment are even more impressive when one considers that 14 of these 18 stroke patients had subtherapeutic protimes at the time of their clinical event. Thus, only 4 of 944 patients (0.4%) treated with warfarin had strokes while receiving adequate anticoagulation, compared with 63 embolic complications that occurred in 946 patients (6.6%) in the control group.

Because the mean age of patients enrolled in these trials was greater than 65 years of age, these studies provide important information about the risk of hemorrhage associated with anticoagulating older groups of patients (29). In each study, the incremental increase in major bleeding (number of events per 100 person-years of follow-up) was less than 1% greater for patients receiving warfarin compared to patients in the control groups. Minor bleeding (number of events per 100 person-years of follow-up) ranged from 1 to 8% greater in the warfarin-treated patients compared to their respective control groups (31).

These studies clearly demonstrate that anticoagulants can be safely administered to an elderly group of patients, but there is room for caution in generalizing these results. First, the risk of bleeding may vary significantly in patients who do not receive the type of regular follow-up and careful monitoring characteristic of these studies. Second, the low risk of hemorrhage noted in these AF patients may not be directly applicable to patients with other indications for anticoagulation such as those with venous thromboembolism or ischemic cerebral vascular disease (Table 2) (32). Third, because the longest follow-up period for any of these clinical trials was only slightly more than 2 years, we can only speculate about the longer term risks of hemorrhage in patients who are chronically receiving oral anticoagulants. Other retrospective studies suggest that the risk of bleeding is greatest in the first several months after the initiation of anticoagulation (33–36), but the long-term risk of bleeding for AF patients on warfarin remains unknown. Last, because all these trials, with the exception of AFASAK, enrolled an overwhelming proportion of male subjects, we should exercise caution in extrapolating these results to elderly female patients.

## Risk Stratification in NVAF Patients

The risks and inconvenience of long-term anticoagulation are considerable. For these reasons, clinicians have attempted to identify high-risk subgroups of NVAF patients who definitely need treatment and low-risk NVAF patients from whom treatment might be safely withheld (30,37,38). Although further analysis of the patient groups enrolled in each of the NVAF clinical trials does not yield a consistent risk profile, some preliminary risk stratification still appears to be feasible (Table 3).

Using techniques of multivariate analysis, the SPAF investigators identified three clinical and two echocardiographic variables that were independently asso-

**Table 2** Relationship of Treatment Indication to Risk of Bleeding

| Indication for treatment | Major bleeding (%) | Fatal bleeding (%) | All bleeding (%) |
|---|---|---|---|
| Ischemic cerebral vascular disease | 7 | 4.8 | 28.7 |
| Venous thrombosis | 8.1 | 0 | 22.6 |
| Ischemic heart disease | 4.7 | 1 | 19.1 |
| Chronic atrial fibrillation | 1.0 | $<1$ | 15.2 |
| Prosthetic heart valves | 2.4 | 1.7 | 5.7 |

*Source*: Adapted from Reference 32.

**Table 3** Predictors of Thromboembolism in Patients with Atrial Fibrillation

| Predictor | AFASAK (5) | SPAFS (6) | BAATAF (7) |
|---|---|---|---|
| Age | No | No | Yes |
| Angina | No | No | Yes |
| Previous MI | Yes | No | No |
| Mitral annular $Ca^{2+}$ | — | No | Yes |
| CHF | No | Yes | No |
| HTN | No | Yes | No |
| Previous embolus | — | Yes | No |
| LV EF decreased | — | Yes | — |
| LA size | No | Yes | No |

AFASAK = Atrial Fibrillation-Aspirin-Anticoagulation Study, BAATAF = Boston Area Anticoagulation Trial for Atrial Fibrillation, SPAFS = Stroke Prevention in Atrial Fibrillation Study, $Ca^{2+}$ = calcification, CHF = congestive heart failure, EF = ejection fraction, HTN = hypertension, LA = left atrial, LV = left ventricle, MI = myocardial infarction.
*Source*: From References 5–7 and 30.

ciated with a substantial risk of thromboembolism (TE) (37). The clinical variables included congestive heart failure within the preceding 3 months, a history of hypertension, and a history of previous arterial embolus. Patients with none of these clinical risk factors had a stroke risk of 2.5% per year, compared to 7.2% per year for patients with one clinical risk factor and 17.2% for patients with two or more of these clinical risk factors. The majority of "at-risk" patients were identified solely on the basis of these clinical variables. Additional findings of global left ventricular dysfunction on two-dimensional echocardiography and left atrial size greater than 2.5 cm/m$^2$ by standard M-mode echocardiography were also found to be independent predictors that contributed to the overall assessment of future thromboembolic risk (38).

Previous studies also demonstrated that patients with nonvalvular atrial fibrillation and a past history of clinically apparent stroke are at high risk for subsequent cerebral infarctions. Szekely found that such patients have a rate of recurrent TE that averages about 9.6% per year (39). Asymptomatic cerebral infarctions have also been found to be disturbingly common in patients with NVAF (40). Feinberg and colleagues evaluated 141 asymptomatic patients with NVAF, 26% of whom were shown to have hypodense areas consistent with cerebral infarctions on unenhanced computed tomographic (CT) scans of the head (40). Increasing age and an enlarged left atrium were the only clinical features associated with these apparently silent CNS events. Patients older than age 65 with left atrial diameters greater than 50 mm had a 52% prevalence of "silent strokes" compared with an 11% prevalence in younger patients (<65 years) with smaller left atrial diameters (<50 mm). The functional and prognostic significance of these presumed silent cerebral infarcts is an area of active investigation. If such hypodense areas are eventually shown to be associated with an increased risk of subsequent clinically apparent strokes, then head CT scans may prove to be a useful means of identifying high-risk AF patients who might be candidates for long-term anticoagulation (40).

## Lone Atrial Fibrillation

The term "lone atrial fibrillation" (LAF) refers to idiopathic atrial fibrillation that is not associated with underlying heart disease. LAF may be chronic or paroxysmal. Its definition generally does not include the type of transient atrial fibrillation that may be precipitated by surgery, trauma, or acute medical illnesses, such as pericarditis, hypoxia, or pneumonia. Lack of a uniformly applied definition has led to some confusion about whether LAF is a significant risk factor for stroke (Table 4).

The Framingham investigators defined LAF as atrial fibrillation that occurred without any preexisting or coexisting evidence of CHD, CHF, rheumatic heart disease, or hypertensive cardiovascular disease (41). At the time of their 30 year follow-up, 376 of 5209 patients (7.2%) were noted to have atrial fibrillation, with 43 of these meeting the definition of LAF. Thus, LAF patients comprised only 0.8% of the entire study population but accounted for 11.4% of all patients with atrial fibrillation. Patients who met the Framingham definition of LAF were found to have an age-adjusted rate of stroke that was about four

**Table 4** Diagnoses Excluded in Patients with Lone Atrial Fibrillation

| | Framingham (41) | Olmsted County (42) |
|---|---|---|
| Coronary artery disease | Excluded | Excluded |
| Congestive heart failure | Excluded | Excluded |
| Rheumatic heart disease | Excluded | Excluded |
| Hypertensive cardiovascular disease | Excluded | Excluded |
| Age > 60 | Included | Excluded |
| Hypertension on medication | Included | Excluded |
| BP average > 140/90 | Included | Excluded |
| COPD | Included | Excluded |
| Thyrotoxicosis | Included | Excluded |
| IDDM | Included | Excluded |

BP = blood pressure, COPD = chronic obstructive pulmonary disease, IDDM = insulin-dependent diabetes mellitus.
*Source*: From References 41 and 42.

times that of an age-matched control (28.2 versus 6.8%). These findings contrast sharply with data from the Mayo Clinic. Investigators from that institution found that a group of LAF patients from Olmsted County, Minnesota had less than half the number of strokes that were expected on a cumulative actuarial basis (3% expected versus 1.3% actual) (42).

Although the Mayo Clinic investigators incorporated more exclusion criteria into their operational definition of LAF (Table 5), significant age differences between Olmsted County and Framingham patients may account for the discordant results of these two studies. Among Framingham LAF patients, 88% were older than age 60, with 56% older than age 70. In the Olmsted County study, Kopecky and colleagues excluded all patients over age 60; the mean age of their subjects at the time of documentation of AF was 44 years of age.

The Stroke Prevention in Atrial Fibrillation Study provides yet a third subset of patients who might be considered to have LAF (37,38). In the SPAF study, 26% of all patients randomized to receive placebo had none of the clinical or echocardiographic predictors of thromboembolism we discussed previously. Such patients were found to have an extremely low risk of primary end points, with a rate of thromboembolism that averaged about 1% per year (38). Moreover, SPAF patients who were younger than 60 years of age and who did not have a history of hypertension, recent congestive heart failure, or evidence of previous systemic embolism experienced no subsequent thromboembolic events (37).

Based on this evidence, we conclude that it is reasonable to withhold long-term anticoagulation from AF patients who are younger than age 60 if there is no clinical or echocardiographic evidence of organic heart disease. AF patients greater than age 60 and younger patients with associated cardiac abnormalities are candidates for long-term treatment with warfarin.

**Table 5** Comparison Between LAF Patients in the Framingham and Olmsted County Studies

| | Framingham (41) | Olmsted County (42) |
|---|---|---|
| Total patients | 5209 | |
| Age | 88% > 60 | None > 60 |
| | 56% > 70 | None > 70 |
| No. patients with AF | 376 (7%) | 3623 |
| No. patients with LAF | 43 | 97 |
| % All AF with LAF | 11.4% | 2.7% |
| LAF a risk factor for stroke? | Yes | No |

AF = atrial fibrillation, LAF = lone atrial fibrillation.
*Source*: From References 41 and 42.

### *Anticoagulation for Elective Cardioversion*

In a study by Bjerkelund and Orning, electrical cardioversion without anticoagulants resulted in a 5.3% incidence of emboli compared with an incidence rate of 0.8% in patients receiving anticoagulants (43). Based on this and several other smaller studies, the ACCP has recommended the following approach to patients with atrial fibrillation who are scheduled for electrical cardioversion on an elective basis (44):

1. Warfarin therapy, in a dose adjusted to maintain the INR between 2.0 and 3.0, should be administered for 3 weeks before the electrical cardioversion of patients who have been in AF for more than 3 days.
2. Anticoagulants should be continued until normal sinus rhythm has been maintained for 2–4 weeks postcardioversion.

### *Quality of Life Issue*

The AF clinical trials have been successful in demonstrating the safety and efficacy of anticoagulation in the elderly, but patient acceptance of long-term treatment with warfarin is an important issue that needs to be addressed. Over one-third of AFASAK patients on warfarin (38% compared to 13–15% in the aspirin and placebo groups) prematurely withdrew from the study for various reasons that included refusal to continue (19%), medication side effects (7%), or noncompliance (7%) (5). Although the number of warfarin and placebo withdrawals from the SPAF (6) (19 versus 10%), BAATAF (10% versus not specified) (7), and CAFA (26 versus 23%) (8) studies was considerably less, lack of long-term patient commitment to this form of treatment raises some concerns.

The need for frequent blood tests, restrictions on the use of alcohol and over-the-counter medications, and concern about the potential for hemorrhagic complications may all contribute to negative perceptions that patients on warfarin have about their health and quality of life. There has also been some concern that healthy patients with AF may somehow feel "labeled" and that this labeling may, in and of itself, have adverse effects. Fortunately, well-validated measures of functional status and health perception have shown that warfarin therapy is not usually associated with a significant decrease in a patient's perceived health status and sense of well-being, unless a bleeding episode has occurred (45).

## Venous Thromboembolic Disease

Although deep venous thrombosis and pulmonary embolism are well recognized as major causes of morbidity and mortality in the elderly, estimates of the exact frequency of these disorders vary considerably. For example, a communitywide study of 16 short-stay hospitals in western Massachusetts determined that 1% of all hospital discharges had a diagnosis of venous thromboembolic disease

(VTE), including both initial and recurrent episodes of deep venous thrombosis and/or pulmonary embolism (46). Based on these data, Anderson and colleagues projected an annual U.S. incidence of about a quarter-million cases of VTE each year. Others believe that the true incidence of VTE may be 20 times higher (47).

There is better agreement that old age is an important risk factor for the development of VTE. Using $I^{125}$ fibrinogen leg scanning, Kakkar et al. found that older patients (61–80 years of age) who were admitted for elective surgery had almost twice the rate of deep vein thrombosis (DVT) as younger patients (<age 60) (48). Based on 1985 U.S. discharge summary diagnoses, Gillum noted a 22-fold increase in the rate of pulmonary embolism (PE) when hospitalized patients older than age 65 were compared to patients between 15 and 44 years old (49). Older patients in this study had a rate of pulmonary embolism that averaged 265 cases per 100,000 population compared with 12 per 100,000 in the younger age group. Samkoff and Comstock noted an overwhelming impact of age upon fatal cases of pulmonary emboli, with mortality rising logarithmically with increasing age, up to age 75 (50).

In their survey of western Massachusetts hospitals, Anderson and associates noted that the mean age of patients admitted with an initial episode of deep venous thrombosis and/or pulmonary embolism was 65 years; they also confirmed that the incidence of VTE increased with advancing age (46). Incidence rates for deep venous thrombosis were 291 per 100,000 in those greater than 80 compared with 43 per 100,000 in those aged 50–59. Patients greater than age 80 had an incidence of pulmonary embolism of 159 per 100,000 population compared to 19 per 100,000 in the 50–59 age group. When Poisson regression methods were used to model the incidence of VTE as a function of age, the relative risk of VTE per 10 year increase in age was found to be 1.9. Analysis of in-hospital case-fatality rates also showed a significant increase with age, an increase that was approximately exponential for age greater than 40 years.

The reason for this high frequency of VTE in elderly patients is uncertain but may be related to the coexistence of age-related comorbidities that serve as predisposing risk factors for thrombosis. For example, decreased mobility due to strokes, recent surgery (particularly orthopedic surgery of the hips and knees), or congestive heart failure may be prominent factors leading to stasis and thrombosis in some elderly patients. In others, hypercoagulable states may be induced by malignancy. Several such predisposing risk factors may frequently be present in the same patient who develops a DVT and/or PE. For example, Anderson et al. found that 80–85% of patients with an initial episode of DVT or PE had at least three factors that placed them at increased risk for the development of VTE (46).

Randomized studies provide solid evidence that treatment with heparin followed by longer term anticoagulation is effective in decreasing mortality in patients with pulmonary emboli (51) and in preventing recurrence in patients with proximal vein thrombosis or symptomatic calf vein thrombosis (52–54). To our knowledge, no prospective studies specifically address the question of whether age alone increases the risk for hemorrhagic complications in elderly VTE patients who are treated with long-term anticoagulants. As noted previously, the low risk of hemorrhagic complications noted in elderly patients enrolled in the NVAF clinical trials may not be directly applicable to patients with VTE (Table 2).

For a more extensive review of pulmonary embolism in the elderly, the reader is referred to Chapter 25.

## Valvular Heart Disease and Prosthetic Heart Valves

### *Native Valve Disease*

Patients with rheumatic mitral valve disease complicated by episodes of systemic embolism, chronic or paroxysmal atrial fibrillation, or echocardiographic evidence of left atrial size greater than 55 mm are candidates for long-term anticoagulation (55). For patients with documented systemic emboli, treatment with warfarin to achieve an INR between 3.0 and 4.5 is recommended for a minimum of 1 year (55). After this time, the intensity of anticoagulation may be reduced to achieve an INR of 2–3 if there has been no subsequent embolic recurrence (55).

Patients with isolated aortic valvular disease usually have a low risk of systemic embolism; routine anticoagulation of such patients is not recommended (55).

### *Prosthetic Heart Valves*

Because many elderly patients with valvular heart disease may eventually be candidates for valve replacement surgery, the subject of anticoagulating patients with either tissue heart valves or mechanical prostheses deserves attention. By obviating the need for long-term anticoagulation, bioprosthetic heart valves (tissue valves) may appear to offer a special advantage over mechanical heart valves in the elderly. However, when making the decision about which type of prosthesis to implant, clinicians must carefully weigh the potential risks of warfarin-induced hemorrhagic complications against the long-term durability of tissue valves. Bioprosthetic valves carry the potential for tissue degeneration, valve dysfunction, and the need for subsequent reoperation to place a second prosthesis (56).

### *Bioprosthetic (Tissue) Valves*

Current recommendations suggest that long-term anticoagulation is not necessary for the majority of patients with bioprosthetic (tissue) valves (57). Long-term anticoagulant use is considered optional in patients who are in sinus rhythm and who have a bioprosthetic valve in the aortic position (57). All patients with a bioprosthesis in the mitral position should be anticoagulated for the first 3 months after valve insertion (2,57). Patients with a bioprosthesis in either position who have a history of thromboembolism, left atrial thrombus at the time of surgery, or atrial fibrillation should be treated with long-term anticoagulation (57).

### *Mechanical Heart Valves*

Despite the lack of firm data from randomized clinical trials, chronic anticoagulation with warfarin is strongly recommended for all patients with mechanical heart valves. Mok et al. showed a relative risk reduction of 60–79% in a prospective study of patients with mechanical heart valves who were randomly assigned to receive warfarin compared to patients who received either dipyramidole-aspirin or pentoxifylline-aspirin to prevent thromboembolism (58).

Although unproven, it is generally accepted that more intense anticoagulant treatment regimens are required to adequately protect patients with mechanical heart valves from developing thromboembolic complications. Current ACCP guidelines recommend that such patients be anticoagulated to achieve an INR between 3.0 and 4.5 (57). One might assume that patients treated with these more intense regimens might experience a higher incidence of bleeding complications, but Levine and colleagues did not find this to be the case (32). When total hemorrhagic episodes are considered, pooled rates of bleeding for patients with prosthetic heart valves appear to be even somewhat lower than the bleeding rates for patients with other indications for treatment (Table 2).

Patients with mechanical heart valves who suffer systemic emboli while adequately anticoagulated should be treated with 400 mg dipyramidole in addition to full-dose warfarin (57,59). Although the addition of low-dose aspirin may also afford additional protection in such patients, there is concern about the increased risk of bleeding in patients being treated with combinations of low-dose aspirin and warfarin.

## Ischemic Heart Disease

As many as 1.5 million Americans suffer myocardial infarctions (MI) each year, with over half these events occurring in patients greater than age 65 years of age (60). The past decade has seen wide acceptance of the critical role that thrombosis plays in the vast majority of MI patients (61), and it seems ironic that no consensus has been reached about the role of long-term anticoagulants as part of a secondary prevention strategy in this setting. Thus, even while more and more acute MI treatment protocols feature the use of thrombolytic agents, the debate of the past 30 years over the role of long-term anticoagulation in the post-MI patient continues.

With the recognition that the treatment goals of anticoagulation for patients with ischemic heart disease remain somewhat unclear, we briefly review here the use of acute and chronic anticoagulants to (1) prevent the progression of unstable angina to myocardial infarction; (2) prevent pulmonary embolism, recurrent MI, stroke, and death in those patients who have suffered a myocardial infarction; and (3) prevent systemic emboli in those patients who develop LV mural thrombi as a complication of their MI.

### *Prevention of the Progression of Unstable Angina to Myocardial Infarction*

Repeated studies have demonstrated that heparin and aspirin are beneficial in treating patients with unstable angina (62–64). Both drugs are effective in reducing the incidence of subsequent myocardial infarction and decreasing cardiovascular mortality, although the relative benefits of heparin versus aspirin in this setting remain unclear (65).

### *Acute Anticoagulation in the Postinfarct Patient*

All patients with an acute myocardial infarction should receive prophylaxis with 5000 units subcutaneous heparin twice daily to prevent deep venous thrombosis and pulmonary embolism. Several recent randomized clinical trials (66,67) and a metaanalysis of 20 acute MI trials (68) showed that heparin-treated patients had impressive decreases in reinfarction and mortality (65). No firm conclusions can be drawn about the relative effectiveness of heparin versus aspirin (or a combination of the two) in acute MI patients because most patients in the control groups of these studies did not receive aspirin. Heparin has also been widely used to prevent early coronary artery reocclusion after successful thrombolysis, and the role of longer term anticoagulation in this setting remains an area of active investigation (66,69,70).

### *Chronic Anticoagulation in the Post–Myocardial Infarction Patient*

Jafri and colleagues recently reviewed the results of 12 large-scale randomized clinical trials that evaluated the role of long-term anticoagulation in the chronic management of post-MI patients (71). Although two-thirds of these studies showed significant decreases in mortality, reinfarction, or embolic events, direct comparisons of patient groups or pooling of study results is not possible because of substantial differences in study design, entry criteria, and treatment protocols. Two of these studies that address issues relevant to the management of elderly post-MI patients are reviewed now in more detail.

The Sixty Plus Reinfarction Trial was a double-blind, multicenter study designed to assess the efficacy of long-term anticoagulation after myocardial infarction in patients over 60 years of age (72,73). In this study, investigators from the Netherlands evaluated 878 patients (mean age of 67.6 years) who had already received oral anticoagulants for at least 6 months following their first transmural MI. Subjects were randomized at entry to an intervention group who were continued on anticoagulation or a control group who were placed on placebo. The 2 year mortality was significantly lower in the group receiving anticoagulation (7.6%) compared to the group receiving placebo (13.4%). The incidence of recurrent myocardial infarction was also significantly lower in the treatment group (5.7%) compared to the control group (15.9%). Although both major and minor bleeding episodes were more frequent in the group receiving anticoagulation, about 75% of these occurred when the prothrombin time was excessively prolonged.

The Norwegian Warfarin Re-Infarction Study (WARIS) was the most recent (and most rigorous) clinical trial designed to evaluate the effect of warfarin on mortality and reinfarction in patients who were recovering from an acute myocardial infarction (71,74). In this double-blind, placebo-controlled trial, Smith and colleagues enrolled over 1200 patients (mean age of 61 years) at a mean interval of 27 days post-MI. Patients were randomized to receive either placebo or warfarin adjusted to achieve a target INR between 2.8 and 4.2 and were followed for an average of 37 months. Using an intention-to-treat analysis, the warfarin-treated group had the following risk reductions compared to placebo: death decreased by 24%, reinfarction decreased by 34%, and cerebrovascular accidents decreased by 55%. These impressive results were all highly significant and were achieved with a combined incidence of major bleeding that was calculated at 0.6% per year. These benefits seem to exceed those expected from low-dose aspirin (75), but further research is needed to directly compare the relative efficacy of aspirin versus warfarin in post-MI patients.

### *Left Ventricular Thrombus*

The risk of systemic embolism (SE) is highest in the first few days following an acute myocardial infarction, with two-thirds of all SE occurring in the first week post-MI (76). Patients at highest risk for the development of SE include those with transmural anterior wall MI who display evidence of akinesis or dyskinesis of the cardiac apex, regardless of whether these findings are associated with a left ventricular mural thrombus.

Johannsen and colleagues studied a large group of patients with anterior wall MI and found that, in addition to thrombus mobility and protuberance, patients older than age 68 years were at significant risk for subsequent embolization (77). Stratton and Resnick also confirmed that thrombus protrusion and mobility were predictive of embolization, but they did not uncover any clinical features, including age, that distinguished those patients with thrombus who were more likely to embolize (78).

The American College of Cardiology and the American Heart Association currently recommend 3 months of warfarin for post-MI patients at high risk for SE. This includes those patients with an anterior or apical infarct, with or without a documented mural thrombus (79). Longer term warfarin therapy is also recommended for survivors of acute myocardial infarction (AMI) with atrial fibrillation, diffusely dilated and poorly contracting left ventricles, significant CHF, venous thromboembolism, or a history of previous systemic embolism (80).

Although approximately 50% of left ventricular aneurysms are noted to contain thrombus, routine anticoagulation of such patients is not recommended unless the course is complicated by a recent myocardial infarction or SE (80).

## Dilated Congestive Cardiomyopathy

Besides the setting of acute myocardial infarctions that involve the cardiac apex, left ventricular thrombi can form and cause emboli in patients with idiopathic dilated cardiomyopathy (IDC). Fuster and colleagues evaluated 104 patients with IDC diagnosed on the basis of clinical and angiographic data (81). Univariate analysis at the time of diagnosis revealed that age greater than 55 was one of three factors that was highly predictive of poor clinical outcome in these patients (the other two being cardiothoracic ratio $> 0.55$ on chest x-ray and cardiac index $< 3.0$ liters/min per $m^2$ measured at the time of cardiac catheterization). The incidence of systemic embolism in patients not receiving long-term anticoagulation was significant, occurring in 19 of 103 patients for an event rate of 3.5 emboli per 100 patient-years of follow-up. Conversely, no embolic events or major hemorrhagic complications were noted in 32 patients who were maintained on anticoagulant agents during 101 patient-years of exposure. A recent decision analysis by Tsevat and colleagues argues that the use of anticoagulation in patients with IDC provides most of its benefit by actually preventing pulmonary embolism, not by reducing systemic embolization (82). In this setting, the benefits of treatment are not as clearly defined as in some of the other conditions we have reviewed. Clinicians and their patients with IDC must therefore decide if the potential benefits are worth the risks, and the sacrifice of life-style changes and restrictions imposed by long-term anticoagulant therapy.

## Ischemic Cerebral Vascular Disease

Disabling stroke is one of the most common and feared illnesses of the elderly (83). Based on the Framingham data, it has been estimated that approximately 500,000 Americans suffer strokes each year (84). Long-term anticoagulation with low-dose warfarin is clearly beneficial in preventing strokes in those patients with atrial fibrillation (5–8), but this subset of patients comprises only a small percentage of the total stroke population (85). Of all acute strokes 85% are attributable to cerebral infarctions, the vast majority secondary to atherothrombotic cerebral vascular disease (84). Even though it is well accepted that thrombosis is an integral part of all pathophysiologic mechanisms that underlie these syndromes of ischemic stroke, the role of antithrombotic therapy in this large group of patients remains uncertain (83).

Although the administration of full-dose heparin therapy to unselected patients with acute ischemic strokes is of questionable benefit, empirical treatment seems to be a reasonable approach in some selected high-risk patients. The decision to anticoagulate patients with ischemic cerebral vascular disease, however, is further complicated by a high rate of serious bleeding events. Using a pooled analysis of the results from multiple published studies, Levine and colleagues found an increased risk of major and fatal bleeding events in patients being anticoagulated for ischemic cerebral vascular disease when they were compared to patients with other indications for anticoagulation (Table 2) (32). Given the magnitude of the stroke problem and the potential hazards of empirical treatment, it is clear that randomized clinical trials are urgently needed to help define the specific role of antithrombotic therapy in cerebral vascular disease.

### *Acute Cardioembolic Stroke*

In the setting of an acute cardioembolic stroke, the use of intravenous heparin to prevent an early recurrent neurological event should be considered empirical and limited to nonhypertensive patients with small to moderately sized emboli (83,85). When anticoagulation is considered, heparinization should probably be delayed at least 48 h until a follow-up CT scan is performed to exclude the possibility of spontaneous hemorrhagic transformation (83,85). Heparin therapy should be followed by warfarin in a dose adjusted to maintain the target INR between 3.0 and 4.5. If there have been no recurrent events after 1 year, the dose of warfarin should be decreased to achieve an INR of 2.0–3.0 and continued indefinitely (85).

### *Unstable or Progressing Thrombotic Stroke*

Although a few small studies have shown trends favoring anticoagulation, there is no convincing evidence from large-scale clinical trials supporting the use of routine anticoagulation in patients with unstable or progressing thrombotic strokes (85). Nonetheless, some clinicians believe that an ischemic stroke that progresses, or one that has a fluctuating clinical course, may be an indication for acute anticoagulation with heparin. Treatment of such "strokes in evolution" is typically reserved for patients who display progressive deterioration within 48 h of stroke onset and who have no other apparent cause to explain their clinical course (83).

### *Acute Transient Ischemic Attack*

The annual U.S. incidence of transient ischemic attacks (TIA) is 1 per 1000 in patients greater than 55 years of age (85). Despite the fact that TIA patients face a 10% annual risk of stroke or death, anticoagulants are not routinely recommended in this setting (85). The few randomized clinical trials that have evaluated the risks and benefits of anticoagulating TIA patients have enrolled small numbers of subjects and produced conflicting results (85).

In the acute setting, treatment with intravenous heparin should probably be restricted to high-risk subgroups of patients with TIA or reversible ischemic neurological deficits. Such high-risk patients might include those with vertebrobasilar TIA or those with crescendo symptoms (86–88). Two common clinical scenarios in which long-term treatment with warfarin is frequently prescribed include (1) patients with nonsurgical disease and recurrent TIA despite adequate antiplatelet therapy and (2) patients with other high-grade, nonsurgical lesions, such as severe basilar artery stenosis (86). We empirically anticoagulate such patients for 3 months using a warfarin dose sufficient to maintain the INR between 2.0 and 3.0. After this time, we reinstitute conventional antiplatelet therapy.

## Peripheral Vascular Disease

Symptomatic occlusive peripheral vascular disease (PVD) occurs in 2–3% of all men and 1% of all women over age 50–65 (89). The decision to anticoagulate such patients should take into account the morbidity directly associated with the PVD, but it should not ignore the fact that such patients are at significant risk for future cardiovascular events. Using a prospective cohort study design, Criqui and colleagues followed 67 patients with PVD over a 10 year period (90). After multivariate adjustments for age, sex, and other risk factors for cardiovascular disease, these investigators noted that the relative risk of dying among subjects with large-vessel peripheral arterial disease was 3.1 times higher compared with those who had no evidence of PVD. Additional analysis showed a 15-fold increase in mortality rates due to cardiovascular disease and CHD among subjects with large-vessel PVD.

At least two studies in the literature lend support to the decision to anticoagulate selected patients with PVD. In the first study, Kretschmer and colleagues randomized 88 patients with reversed autologous saphenous vein femoropopliteal bypasses and demonstrated a significant benefit in maintaining bypass patency in patients receiving warfarin (91). At a mean follow-up of 30 months, 37% of the controls had bypass occlusions compared with only 18% of those on oral anticoagulants. However, 12% of the anticoagulant treatment group had to discontinue warfarin therapy because of major bleeding complications.

In a second study by the same group of investigators, 119 patients (79% male, mean age 63.1 years) who had undergone elective femoropopliteal bypass surgery were randomized to receive treatment with either anticoagulants or placebo (92). During the follow-up period, a total of 30 patients died, 10 in the warfarin group (17%) and 20 in the control group (34%). Graft occlusions occurred in 28 patients, 11 in the warfarin group (18%) and 17 in the control group (29%). Further analysis showed that anticoagulants influenced patient survival irrespective of graft performance, probably by decreasing fatal cardiovascular events. It is premature to recommend long-term anticoagulation for all patients after a femoropopliteal bypass or other vascular reconstruction, but these two studies provide suggestive evidence that anticoagulants may play an important role in such patients. The risks and benefits of such an approach need further study before long-term anticoagulation can be routinely recommended for patients with PVD.

Current ACCP recommendations suggest that patients with PVD who suffer arterial thrombi or emboli may benefit from anticoagulation. Such patients should receive intravenous heparin to prevent clot propagation if surgical revascularization is delayed (93). Warfarin should then be administered in a dose sufficient to prolong the INR to a range between 3.0 and 4.5. If after 1 year of anticoagulation there has been no recurrence, the dose of warfarin should be decreased to achieve a target INR of between 2.0 and 3.0.

## RISK FACTORS FOR ANTICOAGULANT-INDUCED BLEEDING

The risk of developing a hemorrhagic complication from long-term anticoagulation is influenced by multiple variables, including both patient-related and treatment-related factors. Examples of some patient-related risk factors that may be associated with anticoagulant-induced bleeding include demographic variables, such as age and gender, the underlying indication for anticoagulation, presence of comorbid illnesses, use of concurrent medications, and noncompliance with the prescribed treatment program. Examples of some treatment-related risk factors for bleeding include the intensity of therapy, the duration of treatment, and the adequacy of follow-up and monitoring. In the following section we discuss some of these risk factors that have been associated with anticoagulant-induced bleeding.

### Patient-Related Risk Factors for Bleeding

#### *Age*

In a recent comprehensive review of the hemorrhagic complications of long-term anticoagulant therapy, Levine and colleagues sought to establish a relationship between bleeding and age (32). No correlation could be detected because most of the reports in their literature review lacked the necessary information to confirm a definite relationship. Other recent studies that contain information about age as a risk for developing anticoagulant-induced hemorrhage report conflicting results (34–36,94,95).

Gurwitz and colleagues evaluated 321 patients with a mean age of 59 ± 16 years (range 13–92 years) who were followed in the outpatient anticoagulation clinic of a university hospital (34). Over the 8 year period (1978–1986) of this retrospective study, 4.4% of the patients developed major bleeding complications and 19% developed minor bleeding events. No significant differences in the risk of initial minor or major bleeding complications were observed between four age groups (<50, 50–59, 60–69, and ⩾70), despite the fact that these groups differed significantly in the distribution of underlying indications for anticoagulation (AF alone, AF with stroke, PE, or prosthetic heart valve). A multivariate regression analysis confirmed the lack of association between age and bleeding events.

In contradistinction, two other recent, large-scale, retrospective reviews have identified age as the most powerful risk factor for the development of major bleeding episodes in patients on long-term anticoagulation. In the first study, Landefeld and colleagues evaluated an inception cohort of 565 patients (54% female) with a mean age of 61 ± 14 years (range 18–92) who were discharged from a university hospital between 1977 and 1983 after being started on warfarin (35). The treatment indication for these patients included cardiac surgery in 57% and venous thromboembolism in 15%. During 876 patient-years of outpatient therapy with warfarin, the cumulative incidence of major bleeding at 12 months was 11%, with fatal bleeding in 10 patients (2%). Using multivariate regression analysis, age greater than 65 (relative risk of 3.2) was determined to be one of five independent risk factors associated with the development of major bleeding complications. The four other factors and their respective relative risks (RR) included (1) the presence of serious comorbid conditions, such as recent MI, renal insufficiency, or severe anemia (RR 3.0); (2) history of gastrointestinal bleeding (RR 2.9); (3) history of stroke, either past or current (RR 2.5); and (4) atrial fibrillation (RR 2.2).

In the second study, Launbjerg and colleagues reported on 551 Danish patients (60% male) with a mean age of 63 years (range 14–97) who received anticoagulants during the period between 1981 and 1987 (36). The treatment indication for 60% of the patients in this study included either deep venous thrombosis or pulmonary embolism. During 1010 treatment years of follow-up, the incidence of bleeding that necessitated hospital admission was 2.7% per year. Using techniques of multivariate analysis, age > 75 years was found to increase the risk of major bleeding by 10.5%. Other factors that also independently contributed to bleeding risk included current treatment with thiazide diuretics, hypertension (defined as blood pressure greater than 160/95), number of INR values above 7, and the duration of treatment (years).

At the present time, we are not aware of any modern, prospective, clinical trials using less intense treatment regimens that have specifically evaluated the risk of bleeding in elderly patients receiving anticoagulants. The NVAF trials provide important new information about the benefits of anticoagulating older patients, but further work is needed to specifically evaluate the relationship between age and the risk of developing hemorrhagic complications. Because the

SPAF-II trial is stratifying patients with nonvalvular atrial fibrillation into two age groups (<75 years of age versus >75 years of age) before randomization to warfarin or aspirin, this study should eventually provide more direct evidence about the specific risks of anticoagulating older patients (29).

### *Gender*

Earlier studies by Jick and colleagues reported that women may be at particular risk for the hemorrhagic side effects of heparin (96,97). A recent retrospective study also found that the relative risk for hemorrhage was significantly greater in women receiving warfarin (98), but other studies have found no significant differences in bleeding risk between the sexes (36,73).

### *Indication for Treatment*

As noted in Table 2, the risk of anticoagulant-induced hemorrhage does not appear to be uniform across all treatment indications (32). Major bleeding in patients with VTE may frequently be associated with the same risk factors responsible for the development of thrombosis (32). For example, patients with tumor-related hypercoagulability as a predisposing cause leading to the development of deep venous thrombosis may bleed from a friable tumor surface when they are begun on anticoagulation. Likewise, patients being anticoagulated for ischemic cerebral vascular disease may experience higher rates of intracerebral bleeding. Such complications may be related to associated hypertension or underlying cerebrovascular disease per se (32). Differences in the intensity of therapy do not seem to explain the wide range of bleeding rates noted for different treatment indications.

## Treatment-Related Factors

### *Intensity of Treatment*

Hirsh recently summarized the surprisingly small number of prospective studies that have evaluated the relationship between bleeding and the intensity of long-term anticoagulation (16). Randomized clinical trials for patients with deep venous thrombosis (1), tissue heart valves (2), and mechanical heart valves (3,4) have all shown significantly fewer bleeding events when less intense treatment regimens were compared to more intense levels of anticoagulation.

In the treatment of venous thromboembolic disease, Hull and colleagues found that low-dose warfarin provided the same degree of protection as more intense treatment regimens and that low-dose therapy was associated with a lower incidence of hemorrhagic complications (1). A group of 96 consecutive patients (56% > 60 years, 56% male) with proximal vein thrombosis received a standard course of intravenous heparin before being randomized to less intense (INR 2–2.3) or more intense (INR 2.5–4.1) oral anticoagulant treatment regimens. Both treatment groups experienced a similar incidence of recurrent thrombotic events, but only 2 of 47 patients (4%) in the less intense treatment group developed hemorrhagic complications compared to 11 of 49 patients (22%) receiving more intense treatment with warfarin. All patients with major bleeding in this study (2 in each group) had protimes that were prolonged beyond the target treatment range, and each of these 4 patients had an underlying predisposition to hemorrhage; 2 patients who experienced serious bleeding had unsuspected duodenal ulcer disease and the other 2 patients with significant bleeding had recently undergone major surgery.

Turpie and colleagues randomly assigned 284 consecutive patients (mean age 62.3 years, 53% male) with tissue heart valves to receive either less intense or more intense treatment regimens with oral anticoagulants (2). In this study a less intense treatment regimen (INR 2.0–2.3) was just as effective but caused less bleeding than a comparison regimen that employed a more intense level of anticoagulation (INR 2.5–4.0). Although the incidence of embolic complications was the same in each arm of the study, only 6 of 102 patients (6%) in the less intense treatment group experienced hemorrhagic complications compared with 15 of 108 patients (14%) receiving more intense levels of anticoagulation. All 5 patients with major bleeding complications were in the more intense treatment group.

Similar results were reported by Sauor and colleagues, who compared the efficacy and complications of two intensities of warfarin anticoagulation in 247 patients (mean age 52, 55% female) with mechanical heart valves (3). Thromboembolism occurred with equal frequency in both groups. Patients who received the less intense treatment regimen (INR 1.9–3.6) experienced 6.2 total bleeding episodes per 100 patient-years of follow-up compared with 12.1 episodes in a high-intensity treatment group (INR 7.4–10.8). Of the 13 patients with major bleeding complications, 9 (69%) had markedly elevated prothrombin times (greater than three times control) and 8 (62%) had probable predisposing or contributing factors, including trauma, malignancy, peptic ulcer disease, and use of aspirin or nonsteroidal antiinflammatory drugs.

Altman and colleagues evaluated 99 patients (mean age 52, 72% male) with mechanical heart valves and compared groups receiving less intense (INR 2–3) and more intense levels of anticoagulation (INR 3–4.5) for evidence of thromboembolic and hemorrhagic complications (4). A direct comparison of their results with those of other investigators is complicated by the fact that all patients in this study received concurrent treatment with 330 mg aspirin and 75 mg dipyramidole twice each day. The frequency of thromboembolism was equal in both groups. Of 51 patients in the less intense treatment regimen, 2 (3.9%) experienced bleeding complications (3.8 events per 100 patient-years of follow-up) compared with 10 of 48 patients (20.8%) in the more intense treatment group (24.7 events per 100 patient-years of follow-up).

Based on these studies, we conclude that less intense levels of anticoagulation offer equal protection against thromboembolism but are associated with fewer bleeding complications than more intense treatment regimens. At the present time these conclusions should only be applied to patients with venous thromboembolic disease, tissue heart valves, or mechanical heart valves, although data from the NVAF clinical trials also suggests that the protective effect of anticoagulation in AF patients is preserved at less intense treatment levels. For example, the stroke risk reduction in the BAATAF study, which used the least intense treatment regimen (INR 1.5–2.7), was similar (and, in fact, more impressive) to that achieved in the AFASAK study, which employed a moderately intense level of anticoagulation (INR 2.8–4.2). Further research is needed to define the lowest effective dose of anticoagulant necessary to achieve a protective effect (16).

### *Duration of Therapy*

For the most part, current recommendations regarding the duration of oral anticoagulant therapy (Table 6) are based on consensus rather than on data from controlled clinical trials. Several retrospective studies that have attempted to quantitate the relationship between the duration of treatment and the cumulative risk of developing a bleeding complication are now described.

Petitti and colleagues used hospital discharge data collected during a 10 year period (1970–1980) to determine the association between duration of warfarin therapy for venous thromboembolic disease and the cumulative risk of hemorrhage (33). These investigators evaluated the medical records of over 2400 patients with a diagnosis of pulmonary embolism, thrombophlebitis, or both and found that the probability of major hemorrhage increased almost linearly between 1 week and 5 years (10% at 3 months, 18% at 1 year, 26% at 2 years, and 41% at 5 years). Unfortunately, no information was provided regarding the intensity of anticoagulation for the patients in this study.

**Table 6** Duration of Anticoagulation

| | |
|---|---|
| Elective cardioversion | 6–8 weeks |
| Anterior wall MI | 1–3 months |
| Mitral valve bioprosthesis | 3 months |
| DVT/PE (first episode) | 3–6 months |
| DVT/PE (second episode) | 12 months |
| DVT/PE (more than one recurrence) | Lifelong |
| Atrial fibrillation | Lifelong (?) |
| Mechanical heart valves | Lifelong |

DVT = deep venous thrombosis, MI = myocardial infarction, PE = pulmonary embolism.

Landefeld studied an inception cohort of 565 patients (mean age 61 years) who began anticoagulant treatment between 1977 and 1983 and found that the cumulative incidences of major bleeding at 1, 12, and 48 months was 3, 11, and 22%, respectively (35). Using a retrospective chart review of 560 outpatients (mean age 63) who received anticoagulants between 1981 and 1987, Launbjerg determined that each year of treatment increased the risk for major bleeding by 2.0% (36).

Besides the expected cumulative increase in bleeding complications over time, several investigators have also determined that there appears to be a clustering of bleeding events around the time of the initiation of anticoagulation. In their study of 321 patients (mean age 59 ± 16 years) followed over an 8 year period, Gurwitz et al. noted that the risk of minor bleeding was greatest during the first 3 months of therapy (34). Landefeld et al. found that the risk of major bleeding decreased from 3% during the first month of outpatient therapy to 0.3% per month after the first year of treatment (35). Launbjerg determined that, after controlling for the intensity of treatment, there was a relative risk of 1.7 when the incidence of serious bleeding during the first 3 months of anticoagulation was compared with the second 3 months of therapy (36).

The reason for this early clustering of bleeding complications has several possible explanations: (1) suspicion bias on the part of clinicians may lead to more intense monitoring during the early phases of treatment; (2) instability of laboratory values with occasional marked fluctuations of the prothrombin time may lead to episodes of overanticoagulation that provoke bleeding; and (3) clinically "occult" lesions that are predisposed to bleeding may be unmasked by therapeutic levels of anticoagulation (35).

## EVALUATION OF BLEEDING

The question of whether, and how, to evaluate patients with anticoagulant-induced bleeding is important. Should we make a distinction between patients who bleed while their protime is within the therapeutic range versus those who bleed when their protime is excessively prolonged (99)?

Based on the available evidence, it appears that all patients who bleed while being treated with anticoagulants should undergo a thorough diagnostic evaluation. In their study of patients being anticoagulated for proximal vein thrombosis, Hull and colleagues demonstrated predisposing lesions in all patients ($n = 4$) with major hemorrhage and excessive prolongation of the protime (100). In the study by Saour et al., 62% of patients with mechanical heart valves who experienced major bleeding complications had probable predisposing or contributing factors (3). Landefeld et al. reported that, in patients who bled while receiving warfarin for a variety of clinical indications, 38% were found to have important remediable lesions (99). Clinicians were aware of only about half these lesions at the time anticoagulation was initiated. By comparing the intensity of anticoagulation at the time of each bleeding episode, Landefeld concluded that new lesions were more likely to be identified in patients who did not have excessive prothrombin time ratios at the time of the index bleeding event.

In an inception cohort of 565 patients beginning therapy with warfarin, Landefeld et al. identified the five most frequent sites of bleeding (in decreasing order of frequency) as gastrointestinal tract (32%), soft tissue (19%), genitourinary tract (14%), intracranial (8%), and nasopharynx (epistaxis in 8%). Other studies have also found the gastrointestinal (GI) tract to be the most frequent site of bleeding complications in patients on long-term anticoagulation, accounting for about 30% of all serious bleeding episodes (35,94,95).

Wilcox and Truss analyzed 50 anticoagulated patients (mean age 62 years) with gastrointestinal bleeding while receiving anticoagulant therapy (101). The site of bleeding in 23 patients (46%) was the upper GI tract, with gastric and duodenal ulcers the most common lesions (6 patients each). Lower GI bleeding occurred in 20 patients (40%), but a specific diagnosis to account for the bleeding was established in only half of these cases. Adenocarcinoma of the colon was detected in 2 patients and adenomatous polyps were found in 5 others.

Kewenter and colleagues studied the value of stool Hemoccult testing in the diagnosis of colorectal disease in patients receiving anticoagulant therapy by evaluating 849 patients (mean age 67 years) on warfarin (102). A total of 128 patients (15%) had positive stool Hemoccult tests, with 3 patients discovered to have carcinoma and 13 found to have adenomatous polyps on further investigation. No correlation was noted between the intensity of anticoagulation and the occurrence of positive results on stool Hemoccult tests.

Jaffin and associates reported the results of a prospective study designed to determine the effect of anticoagulants on the prevalence of occult GI bleeding (103). These investigators evaluated 249 patients (mean age 64 years) who had received anticoagulants for at least 48 h. Patients on anticoagulants had a 12% positive rate of stool Hemoccult tests compared with a 3% positive rate in the control group. As noted in Kewenter's study, positive stool heme tests were not related to excessive degrees of anticoagulation. Of 16 patients who underwent a diagnostic workup, 15 previously undiagnosed lesions were uncovered, including 3 carcinomas, 1 inflammatory bowel disease, and 2 polyps.

From these studies we conclude that, although anticoagulation may significantly increase the rate of heme-positive stools, occult bleeding should not be attributed to anticoagulation alone. Clinically important but occult lesions of the gastrointestinal tract may frequently be uncovered in such patients by a thorough diagnostic evaluation.

## PRACTICAL CONSIDERATIONS IN USING HEPARIN

### Route of Administration

Because the intensity of therapy is easier to control, continuous intravenous heparin (CIVH) seems to be the preferred route of administration for most patients requiring acute anticoagulation. Alternative routes of heparin administration include intermittent intravenous, fixed subcutaneous dose, and adjusted dose subcutaneous heparin (ADSH).

#### *Continuous Intravenous Heparin (CIVH)*

When administered intravenously, heparin should be given as a loading dose with a bolus of 5000 units followed by a constant intravenous infusion of between 1000 and 1250 units/h (65,105). There are no data to suggest that this dose needs to be adjusted in the elderly.

Laboratory monitoring with an activated partial thromboplastin time (APTT) should be performed at 6 h, with subsequent heparin infusion rates adjusted to achieve an APTT that is 1.5–2.5 times the mean pretreatment or control value (65). Recent nomograms have been published to assist clinicians with the early period of dose adjustment, but variations in the responsiveness of different thromboplastins used to perform the APTT must be taken into account (107).

The risk of recurrent events seems to increase with the amount of time spent with a subtherapeutic APTT (65). Studies by Hull (108) and Basu (109) demonstrated a relative risk of recurrence between 10 and 15 for patients with VTE if the APTT remains subtherapeutic during the first 24 h of heparin administration. Subgroup analysis of two other prospective studies in patients with acute myocardial infarction have demonstrated a relative risk between 6 (110) and 22 (111) for recurrent myocardial infarction (110), angina pectoris (110), or LV mural thrombosis (111) if the lower limit of the therapeutic APTT range was not reached.

Contemporary prospective studies in which heparin was administered by continuous intravenous infusion provide fairly reliable estimates of the incidence of bleeding during heparin therapy. In a recent review of three such studies (100,108,112), Hirsh noted that the incidence of bleeding varied between 1.6 and 7.1% (mean 3.8%) (65).

#### *Intermittent Intravenous Heparin*

Four randomized, unblinded trials have compared intermittent intravenous (IV) heparin to CIVH (113–116). Hirsh found that a pooled analysis of the randomized trials comparing different methods of heparin administration revealed an average incidence of major bleeding of 6.8% in patients receiving CIVH infusions compared with 14.2% among those receiving intermittent IV heparin injections (65). Because the intermittent injection group received higher average doses of heparin, it is difficult to determine if dose alone accounted for the increased rates of bleeding noted in these studies (117).

### *Adjusted Dose Subcutaneous Heparin*

Hull and colleagues reported a higher frequency of recurrent thromboembolism in VTE patients who were treated with ADSH (19.3%) compared with a group receiving CIVH (5.2%). Recurrent thromboses usually occurred in patients who remained subtherapeutic at the beginning of treatment, emphasizing the necessity of maintaining the APTT in the therapeutic range (108). Hommes and colleagues recently published a metanalysis comparing ADSH with CIVH administration in the initial treatment of deep venous thrombosis (118). When the results from six trials with the strongest methodologic study designs were pooled, ADSH was found to be associated with about one-third less extension and recurrence of venous thrombosis than CIVH administration. ADSH also appeared to be at least as safe as CIVH. When the results from all trials were analyzed, the mean incidence of major bleeding was 4.1% in ADSH patients compared with 5.2% in the CIVH group (118). In the acute care setting, ADSH appears to be a reasonable alternative to CIVH, especially in patients with poor venous access or in confused patients who constantly remove intravenous lines (117). For patients requiring long-term anticoagulation, ADSH may provide a reasonable alternative to warfarin. The development of low-molecular-weight heparins with longer biological half lives may make this approach more feasible in the very near future (108).

## How Long Heparin?

Although the optimal duration of IV heparin therapy in the treatment of VTE has not been definitely established, previous clinical recommendations have suggested a period of 7–10 days was necessary (105). This recommendation, which was based on the observation that it takes experimental venous thrombi 5–7 days to become adherent to vessel walls, was recently challenged by two prospective studies that evaluated short and long courses of heparin. In a group of patients with proximal vein thrombosis and submassive pulmonary embolism, Gallus and colleagues initiated therapy with warfarin after 7 days of IV heparin (long course) in 127 patients and compared them to 139 patients who started warfarin within 3 days of initiating heparin (short course) (112). The frequencies of symptomatic VTE recurrence, symptomless new perfusion defects, symptomless proximal extension, and the incidence of major and minor bleeding episodes were similar in both groups.

Hull and associates subsequently designed a randomized, double-blind trial comparing a *short course* of continuous IV heparin (5 days heparin with warfarin begun on day 1) with a *long course* of continuous IV heparin (10 days heparin with warfarin begun on day 5) in the initial treatment of submassive proximal venous thrombosis (100). These investigators found no significant differences in the recurrence rates of thrombosis in either the short (7.1%) or the long (7.0%) treatment arm. The incidence of major bleeding complications (6–7%) also did not differ significantly between the two treatment groups. Thus, warfarin has been found to be both effective and safe when begun shortly after the initiation of heparin therapy. In the Gallus study, early initiation of warfarin significantly shortened hospital stay by an average of almost 4 days (112).

When heparin and warfarin therapy are overlapped it usually takes about 3–4 days to achieve a therapeutic prothrombin time (119). Once the heparin infusion is stopped, the PT should be rechecked 4 h later. The importance of doing so was documented by Lutomski and colleagues, who studied 25 patients receiving overlap therapy with both IV heparin and oral anticoagulants (120). Prothrombin times were measured while patients were receiving a constant heparin infusion and then 4–6 h after the heparin infusion was discontinued. The mean change in the prothrombin time was 1.6 s (range of 0.8 to −5.5 s), with 32% of the patients showing a decrease of greater than 2 s. This change in the prothrombin time was not predictable and correlated poorly with total heparin dose or the previous APTT level. These data strongly suggest that a repeat PT should be checked shortly after discontinuing heparin therapy to avoid allowing the prothrombin time to drop undetected into a subtherapeutic range.

## What Are the Risk Factors for Bleeding in Patients Receiving Heparin?

As noted previously, underlying patient-related risk factors are major determinants of bleeding during treatment with heparin (106). Landefeld et al. identified four factors that were independently related to the development of major bleeding complications in hospitalized patients started on anticoagulation for various reasons (121). These factors included (1) heparin use in patients aged 60 or older; (2) supratherapeutic levels of anticoagulation with maximal prothrombin or partial thromboplastin time greater than two or more times the control value; (3) worsening liver dysfunction on therapy; and (4) the number of specific comorbid conditions (serious cardiac illness, liver dysfunction, renal insufficiency, cancer, or severe anemia).

Hull stratified patients with proximal venous thrombosis into high- or low-risk treatment groups depending on the presence or absence of risk factors for bleeding (100). In this study, high-risk patients had one or more of the following characteristics: (1) surgery within the previous 14 days; (2) history of previous peptic ulcer disease; (3) bleeding into the gastrointestinal or genitourinary tract; (4) disorders predisposing the patient to bleeding; (5) thrombotic stroke within the previous 14 days or; (6) a platelet count less than 150,000. All patients received an IV bolus of 5000 units heparin followed by a continuous IV heparin infusion. Low-risk patients received an intravenous heparin dose of 40,000 units per 24 h, while high-risk patients received 30,000 units per 24 h. Major bleeding occurred in only 1% of the low-risk patients, compared with 11% of the high-risk patients. All patients with major bleeding had an underlying predisposing cause.

Hirsh recently summarized four variables reported to influence bleeding during treatment with heparin (65). These include the dose of heparin, the patient's anticoagulant response, the method of administration, and other patient-related factors, including serious concurrent illnesses, chronic heavy consumption of alcohol, renal failure, age, and sex (96,97,122).

### Heparin-Associated Thrombocytopenia

Although the reported incidence of heparin-associated thrombocytopenia (HAT) varies widely, this complication appears to be two to three times more common in patients receiving heparin derived from bovine lung (15.6%) compared with heparin derived from porcine gut (5.8%) (123). HAT usually begins sometime between 3 and 15 days after the initiation of heparin but may occur as early as several hours into treatment in patients who have been previously exposed (124). To monitor for the development of this reversible complication, platelet counts should be obtained as a baseline at the initiation of heparin therapy and subsequently repeated every 3–4 days as long as heparin is continued (105). Fortunately, less than 0.5% of patients with HAT develop arterial or venous thrombosis secondary to platelet aggregation (124).

## PRACTICAL CONSIDERATIONS IN USING WARFARIN

### Initiating Therapy with Warfarin

For patients who require initial treatment with heparin, warfarin therapy can be initiated on day 1 or 2 either by administering the estimated daily maintenance dose (usually 4–10 mg) or by using a flexible induction protocol like those described by Fennerty et al. (125) and Cosh et al. (126).

There are some theoretical concerns about initiating warfarin therapy without overlapping coverage with heparin. Warfarin causes an early depression of factor VII, resulting in prolongation of the PT; this occurs when the circulating plasma levels of the other three vitamin K-dependent clotting factors are still quite high (Table 7). Warfarin also has an early effect on protein C, a vitamin K-dependent protein with intrinsic anticoagulant and fibrinolytic effects. Because protein C has a short half-life that is similar to that of factor VII, warfa-

**Table 7** Half-life of Vitamin K-Dependent Factors

| Factor | Half-life (h) |
|---|---|
| Factor VII | 4–5 |
| Factor IX | 25 |
| Factor X | 40 |
| Factor II | 60 |
| Protein C | 4–6 |
| Warfarin | 48 |

rin may reduce effective protein C levels to the point that a transient hypercoagulable state is produced during the first 24–48 h of oral anticoagulant therapy. In some patients this early, transient reduction in protein C levels has been thought to be responsible for the syndrome of coumadin necrosis (127–129).

Some clinicians have expressed concern about the possibility of provoking coumadin necrosis in patients with NVAF who are candidates for long-term oral anticoagulation. Unless hemodynamically unstable, such persons usually do not need inpatient hospitalization and most do not require urgent anticoagulation with heparin. Because the NVAF clinical trials did not uncover problems with early strokes or other thrombotic events that might be attributable to protein C-mediated hypercoagulability, we believe that the possibility of coumadin necrosis in such patients is more of a theoretical than a practical concern. It has been our practice to initiate oral anticoagulation in NVAF patients in the outpatient clinic by beginning treatment with the anticipated maintenance dose of warfarin (2.5–5 mg daily) and following prothrombin times at 2–3 day intervals until a stable INR is reached.

## Dose Adjustment

Although most patients on long-term therapy require a daily warfarin dose of about 4–5 mg to maintain a steady state of anticoagulation, there is tremendous dose variation among individual patients. In general, when older patients are compared to younger, the elderly seem to require smaller doses of medication to achieve an equivalent anticoagulant effect (130).

Examples of some conditions that are prevalent in the elderly and known to enhance the prothrombin time response include congestive heart failure, malignancies, malnutrition, and unsuspected vitamin K deficiency (131). Age-related diseases and concurrent drug therapy may account for a major portion of the increased warfarin sensitivity noted in some older patients, but the mechanisms that account for this effect in other elderly patients are not yet fully understood. For example, healthy elderly volunteers taking no other medications still seem to exhibit greater sensitivity to the effects of warfarin than younger patients. Shepherd and colleagues noted that, for a given plasma level of warfarin, older subjects demonstrated greater reductions in the rates of synthesis of coagulation factors than a younger group of controls (132).

## Approach to Patients with Excessive Degrees of Anticoagulation

In patients receiving warfarin, excessive anticoagulation without associated hemorrhage can usually be managed by simply withholding one or several doses of the medication. If vitamin K administration is considered, Shetty and colleagues recommend the use of small doses of vitamin $K_1$ as an effective and convenient method of predictably controlling excessive oral anticoagulation (104). They administered 0.5 mg intravenous vitamin $K_1$ to 21 patients with INR greater than 5.5 (INR range 5.6–25.9) and found that the INR fell below 5.5 in all patients after 24 h. There were no reported instances of overcorrection; the INR did not fall below 2.0 in any patient. No patient had a thrombotic or hemorrhagic complication, and no difficulty was encountered in reestablishing anticoagulant control after 24 h.

## Drug and Dietary Interactions

Drug–drug interactions are among the most frequent problems encountered in the management of elderly persons on long-term anticoagulation. We recommend that physicians routinely caution their patients and other health care providers about the potential for warfarin-drug interactions each time medications are added or deleted from a patient's list of prescriptions. Because of concerns about hemorrhagic gastropathy and inhibition of platelet function, we discourage our patients from using prescription strength or over-the-counter nonsteroidal antiinflammatory drugs or aspirin-containing compounds.

All our patients receive dietary instructions and advice. We do not specifically prohibit the intake of foods high in vitamin K content (133) but instead stress the importance of dietary balance and moderation. We counsel all of our patients about limiting their alcohol intake, and we specifically discuss the increased risk of bleeding associated with binge drinking. Fihn and colleagues noted that elderly patients on warfarin may be at particular risk for alcohol-related bleeding complications (98). In their study, the relative risk for serious warfarin-induced bleeding was 1.4 among binge drinkers and 2.0 among binge drinkers greater than 65 years of age (98).

## Follow-up of Patients on Long-Term Oral Anticoagulants

One prospective British study with a 40 week follow-up found no difference in the degree of control or in the frequency of adverse outcomes in 200 stable outpatients on warfarin who were randomized to follow-up intervals of either 6 or 12 weeks (134). Decreasing the frequency of follow-up may be an option for some stable patients on warfarin, but many of the elderly patients seen in our clinic remain candidates for more frequent monitoring. Age-related comorbidities, the presence of multiple risk factors for serious bleeding complications, and the knowledge that many of our patients have multiple providers who prescribe multiple medications, are all compelling reasons for caution when using anticoagulant drugs in the elderly. Thus, although the potential benefits of routine monthly monitoring have never been shown to justify their cost and inconvenience, we continue to follow our elderly patients on warfarin with monthly determinations of their INR.

## INTERRUPTION OF THERAPY FOR ELECTIVE SURGICAL PROCEDURES

As physicians caring for a large group of patients on oral anticoagulants, we are frequently consulted for advice regarding the appropriate management of anticoagulated patients who are scheduled to undergo elective noncardiac surgery or other invasive procedures. We suggest that patients who need anticoagulation for only a limited period of time should be managed by postponing elective surgical or major dental procedures until the treatment course of anticoagulation is completed. For all others, the decision to continue or interrupt therapy should carefully weigh (1) the thrombotic risk to the patient of allowing the INR to fall below the target treatment threshold; (2) the inherent hemorrhagic risk of the surgery or procedure being considered; and (3) the additional risk of bleeding associated with continuing anticoagulation without modification.

We believe that patients with mechanical heart valves should be considered at relatively high risk for thrombosis if anticoagulants are discontinued for too long. The decision regarding perioperative management of anticoagulation in these patients can be further individualized by considering additional variables that may contribute to thrombotic risk. These variables include the position of the valve, the design and material used for the prosthesis, the presence of atrial fibrillation, and the presence and severity of left ventricular dysfunction (56). An example of a patient with a high thrombotic risk profile is one with congestive heart failure, long-standing atrial fibrillation, and a Starr-Edwards valve in the mitral position. A recent decision analysis examined the cost effectiveness of various strategies for treating patients with mechanical heart valves undergoing noncardiac surgery (135). The authors concluded "that the marginal cost of prolonging hospitalization to administer heparin was prohibitively high compared with most contemporary therapies, except when the patient has the most thrombogenic of valves."

Discontinuation or reduction in the dose of oral anticoagulants does not seem to be necessary for most patients undergoing minor surgical or dental procedures. Benoliel and colleagues recently described their protocol for managing a group of patients with prosthetic heart valves who were having general dental treatment (136). The dose of warfarin was not adjusted when the prothrombin time was less than 2.5 times the control value (the exact level of anticoagulation in these patients was not entirely clear because the thromboplastin reagent was not specified). Only one episode of excessive bleeding occurred during 490 dental procedures, including 87 simple extractions. It has been our practice not to adjust the dose of anticoagulation for patients undergoing routine dental extractions if the INR $< 1.5$. However, we strongly recommend consultation between dentists and primary care physicians to determine whether warfarin dose adjustments are necessary before more complicated dental treatments (such as soft tissue flap reflections) are undertaken.

In a recent review of anticoagulants and anesthesia, Stow and Burrows concluded that the "use of epidural or spinal analgesia in combination with systemic anticoagulation is contraindicated by the standards of most anesthesiologists" (137). The role of regional analgesia in patients receiving anticoagulants is somewhat more controversial and underscores the importance of preoperative consultation among primary care providers, surgeons, and anesthesiologists. For example, routine cataract extraction can be safely recommended in most patients even in the face of systemic anticoagulation because of the relatively avascular field present in cataract surgery (138). The risk of bleeding during other surgical procedures commonly performed in the elderly needs further study so that realistic risk appraisal can replace anecdotal experience.

Thus, the appropriate perioperative strategy for patients on anticoagulants depends on multiple factors, including the underlying indication for anticoagulation, the type of surgical procedure and anesthesia being planned, and a careful and realistic assessment of the risk of thrombosis and/or hemorrhage. Table 8 and the Appendix summarize our approach to these patients.

## FUTURE DIRECTIONS

Further research is needed to define the lowest effective dose of anticoagulant necessary to achieve a protective effect. In doses as low as 1 mg/day, warfarin was effective as prophylaxis against DVT and PE in patients undergoing major gynecological surgery (139). Similar doses have also been shown to prevent

**Table 8** Approach to Patients on Long-Term Anticoagulants Who Require Elective Noncardiac Surgery

Ask the following questions

1. Can the procedure be delayed until the treatment course with anticoagulants is completed?
2. What is the underlying indication for chronic anticoagulation?
3. What is this patient's thrombotic risk if anticoagulents are discontinued?
4. What surgical procedure is being planned?
5. Is this a major or minor procedure?[a]
6. What is the risk of hemorrhage if anticoagulants are continued?
7. Will bleeding compromise or jeopardize the surgical result?
8. What type of anesthesia is being planned?

Talk to the surgeon and/or the referring physician: Identify any special areas of concern

[a]A major procedure is one in which either bone or body cavity is entered.

thrombosis in patients with central venous catheters (140). Future clinical studies need to explore whether such minidoses of warfarin are also effective for other clinical indications.

More work is needed to define high-risk subgroups of NVAF patients who might benefit most from treatment and low-risk subgroups of patients from whom treatment might be safely withheld. Because of the sheer frequency of thrombotic disorders in the elderly, additional clinical trials like SPAF-II are urgently needed to directly compare the risks and benefits of anticoagulating specific subsets of elderly patients (29).

New approaches to patients with cardiac disease are focusing attention on the various roles played by platelets and fibrin in the pathogenesis of clot formation in different clinical settings (cardiac chambers, prosthetic heart valves, and arterial system) (141). Based on an increased understanding of the similarities and differences of clot formation in each of these settings, combination therapies with low-dose warfarin and low-dose aspirin are being clinically evaluated.

Newer antithrombotic agents, such as low-molecular-weight (LMW) heparins (142) and antithrombin III-independent thrombin inhibitors are on the horizon. A recent clinical study with LMW heparin suggested that this agent may be just as effective and safe (but more convenient) than classic intravenous heparin in the treatment of proximal venous thrombosis (143).

Finally, new approaches to monitoring anticoagulant therapy are needed to keep pace with new therapeutic agents and treatment protocols (144). For example, Furie and colleagues demonstrated that the combined rates of bleeding and thrombotic complications were significantly lower in patients monitored with native prothrombin antigen (1.5%) compared to a group of patients monitored with traditional prothrombin times (9.5%) (145). Because the assay for native prothrombin antigen is also sensitive to minidose warfarin regimens, this test may play a much greater role in monitoring future courses of anticoagulant therapy (144).

## APPENDIX: STRATEGIES FOR INTERRUPTING ANTICOAGULATION IN PATIENTS UNDERGOING ELECTIVE NONCARDIAC SURGERY AND MAJOR PROCEDURES

### High Thrombotic Risk → High Hemorrhagic Risk

#### *Example*

A patient with a mechanical mitral valve prosthesis is scheduled to undergo a closed pleural biopsy to diagnose an exudative pleural effusion.

#### *Discussion*

Thrombotic risk is high for a prosthetic valve in this position. Hemorrhagic risk is also high. Hemostasis may be difficult to achieve in the pleural space and other body cavities.

#### *Suggested Strategy*

Discontinue oral anticoagulants before planned procedure. When protime falls to an INR $< 1.3$, hospitalize patient and begin a continuous heparin infusion aiming for a therapeutic APTT of 1.5–2.0 times the control. Discontinue the heparin infusion 4–6 h before the planned procedure. Restart the heparin infusion postprocedure when hemostasis has been achieved. Restart oral anticoagulants when the patient is able to take oral medications.

### High Thrombotic Risk → Low Hemorrhagic Risk

#### *Example*

A patient with a mechanical mitral valve prosthesis is scheduled to undergo a cataract extraction.

#### *Discussion*

This patient's thrombotic risk was just described. Hemorrhagic risk for this procedure is quite low and related to the risk of local (retrobulbar) anesthesia.

#### *Suggested Strategy*

Maintain the patient on warfarin without interruption.

## Low Thrombotic → High Hemorrhagic Risk

### *Example*

A patient with nonvalvular atrial fibrillation being anticoagulated to prevent a cardioembolic stroke is scheduled for colonoscopy and possible polypectomy.

### *Discussion*

The thrombotic risk of interrupting anticoagulant therapy for a brief period of time in patients with nonvalvular atrial fibrillation seems to be quite low. The risk of bleeding in patients undergoing colonoscopic polypectomy is bimodal. One peak occurs at the time of the biopsy; a second window of increased bleeding risk seems to occur about 7–10 days postprocedure.

### *Suggested Strategy*

Discontinue warfarin 2–3 days before the procedure to allow the prothrombin time to normalize. If no biopsy is performed, then resume warfarin at the previous maintenance dose (without a loading dose) on the evening of the procedure. If a biopsy is performed, warfarin is begun at the previous maintenance dose 7–10 days after the procedure. Because it takes several days to achieve a therapeutic protime, there should be adequate time to ensure healing of the biopsy site.

## Low Thrombotic Risk → Low Hemorrhagic Risk

### *Example*

A patient with nonvalvular atrial fibrillation is scheduled for dental extraction.

### *Discussion*

The thrombotic risk of interrupting anticoagulant therapy for a brief period of time in patients with nonvalvular atrial fibrillation seems to be quite low. The risk of significant bleeding from routine dental procedures is quite minimal.

### *Suggested Strategy*

A strategy of no change (or minimal change) seems to be appropriate. Although one might consider withholding a single dose of warfarin before the procedure, this is not routinely necessary. If a dose is withheld, however, warfarin should be resumed in the usual maintenance dose on the night of the procedure.

## NOTE ADDED IN PROOF

Since the submission of this manuscript, the American College of Chest Physicians (ACCP) has published an updated set of recommendations for antithrombotic therapy. For patients with a mechanical heart valve, an INR of 2.5–3.5 is now recommended. An INR of 2–3 remains the recommended intensity of warfarin therapy to prevent thromboembolism in all other patients (146).

## REFERENCES


1. Hull R, Hirsh J, Jay R, Carter C, England C, Gent M, Turpie AGG, McLoughlin D, Dodd P, Thomas M, Raskob G, Ockelford P. Different intensities of oral anticoagulant therapy in the treatment of proximal-vein thrombosis. *N Engl J Med* 1982; 307:1676–1681.
2. Turpie AGG, Gunstensen J, Hirsh J, Nelson H, Gent M. Randomized comparison of two intensities of oral anticoagulant therapy after tissue heart valve replacement. *Lancet* 1988; 1:1242–1245.
3. Saour JN, Sieck JO, Mamo LAR, Gallus AS. Trial of different intensities of anticoagulation in patients with prosthetic heart valves. *N Engl J Med* 1990; 322:428–432.
4. Altman R, Rouvier J, Gurfinkel E, D'Ortencio O, Manzanel R, de la Fuente L, Favaloro RG. Comparison of two levels of anticoagulant therapy in patients with substitute heart valves. *J Thorac Cardiovasc Surg* 1991; 101:427–431.
5. Petersen P, Boysen G, Godtfredsen J, Andersen ED, Andersen B. Placebo-controlled, randomised trial of warfarin and aspirin for prevention of thromboembolic complications in chronic atrial fibrillation: The Copenhagen AFASAK study. *Lancet* 1989; 1:175–178.
6. Stroke Prevention in Atrial Fibrillation investigators. Stroke prevention in atrial fibrillation study: Final results. *Circulation* 1991; 84:527–539.
7. Boston Area Anticoagulation Trial for Atrial Fibrillation investigators. The effect of low-dose warfarin on the risk of stroke in patients with nonrheumatic atrial fibrillation. *N Engl J Med* 1990; 323:1505–1511.
8. Connolly SJ, Laupacis A, Gent M, Roberts RS, Cairns JA, Joyner C. Canadian Atrial Fibrillation Anticoagulation (CAFA) study. *J Am Coll Cardiol* 1991; 18:349–355.
9. Stemerman MB. Coagulation in the elderly. *Clin Geriatr Med* 1985; 1:869–885.
10. Todd M, McDevitt E, McDowell F. Stroke and blood coagulation. *Stroke* 1973; 4:400–405.
11. Hussain S. Disorders of hemostasis and thrombosis in the aged. *Med Clin North Am* 1976; 60:1273–1287.
12. Mansouri A, Bradford DS, Lipschitz DA. Acquired hemostatic abnormalities in the elderly. *J Am Geriatr Soc* 1990; 38:809–816.
13. Robertson BR, Pandolfi M, Nilsson IM. "Fibrinolytic capacity" in healthy volunteers at different ages as studied by standardized venous occlusion of arms and legs. *Acta Med Scand* 1972; 191:199–202.
14. Loeliger EA, Poller L, Samama M, Thomson JM, Van den Besselaar AMHP, Vermylen J, Verstraete M. Questions and answers on prothrombin time standardisation in oral anticoagulant control. *Thromb Haemost* 1985; 54:515–517.
15. Poller L. Progress in standardization in anticoagulant control. *Hematol Rev* 1987; 1:225–241.
16. Hirsh J. Oral anticoagulant drugs. *N Engl J Med* 1991; 324:1865–1875.
17. Hirsh J, Poller L, Deykin D, Levine M, Dalen JE. Optimal therapeutic range for oral anticoagulants. *Chest* 1989; 95:5S–11S.
18. Poller L, Taberner DA. Dosage and control of oral anticoagulants; an international collaborative survey. *Br J Haematol* 1982; 51:479–485.

19. Bussey HI, Force RW, Bianco TM, Leonard AD. Reliance on prothrombin time ratios causes significant errors in anticoagulation therapy. *Arch Intern Med* 1992; 152:278–282.
20. WHO Expert Committee on Biological Standardization. Thirty-third report. Technical report series 687. Geneva: WHO, 1983:81–105.
21. Loeliger EA. ICSH/ICTH Recommendations for reporting prothrombin time in oral anticoagulant control. *Thromb Haemost* 1985; 53:155–156.
22. Loeliger EA, van den Besselaar AMHP, Lewis SM. Reliability and clinical impact of the normalization of the prothrombin times in oral anticoagulant control. *Thromb Haemost* 1985; 54:148–154.
23. Petersen P, Godtfredsen J. Atrial fibrillation—a review of course and prognosis. *Acta Med Scand* 1984; 216:5–9.
24. Kannel WB, Abbott RD, Savage DD, McNamara PM. Epidemiologic features of chronic atrial fibrillation: The Framingham Study. *N Engl J Med* 1982; 306:1018–1022.
25. Aronow WS. Correlation of arrhythmias and conduction defects on the resting electrocardiogram with new cardiac events in 1153 elderly patients. *Am J Noninvas Cardiol* 1991; 5:88–90.
26. Sherman DG, Goldman L, Whiting RB, Jurgensen K, Kaste M, Easton JD. Thromboembolism in patients with atrial fibrillation. *Arch Neurol* 1984; 41:708–710.
27. Wolf PA, Abbott RD, Kannel WB. Atrial fibrillation as an independent risk factor for stroke: The Framingham Study. *Stroke* 1991; 22:983–988.
28. Kutner M, Nixon G, Silverstone F. Physicians' attitudes toward oral anticoagulants and antiplatelet agents for stroke prevention in elderly patients with atrial fibrillation. *Arch Intern Med* 1991; 151:1950–1953.
29. Anderson DC, Progress report of the stroke prevention in atrial fibrillation study. *Stroke* 1990; 21(Suppl. III):12–17.
30. Petersen P, Kastrup J, Helweg-Larsen S, Boysen G, Godtfredsen J. Risk factors for thromboembolic complications in chronic atrial fibrillation: The Copenhagen AFASAK Study. *Arch Intern Med* 1990; 150:819–821.
31. Albers GW, moderator. Stroke prevention in nonvalvular atrial fibrillation. *Ann Intern Med* 1991; 115:727–736.
32. Levine MN, Raskob G, Hirsh J. Hemorrhagic complications of long-term anticoagulant therapy. *Chest* 1989; 95:26s–36s.
33. Petitti DB, Strom BL, Melmon KL. Duration of warfarin anticoagulant therapy and the probabilities of recurrent thromboembolism and hemorrhage. *Am J Med* 1986; 81:255–259.
34. Gurwitz JH, Goldberg RJ, Holden A, Knapic N, Ansell J. Age-related risks of long-term oral anticoagulant therapy. *Arch Intern Med* 1988; 148:1733–1736.
35. Landefeld CS, Goldman L. Major bleeding in outpatients treated with warfarin: incidence and prediction by factors known at the start of outpatient therapy. *Am J Med* 1989; 87:144–152.
36. Launbjerg J, Egeblad H, Heaf J, Nielsen NH, Fugleholm AM, Ladefoged K. Bleeding complications to oral anticoagulant therapy: Multivariate analysis of 1010 treatment years in 551 outpatients. *J Intern Med* 1991; 229:351–355.

37. Stroke Prevention in Atrial Fibrillation investigators. Predictors of thromboembolism in atrial fibrillation. I. Clinical features of patients at risk. *Ann Intern Med* 1992; 116:1–5.
38. Stroke Prevention in Atrial Fibrillation investigators. Predictors of thromboembolism in atrial fibrillation. II. Echocardiographic features of patients at risk. *Ann Intern Med* 1992; 116:6–12.
39. Szekely P. Systemic embolism and anticoagulant prophylaxis in rheumatic heart disease. *Br Med J* 1964; 1:1209–1212.
40. Feinberg WM, Seeger JF, Carmody RF, Anderson DC, Hart RG, Pearce LA. Epidemiologic features of asymptomatic cerebral infarction in patients with nonvalvular atrial fibrillation. *Arch Intern Med* 1990; 150:2340–2344.
41. Brand FN, Abbot RD, Kannel WB, Wolf PA. Characteristics and prognosis of lone atrial fibrillation: 30-Year follow-up in the Framingham study. *JAMA* 1985; 254:3449–3453.
42. Kopecky SL, Gersh BJ, McGoon MD, Whisnant JP, Holmes DR, Ilstrup DM, Frye RI. The natural history of lone atrial fibrillation: A population-based study over three decades. *N Engl J Med* 1987; 317:669–674.
43. Bjerkelund CJ, Orning OM. The efficacy of anticoagulant therapy in preventing embolism related to D.C. electrical conversion of atrial fibrillation. *Am J Cardiol* 1969; 23:208–216.
44. Dunn M, Alexander J, deSilva R, Hildner F. Antithrombotic therapy in atrial fibrillation. *Chest* 1989; 95:118s–127s.
45. Lancaster TR, Singer DE, Sheehan MA, Oertel LB, Maraventano SW, Hughes RA, Kistler JP. The impact of long-term warfarin therapy on quality of life: Evidence from a randomized trial. *Arch Intern Med* 1991; 151:1944–1949.
46. Anderson FA, Wheeler B, Goldberg RJ, Hosmer DW, Patwardhan NA, Jovanovic B, Forcier A, Dalen JE. A population-based perspective of the hospital incidence and case-fatality rates of deep vein thrombosis and pulmonary embolism: The Worcester DVT Study. *Arch Intern Med* 1991; 151:933–938.
47. Moser KM. Venous thromboembolism. *Am Rev Respir Dis* 1990; 141:235–249.
48. Kakkar VV, Howe CT, Nicolaides AN, Renney JTG, Clarke MB. Deep vein thrombosis of the leg; is there a "high risk" group? *Am J Surg* 1970; 120:527–530.
49. Gillum RF. Pulmonary embolism and thrombophlebitis in the United States, 1970–1985. *Am Heart J* 1987; 114:1262–1264.
50. Samkoff JS, Comstock GW. Epidemiology of pulmonary embolism; mortality in a general population. *Am J Epidemiol* 1981; 114:488–496.
51. Barritt DW, Jordan SC. Anticoagulant drugs in the treatment of pulmonary embolism; a controlled trial. *Lancet* 1960; 1:1309–1312.
52. Hull RD, Delmore T, Genton E, Hirsh J, Gent M, Sackett D, McLoughlin D, Armstrong P. Warfarin sodium versus low-dose heparin in the long-term treatment of venous thrombosis. *N Engl J Med* 1979; 301:855–858.
53. Hull R, Delmore T, Carter C, Hirsh J, Genton E, Gent M, Turpie G, McLoughlin D. Adjusted subcutaneous heparin versus warfarin sodium in the long-term treatment of venous thrombosis. *N Engl J Med* 1982; 306:189–194.
54. Lagerstedt CI, Olsson CG, Fagher BO, Oqvist BW, Albrechtsson U. Need for

long-term anticoagulant treatment in symptomatic calf-vein thrombosis. *Lancet* 1985; 2:515–518.

55. Levine HJ, Pauker SG, Salzman EW. Antithrombotic therapy in valvular heart disease. *Chest* 1989; 95:98s–106s.
56. Bodnar AG, Hutter AM. Anticoagulation in valvular heart disease preoperatively and postoperatively. In: Conti CR, ed. Cardiac Drug Therapy. Cardiovascular Clinics. Philadelphia: FA Davis, 1984:247–264.
57. Stein PD, Kantrowitz A. Antithrombotic therapy in mechanical and biological prosthetic heart valves and saphenous vein bypass grafts. *Chest* 1989; 95:107s–117s.
58. Mok CK, Boey J, Wang R, Chan TK, Cheung KL, Lee PK, Chow J, Ng RP, Tse TF. Warfarin versus dipyramidole-aspirin and pentoxifylline-aspirin for the prevention of prosthetic heart valve thromboembolism: A prospective randomized clinical trial. *Circulation* 1985; 72:1059–1063.
59. Sullivan JM, Harken DE, Gorlin R. Effect of dipyramidole on the incidence of arterial emboli after cardiac valve replacement. *Circulation* 1969; 39–40:I–149–153.
60. American Heart Association. Cardiovascular Statistics, 1992. Dallas, Texas
61. DeWood ME, Spores J, Notske R, Mouser LT, Burroughs R, Golden MS, Lang HT. Prevalence of total coronary occlusion during the early hours of transmural myocardial infarction. *N Engl J Med* 1980; 303:897–902.
62. Lewis HD Jr, Davis JW, Archibald DG, Steinke WE, Smitherman TC, Doherty JE III, Schnaper HW, Lewinter MM, Linares E, Pouget JM, Sadharwal SC, Chesler E, Demots H. Protective effects of aspirin against acute myocardial infarction and death in men with unstable angina; results of a Veterans Administration Cooperative Study. *N Engl J Med* 1983; 309:396–403.
63. Theroux P, Ouimet H, McCans J, Latour JG, Joly P, Levy G, Pelletier E, Juneau M, Stasiak J, DeGuise P, Pelletier GB, Rinzler D, Waters DD. Aspirin, heparin, or both to treat acute unstable angina. *N Engl J Med* 1988; 319:1105–1111.
64. RISC Group. Risk of myocardial infarction and death during treatment with low dose aspirin and intravenous heparin in men with unstable coronary artery disease. *Lancet* 1990; 336:827–830.
65. Hirsh J. Heparin. *N Engl J Med* 1991; 324:1565–1574.
66. SCATI group. Randomised controlled trial of subcutaneous calcium-heparin in acute myocardial infarction. *Lancet* 1989; 2:182–186.
67. Neri Serneri GG, Rovelli F, Gensini GF, Pirelli S, Carnovali M, Fortini A. Effectiveness of low-dose heparin in prevention of myocardial reinfarction. *Lancet* 1987; 1:937–942.
68. MacMahon S, Collins R, Knight C, Yusuf S, Peto R. Reduction in major morbidity and mortality by heparin in acute myocardial infarction (abstr). *Circulation* 1988; 78:II–98.
69. International Studies of Infarct Survival Pilot Study investigators. Randomized factorial trial of high-dose intravenous streptokinase, of oral aspirin and of intravenous heparin in acute myocardial infarction. *Eur Heart J* 1987; 8:634–642.
70. International Study group. In-hospital mortality and clinical course of 20,891

patients with suspected acute myocardial infarction randomised between alteplase and streptokinase with or without heparin. *Lancet* 1990; 336:71–75.

71. Jafri SM, Gheorghiade M, Goldstein S. Oral anticoagulation for secondary prevention after myocardial infarction with special reference to the Warfarin Reinfarction Study. *Prog Cardiovasc Dis* 1992; 34:317–324.
72. Sixty Plus Reinfarction Study research group. A double-blind trial to assess long-term oral anticoagulation therapy in elderly patients after myocardial infarction. *Lancet* 1980; 2:989–994.
73. Sixty Plus Reinfarction Study research group. Risks of long-term oral anticoagulation therapy in elderly patients after myocardial infarction. *Lancet* 1982; 1:64–68.
74. Smith P, Arnesen H, Holme I. The effect of warfarin on mortality and reinfarction after myocardial infarction. *N Engl J Med* 1990; 323:147–152.
75. Antiplatelet Trialists' Collaboration. Secondary prevention of vascular disease by prolonged antiplatelet therapy. *Br Med J* 1988; 296:320–331.
76. Ezekowitz MD, Azrin MA. Should patients with large anterior wall myocardial infarction have echocardiography to identify left ventricular thrombus and should they be anticoagulated? In: Cheitlin MD, ed. Dilemmas in Clinical Cardiology. Cardiovascular Clinics. Philadelphia: FA Davis, 1990; 21:105–122.
77. Johannessen KA, Nordrehaug JE, von der Lippe G, Vollset SE. Risk factors for embolisation in patients with left ventricular thrombi and acute myocardial infarction. *Br Heart J* 1988; 60:104–110.
78. Stratton JR, Resnick AD. Increased embolic risk in patients with left ventricular thrombi. *Circulation* 1987; 75:1004–1011.
79. ACC/AHA. Guidelines for the early management of patients with acute myocardial infarction. *Circulation* 1990; 82:664–707.
80. Resnekov L, Chediak J, Hirsh J, Lewis HD. Antithrombotic agents in coronary artery disease. *Chest* 1989; 95:52s–72s.
81. Fuster V, Gersh BJ, Giuliani ER, Tajik AJ, Brandenburg RO, Frye RL. The natural history of idiopathic dilated cardiomyopathy. *Am J Cardiol* 1981; 47:525-531.
82. Tsevat J, Eckman MH, McNutt RA, Pauker SG. Warfarin for dilated cardiomyopathy: A bitter tough pill to swallow? *Med Decis Making* 1989; 9:162–169.
83. Rothrock JF, Hart RG. Antithrombotic therapy in cerebrovascular disease. *Ann Intern Med* 1991; 115:885–895.
84. Cerebral Embolism task force. Cardiogenic brain embolism. *Arch Neurol* 1986; 43:71–84.
85. Sherman DG, Dyken ML, Fisher M, Harrison MJ, Hart RG. Cerebral embolism. *Chest* 1986; 89:82s–98s.
86. Furlan AJ. Transient ischemic attacks: Recognition and management. *Heart Dis Stroke* 1992; 1:33–38.
87. Miller VT. Transient ischemic attacks and ischemic stroke: Indications for anticoagulation. *Clin Cardiol* 1990; 13:29–30.
88. Estol CJ, Pessin MS. Anticoagulation: Is there still a role in atherothrombotic stroke? Current Concepts Cerebrovasc Dis Stroke 1990; 25:1–6.

89. Boobis LH, Bell PR. Can drugs help patients with lower limb ischaemia? *Br J Surg* 1982; 69:s17–s23.
90. Criqui MH, Langer RD, Fronek A, Feigelson HS, Klauber MR, McCann TJ, Browner D. Mortality over a period of 10 years in patients with peripheral arterial disease. *N Engl J Med* 1992; 326:381–386.
91. Kretschmer G, Wenzl E, Piza E, Polterauer P, Ehringer H, Minar E, Schemper M. The influence of anticoagulant treatment on the probability of function in femoropopliteal vein bypass surgery: Analysis of a clinical series (1970 to 1985) and interim evaluation of a controlled clinical trial. *Surgery* 1987; 102:453–459.
92. Kretschmer G, Wenzl E, Schemper M, Polterauer P, Ehringer H, Marcosi L, Minar E. Influence of postoperative anticoagulant treatment on patient survival after femoropopliteal vein bypass surgery. *Lancet* 1988; 1:797–799.
93. Clagett GP, Genton E, Salzman EW. Antithrombotic therapy in peripheral vascular disease. *Chest* 1989; 95:128s–139s.
94. Coon WW, Willis PW. Hemorrhagic complications of anticoagulant therapy. *Arch Intern Med* 1974; 133:386–392.
95. Forfar JC. A 7-year analysis of hemorrhage in patients on long term anticoagulant treatment. *Br Heart J* 1979; 42:128–132.
96. Jick H, Slone D, Borda IT, Shapiro S. Efficacy and toxicity of heparin in relation to age and sex. *N Engl J Med* 1968; 279:284–286.
97. Walker AM, Jick H. Predictors of bleeding during heparin therapy. *JAMA* 1980; 244:1209–1212.
98. Fihn SD, McDonell MB, Vermes D, Kent DL, Henikoff JG, and Warfarin Anticoagulation Study group. Risk factors for complications during chronic anticoagulation. Northwest Field Program HSR&D Newsletter VAMC, Seattle, WA, 1991; 4(3):3.
99. Landefeld CS, Rosenblatt MW, Goldman L. Bleeding in outpatients treated with warfarin: Relation to the prothrombin time and important remediable lesions. *Am J Med* 1989; 87:153–159.
100. Hull RD, Raskob GE, Rosenbloom D, Panju AA, Brill-Edwards P, Ginsberg JS, Hirsh J, Martin GJ, Green D. Heparin for 5 days as compared with 10 days in the initial treatment of proximal venous thrombosis. *N Engl J Med* 1990; 322:1260–1264.
101. Wilcox CM, Truss CD. Gastrointestinal bleeding in patients receiving long-term anticoagulant therapy. *Am J Med* 1988; 84:683–690.
102. Kewenter J, Svanvik J, Svensson C, Wallgren K. The diagnostic value of the hemoccult as a screening test in patients taking anticoagulants. *Cancer* 1984; 54:3054–3058.
103. Jaffin BW, Bliss CM, Lamont JT. Significance of occult gastrointestinal bleeding during anticoagulation therapy. *Am J Med* 1987; 83:269–272.
104. Shetty HGM, Backhouse G, Bentley DP, Routledge PA. Effective reversal of warfarin-induced excessive anticoagulation with low dose vitamin $K_1$. *Thromb Haemost* 1992; 67:13–15.
105. Hyers TM, Hull RD, Weg JG. Antithrombotic therapy for venous thromboembolic disease. *Chest* 1989; 95:37s–51s.

106. Levine MN, Hirsh J. Hemorrhage complications of anticoagulant therapy. *Semin Thromb Hemost* 1986; 12:39–57.
107. Cruickshank MK, Levine MN, Hirsh J, Roberts R, Siguenza M. A standard heparin nomogram for the management of heparin therapy. *Arch Intern Med* 1991; 151:333–337.
108. Hull RD, Raskob GE, Hirsh J, Jay RM, Leclerc JR, Geerts WH, Rosenbloom D, Sackett D, Anderson C, Harrison L, Gent M. Continuous intravenous heparin compared with intermittent subcutaneous heparin in the initial treatment of proximal-vein thrombosis. *N Engl J Med* 1986; 315:1109–1114.
109. Basu D, Gallus A, Hirsh J, Cade JA. Prospective study of the value of monitoring heparin treatment with the activated partial thromboplastin time. *N Engl J Med* 1972; 287:324–327.
110. Kaplan K, Davison R, Parker M, Mayberry B, Feiereisel P, Salinger M. Role of heparin after intravenous thrombolytic therapy for acute myocardial infarction. *Am J Cardiol* 1987; 59:241–244.
111. Turpie AGG, Robinson JG, Doyle DJ, Mulji AS, Mishkel GJ, Sealey BJ, Cairns JA, Skingley L, Hirsh J, Gent M. Comparison of high-dose with low-dose subcutaneous heparin to prevent left ventricular mural thrombosis in patients with acute transmural anterior myocardial infarction. *N Engl J Med* 1989; 320:352–357.
112. Gallus A, Jackaman J, Tillett J, Mills W, Wycherley A. Safety and efficacy of warfarin started early after submassive venous thrombosis or pulmonary embolism. *Lancet* 1986; 2:1293–1296.
113. Salzman EW, Deykin D, Shapiro RM, Rosenberg R. Management of heparin therapy. Controlled prospective trial. *N Engl J Med* 1975; 292:1046–1050.
114. Glazier RL, Crowell EB. Randomized prospective trial of continuous vs intermittent heparin therapy. *JAMA* 1976; 236:1365–1367.
115. Wilson JR, Lampman J. Heparin therapy: A randomized prospective study. *Am Heart J* 1979; 97:155–158.
116. Mant MJ, O'Brien BD, Thong KL, Hammond GW, Birtwhistle RV, Grace MG. Haemorrhagic complications of heparin therapy. *Lancet* 1977; 1:1133–1135.
117. Robitaille D, LeClerc JR, Bravo G. Treatment of venous thromboembolism. In: LeClerc JR, ed. Venous Thromboembolic Disorders. Philadelphia: Lea and Febiger, 1991:267–302.
118. Hommes DW, Bura A, Mazzolai L, Buller HR, ten Cate JW. Subcutaneous heparin compared with continuous intravenous heparin administration in the initial treatment of deep vein thrombosis: A meta-analysis. *Ann Intern Med* 1992; 116:279–284.
119. White RH, Hong R, Venook AP, Daschbach MM, Murray W, Mungall DR, Coleman RW. Initiation of warfarin therapy: Comparison of physician dosing with computer-assisted dosing. *J Gen Intern Med* 1987; 2:141–148.
120. Lutomski DM, Djuric PE, Draeger RW. Warfarin therapy: The effect of heparin on prothrombin times. *Arch Intern Med* 1987; 147:432–433.
121. Landefeld CS, McGuire E III, Rosenblatt MW. A bleeding risk index for estimating the probability of major bleeding in hospitalized patients starting anticoagulant therapy. *Am J Med* 1990; 89:569–578.

122. Landefeld CS, Cook EF, Flatley M, Weisberg M, Goldman L. Identification and preliminary validation of predictors of major bleeding in hospitalized patients starting anticoagulant therapy. *Am J Med* 1987; 82:703–713.
123. King DJ, Kelton JG. Heparin-associated thrombocytopenia. *Ann Intern Med* 1984; 100:535–540.
124. Warkentin TE, Kelton JG. Heparin-induced thrombocytopenia. *Annu Rev Med* 1989; 40:31–44.
125. Fennerty A, Dolben J, Thomas P, Backhouse G, Bentley DP, Campbell IA, Routledge PA. Flexible induction dose regimen for warfarin and prediction of maintenance dose. *Br Med J* 1984; 288:1268–1270.
126. Cosh DG, Dally RJ, Moritz CK, Gallus AS, Ashman KJ. Prospective evaluation of a flexible protocol for starting treatment with warfarin and predicting its maintenance dose. *Aust N Z J Med* 1989; 19:191–197.
127. Scandling J, Walker BK. Extensive tissue necrosis associated with warfarin sodium therapy. *South Med J* 1980; 73:1470–1472.
128. Faraci PA, Deterling RA Jr, Stein AM, Rheinlander HF, Cleveland RJ. Warfarin induced necrosis of the skin. *Surg Gynecol Obstet* 1978; 146:695–700.
129. McGehee WG, Klotz TA, Epstein DJ, Rapaport SI. Coumarin necrosis associated with hereditary protein C deficiency. *Ann Intern Med* 1984; 101:59–60.
130. Redwood M, Taylor C, Bain BJ, Matthews JH. The association of age with dosage requirement for warfarin. *Age Ageing* 1991; 20:217–220.
131. Hazell K, Baloch KH. Vitamin K deficiency in the elderly. *Gerontol Clin* 1970; 12:10–17.
132. Shepherd AMM, Hewick DS, Moreland TA, Stevenson IH. Age as a determinant of sensitivity to warfarin. *Br J Clin Pharmacol* 1977; 4:315–320.
133. Weihrauch JL. Provisional table on the vitamin K content of foods. Human Nutrition Information Service HNIS/PT-104. United States Department of Agriculture, 1986.
134. Howard MR, Milligan DW. Frequency of attendance at anticoagulant clinics: A prospective study. *Br Med J* 1988; 296:898–899.
135. Eckman MH, Beshansky JR, Durand-Zaleski I, Levine HJ, Pauker SG. Anticoagulation for noncardiac procedures in patients with prosthetic heart valves: Does low risk mean high cost? *JAMA* 1990; 263:1513–1521.
136. Benoliel R, Leviner E, Katz J, Tzukert A. Dental treatment for the patient on anticoagulant therapy: Prothrombin time value—what difference does it make? *Oral Surg Oral Med Oral Pathol* 1986; 62:149–151.
137. Stow PJ, Burrows FA. Anticoagulants in anesthesia. *Can J Anaesth* 1987; 34:632–649.
138. Hall DL, Steen WH, Drummond JW. Anticoagulants and cataract surgery. *Ann Ophthalmol* 1980; 12:759–760.
139. Poller L, McKernan A, Thomson JM, Elstein M, Hirsch PJ, Jones JB. Fixed minidose warfarin: A new approach to prophylaxis against venous thrombosis after major surgery. *Br Med J* 1987; 295:1309–1312.
140. Bern MM, Lokich JJ, Wallach SR, Bothe A, Benotti PN, Arkin CF, Greco FA, Huberman M, Moore C. Very low doses of warfarin can prevent thrombosis in

central venous catheters: A randomized prospective trial. *Ann Intern Med* 1990; 112:423–428.

141. Stein B, Fuster V, Halperin L, Cheseboro JH. Antithrombotic therapy in cardiac disease: An emerging approach based on pathogenesis and risk. *Circulation* 1989; 80:1501–1513.
142. Hirsh J, Levine MN. Low molecular weight heparin. *Blood* 1992; 79:1–17.
143. Hull RD, Raskob GE, Pineo GF, Green D, Trowbridge AA, Elliott CG, Lerner RG, Hall J, Sparling T, Brettell HR, Norton J, Carter CJ, George R, Merli G, Ward J, Mayo W, Rosenbloom D, Brant R. Subcutaneous low-molecular weight heparin compared with continuous intravenous heparin in the treatment of proximal-vein thrombosis. *N Engl J Med* 1992; 326:975–982.
144. Furie B, Furie BC. Molecular and cellular biology of blood coagulation. *N Engl J Med* 1992; 326:800–806.
145. Furie B, Diuguid CF, Jacobs M, Diuguid DL, Furie BC. Randomized prospective trial comparing the native prothrombin antigen with the prothrombin time for monitoring oral anticoagulant therapy. *Blood* 1990; 75:344–349.
146. Dalen JE, Hirsh J (ed). Third ACCP consensus conference on antithrombotic therapy. *Chest* 1992; 102:303s–549s.

# 10

# Exercise Training in the Elderly Cardiac Patient

**Mark A. Williams and Dennis J. Esterbrooks**
*Creighton University School of Medicine, Omaha, Nebraska*

## INTRODUCTION

The most critical factor in an elderly cardiac patient's ability to function independently in society is the ability to be mobile without assistance (1). Thus, the overall focus for exercise training should be to enhance health-related fitness components, including cardiorespiratory and muscular endurance, flexibility, strength, and body composition. The cardiorespiratory system of the older cardiac patient is capable of exercise training, and good levels of aerobic fitness are achievable. Regular exercise can also lead to increased strength and muscle mass, a loss of fat, and maintenance of an acceptable level of body composition in this population.

## EFFECTS OF EXERCISE TRAINING IN THE HEALTHY ELDERLY

The cardiovascular benefits of aerobic conditioning are similar in healthy older and younger subjects, although baseline values in older subjects are lower and the elderly may require more time for adaptation (2). Maximal oxygen uptake and physical work capacity can improve as much as 40% in elderly males and females. The amount of improvement depends upon baseline values and the exercise training protocol (3–20). Heart rate, systolic and diastolic blood pressure, and blood lactate are reduced after training at a given submaximal work load. Anaerobic threshold is increased (9,10,15,21–25). Despite these improvements, there is no evidence that myocardial performance is altered with chronic exercise in the elderly (14). Other important changes include increased oxygen pulse (the volume of oxygen consumption with each heart beat), improved cardiovascular recovery, increased duration of submaximal exertion, and lowered resting systolic and diastolic blood pressure (3,4,9,13,14,26–28).

Peripherally, the oxidative capacity of muscle tissue increases, resulting from increased capillarization, increased aerobic enzyme content in the skeletal muscle, and preservation of the size and number of mitochondria (29,30). Conditioning decreases body fat and increases lean mass (31,32). Exercise can benefit carbohydrate and lipid metabolism in younger adults. Although the effects in elderly individuals are less definitive, reductions in total cholesterol and low-density lipoprotein cholesterol, as well as increased high-density lipoprotein concentration, have been reported (10,33).

## Strength Training

The expected improvement in strength from resistance training is difficult to assess. Increases in strength are affected by the initial level of strength and the potential for improvement, which are affected by the presence of chronic disease. In studies of subjects from 60 to 90 years of age, increases in strength following 6–26 weeks of training ranged from 9 to 227%, depending on the muscle group studied. The mean increase for all muscle groups was approximately 75% over an average of 10 weeks (34–41). Strength gains in the elderly have been most often attributed to the improved neural recruitment patterns rather than an actual increase in strength. This is substantiated by the fact that in some studies, no direct correlation has been noted between the degree of hypertrophy and relative strength gains (34,38,40). Strength gains have occurred within the first few weeks of training in these subjects, before hypertrophy would have been a factor. Muscle hypertrophy appears to account for a portion of the strength gains observed in the elderly, however, as assessed by muscle biopsy or cross-sectional computed tomographic scanning (34,37,40,42).

## Flexibility

Flexibility training in the elderly shows improvement in joint flexibility and subjective perception of improved mobility. A sense of well-being is also enhanced in many subjects as a result of improved flexibility, either measured or perceived (43).

## RESPONSES TO TRAINING IN THE CARDIAC ELDERLY

Although the results of studies have been consistent, data are sparse on the effects of aerobic exercise training in cardiac patients over 65 years of age. Investigations have primarily focused on early postdischarge exercise rehabilitation (phase II), with little information from long-term exercise rehabilitation (phase III).

### Short-Term Exercise Training

Studies of the effects of up to 12 weeks of phase II exercise training have demonstrated a variety of training benefits in elderly persons (44–46). Williams and colleagues demonstrated significantly increased maximal exercise tolerance, decreased submaximal exercise myocardial work as estimated by the rate-pressure product, and decreased ratings of perceived effort at standardized work intensities (Table 1). Increased maximal rate-pressure product after training was also observed, suggesting that trained elderly cardiac patients are able to perform at higher levels of myocardial oxygen demand (44). Other investigators have demonstrated similar results (46). These results appear achievable regardless of whether elderly patients are taking $\beta$-blocker medications or are post–acute myocardial infarction (AMI) or post–coronary artery bypass grafting (CABG; Tables 2 and 3). Elderly cardiac patients appear to make modest but significant improvements in weight, percentage of body fat, forced expiratory ventilation in one second, resting heart rate, and resting rate-pressure product. Resting systolic and diastolic blood pressures have not been reported to exhibit a significant training effect.

### Males Versus Females

Although few investigators have compared training effects in elderly males and females, findings suggest that both improve similarly even though females are generally less fit, having nearly a 20% lower maximal oxygen uptake (47–49). Although elderly female cardiac patients are less likely to be referred to cardiac rehabilitation than males, even though they have similar clinical profiles, they improve similarly to elderly male cardiac patients in acute and chronic exercise adaptation.

### The Older Elderly

Results from previously described investigations suggest that elderly cardiac patients as a group are capable of significant increases in maximal exercise tolerance and significant decreases in submaximal exercise myocardial work as

**Table 1** Results of the Evaluation of Elderly Patients Before and After Training

| | Before training | After training |
|---|---|---|
| Body weight, kg | 76.9 ± 12.2 | 75.2 ± 11.9[a] |
| Body fat, % | 22.3 ± 5.7 | 20.8 ± 5.4[a] |
| Vital capacity, liters ($n = 34$) | 3.6 ± 0.6 | 3.6 ± 0.5[a] |
| $FEV_1$, % of vital capacity ($n = 34$) | 73.9 ± 12.1 | 79.4 ± 7.4[a] |
| Before exercise | | |
| HR, beats/min | 77 ± 14 | 68 ± 9[a] |
| Systolic BP, mm Hg | 125 ± 21 | 122 ± 19 |
| Diastolic BP, mm Hg | 76 ± 10 | 73 ± 9 |
| Maximal exercise | | |
| HR | 126 ± 20 | 138 ± 20[a] |
| Systolic BP | 161 ± 27 | 171 ± 24[a] |
| $HR \times BP \times 10^{-2}$ | 205 ± 55 | 234 ± 48[a] |
| Physical work capacity (METs) | 5.3 ± 1.3 | 8.1 ± 1.6[a] |
| Submaximal exercise | | |
| Average $HR \times BP \times 10^{-2}$ (submaximal) | 173 ± 44 | 141 ± 35[a] |
| Average RPE (submaximal) | 12 ± 2 | 10 ± 2[a] |

Data are mean ± standard deviation. $n = 76$, mean age 70.2 ± 3.2 years. BP = blood pressure; $FEV_1$ = formed expiratory ventilation in one second; HR = heart rate; HR × BP = heart rate × systolic blood pressure; METs = multiples of resting oxygen uptake (1 MET = 95 ml of oxygen per kilogram of body weight per minute); RPE = rating of perceived exertion.
[a] $p < 0.05$.
*Source*: From Reference 44.

**Table 2** Test Results Before and After Training in Elderly Patients

| | Before training | After training |
|---|---|---|
| $\beta$ blockade ($n = 25$) | | |
| Physical work capacity (METs) | 5.1 ± 1.5 | 7.8 ± 1.4[a] |
| Average $HR \times BP \times 10^{-2}$ (submaximal) | 155 ± 38 | 125 ± 28[a] |
| Average RPE (submaximal) | 13 ± 2 | 11 ± 2[a] |
| No $\beta$ blockade ($n = 51$) | | |
| Physical work capacity (METs) | 5.4 ± 1.2 | 8.2 ± 1.6[a] |
| Average $HR \times BP \times 10^{-2}$ (submaximal) | 182 ± 44[b] | 149 ± 35[a,b] |
| Average RPE (submaximal) | 12 ± 2 | 10 ± 2[a] |

Abbreviations as in Table 1. Data are mean ± standard deviation.
[a] $p < 0.05$
[b] Significantly different ($p < 0.05$) from $\beta$ blockade group.
*Source*: From Reference 44.

**Table 3** Results of Exercise Tests Before and After Training in Elderly Patients

| | Before training | After training |
|---|---|---|
| After AMI ($n$ = 41) | | |
| Physical work capacity (METs) | 5.4 ± 1.3 | 8.0 ± 1.4[a] |
| Average HR × BP × $10^{-2}$ (submaximal) | 168 ± 43 | 135 ± 33[a] |
| Average RPE (submaximal) | 13 ± 2 | 11 ± 2[a] |
| After CABG ($n$ = 35) | | |
| Physical work capacity (METs) | 5.1 ± 1.3 | 8.1 ± 1.8[a] |
| Average HR × BP × $10^{-2}$ (submaximal) | 179 ± 44 | 148 ± 36[a] |
| Average RPE (submaximal) | 12 ± 2 | 10 ± 2[a] |

Data are mean ± standard deviation. AMI = acute myocardial infarction; CABG = coronary artery bypass grafting; other abbreviations as in Table 1.
[a]$p < 0.05$.
*Source*: From Reference 44.

estimated by lower rate-pressure product following exercise training. Despite these findings, subjective and objective observations have suggested that "older" elderly cardiac patients may not improve as much as "younger" elderly cardiac patients following standard phase II exercise training. The "older" elderly patient group includes those individuals 75 years of age or greater. It has been observed that only limited improvements in submaximal and maximal response to exercise training were exhibited in cardiac patients age 75 years or greater, with even lesser change in patients age 80 years or greater (Table 4) (50).

However, more recent work has suggested that there is a subgroup of this latter patient population that is capable of training benefits similar to that observed in younger elderly patients (Table 5) (51). This subgroup of older elderly cardiac patients was characterized as (1) capable of completing an extended period of exercise training following the standard phase II program; (2) having peak exercise capacity of at least 4–5 METs at the end of the standard phase II program; and (3) capable of increasing exercise training intensity throughout the entire period of early and extended exercise training.

## Long-Term Exercise Training

In many instances, the response to long-term exercise is maintenance of gains previously made. Nevertheless, modest improvements have been reported in weight, resting heart rate, resting systolic blood pressure, and maximal exercise capacity (Table 6) (52). A significant decrease in resting diastolic blood pressure has also been observed, a finding not previously noted with short-term exercise training. Significant improvement has also been observed in physiological and

**Table 4** Exercise Training Results for Elderly Cardiac Patients with Age Subgroups

| Variable | $T_1$ | $T_2$ |
|---|---|---|
| All subjects group ($n = 248$, $\bar{x} = 70.4$ years; 53% post-MI and 47% post-CABG) | | |
| Rest | | |
| Heart rate, bpm | 83 ± 5 | 78 ± 3[a] |
| Systolic pressure, mm Hg | 124 ± 7 | 123 ± 7 |
| Diastolic pressure, mm Hg | 71 ± 4 | 71 ± 3 |
| Submaximal exercise rate-pressure/100 | 144 ± 15 | 123 ± 12[a] |
| Maximal exercise | | |
| Heart rate, bpm | 129 ± 7 | 131 ± 7 |
| Systolic pressure, mm Hg | 167 ± 9 | 172 ± 8[a] |
| Rate-pressure product/100 | 215 ± 19 | 225 ± 16[a] |
| Functional capacity (METs) | 3.2 ± 0.5 | 6.5 ± 0.6[a] |
| Subgroup 1 ($n = 135$, $\bar{x} = 66.9$ years; 52% post-MI and 48% post-CABG) | | |
| Rest heart rate, bpm | 85 ± 7 | 79 ± 5[a] |
| Submaximal exercise rate-pressure product/100 | 148 ± 22 | 126 ± 18[a] |
| Functional capacity (METs) | 3.4 ± 0.7 | 7.0 ± 0.8[a] |
| Subgroup 2 ($n = 70$, $\bar{x} = 72.3$ years; 59% post-MI and 41% post-CABG) | | |
| Rest heart rate, bpm | 81 ± 13 | 74 ± 9 |
| Submaximal exercise rate-pressure product/100 | 143 ± 35 | 120 ± 28 |
| Functional capacity (METs) | 3.2 ± 1.0 | 6.9 ± 1.3[a] |
| Subroup 3 ($n = 28$, $\bar{x} = 76.4$ years; 60% post-MI and 40% post-CABG) | | |
| Rest heart rate, bpm | 85 ± 22 | 80 ± 14 |
| Submaximal exercise rate-pressure product/100 | 142 ± 65 | 123 ± 45 |
| Functional capacity (METs) | 3.1 ± 1.0 | 4.9 ± 2.4 |
| Subgroup 4 ($n = 15$, $\bar{x} = 81.8$ years; 67% post-MI and 33% post-CABG | | |
| Rest heart rate, bpm | 75 ± 21 | 78 ± 16 |
| Submaximal exercise rate-pressure product | 111 ± 86 | 103 ± 67 |
| Functional capacity (METs) | 2.3 ± 1.1 | 2.8 ± 1.8 |

Data are mean ± standard deviation; $\bar{x}$ = mean age.

[a] Significantly different ($p < 0.05$) from $T_1$ value.

*Source*: From Reference 50.

**Table 5** Older Elderly Cardiac Patient ($\geqslant$75 Years of Age) Training Response Following 6 Months of Exercise Training (mean ± standard deviation)

| | $T_1$ | $T_2$ | $T_3$ |
|---|---|---|---|
| Rest heart rate, bpm | 83 ± 17 | 80 ± 13 | 69 ± 7[a] |
| Submaximal exercise rate-pressure product/100 | 137 ± 35 | 118 ± 32 | 77 ± 26[a] |
| Maximal oxygen uptake (METs) | 3.0 ± 9 | 5.1 ± 1.7 | 6.9 ± 1.2[a] |

Data are mean ± standard deviation. $n = 22$. $T_1$ = pretraining data; $T_2$ = data following 3 months of training; and $T_3$ = data following 6 months of training.
[a] Significantly different ($p < 0.05$) from both $T_1$ and $T_2$ values.
*Source*: From Reference 51.

**Table 6** Elderly Cardiac Patient Training Response Following 18 Months of Exercise Training

| | $T_1$ | $T_2$ | $T_3$ |
|---|---|---|---|
| Weight, kg | 79.5 ± 12.3 | 77.5 ± 11.6[a] | 76.1 ± 12.1 |
| Body fat, % | 22.8 ± 5.5 | 20.4 ± 4.8[a] | 20.4 ± 4.6 |
| Resting heart rate, bpm | 83 ± 11 | 77 ± 13[a] | 73 ± 11 |
| Resting systolic blood pressure, mm Hg | 121 ± 17 | 120 ± 16 | 117 ± 15 |
| Resting diastolic blood pressure, mm Hg | 84 ± 9 | 77 ± 11[a] | 69 ± 10[b] |
| Maximal heart rate, bpm | 122 ± 22 | 134 ± 22[a] | 130 ± 18 |
| Maximal systolic blood pressure, mm Hg | 158 ± 27 | 168 ± 27[a] | 166 ± 14 |
| Maximal rate-pressure product/100 | 193 ± 49 | 225 ± 48[a] | 216 ± 33 |
| Maximal exercise capacity (METs) | 4.9 ± 1.7 | 8.1 ± 20[a] | 8.6 ± 2.4 |
| Submaximal average rate-pressure product/100 | 202 ± 49 | 134 ± 26[a] | 113 ± 25[b] |
| Submaximal average rate-pressure product/100 | 12 ± 2 | 10 ± 2 | 9 ± 1[b] |

Data are mean ± standard deviation. $n = 18$. Mean age = 69.3 ± 2.9. $T_1$ = pretraining data; $T_2$ = data following 3 months of training; and $T_3$ = data following 18 months of training.
[a] $p < 0.05$ for $T_1$ versus $T_2$.
[b] $p < 0.05$ for $T_2$ versus $T_3$.
*Source*: From Reference 52.

perceptual responses to standardized submaximal effort, suggesting that continued reduction in submaximal myocardial oxygen demand at standardized work loads is possible. Improvements derived from both short- and long-term exercise rehabilitation will allow elderly patients to function at higher work levels during daily activities and may result in fewer cardiac symptoms and improved quality of life.

## Resistance Training

Although no studies of resistance training in elderly cardiac patients have been reported, indirect evidence suggests that such programs would be of benefit. This evidence includes that (1) resistance training programs are of significant benefit in normal elderly individuals and (2) resistance training has been demonstrated to be practical and safe and to result in significant strength gains of 25–50% in younger cardiac patients (53–55).

## Comparison of Training Adaptation in the Young and Elderly

The aging process has been shown to decrease cardiorespiratory function, which results in diminished physical work capacity. Thus, older patients should not be expected to perform as well as their younger counterparts. However, improvements in endurance and functional capacity can be achieved with exercise training in both healthy and cardiac elderly individuals.

Comparisons of short-term exercise training benefits between young and elderly cardiac patients have provided important information. Results demonstrated that magnitudes of changes and exercise training responses were similar (Table 7) (44). In fact, one observation suggested that elderly cardiac patients might make greater relative improvement in submaximal response to exertion than their younger counterparts (46). A possible explanation for this finding is that regular physical activity has not been a part of elderly patients' lives for many years; hence, improvements may represent a larger percentage change compared with baseline measurements. Additionally, as suggested by Hakki and coworkers, status of left ventricular function may be more important than age in determining exercise capacity in patients with coronary artery disease (56).

There are no studies directly comparing the long-term benefits derived from exercise training between elderly and younger cardiac patients. Studies of long-term exercise training in younger patients have demonstrated significant benefit in anthropometric measurements and cardiovascular measures at rest and in response to submaximal and maximal exertion. Whether a more intense program or a longer period of training in the elderly would result in changes similar to those seen in younger patients has yet to be determined.

**Table 7** Exercise Test Results Before and After Training in Four Age Groups

| | Before training | After training |
|---|---|---|
| Group 1 (mean age 40 ± 4 years) | | |
| Physical work capacity (METs) | 6.3 ± 1.6 | 9.8 ± 1.6[a,b] |
| Average HR × BP × $10^{-2}$ (submaximal) | 170 ± 33 | 143 ± 33[a] |
| Average RPE (submaximal) | 12 ± 2 | 9 ± 2[a,b] |
| Group II (mean age 50 ± 3 years) | | |
| Physical work capacity (METs) | 6.3 ± 1.3[b] | 9.2 ± 1.4[a,b] |
| Average HR × BP × $10^{-2}$ (submaximal) | 168 ± 46 | 134 ± 32[a] |
| Average RPE (submaximal) | 12 ± 2 | 10 ± 2[a] |
| Group III (mean age 59 ± 3 years) | | |
| Physical work capacity (METs) | 6.0 ± 1.7 | 9.0 ± 1.7[a,b] |
| Average HR × BP × $10^{-2}$ (submaximal) | 156 ± 40 | 135 ± 37[a] |
| Average RPE (submaximal) | 12 ± 2 | 10 ± 2[a] |
| Group IV (mean age 70 ± 3 years) | | |
| Physical work capacity (METs) | 5.3 ± 1.3 | 8.1 ± 1.5[a] |
| Average HR × BP × $10^{-2}$ (submaximal) | 173 ± 44 | 141 ± 35[a] |
| Average RPE (submaximal) | 12 ± 2 | 10 ± 2[a] |

Data are mean ± standard deviation. Abbreviations as in Table 3.
[a] Significantly different from before training value ($p < 0.05$).
[b] Absolute value is significantly different from similar value in group IV ($p < 0.05$), although magnitudes of change are not significantly different with the exception of METs in group I versus METs in group IV.
*Source*: From Reference 44.

## SPECIAL CONSIDERATIONS

More than for other age groups, activity programs for the elderly cardiac patient must be tailored to the individual's age, fitness level, and health status, which vary widely within the "older" population (1). Many elderly cardiac patients suffer from one or more chronic diseases that can affect functional capacity. It is not uncommon for elderly cardiac patients to have significant peripheral vascular disease, pulmonary disease, arthritis, and various other problems. Additionally, the altered cardiac structure and functional changes associated with aging, as well as inactivity and deconditioning, may contribute to cardiovascular disability.

## Initial Evaluation

The initial evaluation provides the information for establishing the goals of an exercise training program (57,58). The goals of the program should be established based on the patient's interests and objectives, ensuring that they are realistic, and related to formal and informal exercise programs, activities of daily living, occupational activities, and recreational activities, including hobbies.

The elderly cardiac patient may exhibit a variety of characteristics that require special consideration, including drug and dietary history, evaluation for sensory deficits, and determination of musculoskeletal abnormalities (58). Dietary inadequacies are prevalent and may be compounded by modest increases in caloric expenditure from exercise training (31). The combination of appropriate diet and exercise is an important consideration to achieve several benefits from physical activity (43).

Peripheral neuropathy, gait disturbance, impaired equilibrium, or orthostatic hypotension may increase the potential for falls. Degenerative joint disease is also common in this age group. Assessment of joint stability and range of motion should be performed before exercise training, and when appropriate, activity should be adjusted accordingly (58).

The initial evaluation should also review patient medication regimens for possible interactions with activity programs (1). Diuretics may predispose patients to hypocalcemia, hypokalemia, arrhythmias, and volume depletion. $\beta$-Blocking drugs can alter exercise parameters and reduce exercise tolerance in some elderly individuals, whereas tranquilizers can cause orthostatic dizziness and impair thermal regulation. Patients on insulin or related oral medications may require dose adjustment.

## Aerobic Exercise Prescription

Aerobic exercise involving the large muscles of the body is best to achieve the health and fitness goals of elderly healthy cardiac populations (21,59). Such activities as walking, jogging, rowing, and swimming are good examples. Nonetheless, if an exercise prescription focuses on aerobic exercise involving the lower extremities, such as walking and cycling, a relative weakening of the upper extremity muscles can occur (57). With appropriate precautions and supervision, upper-body aerobic exercise and resistance training can be of significant value in the elderly patient population for maintaining or increasing strength and muscle mass.

General recommendations for exercise training in elderly cardiac patients are presented in Table 8. Some specific comments regarding intensity, frequency,

**Table 8** General Recommendations for the Exercise Prescription

| | |
|---|---|
| Intensity | Maintain at least 50–80% of the peak oxygen uptake attained at the most recent exercise test corresponding to 60–85% of the peak heart rate at same test |
| Frequency | Participation in a formal training program 3 days per week; home exercise (walking or cycle ergometry) 3–5 days per week |
| Duration | 55 min per session, including 10 min warm-up and flexibility exercises, six 5 min periods of activity with 1 min rest periods between stations (35 min), and 10 min cooldown |
| Mode | Alternating arm and leg exercise utilizing treadmill walking, leg ergometry, and arm ergometry |

duration, and modality should be noted, however, because differences among individuals dictate exercise prescription methods.

The exercise prescription should be based on an initial graded exercise test to make appropriate recommendations for heart rate and work load intensity. When exercise testing has not been performed before exercise training, which may apply to as many as 50% of elderly patients, alternative methods can be used to prescribe exercise. These include combinations of reduced exercise work loads and rating of perceived exertion.

### *Intensity and Progression*

The physical work capacity of the elderly cardiac patient, both before and following exercise training, is often significantly lower than that observed in younger cardiac patients (44). Because many elderly patients have been sedentary for a long time, specific muscle groups are often severely deconditioned, particularly those used during arm or leg cycle ergometry. In elderly patients, musculoskeletal limitations may be more important than the cardiac limitations. It is therefore important to prescribe low-level exercise work load intensities, particularly during the first few weeks of exercise training (60).

It is not uncommon that elderly cardiac patients in the exercise program are incapable of exercising within the recommended intensity range (60–85% of maximal heart rate). In these instances, the elderly are encouraged to exercise but at considerably reduced intensities (50–60% of maximal heart rate). When exercise training intensity is low, participants are encouraged to increase the frequency of exercise, perhaps even to several times per day.

Patient progress and consideration for an increase in the exercise training target heart rate should be reviewed periodically. This assessment can be easily accomplished with repeat exercise test, although this may not be possible for all patients. Hence, the updated exercise prescription must be based on data collected during the first few weeks of exercise training to provide a means of safely increasing intensity during the latter weeks of early exercise training. Of course, these increases are made only in patients who have been asymptomatic during training, have not exhibited contraindications to increased exercise intensity, and have shown normal training adaptation (60).

Exercise training intensities are not generally increased beyond 85% of attained maximal heart rate in the elderly patient population because of the potential for musculoskeletal injury (61). Additionally, more recent information regarding the benefit of low-intensity exercise has become available and suggests that high-intensity exercise may not be required to obtain a variety of health benefits (62).

### *Frequency*

Particularly during early exercise training, when low exercise training intensities are dictated by low functional capacities and musculoskeletal limitations, it is important to encourage elderly patients to adhere to "off-day" walking or cycling programs (63). That is, informal exercise is recommended on days when they do not participate in a formal exercise session. This is essential to provide an adequate training stimulus and to increase functional capacity during the initial weeks of the program.

### *Duration*

In general, the duration of the exercise session remains constant for elderly patients during the initial weeks of exercise training (60). Changes in the exercise prescription during this time are primarily made through adjustments in exercise training intensity. However, exercise duration may have to be reduced during the initial weeks of training for patients whose ability to exercise for an entire session is physically or emotionally limited. Patients incapable of sustaining exercise for the recommended duration (20–40 min) are encouraged to exercise more frequently during the day or are provided with longer rest periods during actual training sessions.

As elderly participants move into long-term exercise training, they are encouraged to lengthen the duration of activity (61). This is particularly important for individuals who exercise at low intensity. Lengthening the duration of activity helps to increase caloric expenditure and is associated with improvement of a variety of risk factors, including obesity, lipid abnormalities, hypertension, and elevated blood glucose (62). Increases in exercise duration should be made slowly to allow adaptation.

### *Modalities*

Elderly individuals routinely use the same modalities of exercise utilized by younger patients (60). Many elderly persons have orthopedic problems that have resulted from or may be exacerbated by weight-bearing exercise, however, which lead to added stress to joints and muscles. Thus, special consideration may be important in this patient group.

Bicycling and exercise in the water are excellent modalities of exercise that sustain aerobic activity while decreasing the effects of weight bearing on lower extremities (1). Stationary cycling is recommended for the less healthy patient, particularly for those whose balance, hearing, or vision is impaired. Water exercise, especially for the obese or physically limited patient, allows the patient to become "weightless," thereby decreasing stress in the joints of the lower extremities (1,64).

Many recreational activities, such as golf, dancing, and tennis, provide excellent opportunities for elderly cardiac patients to exercise (65). Participants in a long-term exercise program should be encouraged to resume safe activities that they enjoyed before the cardiac event. Competitive activities, such as tennis and golf, can supplement an exercise program. The level of play should reflect the individual's physical condition, however. Overexertion can lead to adverse consequences, especially when the element of competition causes one to ignore warning symptoms (1). Rhythmic calisthenics and dance exercise can provide both warm-up and sustained activity. Proper counseling is essential to avoid overuse and sudden twisting injuries. Exercises that support the body's weight with the arms, such as push-ups, should be performed with caution, because they may cause an excessive rise in blood pressure and increase the work of the heart.

Although not often considered a part of regular exercise, activities of daily living should also be used to supplement formal training sessions (1). Walking to the store, hedge trimming, painting, and gardening can contribute to improving fitness. Stairways can provide a valuable source of physical training.

## Resistance Training

Resistive strength exercise for cardiac patients, such as weight lifting, has gained acceptance in recent years, although little attention has been placed on its value within the elderly cardiac population. Maintenance and improvement in strength, especially of the upper body, as well as the development of muscle tissue, may facilitate an increase in maximal oxygen uptake as well as being important for many cardiac patients to pursue their occupational or leisure time activities. Thus the role of resistance training for the elderly has important ramifications for exercise program design (34,54,64). Patients should receive instructions in weight training techniques, including proper breathing during these exercises and avoidance of the Valsalva maneuver. Weight training should follow aerobic conditioning in a training session. A minimum of 5–10 min of range of motion activity should be performed before resistance training to prepare for more vigorous activity and prevent injury.

Resistance training must be monitored closely so that overvigorous twisting or excessive strain does not occur. Systemic blood pressure may increase more in response to weight lifting compared to aerobic-type exercise (66). Blood pressure monitoring may be indicated in some individuals (1). Because of a potential increased risk of arrhythmias from resistance activity, electrocardiogram monitoring is recommended during the first few sessions and when increases in weight are made. Resistance exercise has been shown to be safe, and no untoward events have been reported when patients were appropriately screened (67–69).

### *Circuit Weight Training*

Circuit training requires the participant to exercise in short bouts, using light to moderate work loads with frequent repetitions interspersed with short rest periods. This method of exercise challenges the skeletal muscles as well as the cardiovascular system. Guidelines for circuit resistance training in the elderly cardiac patient are found in Table 9 (54). Increases of 5% in work load intensities can be made following reevaluations, performed at 5–6-week intervals.

### *Strength Training*

A traditional strength training program involves four to eight repetitions at each station, with increased total work output a function of increased percentage of one repetition maximum (1RM; 60–80%) (70). In elderly cardiac patients, the use of strength training should be confined to those who have completed a standard phase II exercise training program and circuit training as previously outlined. A recent echocardiogram to evaluate left ventricular function is recom-

**Table 9** Guidelines to Resistance Training

| |
|---|
| Patient characteristics |
| Normal or normalized-controlled blood pressure |
| Free of complex arrhythmias |
| Previous 6–8 weeks of standard cardiac exercise training |
| Minimum 5 METs capacity |
| Testing and circuit training characteristics |
| One repetition maximum (RM) testing |
| 8–12 repetitions |
| 40–60% of 1 RM |
| 30–60 s rests between stations |
| One to three sets |
| Major muscle groups |
| Up to eight stations of upper and lower extremity work |
| Two to three times per week |

mended before initiating strength training. This evaluation may also include an echocardiogram recorded during testing to determine whether maximal resistance effort precipitates any left ventricular wall motion abnormality.

Fewer stations are utilized with strength training because of the relatively high work load outputs at each station and the potential for excessive blood pressure response. Thus, one or two stations of both arm and upper torso and leg exercise are recommended. Updating work load intensities is similar to that used in the circuit training program.

### Flexibility

Flexibility, or range of motion, in most joints is imposed by the soft tissues, including (1) the muscle and its fascial sheaths; (2) the connective tissue, with tendons, ligaments, and joint capsules; and (3) the skin (71,72). Other factors influencing flexibility are the level of recent physical activity and gender, because females are considerably more flexible than males. And, most important for this discussion, increasing age after reaching adulthood is associated with significant decreases in flexibility (72).

Typically, flexibility is assessed by measuring the range of joint motion directly or indirectly. A number of laboratory and field techniques have been devised for assessing flexibility (73,74). Such tests can be very useful in measuring the effectiveness of a flexibility exercise program, and patients generally find the evaluations relatively simple to perform as well as helpful in demonstrating particular limitations. Less emphasis should be placed on the actual classification of flexibility because these apply primarily to younger patients.

Range of motion exercises that use jerking, bobbing, or bouncing invoke the stretch reflex, which actually opposes flexibility. Conversely, static stretch invokes the inverse myotatic reflex, which helps to improve flexibility. Static stretching is safer than ballistic stretching because it does not impose sudden strains upon the tissues involved in the movement. Ballistic stretching frequently causes severe soreness in muscles; conversely, static stretching may help to relieve soreness.

## OTHER CONSIDERATIONS

### Warm-up

Warm-up exercises and careful progression into the aerobic training portion of the program should be performed to reduce the likelihood of exercise-related adverse signs or symptoms or physical injuries (1). These may range from both physical injury, such as muscle strain and joint pain, to signs or symptoms associated with ischemia (75). As a result of aging, sedentary life-style, and arthritis, elderly cardiac patients often show decreases in flexibility. Consequently, they may have to be instructed on how to overcome these limitations and be encouraged to practice regularly various range of motion and flexibility exercises. The inclusion of flexibility training as a part of this pretraining exercise period is strongly recommended. A general preliminary period of stretching and light activity involving the large muscle groups, for 10–15 min, is appropriate for most exercise training programs involving elderly cardiac patients.

### Cooldown

The exercise training session may also require an extended cooldown period following physical activity (1). The cooldown should enhance venous return and reduce the potential for postexercise hypotension, syncopal episodes, or arrhythmias during recovery. A cooldown period also helps remove lactate from the muscles that have been working beyond their anaerobic threshold and decreases the chances that stiffness and muscle pain will develop, particularly early in a training program. The patient should avoid excessively hot showers and prolonged standing in hot and humid areas during the cooldown period.

### Home Exercise

Since formal programs are not always available, some patients must exercise without direct supervision (65). The alternative of denying the benefits of exercise to a patient is unacceptable unless the person is at high risk. Both short- and long-term programs for elderly patients must be developed under specific advice from the patient's primary care physician (65). The exercise prescription can closely follow the recommendations for intensity and progression, frequency, duration, and modality outlined earlier in this chapter. However, patients must take extra care to start an unsupervised exercise program cautiously. It is crucial that patients monitor their own exercise response and potential cardiac symptoms and contact the primary care physician when any changes or symptoms occur. The prescription of home exercise should also provide patients with written material that promotes compliance with the exercise prescription (65). An exercise log book for recording the date, type of exercise, heart rate response, and symptoms should also be provided.

## SUMMARY

Exercise training in the rehabilitation of the elderly cardiac patient will increase functional capacity and enhance personal independence by decreasing the need for assistance in activities of daily life. Moreover, the sense of isolation and depression that often accompanies reduced mobility in the elderly may be averted or offset by the physical improvements associated with exercise training. Exercise training is also associated with improved feelings of well-being and self-esteem. Epidemiological and laboratory studies have also demonstrated that exercise conditioning favorably alters coronary heart disease risk factors. Well-designed individualized exercise training programs that fit the elderly patient's life-style optimize compliance to training. However, providing the elderly cardiac patient with an exercise prescription without support or reinforcement results in low compliance. Prudent cardiac rehabilitation policy suggests that exercise training include strategies for supervision and follow-up (76).

The number of elderly cardiac patients entering outpatient cardiac rehabilitation will continue to escalate. Recent advances in the care of elderly cardiac patients will probably extend longevity an additional 10–20 years following the initial diagnosis of coronary heart disease (77). High-risk patients with myocardial ischemia, arrhythmias, or chronic congestive heart failure will make up a much greater percentage of participants. Many of these will be elderly. The results of life-style changes will improve the quality and perhaps quantity of life. Documenting the value of exercise rehabilitation should increase the number of elderly participants and challenge health care professionals to increase the quantity and quality of programs.

Risk stratification has been described for younger patients but has yet to be evaluated in the elderly cardiac patient (78,79). As the number of elderly cardiac patients increases, there is a need to assess the level of risk of untoward events during exercise (Table 10). Even if risk of morbidity and mortality can be established, however, they may not be as relevant for the elderly as the issue of quality of life.

Program staff must continue to search for the most appropriate training methods for the elderly. Participation will be a function of patient risk and creative programming that center around nonmonitored, less supervised or unsupervised exercise. In some instances, walking programs may be ideal for achieving the benefits associated with physical activity, especially in this age group. The aerobic cost of walking has been documented, and although walking may not provide sufficient intensity for a training benefit in younger subjects, it can be an excellent training modality for those in their seventies, eighties, and nineties (62,80). Walking may also be beneficial for decreasing anxiety and depression and aid in weight control (81).

In summary, the time has long passed for excluding candidates from outpatient cardiac rehabilitation on the basis of age. As the number of elderly patients increases, we are challenged to provide meaningful and valuable programs and to determine ways of making these programs available. Independence is an important concern for the elderly, those who care for them, and those who may be responsible for the costs of health, sickness, and dependence. We must continue to evaluate the specific needs of this group and respond wherever possible with new and innovative approaches to enhance recruitment and maintain adherence to programs of physical activity and life-style management.

**Table 10** Risk Stratification for Elderly Cardiac Patients

| |
|---|
| Low risk |
| Uncomplicated clinical course in the hospital |
| No resting or exertional evidence of myocardial ischemia |
| Functional capacity ⩾ 6 METs |
| Normal left ventricular ejection fraction (>50%) |
| Absence of significant ventricular ectopy |
| Moderate risk |
| Functional capacity 4–5.9 METs |
| Moderately impaired left ventricular ejection fraction (35–49%) |
| High risk |
| Impaired left ventricular ejection fraction (<35%) |
| Exertional hypotension |
| Recurrent angina posthospitalization |
| Functional capacity < 4 METs |
| Exertional myocardial ischemia |
| Reversible thallium defect |
| Congestive heart failure during hospitalization |
| Complex ventricular arrhythmias |

## REFERENCES

1. Elia EA. Exercise and the elderly. *Clin Sports Med* 1991; 10:141–155.
2. Ninimaa Z, Shephard RJ. Training and oxygen conductance in the elderly. II. The cardiovascular system. *J Gerontol* 1978; 33:362–367.
3. Benestad AM. Trainability of old men. *Acta Med Scand* 1965; 178:321–327.
4. Sidney KH, Shepard RJ. Frequency and intensity of exercise training for elderly subjects. *Med Sci Sports* 1978; 10:125–131.
5. Ehsani AA. Cardiovascular adaptations to exercise training in the elderly. *Fed Proc* 1987; 46:1840–1843.
6. Seals DR, Hagberg JM, Hurley BF, Ehsani AA, Holloszy JO. Endurance training in older men and women. I. Cardiovascular responses to exercise. *J Appl Physiol* 1984; 57:1024–1029.
7. Thomas SG, Cunningham DA, Rechnitzer PA, Donner AP, Howard JH. Determinants of the training response in elderly men. *Med Sci Sports Exerc* 1985; 17:667–672.
8. Hagberg JM. Effects of training on the decline of $VO_2$max with aging. *Fed Proc* 1987; 46:1830–1833.
9. Rodahl K. The effects of physical conditioning on older individuals. I. Work capacity, circulatory-respiratory function, and work electrocardiogram. *J Gerontol* 1966; 21:182–191.

10. Cunningham DA, Rechnitzer PA, Howard JH, Donner AP. *J Gerontol* 1987; 42:17–23.
11. Blumenthal JA, Emery CF, Madden DJ, Coleman RE, Riddle MW, Schniebolk S, Cobb FR, Sullivan MJ, Higginbotham MB. Effects of exercise training on cardiorespiratory function in men and women > 60 years of age. *Am J Cardiol* 1991; 67:633–639.
12. Niinimaa V, Shephard RJ. Training and oxygen conductance in the elderly. I. The respiratory system. *J Gerontol* 1978; 33:354–361.
13. DeVries HA. Physiological effects of an exercise training regimen upon men aged 52 to 88. *J Gerontol* 1970; 25:325–336.
14. Posner JD, Gorman KM, Klein HS, Woldow A. Exercise capacity in the elderly. *Am J Cardiol* 1986; 57:52C–58C.
15. Adams GM, deVries HA. Physiological effects of an exercise training regimen upon women aged 42 to 79. *J Gerontol* 1973; 28:50–55.
16. Astrand PO. Quantification of exercise capability and evaluation of physical capacity in men. *Prog Cardiovasc Dis* 1976; 19:51–67.
17. Astrand I, Astrand PO. Aerobic work performance: A review. In: Folinsbee LB, ed. Environmental Stress: Individual Human Adaptations. New York: Academic Press, 1978:1149–163.
18. Ekblom B, Astrand PO, Saltin B, Stenberg J, Wallstrom B. Effective training on circulatory response to exercise. *J Appl Physiol* 1968; 24:518–528.
19. Ekblom B. Effective physical training on the oxygen transport system in man. *Acta Physiol Scand* Suppl 1969; 328:9–45.
20. Blumenthal JA, Schocker DD, Needels TL, Hindle P. Psychological and physiological effects of physical conditioning on the elderly. *J Psychomotor Res* 1982; 26:505–510.
21. Preventive and Rehabilitative Exercise Committee, American College of Sports Medicine. Guidelines for Exercise Testing and Prescription, 4th ed. Philadelphia: Lea & Febiger, 1991.
22. Boyer JL, Kasch FW. Exercise therapy in hypertension. *JAMA* 1970; 211:1168–1671.
23. Seals DR, Hurley BF, Schultz J, Hagberg JM. Endurance training in older men and women. II. Blood lactate responses to submaximal exercise. *J Appl Physiol* 1984; 57:1030–1031.
24. Davis JA, Frank MH, Whipp BJ, Wassman K. Anaerobic threshold alterations caused by endurance training in middle-aged men. *J Appl Physiol* 1979; 46:1039–1046.
25. Montgomery DL, Ismail AH. The effect of a four-month physical fitness program on high-and-low fit groups matched for age. *J Sports Med* 1977; 17:327–333.
26. DeVries HA, Adams GM. Comparison of exercise responses in old and young men. *J Gerontol* 1972; 27:344–348.
27. Stamford BA. Physiologic effects of training upon institutionalized geriatric men. *J Gerontol* 1972; 27:451–455.
28. Cononie CC, Graves JE, Pollock ML, Phillips MI, Sumners C, Hagberg JM. Effective exercise training on blood pressure in 70- to 79-yr-old men and women. *Med Sci Sports Exerc* 1991; 23:505–511.

29. Shock NW. Physiological aspects of aging in man. *Annu Rev Physiol* 1961; 23:97–122.
30. Saltin B. The aging endurance athlete. In: Sutton JR, Brock R, eds. Sports Medicine for the Mature Athlete. Indianapolis, IN: Benchmark Press, 1986:59–80.
31. Shephard RJ. Physical Activity and Aging, 2nd ed. Rockville, MD: Aspen Publishers, 1987.
32. Sidney KH, Shephard RJ, Harrison J. Endurance training and body composition of the elderly. *Am J Clin Nutr* 1977; 30:326–333.
33. Saltin B, Lingarde F, Houston M, Horlin R, Nugaard E, Gad P. Physical training and glucose tolerance in middle-aged men with chemical diabetes. *Diabetes* 1979; 28:30–32.
34. Fiatarone MA, Marks EC, Ryan ND, Meredith CN, Lipsitz LA, Evans WJ. High intensity strength training in nonagenarians. Effects on skeletal muscle. *JAMA* 1990; 263:3029–3034.
35. Perkins LC, Kaiser HL. Results of short-term isotonic and isometric exercise programs in persons over 60. *Phys Ther Rev* 1961; 41:633–635.
36. Liemohn WP. Strength in aging: An exploratory study. *Int J Aging Hum Dev* 1975; 6:347–357.
37. Aniansson A, Gustafsson E. Physical training in elderly men with special reference to quadriceps, muscle, strength, and morphology. *Clin Physiol* 1981; 1:87–98.
38. Moritani T, deVries HA. Potential for gross muscle hypertrophy in older men. *J Gerontol* 1980; 35:672–682.
39. Kauffman TL. Strength training effect in young and aged women. *Arch Phys Med Rehabil* 1985; 65:223–226.
40. Frontera WR, Meredith CN, O'Reilly KP, Knuttgen HG, Evans WJ. Strength conditioning in older men: Skeletal muscle hypertrophy and improved function. *J Appl. Physiol* 1988; 64:1038–1044.
41. Hagberg JM, Graves JE, Limacher M, Woods DR, Leggett SH, Cononie C, Gruber JJ, Pollock ML. Cardiovascular responses of 70–79-yr-old men and women to exercise training. *J Appl Physiol* 1989; 66:2589–2594.
42. Larsson L. Physical training effects on muscle morphology in sedentary males at different ages. *Med Sci Sports Exerc* 1982; 14:203–206.
43. Smith EL, Serfass RC. Exercise and Aging: The Scientific Basis. Hillside, NJ: Enslow Publishers, 1981.
44. Williams MA, Maresh CM, Esterbrooks DJ, Harbrecht JJ, Sketch MH Sr. Early exercise training in patients older than age 65 years compared with that in younger patients after acute myocardial infarction or coronary artery bypass grafting. *Am J Cardiol* 1985; 55:263–266.
45. Ades PA, Grunvald MH. Cardiopulmonary exercise testing before and after conditioning in older coronary patients. *Am Heart J* 1990; 120:585–589.
46. Ades PA, Hanson JS, Gunther JGS, Tonino RP. Exercise conditioning in the elderly coronary patient. *J Am Geriatr Soc* 1987; 35:121–124.
47. Ades P, Waldmann M, Polk D, Coflesky J. Referral patterns and exercise response in the rehabilitation of female coronary patients aged $\geqslant$ 62 years. *Am J Cardiol* 1992; 69:1422–1425.

48. Oldridge NB, LaSalle D, Jones NL. Exercise rehabilitation of female patients with coronary artery disease. *Am Heart J* 1980; 100:755–757.
49. Petratis MM, Williams MA, Fogland TL, Esterbrooks DJ. The benefits of early exercise training in female cardiac patients. abstr. *J Cardiac Rehabil* 1987; 7:503.
50. Williams MA, Esterbrooks DJ, Sketch MH Sr. Limitations of phase II exercise training in the "older" elderly cardiac patient. abstr. *Circulation* 1990; 82:III–576.
51. Williams MA, Esterbrooks DJ, Sketch MH Sr. Extension of phase II exercise training produces significant benefit in the older elderly participant. abstr. *J Cardiopulm Rehabil* 1991; 11:312.
52. Williams MA, Maresh CM, Esterbrooks DJ, Sketch MH Sr. abstr. *J Am Geriatr Soc* 1987; 35:904.
53. Kelemen MH, Stewart KJ, Gillilan RE, Ewart CK, Valenti SA, Manley JD, Kellemen MD. Circuit weight training in cardiac patients. *J Am Coll Cardiol* 1986; 7:38–42.
54. Vander LB, Franklin BA, Wrisley D, Rubenfire M. Acute cardiovascular responses to Nautilus exercise in cardiac patients: Implications for exercise training. *Ann Sports Med* 1986; 2:165–169.
55. Butler RM, Beierwaltes WH, Rodgers FJ. The cardiovascular response to circuit weight training in patients with coronary diseases. *J Cardiopulm Rehabil* 1987; 7:402–409.
56. Hakki AH, DePace NL, Iskandrian AS. Effect of age on left ventricular function during exercise in patients with coronary artery disease. *J Am Coll Cardiol* 1983; 2:645–651.
57. Smith EL, Gilligan C. Physical activity prescription for the older adult. *Physician Sportsmed* 1983; 11(8):91–101.
58. Fitzgerald PL. Exercise for the elderly. *Med Clin North Am* 1985; 69:189–196.
59. Shephard RJ. Prescribing Exercise for the Senior Citizen: Some Simple Guidelines. Chicago: Year Book, 1989.
60. Williams MA, Esterbrooks DJ, Sketch MH. Guidelines to exercise therapy of the elderly after myocardial infarction. *Eur Heart J* 1984; 5(Suppl E):121–123.
61. Williams MA, Sketch MH. Guidelines for exercise training of elderly patients following myocardial infarction and coronary bypass graft surgery. *Geriatr Cardiovasc Med* 1988; 1:107–110.
62. Blair SN, Kohl HW, Paffenbarger DR Jr, Clark DG, Cooper KH, Bibbons LW. Physical fitness and all-cause mortality: A prospective study of healthy men and women. *JAMA* 1989; 262:2395–2401.
63. Pollock ML, Ward A, Foster C. Exercise prescription for rehabilitation of the cardiac patient. In: Pollock ML, Schmidt DH, eds. Heart Disease and Rehabilitation. Boston: Houghton-Mifflin, 1979:413–445.
64. Shephard RJ. Physical training for the elderly. *Clin Sports Med* 1986; 5:515–533.
65. Williams MA, Sketch MH Sr. After a heart attack: Prescribing exercise to speed recovery. *Senior Patient* 1990; 2:16–20.
66. Lind AR, McNichol GW. Muscular forces which determine the cardiovascular responses to sustained and rhythmic exercise. *Can Med Assoc J* 1967; 96:706–713.
67. Lewis SF, Snell PG, Taylor WF, Hamra M, Graham RM, Pettinger WA,

Blomqvist CG. Role of muscle mass and mode of contraction in circulatory response to exercise. *J Appl Physiol* 1985; 58:46–151.

68. DeBusk RF, Baldez R, Houston N, Haskell W. Cardiovascular responses to dynamic and static efforts soon after myocardial infarction. Application to occupational work assessment. *Circulation* 1978; 58:368–375.
69. Ferguson RJ, Cote P, Bourassa MG, Corbara F. Coronary blood flow during isometric and dynamic exercise in angina pectoris patients. *J Cardiac Rehabil* 1981; 1:21–27.
70. Baechle TR, Groves BR. Weight Training. Champaign, IL: Leisure Press, 1992:141–151.
71. Pollock ML, Wilmore JH. Exercise in health and disease. Evaluation and Prescription for Prevention and Rehabilitation, 2nd ed. Philadelphia: W. B. Saunders, 1990:202–236.
72. deVries HA. Physiology of Exercise for Physical Education and Athletics, 4th ed. Dubuque, IA: William C. Brown, 1986.
73. Heyward VH. Designs for Fitness. New York: Macmillan, 1984:140–150.
74. Wear CL. The relationship of flexibility measurements to length of body segments. *Res Q* 1963; 34:234–238.
75. Barnard RJ, MacAlpin R, Kattus AA, Buckberg GD. Ischemic response to sudden strenuous exercise in healthy men. *Circulation* 1973; 48:936–942.
76. Lampman RM. Evaluating and prescribing exercise for elderly patients. *Geriatrics* 1987; 42:63–76.
77. Guralnik JM, FitzSimmons SC. Aging in America: A demographic perspective. *Cardiol Clin* 1986; 4:175–183.
78. DeBusk RF, Haskell WL, Miller NH, Berra K, Taylor CB, Berger WE, Lew H. Medically directed at-home. Rehabilitation soon after clinically uncomplicated acute myocardial infarction: A new model for patient care. *Am J Cardiol* 1985; 55:251–257.
79. American Association of Cardiovascular and Pulmonary Rehabilitation. Guidelines for Cardiac Rehabilitation Programs. Champaign, IL: Human Kinetics Books, 1991:1–8.
80. Bruce RA, Larson EB, Stratton J. Physical fitness, functional aerobic capacity, and responses to physical training or bypass surgery in coronary patients. *J Cardiopulm Rehabil* 1989; 9:24–34.
81. Wenger NK. Rehabilitation of the coronary patient in the 21st century: Challenges and opportunities. In: Wenger NK, Hellerstein HK, eds. Rehabilitation of the Coronary Patient. New York: Churchill Livingstone, 1992:581–592.

# 11

# Recognition and Diagnosis of Coronary Artery Disease in the Elderly

**Donald D. Tresch**
*Medical College of Wisconsin and University of Wisconsin, Milwaukee, Wisconsin*

**Wilbert S. Aronow**
*Mount Sinai School of Medicine, New York, New York and Hebrew Hospital Home, Bronx, New York*

## INTRODUCTION

Autopsy studies (1,2) demonstrate that approximately 70% of persons between 70 and 80 years have coronary atherosclerosis, with the prevalence increasing to 80% in persons older than 80 years. The autopsy finding may be coincidental, with the disease process clinically silent throughout the person's life and the person's death unrelated to coronary artery disease. At least 20–30% of persons over the age of 65 years, however, clinically demonstrate coronary artery disease (CAD) and many are functionally impaired by the disease (3,4). Furthermore, CAD is the number one cause of death in patients older than 65 years (5,6). Women appear protected from CAD in their youth and middle years, with the mortality from CAD in women of middle age approximately only half that in men of the same age range, although after 65 years the morbidity from CAD markedly increases, until at age 75, coronary morbidity is equal for men and for women (7). Even though so prevalent, clinical manifestations of CAD are often clinically missed or misdiagnosed as caused by another disease in the elderly. This difficulty in diagnosing CAD in the elderly may be because the clinical manifestations can be significantly different from those in the younger patient with the disorder. Such differences may reflect a difference in the disease process between the age groups, or it may be related to the superimposition of normal physiological aging changes and the presence of concomitant diseases that mask the usual clinical manifestations.

Coronary artery disease in the elderly is diagnosed if the patient has angiographic evidence of significant CAD, a documented myocardial infarction (MI), or clinical findings of myocardial ischemia.

## MYOCARDIAL ISCHEMIA

Myocardial ischemia presenting as angina pectoris is commonly the first clinical manifestation of CAD in middle-aged persons and is usually readily recognized. This may not be the case in the elderly person with CAD, and not infrequently, typical angina may not be present. Because of limited activity, many elderly persons with CAD do not experience the exertional angina so common in younger patients with the disease. Ischemia, when manifesting as pain in the back or shoulders, is often in the elderly misinterpreted as related to degenerative joint disease. If the ischemia is nocturnal, and particularly if it has an epigastric location or is relieved with antacids, it may be misdiagnosed as ulcer disease. The postprandial epigastric chest pain that is burning in quality is often considered hiatus hernia reflux, not CAD. In addition, the pain of ischemia in the elderly person not uncommonly may be described as less severe and of shorter duration in the elderly because of mental confusion.

Frequently, instead of angina, a common manifestation of myocardial ischemia in the elderly is dyspnea. In many elderly persons the dyspnea is exertional, although in certain elderly persons acute pulmonary edema occurs. Acute pulmonary edema may even be the first manifestation of the disease. Siegel and associates (8) reported 23 patients presenting with acute pulmonary edema secondary to CAD without an associated acute myocardial infarction. The mean age of the group was 69 ± 9 years. Only 25% of the patients had a past history of myocardial infarction; however, a history of hypertension was present in 90% of the patients. As demonstrated by angiography, three-vessel disease was common (70%), although left ventricular systolic function was only moderately abnormal (mean left ventricular ejection fraction 43 ± 12%). Of the elderly patients 65% were treated with interventional therapy (coronary artery bypass surgery or percutaneous coronary angioplasty). Prognosis was excellent in this elderly group of patients; all patients survived the acute hospitalization, and at 23 months follow-up 73% of the patients were still alive. Stone and associates (9) also studied acute pulmonary edema secondary to CAD and reported findings similar to those in Siegel's study; the mean age of patients in the Stone group's study was 76 years, 70% had a history of hypertension, and the mean left ventricular ejection fraction was 43%. Kuris (10) reported 4 elderly patients (mean age 80) with documented CAD who had recurrent pulmonary edema that could not be controlled with medical therapy. Severe left main or three-vessel disease was present in all patients, although left ventricular systolic function was essentially normal. Only after coronary bypass surgery was recurrent pulmonary edema prevented.

Cardiac arrhythmias can be a manifestation of myocardial ischemia in all age groups and is a common problem in the elderly patient with CAD. Sudden death as an initial manifestation of CAD increases with age (11,12). Tresch and associates (13), in a study of initial manifestations of CAD, reported 9 of 66 elderly patients with the initial manifestation of CAD demonstrated cardiac arrhythmias; 2% of the 66 elderly patients experienced out-of-hospital cardiac arrest.

As in younger patients, myocardial ischemia may be silent and completely unrecognized in elderly patients with CAD. In the Tresch's study (13), approximately 15% of patients older than 65 years of age were asymptomatic, and myocardial ischemia was detected by an exercise stress test during a preoperative evaluation. All patients had CAD documented by coronary angiographic studies, and greater than 65% of the elderly patients demonstrated multiple-vessel disease. Aronow and associates (14) demonstrated silent ischemia detected by Holter monitoring in 34% of 185 nursing home patients with CAD whose mean age was 82 ± 8 years. Hedblad and associates (15) reported similar findings; silent ischemia was documented by Holtor monitoring in 36% of 53 patients age 68 years with stable CAD.

## MYOCARDIAL INFARCTION

Q-wave myocardial infarction may be diagnosed in a patient with clinical symptoms by the development on serial electrocardiograms of pathological Q waves with a duration of at least 0.04 s and a depth of at least 0.2 mV. If the pathological Q waves seen on a resting electrocardiogram are unassociated with clinical symptoms of MI, the Q-wave MI is classified as a silent infarction. Non–Q-wave infarction may be diagnosed in a patient with clinical symptoms if serial electrocardiograms show the development of new ST segment elevation or depression of at least 0.1 mV (ST segment elevations are measured 0.02 s after the J point and ST segment depression 0.08 s after the J point) or new T-wave inversion of at least 0.1 mV in leads II, III, and aVF in at least two of the six precordial leads, or in leads I and aVL plus increased plasma levels of MB isoenzyme of creatinine kinase (≥5%). In a percentage of patients with non–Q-wave MI, as in the case of Q-MI, the patients may be without clinical symptoms (silent).

Clinically, an acute MI may be even more difficult to diagnose than myocardial ischemia in elderly patients. The Framingham Heart Study (16,17) demonstrated by electrocardiography that in the general population approximately 25% of acute MI are unrecognized or silent. Of these, 48% were truly silent; in the remainder some atypical symptoms were present but were not sufficient for

**Table 1** Prevalence of Incidence of Silent or Unrecognized Q-Wave Myocardial Infarction (MI) in Elderly Patients

| Study | Age (years) | Results |
|---|---|---|
| Rodstein (19) | >60 | Unrecognized MI in 16 of 52 MI (31%) |
| Aronow et al. (20) | >64 | Unrecognized MI in 78 of 115 MI (68%) |
| Aronow (18) | >62 | Unrecognized MI in 23 of 110 MI (21%) |
| Vokonas et al. (21) | >65 | Unrecognized MI in 33% of 199 MI in men and in 36% of 162 MI in women |
| Muller et al. (22) | >65 | Painless MI in 14 of 46 MI in men (30%) and in 34 of 67 MI in women (51%) |
| Nadelmann et al. (23) | >75 | Unrecognized MI in 50 of 115 MI (43%) |

either the patient or physician to consider that an infarction was occurring. The incidence of silent MI in men increased from 18% in those aged 45–54 to 42% in those aged 75–84; the incidence was 33% in males aged 85–94. A significant age difference was not noted in women, although the proportion of unrecognized myocardial infarctions was more common in women.

In addition to the Framingham Study, other investigators have noted the high occurrence of unrecognized or silent MI in the elderly population (18–24). Table 1 shows that the prevalence or incidence of unrecognized Q-wave MI in elderly patients ranges from 21 to 68% (18–23). Unrecognized MI are just as likely as MI with clinical symptoms to be associated with increased incidences of new coronary events (21–26). Table 2 reveals that the incidences of recurrent MI, primary ventricular fibrillation, sudden coronary death, and new coronary events were not significantly different in elderly patients with recognized or unrecognized MI (25).

**Table 2** Incidences of Recurrent Myocardial Infarction, Primary Ventricular Fibrillation, Sudden Coronary Death, or New Coronary Events at 4 Years Follow-up in Elderly Patients with Recognized or Unrecognized Myocardial Infarction

| | New MI | | Primary VF | | SCD | | Coronary events | |
|---|---|---|---|---|---|---|---|---|
| | *n* | % | *n* | % | *n* | % | *n* | % |
| Recognized MI | 12/37 | 32 | 5/37 | 14 | 7/37 | 19 | 24/37 | 65 |
| Unrecognized MI | 24/78 | 31 | 8/78 | 10 | 12/78 | 15 | 44/78 | 56 |

MI = myocardial infarction; VF = ventricular fibrillation; SCD = sudden coronary death.
*Source*: Adapted from Aronow (25).

Symptoms in the elderly patient with an acute MI can be extremely variable, and the diagnosis is easily overlooked. Instead of the classic feature of chest pain, many investigators (18,19,27–33) have found, as in myocardial ischemia, dyspnea to be a common presenting symptom of an acute MI in the elderly patient. This frequent complaint of dyspnea associated with coronary artery insufficiency in the elderly has been explained by an elevated end-diastolic left ventricular pressure secondary to an ischemia-induced decrease in ventricular compliance superimposed on the diminished compliance that occurs secondary to normal aging.

Table 3 lists the prevalence of chest pain, dyspnea, and neurological symptoms in various studies of elderly patients with documented acute MI (9,18,29–31). The prevalence of chest pain associated with acute MI ranged from 19 to 66%, the prevalence of dyspnea was from 20 to 42%, and the prevalence of neurological symptoms was from 16 to 33% (27–33). Other clinical features associated with acute MI in these studies were gastrointestinal symptoms, sudden death, peripheral gangrene or increased claudication, palpitations, renal failure, weakness, pulmonary embolism, restlessness, and sweating.

The reason for the frequent absence of typical chest pain in elderly patients with CAD is unclear. Various speculations have included (1) mental deterioration with inability to verbalize a sensation of pain; (2) better myocardial collateral circulation related to gradual progressive coronary artery narrowing; and (3) a decreased sensitivity to pain due to aging changes. Another theory has suggested that the increase in silent myocardial ischemia and infarction in elderly patients with CAD is related to increased levels of, or receptor sensitivity to, endogenous opioids (34). This explanation does not appear likely, since studies have demonstrated similar increase response in $\beta$-endorphin levels to exercise in both elderly and younger subjects (35) and animal studies show a decrease in opioid receptor responsivity with advancing age (36).

**Table 3** Prevalence of Chest Pain, Dyspnea, and Neurological Symptoms Associated with Acute Myocardial Infarction in Elderly Patients

| | Chest pain | | Dyspnea | | Neurological symptoms | |
|---|---|---|---|---|---|---|
| | *n* | % | *n* | % | *n* | % |
| Rodstein (19) | 15/52 | 29 | —[a] | | —[a] | |
| Pathy (29) | 75/387 | 19 | 77/387 | 20 | 126/387 | 33 |
| Tinker (30) | 51/87 | 59 | 19/87 | 22 | 14/87 | 16 |
| Bayer et al. (31) | 515/777 | 66 | 329/777 | 42 | 232/777 | 30 |
| Aronow (18) | 24/110 | 22 | 38/110 | 35 | 20/110 | 18 |

[a] Symptom present but number and percentage not stated.

Elderly patients with MI are more likely to have complications from the acute MI and are more likely to die from the MI than patients under 70 years of age with acute MI. Fedullo and Swinburne (37) reported that chest x-ray evidence of interstitial or alveolar edema occurred in 37% of 104 patients 70 years of age or older with acute MI, compared to only 11% of 157 younger patients with acute MI. Peripheral edema was also more common in the elderly patients. Table 4 lists and compares other major complications of acute MI between the younger and older patients in the Fedullo and Swinburne study. Older patients had a significantly higher mortality and a significantly higher incidence of cardiogenic shock. Congestive heart failure was also more common in older patients with pulmonary edema, occurring in almost 20% of the older patients compared to only 4% of the patients under 70 years of age.

Rich (38) reviewed the incidence of complications in the elderly patients versus younger patients with acute MI in various studies reported in the literature (Table 5). Older patients with MI had an increased incidence of cardiogenic shock, rupture of the left ventricular free wall, septum, or papillary muscle, congestive heart failure, and atrial fibrillation or flutter and a decreased incidence of ventricular fibrillation.

This increased mortality associated with an acute MI in elderly patients was recently substantiated by the result of thrombolytic studies. The GISSI-1 study reported that the mortality from acute MI was 8% in patients 65 years of age or younger, 18% in patients 66–75 years of age, and 33% in patients 76 years of age or older (39).

**Table 4** Complications of Myocardial Infarction in 104 Elderly Patients and in 157 Younger Patients with Acute Myocardial Infarction

| Complications | <70 years (%) | 70+ Years (%) |
|---|---|---|
| Mortality | 5 | 22[a] |
| Cardiogenic shock | 1 | 7[a] |
| Ventricular tachycardia or fibrillation | 10 | 12 |
| Pulmonary edema | 4 | 18[a] |
| Congestive heart failure | 14 | 29[a] |
| Rhythm disturbance requiring pacemaker | 1 | 5 |
| Pericarditis | 5 | 2 |

[a] Significantly higher in older group.
*Source*: Adapted from Fedullo and Swinburne (37).

**Table 5** Relative Incidence of Complications from Acute Myocardial Infarction in Elderly Versus Younger Patients

| Complications | Elderly versus younger |
|---|---|
| Cardiogenic shock | Increased two times |
| Ventricular fibrillation | Decreased two times |
| Rupture of left ventricular free wall, septum, or papillary muscle | Increased incidence |
| Congestive heart failure | Increased two to three times |
| Atrial fibrillation or flutter | Increased two to three times |
| Conduction disturbances | Similar incidence |
| Pericarditis | Similar incidence |

*Source*: Adapted from Rich (38).

# DIAGNOSTIC TECHNIQUES

## Resting Electrocardiogram

In addition to diagnosing recent or old myocardial infarction, the resting electrocardiogram may show ischemic ST segment depression, arrhythmias, conduction defects, and left ventricular hypertrophy, which may predict subsequent coronary events. In the Coronary Drug Project, men postmyocardial infarction with $\geqslant$1.0 mm ischemic ST segment depression on the resting electrocardiogram were 3.9 times more likely to die during 3 year follow-up than men postmyocardial infarction with no ST segment depression (40). Chronic atrial fibrillation, premature ventricular complexes, left bundle branch block, and intraventricular conduction defect were also risk factors for mortality in the Coronary Drug Project (40).

In a study of nursing home patients in which resting electrocardiographic findings were assessed as predictors of mortality and new coronary events, Aronow (41) found that at 37 months mean follow-up elderly patients (mean age 82 $\pm$ 8 years, range 62–103) with ischemic ST segment depression $\geqslant$ 1.0 mm on the resting electrocardiogram were 3.1 times more likely to develop new coronary events (myocardial infarction, primary ventricular fibrillation, or sudden cardiac death) than elderly patients with no significant ST segment depression. Elderly patients with an ischemic ST segment depression of 0.5–0.9 mm on the resting electrocardiogram were 1.9 times more likely to develop new coronary events than elderly patients with no significant ST segment depression (41). At 45 months mean follow-up, pacemaker rhythm, atrial fibrillation, premature ventricular complexes, left bundle branch block, intraventricular conduction defect, and type II second-degree atrioventricular block documented on a resting electrocardiogram were associated with a higher incidence of new coronary events in elderly patients with CAD (42).

Numerous studies have documented that patients with electrocardiographic left ventricular hypertrophy have an increased incidence of new cardiovascular events. Table 6 shows that men and women 65–94 years of age in the Framingham Heart Study with electrocardiographic left ventricular hypertrophy had an increased incidence of coronary events, atherothrombotic brain infarction, congestive heart failure, and peripheral arterial disease (43).

Similar results were reported by Aronow and associates (44). Elderly nursing home patients with hypertension or CAD and electrocardiographic left ventricular hypertrophy had an increased incidence of new coronary events and atherothrombotic brain infarctions at 37 months mean follow-up (Table 6). The increased incidence of cardiovascular morbidity was not different between black and white elderly nursing home patients who had hypertension and demonstrated electrocardiographic findings of left ventricular hypertrophy (Table 6) (45).

**Table 6** Increased Incidence of Cardiovascular Events in Prospective Studies of Elderly Patients with Electrocardiographic Left Ventricular Hypertrophy

| | Increased incidence of cardiovascular events | | | | |
|---|---|---|---|---|---|
| Study | Follow-up | Coronary events | ABI | CHF | PAD |
| Elderly men in Framingham Study (43) | 30 years | 3.0 | 3.2 | 9.0 | 1.9 |
| Elderly women in Framingham Study (43) | 30 years | 3.7 | 6.5 | 6.0 | 2.7 |
| 360 Elderly patients with hypertension or CAD (44) | 37 months | 1.4 | 1.7 | | |
| 84 Elderly blacks with hypertension (45) | 37 months | 1.5 | 1.8 | 1.3 | |
| 326 Elderly whites with hypertension (45) | 43 months | 1.4 | 1.9 | 1.6 | |

ECG = electrocardiographic; LVH = left ventricular hypertrophy; ABI = atherothrombotic brain infarction; CAD = coronary artery disease; CHF = congestive heart failure; PAD = peripheral arterial disease.

## Exercise Electrocardiogram (Exercise Stress Testing)

Exercise electrocardiography using either a treadmill or bicycle ergometer is useful in diagnosing and evaluating elderly patients with suspected or documented CAD (46,47). Exercise electrocardiography may also be a useful prognostic indicator of subsequent coronary events in elderly patients with documented CAD, with and without prior MI (46,47). Exercise testing in elderly patients should evaluate symptoms developing during exercise (especially angina pectoris or dyspnea, which may be an anginal equivalent), the duration and degree of exercise, the heart rate and blood pressure response to exercise, the presence of ischemic ST segment depression or elevation, and the presence of exercise-induced arrhythmias.

Some studies have suggested that exercise electrocardiographic stress testing may be more sensitive in diagnosing CAD in elderly patients compared to younger patients, although the sensitivity may be decreased. Hlatky and associates (48) demonstrated in patients 60 years of age or older a sensitivity of 84% and a specificity of 70% for the exercise electrocardiogram in diagnosing CAD. Newman and Phillips (49) found in patients 65 years of age or older a sensitivity of 85%, a specificity of 56%, and a positive predictive value of 86% for the exercise electrocardiogram in diagnosing CAD. This increased sensitivity and decreased specificity of the exercise electrocardiogram with increasing age is thought to be due to the increased prevalence and severity of CAD in elderly persons (50).

In contrast to the findings of Hlatky and Newman, Martinez-Caro and associates (51), using symptom-limited upright bicycle exercise testing, demonstrated in patients 65 years of age or older a sensitivity of 62% and a specificity of 93% for the exercise electrocardiogram in diagnosing CAD, values similar to those found in younger patients. Gaul (52) also found with symptom-limited semisupine bicycle exercise testing that the sensitivity and specificity for the exercise electrocardiogram in diagnosing CAD in patients older than 65 years of age were almost identical to those in younger patients. Samek and associates (53), using supine bicycle exercise testing, demonstrated by multivariate analysis in patients older than 65 years of age that the magnitude of ST segment depression plus the resting pulmonary capillary wedge pressure correctly predicted 90% of patients with significant three-vessel CAD and 32% of patients with significant one- and two-vessel CAD.

In assessing the value of exercise stress testing in predicting future coronary events in elderly patients, many studies have found it a useful tool (54–58). Using symptom-limited exercise stress testing with either a treadmill or an upright bicycle ergometer in patients with chronic stable CAD older than 65 years of age, Glover and associates (54) observed at 2 years follow-up that cardiac death occurred in 8 of 47 patients (17%) with exercise-induced ischemic ST segment depression; in comparison, only 1 of 51 patients (2%) with negative or equivocal ST segment responses died of a cardiac etiology. Saunamaki (55) found similar results when studying bicycle exercise stress testing in 62 patients 70 years of age or older in the third week after an acute MI. At 4.5 years follow-up, only 8 of 32 patients (25%) who had exercise-induced ventricular arrhythmias or failed to increase the pressure-rate product from rest to peak exercise greater than 1500 were alive, compared to 23 of 30 patients (77%) without either of these two prognostic variables. In a similar study, Fioretti and associates (56) obtained bicycle exercise stress tests in 48 patients 65 years of age or older and in 109 patients 55–64 years of age at a median time of 12 days after acute MI. The 1 year mortality was 2% (2 of 110 patients) in patients with a systolic blood pressure increase during exercise of greater than 30 mm Hg, compared to a 15% mortality (7 of 47 patients) in patients who had a lesser rise in systolic blood pressure during exercise.

Deckers and associates (57) demonstrated that the 1 year mortality following an acute MI was 4% for the 48 patients 65 years of age or older who were able to perform a bicycle exercise stress test and 37% for the 63 elderly patients excluded from this study. The inability to perform a predischarge exercise stress test after acute MI has also been associated with a poor prognosis in younger populations. In the Multicenter Postinfarction Research Group study, the 1 year cardiac mortality was 14% in the 192 patients who did not perform a low-level treadmill exercise test early after acute MI (150 for medical reasons and 42 for logistic reasons) and 5% in 667 patients who performed the low-level treadmill exercise test (58).

Exercise stress testing using thallium perfusion scintigraphy (59), radionuclide ventriculography (60), and echocardiography (61) may also be useful in the diagnosis and prognosis of CAD, and the benefit applies to elderly patients as well as younger patients. Iskandrian and associates (59) demonstrated that exercise thallium 201 imaging can be used for risk stratification of elderly patients with CAD. The risk of cardiac death or nonfatal MI at 25 months follow-up in 449 patients 60 years of age or older was less than 1% in patients with normal images, 5% in patients with one-vessel thallium 201 abnormality, and 13% in patients with multivessel thallium 201 abnormality.

Because of musculoskeletal disorders or general debilitation, many elderly patients are not able to perform exercise stress testing. In such patients right atrial pacing has been shown to be useful to stratify postinfarction patients into high- and low-risk groups (62). More recently, and more generally accepted than atrial pacing, intravenous dipyridamole-thallium imaging has been used to determine the presence of CAD in elderly patients unable to undergo treadmill or bicycle exercise stress testing. In 101 patients 70 years of age or older, the sensitivity of intravenous dipyridamole-thallium imaging for diagnosing significant CAD was 86% and the specificity 75%, which was similar to the sensitivity and specificity of the test in patients younger than 70 years of age (63).

## Ambulatory Electrocardiography (Holter Monitoring)

Elderly patients with CAD who have ventricular tachycardia or complex ventricular arrhythmias detected by 24 h ambulatory electrocardiography are at increased risk for developing new coronary events (64–66). Ambulatory electrocardiography performed for 24 h may also be useful in detecting silent myocardial ischemia in elderly patients with suspected CAD who cannot perform treadmill or bicycle exercise stress testing because of advanced age, intermittent claudication, musculoskeletal disorders, congestive heart failure, or pulmonary disease. It has been shown that both younger and older patients with stable CAD (14,15,66–72), unstable angina pectoris (73–75), and high-risk post-MI patients (76) who have silent myocardial ischemia detected by 24 h ambulatory electrocardiography are at increased risk for new coronary events.

Aronow and Epstein (14) detected silent myocardial ischemia by 24 h ambulatory electrocardiography in 62 of 185 patients (34%) older than 62 years, mean age 82 ± 8 years, with stable CAD. At 26 months mean follow-up (range 8–34 months), new coronary events (nonfatal or fatal MI, primary ventricular fibrillation, or sudden coronary death) developed in twice as many elderly patients with silent myocardial ischemia as in elderly patients without silent myocardial ischemia (Table 7). In a similar study, Hedblad and associates (15) detected myocardial ischemia by 24 h ambulatory electrocardiography in 19 of 53 patients (36%) age 68 years with stable CAD. At 43 months follow-up, elderly patients with myocardial ischemia had 6.2 times the incidence of nonfatal MI or death from CAD as elderly patients without myocardial ischemia (Table 7). In the Baltimore Longitudinal Study of Aging, silent myocardial ischemia was detected by 24 h ambulatory electrocardiography in 5 of 98 healthy elderly persons (5%) (77). At 10 years mean follow-up, coronary events developed in 2 of the 5 persons (40%) with silent ischemia, compared to 8 of 93 persons (9%) without myocardial ischemia (relative risk 4.4).

## Echocardiography

Echocardiography can be useful in detecting regional left ventricular wall motion abnormalities, acute myocardial ischemia and complications secondary to acute MI, left ventricular aneurysm, cardiac thrombus, left main CAD, left ventricular hypertrophy, and associated valvular heart disease and in evaluating left ventricular function and cardiac chamber size in elderly patients with CAD (78). Specifically, the echocardiogram can be very useful in diagnosing diastolic

**Table 7** Increased Incidence of Coronary Events in Elderly Patients with Stable Coronary Artery Disease and Myocardial Ischemia During 24 h Ambulatory Electrocardiographic Monitoring

| | | | New coronary events | |
|---|---|---|---|---|
| Study | Number patients (%) | Follow-up (months) | Number patients (%) | Relative risk |
| Aronow and Epstein (14) | | | | |
| Total patients (82 years)[a] | 185 | 26 | | |
| Patients with ischemia | 62 (34)[b] | | 40 (65) | 2.0 |
| Patients without ischemia | 123 (66) | | 39 (32) | |
| Hedblad et al. (15) | | | | |
| Total patients (68 years)[a] | 53 | 43 | | |
| Patients with ischemia | 19 (36) | | 7 (37) | 6.2 |
| Patients without ischemia | 34 (64) | | 2 (6) | |

[a] Mean age.
[b] Silent ischemia.

dysfunction (excluding systolic dysfunction) in patients with left ventricular failure, which some studies have demonstrated to be so prevalent in elderly patients (79–81). The echocardiogram may also be of value in predicting prognosis in elderly patients with CAD. Aronow and associates (64), in a study of nursing home patients over age 62, found that new coronary events developed at 2 years follow-up in 30 of 45 elderly patients (67%) with CAD and abnormal left ventricular ejection fractions (<50%) demonstrated by echocardiography, compared to 24 of 90 elderly patients (27%) with CAD and normal left ventricular ejection fraction (≥50%; relative risk 2.5). Comparing elderly nursing home patients with CAD and clinical heart failure, Aronow and associates (82) found mortality to be higher in elderly patients with CAD and congestive heart failure and abnormal left ventricular ejection fraction than in elderly patients with CAD and congestive heart failure and normal left ventricular ejection fraction. Multivariate analysis showed that the left ventricular ejection fraction was the most important prognostic variable for mortality in elderly patients with congestive heart failure associated with CAD.

Many studies have demonstrated that elderly patients with CAD and echocardiographic left ventricular hypertrophy have an increased incidence of new cardiovascular events (44,45,65,72,83–86). Elderly men and women in the Framingham Heart Study with echocardiographic left ventricular hypertrophy had at 4 years follow-up a relative risk for coronary events of 1.67 for men and 1.60 for women per 50 g/m increase in left ventricular mass/height (Table 8) (83). In

**Table 8** Increased Incidence of Cardiovascular Events in Prospective Studies of Elderly Patients with Echocardiographic Left Ventricular Hypertrophy

| Study | Increased incidence of cardiovascular events | | | | |
|---|---|---|---|---|---|
| | Follow-up | Coronary events | ABI | CHF | V Fib or SCD |
| 406 Elderly men in Framingham Study (82) | 4 years | 1.67[a] | | | |
| 735 Elderly women in Framingham Study (82) | 4 years | 1.60[a] | | | |
| 196 Elderly patients with CAD (85) | 27 months | 2.2 | | | |
| 360 Elderly patients with hypertension or CAD (44) | 37 months | 2.0 | 2.8 | | |
| 468 Elderly patients with heart disease (65) | 27 months | | | | 3.3 |
| 84 Elderly blacks with hypertension (45) | 37 months | 3.3 | 2.8 | 3.7 | |
| 326 Elderly whites with hypertension (45) | 43 months | 2.7 | 3.3 | 3.5 | |

ABI = atherothrombotic brain infarction; CHF = congestive heart failure; V Fib = ventricular fibrillation; SCD = sudden cardiac death.

[a] Relative risk for coronary events per 50 g/m increase in left ventricular mass/height.

this study, echocardiographic left ventricular hypertrophy was a predictor of coronary events independently of standard coronary risk factors. Echocardiographic left ventricular hypertrophy was 15.3 times more sensitive in predicting coronary events in elderly men and 4.3 times more sensitive in predicting coronary events in elderly women than electrocardiographic left ventricular hypertrophy. In a study of nursing home patients with CAD, Aronow and associates (85) reported at 27 months mean follow-up a 2.2 times higher incidence of new coronary events in elderly patients with echocardiographic left ventricular hypertrophy than in elderly patients with CAD and no echocardiographic left ventricular hypertrophy (Table 8). Elderly patients with a history of hypertension or CAD and echocardiographic left ventricular hypertrophy had at 37 months mean follow-up a 2.0 times higher incidence of new coronary events and a 2.8 times higher incidence of new atherothrombotic brain infarction than elderly patients with hypertension or CAD and no echocardiographic left ventricular hypertrophy (Table 8) (44). As in the Framingham Heart Study (83), echocardiographic findings of left ventricular hypertrophy was 4.3 times more sensitive in predicting new coronary events and 4.0 times more sensitive in predicting new atherothrombotic brain infarction than electrocardiographic left ventricular hypertrophy (44). In assessing predictors of primary ventricular fibrillation or sudden death, Aronow and associates (65) reported that the incidence of primary ventricular fibrillation or sudden cardiac death at 27 months mean follow-up in elderly nursing home patients with heart disease was 3.3 times greater in elderly patients with echocardiographic left ventricular hypertrophy than in elderly patients without echocardiographic left ventricular hypertrophy (Table 8). Elderly black patients with hypertension and echocardiographic left ventricular hypertrophy had at 37 months mean follow-up a 3.3 times higher incidence of new coronary events, a 2.8 times higher incidence of new atherothrombotic brain infarction, and a 3.7 times higher incidence of congestive heart failure than elderly black patients with hypertension and no echocardiographic left ventricular hypertrophy (Table 8) (45). Elderly white patients with hypertension and echocardiographic left ventricular hypertrophy had similar findings; at 43 months mean follow-up, a 2.7 times greater incidence of new coronary events, a 3.3 times higher incidence of new atherothrombotic brain infarction, and a 3.5 times higher incidence of congestive heart failure was found in elderly white patients with hypertension and echocardiographic left ventricular hypertrophy compared to elderly white patients with hypertension and no echocardiographic left ventricular hypertrophy (Table 8) (45). Using logistic regression models with 15 variables, the odds ratios, 95% confidence limits, for echocardiographic left ventricular hypertrophy in elderly black patients and white patients with hypertension were 3.21 (1.67–6.15) for new coronary events, 4.17 (1.91–9.13) for new atherothrombotic brain infarction, and 2.57 (1.18–5.6) for congestive heart failure.

## REFERENCES


1. Monroe RT. Diseases in old age. Cambridge, MA: Harvard University Press, 1951.
2. McKeown F. Pathology of the Aged. London: Butterworths, 1965:5,44–45.
3. Kennedy RO, Andrews GR, Caird FI. Ischemic heart disease in the elderly. *Br Heart J* 1977; 39:1121.
4. Akhtar AJ, Broe GA, Crombie A, McLean WMR, Andrews GR, Caird FI. Disability and dependence in the elderly at home. *Age Aging* 1973; 2:102–110.
5. O'Rourke RA, Chatterjee K, Wei JY. Coronary heart disease. *J Am Coll Cardiol* 1987; 10(2 Suppl. A):52–56.
6. World Health Organization. The ten leading causes of death for selected countries in North America, Europe and Oceania, 1970 and 1971. *World Health Stat Rep* 1974; 27:563.

7. Wenger NK. Coronary heart disease in women: Clinical syndromes, prognosis, and diagnostic testing. In: Douglas PS, ed. Heart Disease in Women. Philadelphia: F. A. Davis, 1989:173–186.
8. Siegel R, Clemens T, Wingo M, Tresch DD. Acute heart failure in elderly: Another manifestation of unstable "angina." *J Am Coll Cardiol* 1991; 17:149A.
9. Stone GW, Griffin B, Shah PK, Berman DS, Siegel RJ, Cook SL, Maurer G. Prevalence of unsuspected mitral regurgitation and left ventricular diastolic dysfunction in patients with coronary artery disease and acute pulmonary edema associated with normal or depressed left ventricular systolic function. *Am J Cardiol* 1991; 67:37–41.
10. Kunis R, Greenberg H, Yeoh CB, Garfein OB, Pepe AJ, Pinkernes BH, Sherrid MV, Dwyer EM. Coronary revascularization for recurrent pulmonary edema in elderly patients with ischemic heart disease and preserved ventricular function. *N Engl J Med* 1985; 313:1207–1210.
11. Kannel WB, Schatzkin A. Sudden death: Lesions from subsets in population studies. *J Am Coll Cardiol* 1985; 5:141B–149B.
12. Elveback LR, Connelly DC, Kurland LT. Coronary heart disease in residents of Rochester, Minnesota. II. Mortality, incidence, and survivorship, 1950–1975. *Mayo Clin Proc* 1981; 56:665–672.
13. Tresch DD, Saein K, Hoffman R. Elderly patients with late onset of coronary artery disease: Clinical and angiographic findings. Am J Geriatr Cardiol 1992: 14–25.
14. Aronow WS, Epstein S. Usefulness of silent myocardial ischemia detected by ambulatory electrocardiographic monitoring in predicting new coronary events in elderly patients. *Am J Cardiol* 1988; 62:1295–1296.
15. Hedblad B, Juul-Moller S, Svensson K, Hanson BS, Isacsson S-O, Janzon L, Lindell S-E, Steen B, Johansson BW. Increased mortality in men with ST segment depression during 24 h ambulatory long-term ECG recording. Results from prospective population study "Men born in 1914," from Malmo Sweden. *Eur Heart J* 1989; 10:149–158.
16. Kannel WB, Abbott RD. Incidence and prognosis of unrecognized myocardial infarction: An update on the Framingham Study. *N Engl J Med* 1984; 311:1144–1147.
17. Kannel WB, Abbott RD. Incidence and progress of unrecognized myocardial infarction: Based on 26 years follow-up in Framingham Study. In: Rutishouser W, Raskamm H, eds. Silent Myocardial Ischemia. Berlin: Springer-Verlag, 1984:131–137.
18. Aronow WS. Prevalence of presenting symptoms of recognized acute myocardial infarction and of unrecognized healed myocardial infarction in elderly patients. *Am J Cardiol* 1987; 60:1182.
19. Rodstein M. The characteristics of non-fatal myocardial infarction in the aged. *Arch Intern Med* 1956; 98:84–90.
20. Aronow WS, Starling L, Etienne F, D'Alba P, Edwards M, Lee NH, Parungao RF. Unrecognized Q-wave myocardial infarction in patients older than 64 years in a long-term health-care facility. *Am J Cardiol* 1985; 56:483.

21. Vokanas PS, Kannel WB, Cupples LA. Incidence and prognosis of unrecognized myocardial infarction in the elderly. The Framingham Study (abstract). *J Am Coll Cardiol* 1988; 11:51A.
22. Muller RT, Gould LA, Betzu R, Racek T, Pradeep V. Painless myocardial infarction in the elderly. *Am Heart J* 1990; 119:202–204.
23. Nadelmann J, Frishman WH, Ooi WL, Tepper D, Greenberg S, Guzik H, Lazar EJ, Heiman M, Aronson M. Prevalence, incidence, and prognosis of recognized and unrecognized myocardial infarction in persons aged 75 years or older: The Bronx Aging Study. *Am J Cardiol* 1990; 66:533–537.
24. Grimm RH, Tillinghast S, Daniels K, Neaton JD, Mascioli S, Crow R, Pritzker M, Prineas RB. Unrecognized myocardial infarction: Experience in the multiple risk factor intervention trial (MRFIT). *Circulation* 1987; 759(Suppl.II):6–8.
25. Aronow WS. New coronary events at four-year follow-up in elderly patients with recognized or unrecognized myocardial infarction. *Am J Cardiol* 1989; 63:621–622.
26. Yano K, MacLean CJ. The incidence and prognosis of unrecognized myocardial infarction in the Honolulu, Hawaii, Heart Program. *Arch Intern Med* 1989; 149:1528–1532.
27. Solomon CG, Lee TH, Cook EF, Weisberg MC, Brand DA, Rouan GW, Goldman L. Comparison of clinical presentation of acute myocardial infarction in patients older than 65 years of age to younger patients: The multicenter chest pain study experience. *Am J Cardiol* 1989; 63:772–776.
28. Wroblewski M, Mikulowski P, Steen B. Symptoms of myocardial infarction in old age: Clinical case, retrospective and prospective studies. *Age Aging* 1986; 15:99–104.
29. Pathy MS. Clinical presentation of myocardial infarction in the elderly. *Br Heart J* 1967; 29:190–199.
30. Tinker GM. Clinical presentation of myocardial infarction in the elderly. *Age Aging* 1981; 10:237–240.
31. Bayer AJ, Chadha JS, Farag RR, Pathy MSJ. Changing presentation of myocardial infarction with increasing old age. *J Am Geriatr Soc* 1986; 23:263–266.
32. MacDonald JB. Presentation of acute myocardial infarction in the elderly. A review. *Age Ageing* 1980; 13:196–204.
33. Sugura M, Ohkawa S, Hiroaka Y, et al. Clinicopathologic aspects of ischemic heart disease in the elderly. *Jpn Heart J* 1981; 22:15–30.
34. Ellestad MH, Kuan P. Naloxone and asymptomatic ischemia: Failure to induce angina during exercise testing. *Am J Cardiol* 1984; 54:982–984.
35. Hatfield BD, Goldfarb AH, Sporzo GA, Flynn MG. Serum beta-endorphin and affective responses to graded exercise in young and elderly men. *J Gerontol* 1987; 42:429–431.
36. Morley JE. Neuropeptides, behavior and aging. *J Am Geriatr Soc* 1986; 34:52–61.
37. Fedullo AJ, Swinburne AJ. Intensive care of elderly patients with myocardial infarction: Age-related comparison of clinical features and outcome. *J Intens Care Med* 1988; 3:265–271.

38. Rich MW. The geriatric patient in the coronary care unit. In: Coronary Care for the House Officer. Baltimore: Williams & Wilkins, 1989:202–208.
39. Gruppo Italiano per lo Studio della Streptochinasi nell'Infarto Miocardico (GISSI). Effectiveness of intravenous thrombolytic treatment in acute myocardial infarction. *Lancet* 1986; 1:397–402.
40. Coronary Drug Project Research Group. The prognostic importance of the electrocardiogram after myocardial infarction. Experience in the Coronary Drug Project. *Ann Intern Med* 1972; 77:677–689.
41. Aronow WS. Correlation of ischemic ST-segment depression on the resting electrocardiogram with new cardiac events in 1,106 patients over 62 years of age. *Am J Cardiol* 1989; 64:232–233.
42. Aronow WS. Correlation of arrhythmias and conduction defects on the resting electrocardiogram with new cardiac events in 1,153 elderly patients. *Am J Noninvas Cardiol* 1991; 5:88–90.
43. Kannel WB, Dannenberg AL, Levy D. Population implications of electrocardiographic left ventricular hypertrophy. *Am J Cardiol* 1987; 60:851–931.
44. Aronow WS, Koenigsberg M, Schwartz KS. Usefulness of echocardiographic and electrocardiographic left ventricular hypertrophy in predicting new cardiac events and atherothrombotic brain infarction in elderly patients with systemic hypertension or coronary artery disease. *Am J Noninvas Cardiol* 1989; 3:367–370.
45. Aronow WS, Ahn C, Kronzon I, Koenigsberg M. Congestive heart failure, coronary events, and atherothrombotic brain infarction in elderly blacks and whites with systemic hypertension and with and without electrocardiographic and electrocardiographic evidence of left ventricular hypertrophy. *Am J Cardiol* 1991; 67:295–299.
46. Aronow WS. Diagnostic and prognostic value of exercise electrocardiography for coronary artery disease. *Comp Ther* 1989; 15(11):20–26.
47. Fleg JL. Exercise testing of elderly patients. *Cardiology* 1989; 3:105–109.
48. Hlatky MA, Pryor DB, Harrell FE Jr, Califf RM, Mark DB, Rasati RA. Factors affecting sensitivity and specificity of exercise electrocardiography. Multivariate analysis. *Am J Med* 1984; 77:64–71.
49. Newman KP, Phillips JH. Graded exercise testing for diagnosis of coronary artery disease in elderly patients. *South Med J* 1988; 81:430–432.
50. Chaitman BR, Bourassa MG, Davis K, Rogers WJ, Tyras DH, Berger R, Kennedy JW, Fisher L, Judkins MP, Mock MB, Killip T. Angiographic prevalence of high-risk coronary artery disease in patient subsets (CASS). *Circulation* 1981; 64:360–367.
51. Martinez-Caro D, Alegria E, Lorente D, Azpilicueta J, Calabuig J, Ancin R. Diagnostic value of stress testing in the elderly. *Eur Heart J* 1984; 5(Suppl.E):63–67.
52. Gaul G. Stress testing in persons above the age of 65 years: Applicability and diagnostic value of a standardized maximal symptom-limited testing protocol. *Eur Heart J* 1984; 5(Suppl.E):51–53.
53. Samek L, Betz P, Schnellbacher K. Exercise testing in elderly patients with coronary artery disease. *Eur Heart J* 1984; 5(Suppl.E):69–73.

54. Glover DR, Robinson CS, Murray RG. Diagnostic exercise testing in 104 patients over 65 years of age. *Eur Heart J* 1984; 5(Suppl.E):59–61.
55. Saunamaki KI. Early post-myocardial infarction exercise in subjects 70 years or more of age. Functional and prognostic evaluation. *Eur Heart J* 1984; 5(Suppl.E):93–96.
56. Fioretti P, Deckers JW, Brower RW, Simoons ML, Beelen JA, Hugenholtz PG. Predischarge stress test after myocardial infarction in the old age: Results and prognostic value. *Eur Heart J* 1984; 5(Suppl.E):101–104.
57. Deckers JW, Fioretti P, Brower RW, Simoons ML, Baardman T, Hugenholtz PG. Inability for predischarge exercise testing after myocardial infarction in the elderly: Implications for prognosis. *Eur Heart J* 1984; 5(Suppl.E):97–100.
58. Krone RJ, Gillespie JA, Weld FM, Miller JP, Moss AJ, Multicenter Postinfarction Research Group. Low-level exercise testing after myocardial infarction: Usefulness in enhancing clinical risk stratification. *Circulation* 1985; 71:80–89.
59. Iskandrian AS, Heo J, Decoskey D, Askenase A, Segal BL. Use of exercise thallium-201 imaging for risk stratification of elderly patients with coronary artery disease. *Am J Cardiol* 1988; 61:269–272.
60. Johnson SH, Bigelow C, Lee KL, Pryor DB, Jones RH. Prediction of death and myocardial infarction by radionuclide angiocardiography in patients with suspected coronary artery disease. *Am J Cardiol* 1991; 67:919–926.
61. Ryan T, Vasey CG, Presti CF, O'Donnell JA, Feigenbaum H, Armstrong WF. Exercise echocardiography: Detection of coronary artery disease in patients with normal left ventricular wall motion at rest. *J Am Coll Cardiol* 1988; 11:993–999.
62. Tzivoni D, Gottlieb S, Keren A, Behorin J, Chenzbraun A, Waksman R, Stern S. Early right atrial pacing after myocardial infarction. I. Comparison with early treadmill testing. *Am J Cardiol* 1984; 53:414–417.
63. Lam JYT, Chaitman BR, Glaenzer M, Byers S, Fite J, Shah Y, Goodgold H, Samuels L. Safety and diagnostic accuracy of dipyridamole-thallium imaging in the elderly. *J Am Coll Cardiol* 1988; 11:585–589.
64. Aronow WS, Epstein S, Koenigsberg M, Schwartz KS. Usefulness of echocardiographic abnormal left ventricular ejection fraction, paroxysmal ventricular tachycardia and complex ventricular arrhythmias in predicting new coronary events in patients over 62 years of age. *Am J Cardiol* 1988; 61:1349–1351.
65. Aronow WS, Epstein S, Koenigsberg M, Schwartz KS. Usefulness of echocardiographic left ventricular hypertrophy, ventricular tachycardia and complex ventricular arrhythmias in predicting ventricular fibrillation or sudden cardiac death in elderly patients. *Am J Cardiol* 1988; 62:1124–1125.
66. Aronow WS, Epstein S. Usefulness of silent ischemia, ventricular tachycardia, and complex ventricular arrhythmias in predicting new coronary events in elderly patients with coronary artery disease or systemic hypertension. *Am J Cardiol* 1990; 65:511–512.
67. Rocco MB, Nabel EG, Campbell S, Goldman L, Barry J, Mead K, Selwyn AP. Prognostic importance of myocardial ischemia detected by ambulatory monitoring in patients with stable coronary artery disease. *Circulation* 1988; 78:877–884.

68. Tzivoni D, Gavish A, Zin D, Gottlieb S, Moriel M, Keren A, Banai S, Stern S. Prognostic significance of ischemic episodes in patients with previous myocardial infarction. *Am J Cardiol* 1988; 62:661–664.
69. Tzivoni D, Weisz G, Gavish A, Zin D, Keren A, Stern S. Comparison of mortality and myocardial infarction rates in stable angina pectoris with and without ischemic episodes during daily activities. *Am J Cardiol* 1989; 63:273–276.
70. Deedwania PC, Carbajal EV. Silent ischemia during daily life is an independent predictor of mortality in stable angina. *Circulation* 1990; 81:748–756.
71. Aronow WS, Epstein S, Koenigsberg M. Usefulness of echocardiographic left ventricular ejection fraction and silent myocardial ischemia in predicting new coronary events in elderly patients with coronary artery disease or systemic hypertension. *Am J Cardiol* 1990; 65:811–812.
72. Aronow WS, Epstein S, Koenigsberg M. Usefulness of echocardiographic left ventricular hypertrophy and silent ischemia in predicting new cardiac events in elderly patients with systemic hypertension or coronary artery disease. *Angiology* 1990; 41:189–193.
73. Gottlieb SO, Weisfeldt ML, Ouyang P, Mellits ED, Gerstenblith G. Silent ischemia as a marker for early unfavorable outcomes in patients with unstable angina. *N Engl J Med* 1986; 314:1214–1219.
74. Gottlieb SO, Weisfeldt ML, Ouyang P, Millets ED, Gerstenblith G. Silent ischemia predicts infarction and death during 2 year follow-up of unstable angina. *J Am Coll Cardiol* 1987; 10:756–760.
75. Nademanee K, Intarachot V, Josephson MA, Rieders D, Mody FV, Singh BN. Prognostic significance of silent myocardial ischemia in patients with unstable angina. *J Am Coll Cardiol* 1987; 10:1–9.
76. Gottlieb SO, Gottlieb SH, Achuff SC, Baumgardner R, Mellits ED, Weisfeldt ML, Gerstenblith G. Silent ischemia on Holter monitoring predicts mortality in high-risk postinfarction patients. *JAMA* 1988; 259:1030–1035.
77. Fleg JL, Kennedy HL. Long-term prognostic significance of ambulatory electrocardiographic findings in apparently healthy subjects ⩾60 years of age. *J Am Coll Cardiol* 1992; 70:748–751.
78. Aronow WS. Echo in the elderly. *Cardio* 1990; 8:81–90.
79. Luchi RJ, Taffet GE, Teasdale TA. Congestive heart failure in the elderly. *J Am Geriatr Soc* 1991; 39:810–825.
80. Wong WF, God S, Fukuyama O, Blanchette PL. Diastolic dysfunction in elderly patients with congestive heart failure. *Am J Cardiol* 1989; 63:1526–1528.
81. Taffet GE, Teasdale TA, Bleyer AJ, Kutka NJ, Luchi RJ. Survival of elderly men with congestive heart failure. *Age Aging* 1992; 21:49–55.
82. Aronow WS, Ahn C, Kronzon I. Prognosis of congestive heart failure in elderly patients with normal versus abnormal left ventricular systolic function associated with coronary artery disease. *Am J Cardiol* 1990; 66:1257–1259.
83. Levy D, Garrison RJ, Savage DD, Kannel WB, Castelli WP. Left ventricular mass and incidence of coronary heart disease in an elderly cohort. The Framingham Heart Study. *Ann Intern Med* 1989; 110:101–107.

84. Levy D, Plehn JF, Wolf PA, Garrison RJ, Kase CS, Abbott RD, Kannel WB, Castelli WP. Left ventricular mass and risk of stroke in men (abstract). *Circulation* 1987; 76(Suppl.IV):IV–143.
85. Aronow WS, Koenigsberg M, Schwartz KS. Usefulness of echocardiographic left ventricular hypertrophy in predicting new coronary events and atherothrombotic brain infarction in patients over 62 years of age. *Am J Cardiol* 1988; 61:1130–1132.
86. Aronow WS, Gutstein H, Hsieh FY. Risk factors for thromboembolic stroke in elderly patients with chronic atrial fibrillation. *Am J Cardiol* 1989; 63:366–367.

# 12

# Medical Therapy for Acute Myocardial Infarction in the Elderly

**Robert Forman and William H. Frishman**
*Albert Einstein College of Medicine and Montefiore Medical Center, Bronx, New York*

## INTRODUCTION

Myocardial infarction is the leading cause of death in the elderly; 60% of all deaths from acute myocardial infarction occur in patients over the age of 75 years (1) and 88% in patients over the age of 65 (2). Of all patients hospitalized for acute myocardial infarction in the Seattle area, 57% were older than 65 years and 28% older than 75 years (2). The mortality for acute myocardial infarction increases significantly with age. The mortality rate in groups of patients not treated with thrombolytic agents has been described as ranging from 3.4 to 7.7% (2,3) in patients less than 65 years of age, 12.2–18.1% (2–4) in patients 66–75 years of age, and 17.8–33% in patients older than 75 years of age. The greater mortality rate in the elderly is presumably related to a high incidence of preexisting heart failure and the presence of multivessel coronary artery disease (5,6). Thus, there is a greater potential for improving the mortality rate and, more importantly, the number of lives saved, in elderly patients treated with optimal and appropriate therapy for acute myocardial infarction.

Unfortunately, the diagnosis of acute myocardial infarction is often more difficult in the elderly: a far greater percentage of these patients present with atypical symptoms (7,8) and arrive significantly later in the emergency room (2) (see Chap. 11).

## THROMBOLYTIC AGENTS

It is standard practice to administer thrombolytic agents in younger patients with acute myocardial infarction, whereas there is a general reluctance to use these agents in the elderly because of the generally perceived notions that the complication rate from their use is higher and they are less effective in this age group. Thus, in recent surveys, only 1–5% (2,4) of patients older than 75 years of age with acute myocardial infarction received thrombolytic agents, in contrast to 20% (9) of patients younger than 75 years of age. However, a higher percentage of elderly patients have contraindications to thrombolytic therapy, including severe hypertension, recent cerebrovascular accident, and bleeding disorder, or arrive too late in the emergency room. Unfortunately, elderly patients have specifically been excluded from many of the randomized trials of thrombolytic agents conducted in the United States but have been enrolled in the European trials, particularly when streptokinase has been studied.

The mortality rates for the major placebo-controlled trials of thrombolytic agents for acute myocardial infarction have been tabulated according to age (Table 1). Although streptokinase is the only thrombolytic agent that was administered to patients older than 75 years in these trials, we have no reason to believe that other agents will be less effective in this age group. In the Gruppo Italiano per lo Studio della Streptochinasi nell'Infarcto Miocardico (GISSI-1) (3), a significant reduction in mortality was seen in patients younger than 66 years treated with streptokinase compared to controls. Whereas the mortality rate was lower in patients older than 65 and 75 years who received streptokinase, the reduction in mortality was not statistically significant. However, the number of lives saved was more than 4 patients per 100 treated in the elderly and only 2 in the younger group. The Intravenous Streptokinase in Acute Myocardial Infarction (ISAM) (10) trial was the only study in which a greater mortality in the elderly was reported, but the total number of patients in this age group was small and the results were not statistically significant. By far the largest number of elderly patients were randomized to streptokinase or placebo in the Second International Study of Infarct Survival (ISIS-2) (11). In this study, which had four arms (streptokinase, streptokinase with aspirin, aspirin, and placebo), the mortality rate was significantly reduced in the elderly in all three active treatment groups, but particularly when aspirin was combined with streptokinase.

In the Anglo–Scandinavian Study of Early Thrombolysis (ASSET) (12), in which patients were randomized to tissue plasminogen activator (tPA) or placebo and heparin was given to both groups, all patients were less than 75 years of age. In this trial, the reduction in mortality for patients less than 66 years of age was not significant but was highly significant for those patients older than 65 years. The results of the APSAC International Mortality Study (AIMS) trial (13)

**Table 1** Effect of Age on Early Mortality Following Thrombolysis

| Trial | *N* | Active/placebo (%) | | Reduction in mortality (%) | *p* Value | Lives saved per 1000 |
|---|---|---|---|---|---|---|
| Streptokinase | | | | | | |
| GISSI-I (3) | | | | | | |
| ⩽75 years | 10,494 | 8.7 | 10.6 | 18 | 0.001 | 19 |
| >75 years | 1,215 | 28.9 | 33.1 | | | |
| ISAM (10) | | | | | | |
| <70 years | 1,454 | 5.1 | 6.6 | 23 | 0.21 | 15 |
| 70–75 years | 287 | 13.0 | 9.6 | (35) | 0.37 | (34) |
| ISIS-2 (11) | | | | | | |
| <70 years | 13,776 | 7.0 | 9.6 | 27 | 0.001 | 26 |
| ⩾70 years | 3,812 | 18.2 | 21.6 | 16 | 0.01 | 34 |
| tPa | | | | | | |
| ASSET (12) | | | | | | |
| ⩽65 years | 3,352 | 5.4 | 6.3 | 14 | 0.24 | 11 |
| 66–75 years | 1,679 | 10.8 | 16.4 | 34 | 0.001 | 56 |
| APSAC | | | | | | |
| AIMS (13) | | | | | | |
| <60 years | 1,257 | 5.2 | 8.5 | 39 | 0.06 | 32 |
| 60–70 years | 751 | 12.2 | 30.2 | 60 | 0.003 | 180 |

GISSI = Gruppo Italiano per lo Studio della Streptochinasi nell'Infarcto Miocardio; ISAM = Intravenous Streptokinase in Acute Myocardial Infarction; ISIS-2 = Second International Study of Infarct Survival; tPA = tissue plasminogen activator; ASSET = Anglo-Scandinavian Study of Early Thrombolysis; APSAC = anisoylated plasminogen–streptokinase activator complex; AIMS = APSAC International Mortality Study.

were similar to those from ASSET in that the mortality rate was reduced in patients randomized to receive anisoylated plasminogen-streptokinase activator complex but was only significant in the older patients. In this latter trial, however, all patients were less than 70 years of age and the numbers were relatively small.

A post hoc subgroup analysis always has the potential danger of producing misleading results, and in none of these studies were patients specifically randomized according to age. However, the consistent results showing improved short-term mortality in the elderly strongly suggest that this group should not be denied thrombolytic therapy because of age alone.

It may be argued that by administering thrombolytic agents in the elderly, one may necessarily be pursuing a more aggressive approach, resulting in cardiac catherterization, coronary angioplasty, and bypass surgery. However, these interventions may only be necessary when postthrombolytic ischemia occurs spontaneously or is provoked (14). Even with a conservative approach, however, one expects a greater percentage of patients treated with thrombolytic agents to undergo subsequent revascularization procedures.

The fear of causing significant hemorrhage undoubtedly has been a deterrent in the use of thrombolytic treatment in the elderly. In one frequently quoted series (15), 25% of the patients above 75 years of age had serious hemorrhagic complications, but there were only 24 patients in this group and the difference in hemorrhagic complications between the older and younger groups in this series was not significant. Hemorrhagic complications were significantly greater in elderly patients in the Thrombolysis in Myocardial Infarction (TIMI-I and TIMI-IIA) trials (16). However, these patients had invasive procedures within 36 h of thrombolysis. Probably more relevant was that in the GISSI-1 and ISIS-2 (3,11) trials, in which angiography was not routinely performed, there was a remarkably low incidence of major bleeding complications in the elderly.

The most serious hemorrhagic complication following thrombolytic therapy is the occurrence of a cerebral hemorrhage and its dire consequences. The overall incidence of cerebral hemorrhage using conventional doses of thrombolytic agents is reported to be between 0.3 and 0.6% but is higher in older patients (17,18). This rate may be lower than that encountered in the general population receiving thrombolytics, however, because of a more careful selection and exclusion of higher risk patients from the trials. A truer rate of cerebral hemorrhage was reported as 1% in a registry of patients less highly selected than in the randomized trials (19) and probably more accurately reflects its occurrence. However, it should be remembered that the stroke rate reported to complicate acute myocardial infarction in a prethrombolytic era of 1.7–2.4% (20,21) mostly occurred as a result of thromboembolism. The exact role of heparin in the genesis of these hemorrhagic strokes is not clear. Whereas it can be generally stated that the incidence of thromboembolism is reduced in patients treated with thrombolysis, aspirin, and subsequent heparin therapy, the incidence of cerebral hemorrhage has increased.

## ASPIRIN

Aspirin is given to patients following acute myocardial infarction to reduce the increased platelet aggregation resulting from the infarct itself and as a consequence of fibrinolytic therapy.

As a result of cyclooxygenase inhibition by aspirin, the platelets of treated patients fail to synthesize thromboxane $A_2$ and thus show reduced platelet aggregation in response to many stimuli, such as collagen, epinephrine, adenosine diphosphate, and arachidonate (22,23). Second-phase aggregation in response to adenosine diphosphate and epinephrine is abolished altogether. Bleeding time roughly doubles from baseline values for at least 24 h.

Inhibition of cyclooxygenase does not fully account for aspirin's antithrombotic activity. Possible additional mechanisms include the inhibition of vitamin D-dependent clotting factor synthesis, stimulation of fibrinolysis, and antagonism of the lipooxygenase pathway of arachidonic acid metabolism in platelets and leukocytes (24). Aspirin may also possess antiarrhythmic properties (25) and may augment collateral blood flow to ischemic myocardial (26), both by mechanisms independent of platelet inhibition.

The dose of aspirin required to produce clinical antiplatelet effects is very small (27,28). Ingestion of a single adult aspirin tablet (325 mg) produces almost total inhibition of thromboxane $A_2$ synthesis and inhibits platelet aggregation (22,23). The inhibition lasts for 48 h, followed by a slow return to normal over a week to 10 days. Even a daily 20 mg dose of aspirin has been shown to inhibit platelet aggregation responses markedly and to reduce thromboxane $A_2$ generation by greater than 90% (27).

In the ISIS-2 trial (11), the use of aspirin was tested for the first time during the acute phase of myocardial infarction. Administration of 160 mg aspirin daily with initiation of treatment proved highly successful in reducing 5 week mortality by 21% and, when given together with streptokinase, reduced mortality a further 25%. The benefits of aspirin were still evident 15 months later. The addition of aspirin to streptokinase or placebo in patients 70 years or older resulted in a significant reduction in mortality to 17.6%, compared to 22.3% in the group of patients who did not receive aspirin. No increase in cerebral hemorrhage was found in the aspirin-treated patients. Aspirin therapy was also successful in reducing the reinfarction rate, from 3.7% in patients receiving streptokinase alone to 1.8% in those patients receiving aspirin and streptokinase (11).

Immediate administration of 160 mg aspirin and its continuation daily thereafter, provided there are no contraindications, is now accepted as standard therapy in the management of acute myocardial infarction.

Aspirin should be continued for at least 2 years and probably indefinitely. There are no data as yet to suggest that the new platelet agent ticlopidine (29) or dipyridamole and sulfinpyrazone have any greater clinical efficacy than aspirin in acute myocardial infarction.

## HEPARIN

It has become standard practice in North America to administer intravenous heparin together with or immediately following the infusion of a thrombolytic agent during acute myocardial infarction. Heparin is usually started as an intravenous bolus of 5000 units, followed by a maintenance infusion, keeping the partial thromboplastin time more than twice control level and continuing for 3–7 days. Heparin has been shown to inhibit the systemic thrombin activity occurring during and following a thrombolysis (30,31), resulting in a reduced early coronary reocclusion rate (32,33). In the ISIS-2 trial (11), early mortality was significantly lower in the group of patients who received intravenous heparin, but heparin therapy was not randomized in this part of the trial. There was a small increase in bleeding complications in the patients receiving heparin (1.1%) compared to those who did not receive heparin (0.3%). In none of these reports was the effect of age on heparin studied. Although subcutaneous heparin has been used extensively in European trials, it is not generally recommended for the prevention of coronary reocclusion following thrombolysis because it takes 12–24 h for heparin to reach therapeutic levels.

In the HART study (32), heparin (5000 unit bolus followed by a continuous infusion) appeared to be a more effective antithrombotic agent than low-dose (80 mg) aspirin when they were given in conjunction with tPA for thrombolysis. Angiograms obtained 7–24 h after thrombolysis showed a 82% patency rate in the patients assigned to heparin group compared to 52% in the aspirin group. In contrast, aspirin was at least as effective as heparin in preventing reocclusion between days 1 and 7 postthrombolysis. Questions were raised about whether an adequate dose of aspirin was used at the onset of the fibrinolytic therapy. In a recently published metaanalysis of 32 studies that assessed the effects of aspirin on coronary reocclusion and recurrent ischemia after thrombolysis (34), it was concluded that aspirin in the presence of heparin prevents reocclusion.

Systemic embolism has been recorded in approximately 5% of patients who have large anterior and apical Q-wave myocardial infarctions. Thus, it is advisable to anticoagulate these patients with heparin at the time of the infarction, whether or not a left ventricular apical thrombus is seen. Heparin should be switched to sodium warfarin before discharge and continued for an additional 6–12 weeks.

All patients, particularly the elderly (35) and those with congestive heart failure, are at risk for venous thromboembolism and should be anticoagulated with subcutaneous heparin if they are not fully anticoagulated and maintained on heparin until they are fully mobilized.

## PHARMACOLOGICAL CONSIDERATIONS IN THE ELDERLY PATIENT WITH ACUTE MYOCARDIAL INFARCTION

There are nonpathological human conditions that alter the interactions between drugs and human beings, particularly the extremes of age (36–39).

Although there is slowing of gastric emptying, reduced secretion of hydrochloric acid, and reduction in gastrointestinal motility, there are few data indicating significant changes in drug absorption in the elderly (36).

Changes in body composition, however, that is, reduction in lean body mass and water and a relative increase in body fat, lead to alteration in volume of distribution (36,37). Increases occur for lipid-soluble drugs, such as diazepam and lidocaine, thereby prolonging their pharmacological half-lives (38,39). Reduction in plasma albumin may lead to higher free concentrations of highly protein bound agents, such as warfarin (38,39).

The usual indices of liver function do not change with age, despite reduction in hepatic blood flow and in the activity of the microsomal mixed-function oxidative system (phase I). A few changes in conjugative processes (phase II) have been described. Dealkylation (amitriptyline and diltiazem) may be slightly impaired (38,39). It appears that the elimination of benzodiazepines that undergo phase I oxidative metabolism (diazepam, flurazepam, chlordiazepoxide, and alprazolam) is decreased in old age (38,39). Therefore, such agents as lorazepam, oxazepam, and temazepam, which are predominantly eliminated by conjugation, are preferred (38).

Beginning in the fourth decade, there is a 0.5–1% annual reduction in glomerular filtration rate and in renal plasma flow (36,37). Additionally, a 70-year-old man may have a 40–50% reduction in renal function, excluding any effects of concomitant disease processes (36). Thus, dose modifications are necessary for drugs that are eliminated predominantly by the kidney or whose active metabolites are excreted in the urine (digoxin) (38,39). Decreased loading and maintenance doses of digoxin are generally required in older patients because of age-related reductions in volume of distribution and clearance, respectively (36,38,39).

## β-ADRENERGIC BLOCKERS

Since 1974, the overall results of 15 major randomized, long-term, placebo-controlled clinical trials with β-adrenergic blockers in postmyocardial infarction patients have documented reductions in total mortality, cardiovascular mortality, sudden death, and nonfatal reinfarction with active treatment; mean follow-up extended from 9 months to 6 years (22). Retrospective analyses of the trials suggest that patients with non-Q-wave myocardial infarction should benefit from β-blockade similarly to patients with Q-wave myocardial infarction (40). Diabetic patients also appear to gain benefit from β-blockade postmyocardial infarction (41). Although β-blockers have been used in the extremely elderly for many years in clinical practice, there are no data from any long-term postinfarction trials regarding the safety and efficacy of treating patients over 75 years of age with these drugs.

The role of β-blockers in the hyperacute phase of myocardial infarction in an elderly population has also not been resolved. In deciding to use β-blockers in elderly patients with acute myocardial infarction, one must consider that adverse effects (e.g., congestive heart failure, heart block, and bradycardia) are more common than in younger patients (42).

$\beta$-Adrenergic blockers have been considered for use as therapy in patients with hyperacute myocardial infarction to prevent the undesirable consequences of increased sympathoadrenal discharge, coronary artery rethrombosis, arrhythmias, and extension of myocardial injury (43–46). In clinical trials using intravenous atenolol (47) or metoprolol (48,49) in selected patients during the first 24 h of myocardial infarction followed by oral dosing, early mortality was reduced by approximately 15% compared to control, with the greatest benefit seen in the first 36 h of myocardial infarction. The continued benefits of oral $\beta$-blocker therapy with metoprolol were seen for up to 2 years (50).

In one metoprolol trial (intravenous therapy followed by oral therapy), the 3 month mortality with active treatment was reduced by 36% compared with placebo (in those aged 40–64 years by 27% and in those aged 65–74 years by 45%) (42,48). The difference in total mortality after 3 months remained the same after 1 year and also at 2 years after randomization, despite that both groups were treated similarly during long-term follow-up (42). The reduction in mortality seemed confined to patients with definite myocardial infarction, with no difference in patients with possible or no myocardial infarction (42,48). There was a reduction both in lactic acid dehydrogenase (LDH) isoenzymes and in the frequency of ventricular fibrillation in patients treated within 12 h of infarction (42,48). Both variables were reduced in patients aged 40–64 years, as well as in patients aged 65–74 years, although not significantly in the older group (42,48).

Results from the Metoprolol in Acute Myocardial Infarction Study (MIAMI) showed a modest but insignificant effect of metoprolol versus placebo on total mortality (49). Patients over age 60 appeared to benefit the most, with an 18% reduction in mortality compared with placebo; patients under age 60 seemed to derive no benefit from therapy (42,49).

The addition of $\beta$-blockers to acute thrombolytic therapy in myocardial infarction may improve patient outcome to a greater extent than either treatment used alone. This was suggested by the favorable findings of TIMI-II, in which metoprolol was combined with tPA in patients with myocardial infarction (14,43).

It has been demonstrated conclusively that $\beta$-blockers can prolong life in patients who have had myocardial infarction. It has also been shown that $\beta$-adrenergic blockade can be initiated early and safely to infarct patients under 75 years of age with and without thrombolysis. Caution should be given in administering $\beta$-blockers to patients with transmural inferior wall myocardial infarction, in whom the hemodynamic complications of a right ventricular infarction may be unmasked (43). Intravenous metoprolol and atenolol are currently approved for intravenous use in patients with myocardial infarction. Oral atenolol, metoprolol, propranolol, and timolol are approved for long-term use in survivors of acute myocardial infarction to reduce the risk of mortality and nonfatal reinfarction. In long-term studies, the benefits of $\beta$-blockade in patients older than 65 years of age are at least as favorable as in the younger patients (Table 2) (48,51,52). In clinical trials, the incidence of side effects, the number of withdrawals, and reasons for withdrawal from $\beta$-blocker therapy appear to be similar in older and younger patients (51,52). It is concluded that age itself should not be a decision-making factor concerning $\beta$-blocker therapy in older patients with myocardial infarction.

## ANTIARRHYTHMIC DRUG THERAPY

In acute myocardial infarction, class II–III ventricular ectopic activity, especially when associated with a low left ventricular ejection fraction, is associated with a poor prognosis. There is controversy, however, about whether ventricular arrhythmia suppression with antiarrhythmic drugs other than $\beta$-blockers will alter this prognosis.

In older patients, the clearance of the antiarrhythmic drugs quinidine and procainamide (and its active metabolite *n*-acetylprocainamide) is reduced, requiring close monitoring of drug levels. Although lidocaine is associated with only minor age-related changes in pharmacokinetics, the clearance of the drug is decreased in the presence of congestive heart failure, a complication of acute myocardial infarction that occurs more commonly in older patients (53). The incidence of side effects with lidocaine, such as drowsiness, slurred speech, confusion, and paresthesias, is also increased in elderly patients (53). It is therefore advised that the loading and maintenance doses of lidocaine be reduced by one-half and should be discontinued after 24 h in patients who are older than 70 to reduce the risk of toxicity.

Prophylactic utilization of lidocaine to reduce the risk of ventricular fibrillation in patients with acute myocardial infarction is a controversial issue (54). Recent metaanalysis suggested that prophylactic lidocaine may in fact not be beneficial (55). Our group, however, believes this issue has not been resolved (56). In patients over 75 years of age with acute myocardial infarction, prophylactic lidocaine is usually not administered because of the risk of drug toxicity.

## CALCIUM CHANNEL BLOCKERS

The clinical trials with the calcium channel blockers have demonstrated less benefit than that reported with $\beta$-blockers or aspirin in myocardial infarction survivors (43). Patients up to the age of 75 years were evaluated in these studies. Some data suggest a role for diltiazem therapy in reducing the development of transmural myocardial infarction and angina pectoris in those patients sustaining

**Table 2** Results of Long-Term β-Blocker Trials in Survivors of Acute Myocardial Infarction: Examining the Influence of Age upon Treatment Effect

| | | | | | Randomization ($n$) | | Mortality (%) | | |
|---|---|---|---|---|---|---|---|---|---|
| Trial | Drug | Age limit | Follow-up | Age | C | I | C | I | $p$ |
| Goteborg (48) | MET | <75 | 3 months | <65 | 453 | 464 | 5.7 | 4.5 | NS |
| | | | | ≥65 | 244 | 234 | 14.8 | 8.1 | <0.032 |
| BHAT (51) | PROP | <70 | up to 3 years | <60 | 1288 | 1301 | 7.4 | 6.0 | |
| | | | | ≥60 | 633 | 615 | 14.7 | 9.8 | |
| Norwegian Multicenter (52) | TIM | <75 | 12–33 months | <65 | 555 | 597 | 12.4 | 7.7 | <0.01 |
| | | | | ≥65 | 384 | 348 | 21.6 | 14.9 | <0.05 |

C = control; I = intervention; BHAT = Beta Blocker Heart Attack Trial; MET = metoprolol; PROP = propranolol; TIM = timolol.
*Source*: From Frishman et al. Treatment of ischemic heart disease in the elderly. Beta-adrenergic blockade and coronary artery bypass surgery. In: Wenger NK, Furberg CD, Pitt E, eds. Coronary Heart Disease in the Elderly. New York: Elsevier, 1986.

non-Q-wave infarctions (57,58). More recent studies with verapamil demonstrate a modest effect in reducing deaths and reinfarctions in survivors of myocardial infarction (59). There is a lesser incidence of transient myocardial ischemia assessed by ambulatory electrocardiographic (ECG) monitoring in verapamil-treated patients compared to placebo (60). There also appears to be less benefit or even potential danger when using calcium channel blockers in patients with myocardial infarction and left ventricular dysfunction (59,61,62).

There have been no specific studies assessing the effects of calcium channel blockers in elderly patients with myocardial infarction. Based on the available information, it is recommended that in the elderly, rate-lowering calcium channel blockers (diltiazem or verapamil) be considered in infarction survivors with or without aspirin if $\beta$-blockers are not tolerated or contraindicated and patients do not have left ventricular dysfunction.

## ANGIOTENSIN CONVERTING ENZYME INHIBITORS

Recognition of the importance of the renin-angiotensin-aldosterone system in heart failure, along with an appreciation of the hemodynamic benefits of vasodilator therapy, has led to the widespread use of angiotensin converting enzyme (ACE) inhibitors in the treatment of heart failure, resulting in symptomatic improvement and improved survival (63,64).

A recently completed trial demonstrated the benefit of long-term captopril therapy in reducing the mortality of patients who survived an acute myocardial infarction (65). Other studies have also demonstrated that early utilization of ACE inhibitors in patients with myocardial infarction might facilitate successful ventricular remodeling and preserve left ventricular function (66). Our group has participated in a recently completed multicenter study that utilized captopril in conjunction with thrombolytic therapy in the hyperacute phase of myocardial infarction to assess the effects of therapy on short-term and long-term left ventricular function.

Until the data from some of the studies are analyzed, with particular attention to the effects of ACE inhibition in the elderly, it would be prudent not to routinely administer ACE inhibitors during the acute phase of myocardial infarction. However, there are good data to support their long-term use in patients with left ventricular dysfunction who survive an acute myocardial infarction.

## EXERCISE TESTING

Exercise testing can be done in the elderly patient following an acute myocardial infarction to assess ischemic heart disease and left ventricular function (67,68) despite the decline in maximal aerobic capacity with age (67–69). Often, however, the ability to test patients on a treadmill or bicycle may be limited by arthritis and musculoskeletal disorders (70). The ability to interpret the exercise ECG may also be limited by concurrent diseases, drugs, or both (67,68). Exercise or dipyridamole (71) radionuclide myocardial imaging may be useful in detecting myocardial ischemia when the exercise ECG is inconclusive because of rest ECG abnormalities, such as bundle branch block, or when patients are unable to exercise (see Chapter 11).

## CONCLUSION

Medical therapy has thus been shown to be highly effective in treating acute myocardial infarction in the elderly. Because of the higher mortality and morbidity rates in this age group, the number of lives saved is frequently greater and the results more beneficial. Thus, old age, per se, is not a contraindication to institute aggressive medical management for acute myocardial infarction.

## REFERENCES

1. Kapantis G, Powel-Griner E. Characteristics of persons dying of diseases of the heart: Preliminary data from the 1986 National Mortality Followback Survey. Hyattsville, MD: National Center for Health Statistics, Advanced Data, 1989:172.
2. Weaver WD, Litwin PE, Martin JS, Kundenchuk PS, Maynard C, Eisenberg MS, Ho MT, Cobb LA, Kennedy JW, Wirkus MS, MITI Project Group. Effect of age on use of thrombolytic therapy and mortality in acute myocardial infarction. *J Am Coll Cardiol* 1991; 18:657–662.
3. Gruppo Italiano per lo Studio della Streptochinasi nell'Infarcto Miocardio (GISSI). Effectiveness of intravenous thrombolytic treatment in acute myocardial infarction. *Lancet* 1986; 1:397–401.
4. Smith SC, Gilpin E, Ahnve S, Dittrich H, Nicok P, Henning H, Ross J. Outlook after acute myocardial infarction in the very elderly compared with that in patients aged 65 to 75 years. *J Am Coll Cardiol* 1990; 16:784–792.
5. Wilcox RG, Hampton JR. Importance of age in prehospital and hospital mortality of heart attack. *Br Heart J* 1980; 44:503–507.
6. Toffler GH, Muller FE, Stone PH, Willich SN, Davis VG, Poole WK, Braunwald E, MILIS Study Group. Factors leading to shorter survival after acute myocardial infarction in patients aged 65 to 75 years compared with younger patients. *Am J Cardiol* 1988; 62:860–867.
7. Nadelman J, Frishman WH, Ooi WL, Tepper D, Greenberg S, Guzik H, Lazar EJ, Heiman M, Aronson M. Prevalence, incidence and prognosis of recognized and unrecognized myocardial infarction in persons aged 75 years and older: The Bronx Aging Study. *Am J Cardiol* 1990; 66:533–537.
8. Bayer AJ, Chadha JS, Farag RR, Pathy MSJ. Changing presentation of myocardial infarction with increasing old age. *J Am Geriatr Soc* 1986; 34:263–266.

9. Muller DWM, Topol EJ. Selection of patients with acute myocardial infarction for thrombolytic therapy. *Ann Intern Med* 1990; 113:949–960.
10. ISAM Study Group. A perspective trial of intravenous streptokinase in acute myocardial infarction (ISAM). *N Engl J Med* 1986; 314:1465–1471.
11. ISIS-2 (Second International Study of Infarct Survival) Collaborative Group. Randomized trial of intravenous streptokinase, oral aspirin, both or neither among 17,187 cases of suspected acute myocardial infarction. ISIS-2. *Lancet* 1988; 2:349–360.
12. Wilcox RG, Olsson CG, Skene AM, von der Lippe G, Jensen G, Hampton JR. Trial of tissue plasminogen activator for mortality reduction in acute myocardial infarction: Anglo-Scandinavian Study of Early Thrombolysis (ASSET). *Lancet* 1988; 2:825–830.
13. AIMS Trial Study Group. Effect of intravenous APSAC on mortality after acute myocardial infarction: Preliminary report of a placebo-controlled clinical trial. *Lancet* 1988; 1:545–549.
14. TIMI Study Group. Comparison of invasive and conservative strategies after treatment with intravenous tissue plasminogen activator in acute myocardial infarction: results of the Thrombolysis in Myocardial Infarction (TIMI) Phase II trial. *N Engl J Med* 1989; 320:618–627.
15. Lew AS, Hanock H, Cercek B, Shah PK, Ganz W. Mortality and morbidity rates of patients older and younger than 75 years with acute myocardial infarction treated with intravenous streptokinase. *Am J Cardiol* 1987; 59:1–5.
16. Chaitman BR, Thompson B, Wittry MD, Stump D, Hamilton WP, Hillis LD, Dwyer JG, Solomon RE, Knatterud GL, TIMI Investigators. The use of tissue-type plasminogen activator for acute infarction in the elderly: Results from Thrombolysis in Myocardial Infarction Phase I Open Label Studies and the Thrombolysis in Myocardial Infarction Phase II Pilot Study. *J Am Coll Cardiol* 1989; 14:1159–1165.
17. Gore JM, Sloan MS, Price TR. Intracerebral hemorrhage, cerebral infarction and subdural hematoma after acute myocardial infarction and thrombolytic therapy in Thrombolysis in Myocardial Infarction Study. Thrombolysis in Myocardial Infarction Phase II Pilot and Clinical Trial. *Circulation* 1991; 83:448–459.
18. O'Connor CM, Califf RM, Masey EW, Mark DB, Kereiakes DJ, Candela RJ, Abbottsmith C, George B, Stack RS, Aronson L, Mantell S, Topol EJ. Stroke and acute myocardial infarction in the thrombolytic era: Clinical correlates and long-term prognosis. *J Am Coll Cardiol* 1990; 16:533–540.
19. DeJaegere PP, Arnold AA, Balk AH, Simmons ML. Intracranial hemorrhage in association with thrombolytic therapy: Incidence and clinical predictive factors. *J Am Coll Cardiol* 1992; 19:289–294.
20. Thompson PL, Robinson JS. Stroke after acute myocardial infarction: Relation to infarct size. *Br Med J* 1978; 2:457–459.
21. Komrad MS, Coffey CE, Coffey MS, McKinnis R, Massey EW, Califf RM. Myocardial infarction and stroke. *Neurology* 1984; 34:1403–1409.
22. Frishman WH. Secondary prevention: Beta-adrenergic blockers and aspirin. *Curr Opin Cardiol* 1991; 6:567–573.

23. Miller KP, Frishman WH. Platelets and anti-platelet therapy in ischemic heart disease. *Med Clin North Am* 1988; 72:117–184.
24. DeGaetano G, Cerletti C, Dejana E, Latini R. Pharmacology of platelet inhibition in humans. Implications of the salicylate-aspirin interaction. *Circulation* 1985; 72:1185–1193.
25. Moschos CB, Haider B, DelaCruz C, Lyons MM, Regan TJ. Antiarrhythmic effects of aspirin during nonthrombotic coronary occlusion. *Circulation* 1978; 57:681–684.
26. Capurro NL, Marr KC, Aamodt R, Goldstein RE, Epstein SE. Aspirin-induced increase in collateral flow after acute coronary occlusion in dogs. *Circulation* 1979; 59:744–747.
27. Weksler BB, Tack-Goldman K, Subramanian VA, Gay WA Jr. Cumulative inhibitor effect of low dose aspirin on vascular prostacyclin and platelet thromboxane production in patients with atherosclerosis. *Circulation* 1985; 71:332–340.
28. Dutch TIA Trial Study Group. A comparison of two doses of aspirin (30 mg vs 283 mg a day) in patients after a transient ischemic attack or minor ischemic stroke. *N Engl J Med* 1991; 325:1261–1266.
29. Editorial. Ticlopidine. *Lancet* 1991; 337:459–460.
30. Eisenberg PR, Sherman LA, Jaffe AS. Paradoxic elevation of fibrinopeptide A after streptokinase: Evidence of continued thrombosis despite intense fibrinolysis. *J Am Coll Cardiol* 1987; 10:527–530.
31. Rapold HJ, deBono D, Arnold AER, Arnout J, DeCock F, Collen D, Verstraete M. Plasma fibrinopeptide A levels in patients with acute myocardial infarction treated with altephase: Correlation with concomitant heparin, coronary artery patency, and recurrent ischemia. *Circulation* 1992; 85:928–934.
32. Hsia J, Hamilton WP, Kleinman N, Roberts R, Chaitman BR, Ross AM. A comparison between heparin and low dose aspirin as adjunctive therapy with tissue plasminogen activator for acute myocardial infarction. *N Engl J Med* 1990; 323:1433–1437.
33. Bleich SD, Nichols TC, Schumaker RR, Cooke DH, Tate DA, Teichman SL. Effect of heparin on coronary artery patency after thrombolysis with tissue plasminogen activator in acute myocardial infarction. *Am J Cardiol* 1990; 66:1412–1417.
34. Roux S, Christeller E, Ludin E. Effects of aspirin on coronary reocclusion and recurrent ischemia after thrombolysis: A meta-analysis. *J Am Coll Cardiol* 1992; 19:671–677.
35. Simmons AV, Sheppard MA, Cox AF. Deep venous thrombosis after acute myocardial infarction: Predisposing factors. *Br Heart J* 1973; 35:623–625.
36. Avorn J, Gurwitz J. Principles of pharmacology. In: Cassel CK, Riesenberg DE, Sorensen LB, Walsh JR, eds. Geriatric Medicine. New York: Springer-Verlag, 1990.
37. Greenblatt DJ. Disposition of cardiovascular drugs in the elderly. *Med Clin North Am* 1989; 73:487–494.
38. Montamat SC, Cusack BJ, Vestal RE. Management of drug therapy in the elderly. *N Engl J Med* 1989; 321:303–309.

39. Yuen FJ. Altered pharmacokinetics in the elderly. *Clin Geriatr Med* 1990; 6:257–269.
40. Yusuf S, Wittes J, Probstfield J. Evaluating effects of treatment in subgroups of patients within a clinical trial: The case of non-Q-wave myocardial infarction and beta blockers (editorial). *Am J Cardiol* 1990; 66:220–222.
41. Kjekshus J, Gilpin E, Cali G, Blackey AR, Henning H, Ross J Jr. Diabetic patients and beta blockers after myocardial infarction. *Eur Heart J* 1990; 11:43–50.
42. Frishman WH, Bauman J, Soberman J, Nadelmann J, Wurzelmann, J, Aronson M. Treatment of ischemic heart disease in the elderly: Beta-adrenergic blockade and coronary artery bypass surgery. In: Wenger NK, Furberg CD, Pitt E, eds. Coronary Heart Disease in the Elderly. New York: Elsevier, 1986:153–193.
43. Frishman WH, Skolnick AE, Miller KP. Secondary prevention postinfarction: The role of $\beta$-adrenergic blockers, calcium channel blockers, and aspirin. In: Gersh BJ, Rahimtoola SH, eds. Acute Myocardial Infarction. New York: Elsevier, 1991:469–492.
44. Frishman WH, Furberg CD, Friedewald WT. $\beta$-Adrenergic blockade for survivors of acute myocardial infarction. *N Engl J Med* 1984; 310:830–837.
45. Frishman WH, Lazar EJ. Reduction of mortality, sudden death and non-fatal reinfarction with beta-adrenergic blockers in survivors of acute myocardial infarction: A new hypothesis regarding the cardioprotective action of beta-adrenergic blockade. *Am J Cardiol* 1990; 66:66G–70G.
46. Frishman WH. Multifactorial actions of $\beta$-adrenergic blocking drugs in ischemic heart disease. Current concepts. *Circulation* 1983; 67(6 Part 2):I11–I18.
47. ISIS-I (First International Study of Infarct Survival) Collaborative Group. Randomized trial of intravenous atenolol among 16,027 cases of suspected acute myocardial infarction. ISIS-I. *Lancet* 1986; 2:57–66.
48. Hjalmarson A, Elmfeldt D, Herlitz J, et al. Effect on mortality of metoprolol in acute myocardial infarction: A double-blind randomized trial. *Lancet* 1981; 2:823–827.
49. MIAMI Trial Research Group. Metoprolol in acute myocardial infarction (MISMI): A randomized placebo-controlled international trial. *Eur Heart J* 1985; 6:199–226.
50. Herlitz J, Holmberg S, Pennert K, et al. Gotebord Metoprolol Trial: Design, patient characteristics and conduct. *Am J Cardiol* 1984; 53:3D–8D.
51. Hawkins CM, Richardson DW, Vokonas PS. Effect of propranolol in reducing mortality in old myocardial infarction patients: The Beta-Blocker Heart Attack Trial Experience. *Circulation* 1983; 67(Suppl. I):I-94–97.
52. Gundersen T, Abrahamsen M, Kjekshus J, et al. Timolol-related reduction in mortality and reinfarction in patients ages 65–75 years surviving acute myocardial infarction. *Circulation* 1982; 66:1179–1184.
53. Ribner HS, Isaacs ES, Frishman WH. Lidocaine prophylaxis against ventricular fibrillation. *Prog Cardiovasc Dis* 1979; 21:287–313.
54. Da Silva RA, Henneckens CH, Lown B, Casscells W. Lignocaine prophylaxis in acute myocardial infarction: An evaluation of randomized trials. *Lancet* 1981; 2:855–858.

55. Hine LK, Laird N, Hewitt P, Chalmers TC. Meta-analytic evidence against prophylactic use of lidocaine in acute myocardial infarction. *Arch Intern Med* 1989; 149:2694–2698.
56. Ribner HS, Frishman WH. Prophylactic lidocaine therapy in acute myocardial infarction. *Cardiovasc Rev Rep* 1990; 11(9):53–60.
57. Gibson RS, Boden WE, Theroux P, et al. Diltiazem and reinfarction in patients with non-Q-wave myocardial infarction: Results of a double-blind, randomized multicenter trial. *N Engl J Med* 1986; 315:423–429.
58. Gibson RS, Young PM, Boden WE, et al. Prognostic significance and beneficial effect of diltiazem on the incidence of early recurrent ischemia after non-Q-wave myocardial infarction: Results from the multicenter diltiazem reinfarction study. *Am J Cardiol* 1987; 60:203–209.
59. Hansen JP. Treatment with verapamil during and after an acute myocardial infarction: A review based on the Danish Verapamil Infarction Trials I and II. *J Cardiovasc Pharmacol* 1991; 18(Suppl. 6):S20–S25.
60. Vaage-Nilsen M, Rasmussen V, Hansen JF, Hagerup L, Sorensen MB, Bjergaard OP, Mellemgaard K, Hollander NH, Nielsen I, Sigurd B. Effect of verapamil on ischemia and ventricular arrhythmias after an acute myocardial infarction: prognostic implications. *J Cardiovasc Pharmacol* 1991; 18(Suppl.6):S26–S29.
61. Skolnick AE, Frishman WH. Calcium channel blockers in myocardial infarction. *Arch Intern Med* 1989; 149:1669–1677.
62. Multicenter Diltiazem Post-Infarction Trial Research Group. The effect of diltiazem on mortality and reinfarction after myocardial infarction. *N Engl J Med* 1988; 319:385–392.
63. CONSENSUS Trial Study Group. Effects of enalapril on mortality in severe congestive heart failure: Results of the Cooperative North Scandinavian Enalapril Survival Study. *N Engl J Med* 1987; 316:1429–1435.
64. SOLVD Investigators. Effect of angiotensin converting enzyme inhibitor enalapril on survival in patients with reduced left ventricular ejection fraction and congestive heart failure. *N Engl J Med* 1991; 325:293–302.
65. St John Sutton M, Pfeffer MA, Plappert T, Arnold JMO, Basta LL, Bittar N, Goldman S, Gottlieb SS, Klein M, Lamas GA, Moyé LA, Rouleau JL, Braunwald E. Survival and ventricular enlargement (SAVE) quantitative 2D echo substudy: Effects of ACE inhibition therapy on ventricular enlargement. *J Am Coll Cardiol* 1992; 19(3):205A.
66. Pfeffer MA, Lamas GA, Vaughan DE, et al. Effect of captopril on progressive ventricular dilatation after anterior myocardial infarction. *N Engl J Med* 1988; 319:80–86.
67. Frishman WH, DeMaria AN, Ewy GA. Clinical assessment (18th Bethesda Conference—Cardiovascular Disease in the Elderly). *J Am Coll Cardiol* 1987; 10:48A–51A.
68. Samek L, Betz P, Schnellbacher K. Exercise testing in elderly patients with coronary artery disease. *Eur Heart J* 1984; 5(Suppl. E):69–73.
69. Lakatta EG. Determinants of cardiovascular performance: Modification due to aging. *J Chron Dis* 1983; 36:15–30.

70. Saunamaki KI. Early post-myocardial infarction exercise testing in subjects 70 years or more of age. Functional and prognostic evaluation. *Eur Heart J* 1984; 5(Suppl.E):41–45.
71. Boucher CA, Brester DC, Darling RC, Okada RD, Strauss HW, Pohost GM. Determination of cardiac risk by dipyridamole-thallium imaging before peripheral vascular surgery. *N Engl J Med* 1985; 312:389–394.

# 13

# Coronary Artery Bypass Surgery and Percutaneous Transluminal Coronary Angioplasty in the Elderly Patient with Ischemic Heart Disease

**Thomas M. Shimshak and Ben D. McCallister**
*Mid-America Heart Institute and University of Missouri,*
*Kansas City, Missouri*

## INTRODUCTION

Symptomatic coronary artery disease is common in the elderly and is the most common cause of death in persons older than 65 years of age. Based on the Framingham Heart Study, more than half of all patients currently hospitalized for an acute myocardial infarction are older than 65 (1). Although overall mortality due to coronary heart disease in this country declined significantly during the 1970s, mortality rates for patients > 65 years have not shown the same rate of decline observed in younger patients (1). Current therapeutic options for elderly patients with coronary artery disease include medical management, coronary artery bypass grafting (CABG), and percutaneous transluminal coronary angioplasty (PTCA). This chapter will, we hope, facilitate the decision-making process for the clinician by a review of the pertinent literature and the data base at one institution (Mid-America Heart Institute, MHI).

## CORONARY ARTERY BYPASS SURGERY

Approximately 370,000 coronary bypass procedures were performed in the United States in 1989, including 191,000 patients over the age of 65 years (2). Appropriate indications for CABG in patients of all ages have been well outlined in the American College of Cardiology/American Heart Association

(ACC/AHA) Task Force Guidelines for CABG (3). Objective evidence of myocardial ischemia as demonstrated by noninvasive stress testing, significant symptoms of angina pectoris, the presence of multivessel disease, and abnormal left ventricular function support a decision to advise CABG (3).

Coronary artery bypass grafting has been demonstrated in many studies on older patients to be effective in the treatment of angina pectoris. Benefits have been comparable to those seen in younger patients, but multivariate analyses have identified advancing age as a strong adverse predictor of short- and long-term outcome and complications. Patients over 65 are also more likely to have other associated conditions, such as diabetes, peripheral vascular disease, cerebrovascular disease, and chronic pulmonary or renal insufficiency, which may adversely affect immediate or long-term results.

In the older patient specific considerations are important, including the patient's physical and mental age and personal expectations, the presence of other medical illness, the expected mortality and morbidity with and without surgery, and the expected advantages and disadvantages over other therapeutic options (PTCA or medical therapy). An increasing number of patients in the older age group have had prior CABG, with an expected increased risk for reoperation, primarily because of an increase in associated risk factors other than the reoperation procedure. An increasing percentage of women in the older age group require operation versus patients less than 65 years, as the coronary risk factor profile increases after menopause. Female gender has been identified as an increased risk factor for morbidity and mortality following coronary bypass surgery, in part related to smaller coronary arteries, which make revascularization more technically difficult, and the presence of other associated diseases, such as hypertension and diabetes mellitus.

Table 1 summarizes the results of individual studies of CABG in elderly patients published in the past two decades (4–32).

The presence of unstable angina, the need for other associated cardiac surgery (valve replacement of aneurysm resection), the need for urgent or emergency surgery, LMCA disease, cigarette smoking, pulmonary rales, one or more associated medical illnesses, female sex, decreased LV function, prior CABG, and an increased extent of coronary artery disease (CAD), have all been reported to substantially increase the risk of surgery in this age group (5,8,12).

The profile of perioperative complications following CABG in the elderly patient is similar to that seen in younger patients, although serious complications are more frequent, occurring in 37–75% of elderly patients (8,13,14). In particular, there is an increased incidence of stroke (1.7–8.5%; Table 1) and other neurological disorders (8,9,12,13,16). Other nonfatal complications include perioperative myocardial infarction, the need for prolonged ventilatory support, atrial and ventricular arrhythmias, need for intraaortic balloon pumping, oliguric renal failure, and increased duration of intensive care. Previous studies

**Table 1** Coronary Artery Bypass Surgery in the Elderly

| Authors | References | Year | Number patients | Age | Perioperative MI (%) | Overall operative mortality (%) | CVA (%) | Mortality in nonelderly patients (%) | % survival, ($\bar{x}$ follow-up years) | Mortality elective versus urgent surgery (%) |
|---|---|---|---|---|---|---|---|---|---|---|
| Ashor et al. | 4 | 1973 | 78 | >65 | | 3 | | | | |
| Gersh et al. | 5, 6, 32 | 1983, 1985 | 1086 | >65 | | 5.2 | | 1.9 | 83 (5) | 3.9/7.7 |
| Rahimtoola et al. | 7 | 1986 | 1126 | 65–74 | | 3 | | 2. | 83 (5)/66 (10) | |
| Loop et al. | 8 | 1988 | 5070 | 65–74 | | 2 | 2.7 | 0.7 | | |
| Faro et al. | 9 | 1983 | 105 | >72 | | 10.5 | 8.5 | 3.5 | | |
| McCallister et al. | 10 | 1975 | 48 | >70 | | 6 | | | | |
| Killen | 11 | 1988 | 817 | 70–75 | | 6.1 | | 1.0 | 78 (5)/55 (10) | |
| Meyer et al. | 12 | 1975 | 95 | >70 | 7.9 | 12.6 | 4 | | | |
| Rose et al. | 13 | 1985 | 201 | >70 | | 5.9 | 4 | 1.9 | | |
| Knapp et al. | 14 | 1981 | 121 | ≥70 | 3.3 | 1.6 | 2.5 | 1.1 | 95 (5) | |
| Edwards et al. | 15 | 1991 | 121 | >70 | | 7.4 | | | | 2.9/8.6 |
| Horneffer et al. | 16 | 1987 | 201 | >70 | 7.9 | 5.9 | 4 | | | |
| Hochberg et al. | 17 | 1982 | 75 | >70 | | 12 | 2.6 | 4. | | |
| Pelletier et al. | 18 | 1983 | 71 | >70 | 1.4 | 7.0 | 0 | | | |
| Dorros et al. | 19 | 1987 | 121 | >70 | 7.1 | 1.6 | 4.2 | | 64(7) | |
| Elayda et al. | 20 | 1984 | 674 | >70 | 7.1 | 7.4 | 4.2 | | | |
| Berry et al. | 21 | 1981 | 23 | >70 | 4.0 | | | | 76 (5) | |
| Bhattacharya et al. | 22 | 1984 | 597 | >70 | 1.5 | 2.7 | | | | |
| Montague et al. | 23 | 1985 | 228 | >70 | | 9.3 | 7.5 | | | |
| Sutton et al. | 24 | 1992 | 195 | >70 | 6.2 | 8.7 | 5 | | 65 (5) | |
| Loop et al. | 8 | 1988 | 467 | >75 | | 4.7 | 2.4 | 0.7 | | |
| Salomon et al. | 25 | 1991 | 469 | >75 | 5.1 | 6.8 | 4.1 | 2.1 | 80 (5)/55 (10) | 1.7/9.6 |
| Horvath et al. | 26 | 1990 | 222 | >75 | | 10.8 | | 3.1 | 75 (4) | |
| Rich et al. | 27 | 1988 | 60 | >75 | | 3.3 | 1.7 | | | |
| Killen | 11 | 1988 | 279 | 75–79 | | 6.5 | | 1.0 | | |
| Rahimtoola et al. | 7 | 1986 | 178 | 75–84 | | 3 | | 2. | 73 (5)/65 (10) | |
| Naunheim et al. | 28 | 1987 | 16 | ≥80 | | 12.5 | | | 82 (2) | |
| Edmunds et al. | 29 | 1988 | 41 | ≥80 | | 24 | | | 54 (5) | 50/— |
| Mullany et al. | 30 | 1990 | 159 | ≥80 | 5.6 | 10.7 | 4.4 | | 71 (5) | |
| Ko et al. | 31 | 1991 | 100 | ≥80 | 5 | 12 | 3 | | | 2.8/33 |
| Killen | 11 | 1988 | 60 | 80–89 | | 6.6 | | 1.0 | | |

have demonstrated that with each decade of increasing age, hospital stay, costs, and operative mortality increase and long-term survival decreases (5,14,25).

Transient mental confusion and symptoms of hypoxic encephalopathy can complicate the care in the postoperative period but are usually reversible. The management of patients with known cerebrovascular disease (either the patient with prior symptoms or those with identified carotid lesions on duplex scan or angiography) is difficult, and complications are not always predictable. Combined endarterectomy and CABG is no longer performed in most centers. Carotid endarterectomy may be indicated in some patients before CABG, particularly if the carotid disease is symptomatic, but in other patients, myocardial revascularization should take precedence. Each case requires individual management decisions and consultation with neurology colleagues.

Long-term survival studies have been encouraging and have approached that expected from life tables from the general population, although no randomized trials comparing PTCA, medical, or CABG therapy in older patients have been reported (Table 1). However, in the Coronary Artery Surgery Study (CASS) nonrandomized studies, CABG appeared to improve survival and symptoms compared with medical therapy alone (realizing a difference in important baseline characteristics) (32). Gersh reported a 6 year survival of 79% in 861 patients 65 years or older treated surgically versus 64% for the 630 medically treated nonrandomized patients 65 years of age or older in the CASS registry ($P = < 0.0001$). At 5 years, chest pain was absent in 62% of the surgical group and 29% of the medical group ($P < 0.0001$) (32).

In summary, in selected elderly patients CABG is a highly effective form of revascularization therapy. However, the clinician should perform a careful preoperative assessment of the relative risk of surgery and determine the potential for each patient to return to a meaningful, functional level of activity. Factors associated with increased operative risk among elderly patients undergoing CABG include female sex, advanced age, unstable angina, severe three-vessel disease, left ventricular dysfunction, and nonelective surgery. Compared to medical therapy, those patients at highest risk may benefit most from surgery. Despite an increased risk profile in the older patient, late results demonstrate improvement in symptoms in the majority of patients and satifactory late and event-free survival.

## PERCUTANEOUS TRANSLUMINAL CORONARY ANGIOPLASTY IN THE ELDERLY

Percutaneous transluminal coronary angioplasty has revolutionalized the treatment of atherosclerotic coronary artery disease since its introduction in 1977. Initially, this nonsurgical treatment was limited primarily to younger, symptomatic patients with noncalcific, discrete stenoses in the proximal portion of the coronary artery. Over the last 15 years, increased operator experience and technical advancements in equipment have resulted in an increase in procedural success with lower complication rates. In 1989, approximately 259,000 PTCA were performed in the United States, including 107,000 in patients 65 years of age or older (2). In experienced angioplasty centers, PTCA is now routinely performed in many "high-risk" patients previously considered ineligible because of concerns regarding procedural outcome, including patients with advanced age.

Between January 1981 and June 1992, we performed 12,110 elective PTCA at the Mid-America Heart Institute, including 4852 procedures (40%) in patients 65 years of age or older. Figure 1 shows the increasing number of elderly patients undergoing elective PTCA at the Mid-America Heart Institute each year between 1980 and 1992 (33). In the last 2 years, more than 50% of the total elective PTCAs at the Mid-America Heart Institute were performed in patients 65 years of age or older (33).

## Procedural Results

Several authors have described the procedural results of PTCA in elderly and ultraelderly patients (33–44). Table 2 summarizes the procedural results of elec-

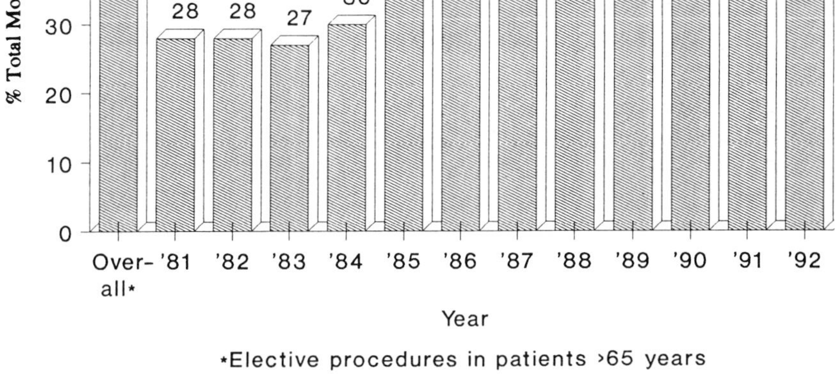


**Figure 1** Trends in PTCA in the elderly: MHI experience, January 1981 through June 1992. Total elective procedures 12,110.

**Table 2** Procedural Results of Elective PTCA in the Elderly

| Authors | Reference | Age | $N$ | Success (%) | Complications MI (%) | CABG (%) | Death (%) |
|---|---|---|---|---|---|---|---|
| Mock et al. | 34 | <65 | 2709 | 62 | 4.9 | 6.5 | 0.7 |
| | | >65 | 370 | 53 | 5.6 | 6.8 | 2.2 |
| Dorros et al. | 35 | >70 | 109 | 89 | 2.8 | 0.9 | 1.8 |
| Raizner et al. | 36 | <65 | 518 | 80 | 2.9 | 4.7 | 0 |
| | | >65 | 121 | 81 | 2.5 | 4.1 | 0.8 |
| Holt et al. | 37 | >70 | 54 | 80 | 3.7 | 5.5 | 0 |
| Simpendorfer et al. | 38 | >70 | 366 | 91 | 0.9 | 3.3 | 0.6 |
| Urban et al. | 39 | >65 | 51 | 68 | 4.6 | 4.6 | 4.6 |
| Mills et al. | 40 | <65 | 1177 | 84 | — | — | 0.3 |
| | | >65 | 644 | 83 | — | — | 0.9 |
| Jeroudi et al. | 41 | <80 | 2085 | 92 | 1.1 | 3.7 | 0.4 |
| | | >80 | 54 | 91 | 4.0 | 0 | 4.0 |
| Hartzler et al. | 42 | >70 | 1038 | 94 | 0.8 | 1.3 | 1.4 |
| Good et al. | 43 | >80 | 75 | 89 | 1.2 | 0 | 3.5 |
| Shimshak et al. | 44 | >70 | 1847 | 95 | 1.8 | 1.5 | 2.2 |

MI = periprocedural myocardial infarction; CABG = emergency coronary artery bypass surgery.

tive PTCA in elderly patients from a number of institutions over the last 10 years. The procedural success rate of PTCA in patients with advanced age has increased significantly since the early reports from the National Heart, Lung, and Blood Institute Registry in which Mock et al. reported a success rate of 62% in patients < 65 years of age and 53% in patients older than 65 years of age ($p < 0.01$) (34). Subsequent investigators have reported PTCA success rates in the elderly ranging from 68 to 96% (33–44). With continued improvements in equipment and increased operator experience, the procedural success rate of PTCA in the elderly can now be expected to approach that in younger patients. Analysis of the first 10,000 PTCAs from our institution performed between 1980 and 1990 revealed a success rate of 95% overall, as well as in the nearly 2000 PTCA patients who were 70 years of age or older (44). We recently described the results of elective, multivessel PTCA in 1373 elderly patients at the Mid-America Heart Institute. The procedural success rate in this group of patients with advanced age was 96% (33).

## Procedural Complications

Percutaneous transluminal coronary angioplasty in the elderly and ultraelderly is generally associated with an increased incidence of major complications, including Q-wave myocardial infarction, urgent or emergent coronary artery bypass surgery, and death (Table 2). Previous reports of PTCA in the elderly demonstrated major complication rates, ranging from 0.8 to 6.0% for myocardial infarction, from 0 to 6.0% for need for emergency bypass surgery, and from 0 to 4.6% for procedure-related death (34–44). In comparison, the complication rate for all elective procedures in our first 10,000 PTCA was 3.4% and included Q-wave myocardial infarction (1.3%), emergency CABG (1.7%), and death (0.9%) (44). This series also included 1847 patients age 70 years or older who had elective PTCA. The incidence of major complications in this elderly cohort included Q-wave myocardial infarction (1.8%), emergent CABG (1.5%), and in-hospital mortality (2.2%). In our experience, univariate and multivariate stepwise regression analysis identified high-risk subgroups based on procedural mortality and risk ratios. The most significant high-risk subgroups included age of 70 years or more, impaired left ventricular function (ejection fraction < 40%), unstable angina, and three-vessel disease. Procedural mortality increased with an increasing number of risk factors, ranging from 0.3% if no risk factors were present to 13.1% if all four risk factors were present (Fig. 2). Although procedural mortality correlated with these risk factors, advanced age alone was a univariate predictor of procedural mortality, particularly for patients older than 80 years of age (45).

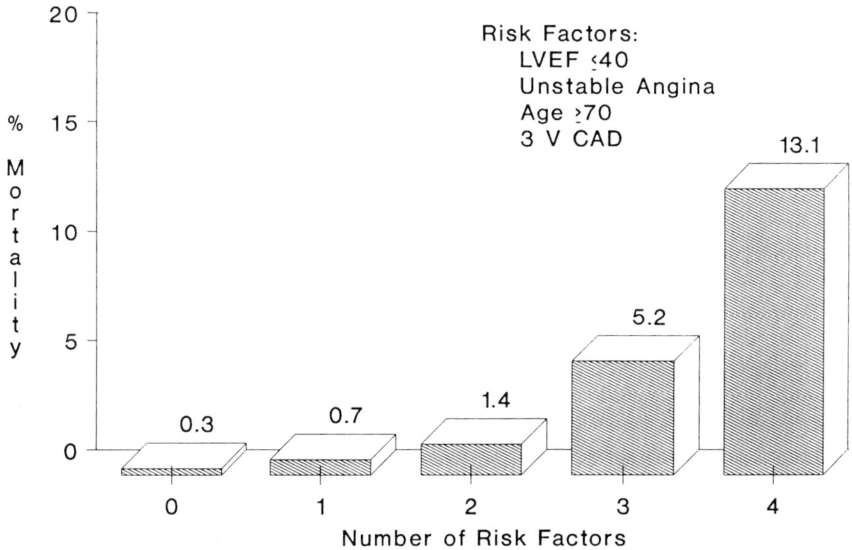


**Figure 2** In-hospital mortality related to number of risk factors. LVEF = left ventricular ejection fraction; 3 V CAD = three-vessel coronary artery disease.

In the Bedotto report from our institution summarizing the results of elective, multivessel PTCA in the elderly (33), the overall complication rate was 3.2% and included myocardial infarction (1.4%), emergent CABG (0.8%), and death (1.6%). In this report, independent predictors of in-hospital mortality were ejection fraction < 40%, three-vessel disease, female gender, and PTCA performed between 1981 and 1985 (i.e., in our early experience).

## Long-Term Follow-up

Table 3 summarizes the reported long-term results of PTCA in the elderly from a number of different institutions (33–38,41,43,46,47). The duration of follow-up was variable, ranging from 12 months to 36 months. At late follow-up between 55 and 93% of patients were free of angina. The late myocardial infarction rate ranged from 1.4 to 8.3%.

Although PTCA improves symptoms in the majority of patients, late revascularization is often required. In previous reports rates of late revascularization ranged from 6.4 to 36.3% for repeat PTCA and 2.8 to 41.5% for CABG (Table 3). Despite this limitation, however, the long-term survival of elderly patients is

**Table 3** Late Results of PTCA in the Elderly

| | | | | Events | | | | |
|---|---|---|---|---|---|---|---|---|
| Authors | Reference | Duration of follow-up (months) | Incidence of angina (%) | MI (%) | Repeat PTCA (%) | CABG (%) | Survival (%) | % E-F survival (years) |
| Mock et al. | 34 | 12 | 74 | 8.3 | 6.4 | 41.5 | 95 | |
| Dorros et al. | 35 | 23 | 65 | 1.8 | 12.8 | 2.8 | 97 | |
| Raizner et al. | 36 | 18 | 55 | — | — | — | 98 | |
| Holt et al. | 37 | | | 2.3 | 11.6 | 4.6 | 91 | |
| Simpendorfer et al. | 38 | 28 | 77 | 1.9 | 21 | 12 | 94 | 4 (75) |
| Jeroudi et al. | 41 | 19 | 93 | 3.7 | 12.9 | 5.5 | 87 | 1 (81) |
| | | | | | | | | 3 (78) |
| Good et al. | 43 | 20 | | 1.4 | | 13 | 76 | |
| Hartzler et al. | 46 | 36 | | | | | 80 | |
| McCallister et al. | 47 | 33 | 60 | | | | 90 | 1 (79) |
| | | | | | | | 81 | 3 (66) |
| | | | | | | | 72 | 5 (54) |

MI = myocardial infarction; PTCA = percutaneous transluminal coronary angioplasty; CABG = coronary artery bypass surgery; E-F survival = event-free survival (freedom from myocardial infarction, coronary artery bypass surgery, or death).

quite favorable. In addition, the 1, 3, and 5 year event-free survival (freedom from late myocardial infarction, CABG, or death) ranged from 79 to 81%, from 66 to 78%, and from 54 to 56%, respectively.

Figure 3 summarizes the 5 year mortality rates following PTCA for various subsets of patients from our data base. The 5 year mortality rate for all patients was 15% and ranged from 6% in patients with no risk to 65% for patients in the high-risk subgroup (i.e., patients with the combined risk factors of > 70 years of age, LVEF < 40%, three-vessel coronary artery disease, and unstable angina).

Figure 4 shows the actuarial survival and event-free survival (freedom from MI, CABG, or death) of patients aged 70 years or older who have had PTCA at our institution. The 1, 3, and 5 year survival was 90, 81, and 72%, respectively. The event-free survival at 1, 3, and 5 years was 79, 66, and 54%, respectively.

In general, PTCA in the elderly resulted in sustained improvement in symptoms in the majority of patients and favorable late survival. However, the event-free survival following PTCA was adversely affected by the need for repeat revascularization procedures, either PTCA or CABG. The 1 and 5 year need for repeat revascularization rates was 30 and 47%, respectively.

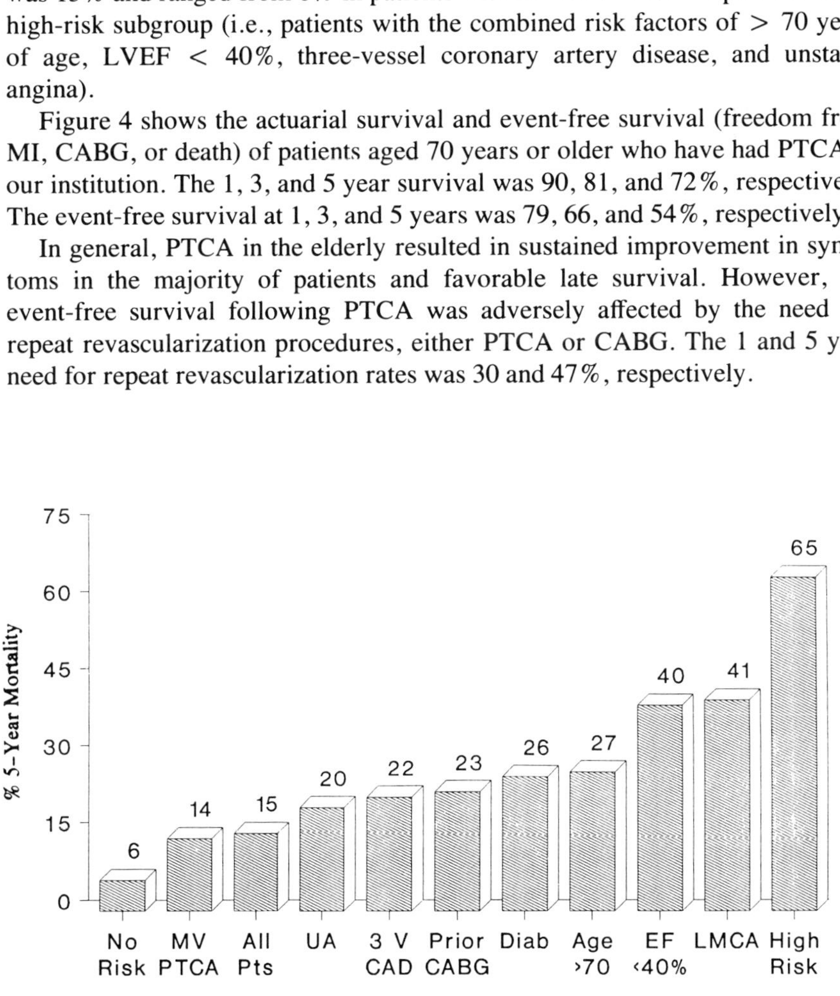


**Figure 3** PTCA, 1980–1991: 5 year mortality.
MV PTCA = multivessel PTCA; UA = unstable angina; 3 V CAD = three-vessel coronary artery disease; prior CABG = prior coronary artery bypass graft; diab = diabetes; EF = ejection fraction; LMCA = left main coronary artery.

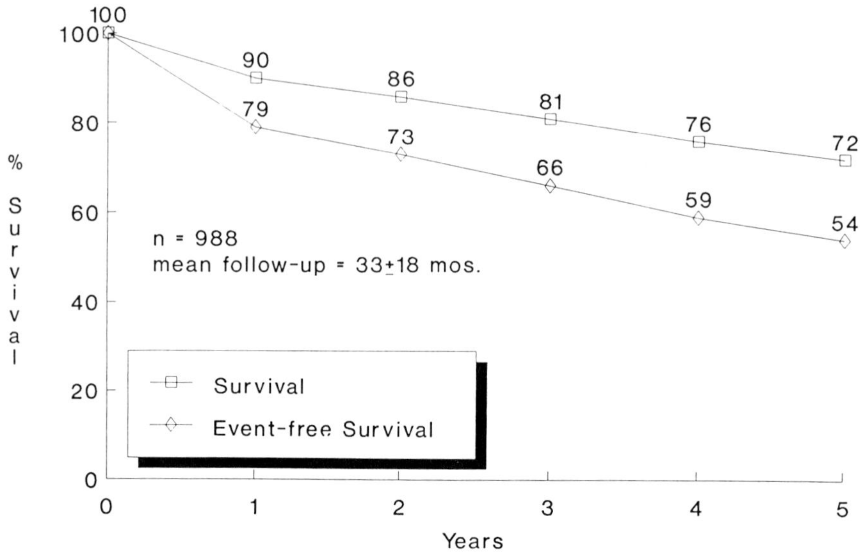


**Figure 4** Survival in the elderly following PTCA: MHI experience.

## Emergency PTCA for Acute Myocardial Infarction

During the last decade, several studies demonstrated that thrombolytic reperfusion therapy for acute myocardial infarction resulted in limitation of infarct size and a decrease in early mortality. Despite the proven benefit of this treatment, however, the use of intravenous thrombolytic therapy has been limited in the elderly patient. All the thrombolytic agents currently available have a reperfusion plateau of 70–85%. In addition, current eligibility criteria restrict this form of treatment to a minority of infarct patients. In fact, elderly patients with an acute myocardial infarction have been excluded from many large thrombolytic trials. Although these agents are capable of restoring patency of the infarcted artery, the underlying stenosis usually persists and recurrent ischemic events are common. In addition, several thrombolytic trials have demonstrated an increased incidence of stroke and hemorrhagic complications, particularly in older patients.

Three large randomized trials have demonstrated that immediate PTCA following intravenous rtPA resulted in a higher complication rate and early mortality compared to a deferred strategy (48–51). However, the Thrombolysis in Acute Myocardial Infarction (TAMI) trial showed that "salvage" PTCA for patients who failed to reperfuse with intravenous rtPA resulted in improved clinical outcomes (49,50).

We have performed direct PTCA as a primary treatment for patients with an acute myocardial infarction since 1980. This treatment strategy consists of emergent coronary angiography and PTCA of the infarct artery without antecedent thrombolytic therapy. Compared to intravenous thrombolysis, direct PTCA for acute myocardial infarction has a number of theoretical advantages. Direct PTCA for acute myocardial infarction has the potential to surpass the 70–85% reperfusion plateau associated with intravenous thrombolytic therapy; i.e., ±95% of patients will have a successful PTCA with a residual luminal narrowing < 50%. In addition, direct PTCA is possible in most patients with an acute myocardial infarction, including patients traditionally excluded from thrombolytic trials (elderly, cardiogenic shock, a history of prior bypass surgery, and recent cardiopulmonary resuscitation, CPR).

In 1989 we reported the procedural and late results from the Mid-America Heart Institute of direct PTCA in acute myocardial infarction without prior thrombolytic therapy in 500 consecutive patients (52). This experience has now been extended to over 900 patients. In our first 879 patients of all ages, the overall procedural success rate of direct PTCA for acute myocardial infarction was 94%. The procedural success rate was lower for patients with three-vessel disease (88%) and cardiogenic shock (84%). The overall in-hospital mortality rate was 7.8% and ranged from 1% for patients with single-vessel disease to 41% for patients presenting in cardiogenic shock. The early mortality rate for patients who would have been eligible for thrombolytic therapy (age < 70 years, ejection fraction > 40%, and no shock or prior bypass surgery) was 4–6% and compared favorably with results from large thrombolytic trials. Although the early mortality rate for patients in cardiogenic shock treated with direct PTCA was high (41%), this represents a considerable improvement from the traditional mortality of ±80% for this high-risk subset treated medically.

Holland et al. summarized the results from the University of Michigan of emergency infarct PTCA in 35 patients older than 70 years of age (53). Of these patients 49% also received intravenous steptokinase, tissue plasminogen activator, or combination lytic therapy. Patency of the infarct-related artery was achieved in 74% of patients, and the total in-hospital mortality was 34% (versus 6% in patients < 70 years). In-hospital mortality was much higher in patients with an occluded infarct-related artery after failed PTCA compared to patients with a patent artery (78 versus 19%). In 1990, Lee et al. reported the results of direct infarct angioplasty without prior thrombolytic therapy in 105 consecutive elderly patients from the Mid-America Heart Institute (54). The mean age of patients in this retrospective series was 74 years. Multivessel disease was present in 67% and cardiogenic shock in 11% of patients. The primary success of PTCA of the infarct-related artery was 91%. The most significant predictors of in-hospital death in this series were three-vessel disease and cardiogenic shock. PTCA resulted in significant improvement in global ejection fraction. The 1 and 5 year survival rates were 73 and 67%, respectively (54).

Recently the results of the PAMI (Primary Angioplasty in Myocardial Infarction) trial were published (66). This study was the first randomized trial comparing the results of direct PTCA without antecedent thrombolytic therapy to intravenous tissue plasminogen activator (t-PA) in patients with an acute myocardial infarction. This multicenter study enrolled 395 patients presenting within 12 h of the onset of an acute myocardial infarction and randomized patients to receive either immediate PTCA without prior thrombolytic therapy (195 patients) or t-PA (200 patients). The success rate was 97% in patients randomized to PTCA and no patient required emergency coronary artery bypass surgery. The in-hospital mortality rates in the t-PA and PTCA groups were 6.5% and 2.6%, respectively ($p = 0.06$). The corresponding mortality rates in the "not low risk" subgroups were 10.4% and 2.0%, respectively ($p = 0.01$). The not low risk category included persons older than 70 years of age, who had an anterior infarction or a heart rate of greater than 100 beats per minute on admission. Reinfarction or death in-hospital occurred in 12.0% of t-PA treated patients and 5.1% in patients treated with PTCA ($p = 0.02$). The rate of intracranial bleeding was significantly higher in patients treated with t-PA compared to PTCA (2.0% vs 0%) ($p = 0.05$). At 6 weeks, the mean left ventricular ejection fraction at rest and with exercise was similar in the two treatment groups. However, at 6 months, significant differences in the rate of reinfarction or death were observed in the two treatment groups (16.8% in t-PA treated patients compared to 8.5% in patients treated with PTCA) ($p = 0.02$). Thus, compared to t-PA, immediate PTCA for patients with an acute myocardial infarction resulted in a reduction in the combined occurrence of nonfatal reinfarction or death, a lower rate of intracranial hemorrhage, and similar left ventricular systolic function.

The PAMI trial also demonstrated an early survival advantage of PTCA compared to t-PA in women (4.0% vs 14.0%) ($p = 0.06$) and in patients 65 years of age or older (5.7% vs 15.0%) ($p = 0.066$). The incidence of stroke in patients $\geqslant$ 65 years of age was 6.7% in the t-PA group and 0% in the PTCA group ($p = .03$) (67). Finally, compared to t-PA, patients with an anterior infarction treated with direct PTCA had a reduced rate of in-hospital mortality (11.9% vs 1.4%) ($p = 0.01$) and stroke (6.0% vs 0%) ($p = 0.037$) (68).

Thus, coronary angioplasty is an effective alternative form of reperfusion for elderly patients with an acute myocardial infarction, particularly in those patients ineligible for the thrombolysis. The procedural success rate is high (89–91%), and the in-hospital mortality is comparable to that reported following thrombolytic therapy.

## OTHER ISSUES RELATED TO PTCA IN THE ELDERLY

### Complete Versus Incomplete Revascularization

Although, in general, the objective of multivessel PTCA should be complete revascularization, in selected patients incomplete revascularization may be an acceptable end point. In symptomatic patients with advanced age and complex coronary artery disease, it may be appropriate to dilate only the "culprit" lesion, that is, the most critical stenosis in a vessel supplying the largest amount of myocardium and felt to be responsible for the patients' symptoms. Although this strategy may not favorably impact survival, it often palliates symptoms and thereby improve the patient's quality of life.

### Recommended Follow-up Management Following PTCA

1. Continued aspirin therapy as an antiplatelet drug.
2. Risk factor management, including weight loss, an exercise program, cessation of smoking, and lipid control when appropriate.
3. Prompt repeat angiography and angioplasty if the patient develops significant recurrent angina.
4. If the patient does not develop angina, an exercise electrocardiographic (ECG) test is usually done at 3–4 months and thallium stress test (treadmill or adenosine) at 6 months post-PTCA.
5. If significant evidence of stenosis is evident on the scintigraphic studies, repeat PTCA may be advisable in certain cases even in the absence of recurrent angina. In general, the absence of a significant redistribution defect on a tomographic thallium study has correlated well with the absence of significant stenosis.
6. Repeat PTCA may be utilized one to three times if necessary before a decision is made to abandon further attempts at PTCA and to proceed with medical or CABG therapy.

### Restenosis

Although PTCA is a highly effective form of treatment for ischemic heart disease, restenosis remains as the major limitation. Approximately 25–30% of patients develop either clinical or angiographic evidence of restenosis within the first 4–6 months after PTCA. Restenosis is a complex process involving a number of factors, including suboptimal dilatation, elastic vessel wall recoil, residual plaque, thrombus, and, ultimately, neointimal smooth muscle cell proliferation. Clinical factors associated with higher rates of restenosis include male sex, diabetes mellitus, hypercholesterolemia, cigarette smoking, recent myocardial infarction, and unstable angina. Thus far, no single pharmacological agent has been shown consistently to prevent restenosis. Although a number of alternative interventional devices (atherectomy, laser, and stents) have achieved initial results comparable to balloon angioplasty, they have been generally disappointing in terms of their ability to limit restenosis. Elderly patients with restenosis should not be denied repeat angioplasty by virtue of age alone, because repeat angioplasty may be the most prudent therapeutic option. Selected patients at the initial procedure or with restenosis may benefit from alternative interventional technologies. To date, however, other techniques such as stents, laser, or atherectomy devices have not had a substantial impact on balloon angioplasty, except for certain "niche" indications.

## SUMMARY

Percutaneous transluminal coronary angioplasty is a highly effective form of treatment for selected patients with atherosclerotic heart disease. Selection criteria for this procedure now include many traditional high-risk subgroups, including the elderly and ultraelderly. PTCA in the elderly is associated with a high procedural success rate; however, major procedural complications (myocardial infarction, coronary artery bypass surgery, and death) are more common in the elderly than in younger patients. Procedural mortality, late survival, and event-free survival are related to preprocedural clinical variables that have a cumulative adverse effect. These same preprocedural clinical variables have been shown to affect long-term survival adversely (55). Although repeat revascularization is frequently required, the majority of patients are clinically improved by coronary angioplasty and approximately 70–80% of patients can be managed without the need for subsequent CABG. PTCA is also effective, can be performed with an acceptable risk in certain patients with multivessel disease, and can be used as an alternative to thrombolytic therapy for reperfusion in patients with an acute myocardial infarction. Studies have indicated that in-hospital mortality is comparable in patients treated with PTCA versus thrombolytic therapy, yet PTCA is associated with a minimal risk of intracranial hemorrhage, certainly a potential advantage in the elderly patient.

## COMPARATIVE STUDIES: CABG VERSUS PTCA

There are currently no published randomized studies comparing CABG to PTCA in elderly patients.

In a recent study from our institution comparing nonrandomized consecutive PTCA versus CABG in patients of all ages with multivessel disease and left ventricular dysfunction, early results favored PTCA; late follow-up, however, tended to favor CABG (56). In-hospital mortality rates were similar in the CABG (5%) and angioplasty groups (3%; *P* NS, not significant). Stroke was seen more significantly in the bypass group (7 versus 0%). During the 5 year follow-up, improved relief from angina 99 versus 89% ($P = 0.01$) and a trend toward improved survival (76 versus 67%) ($P = 0.09$) were observed in the CABG versus PTCA group, respectively. Multivariate analysis correlates of late mortality included age and incomplete revascularization, but not mode of revascularization (56).

In another study from our institution, McCallister et al. reviewed 100 consecutive patients in each of two groups having either PTCA or CABG between the years 1986 and 1987 (57). The average age was 64 versus 65 years for the PTCA and CABG groups, respectively; the incidence of postoperative cardiovascular accident (CVA) was 0 versus 3%, and in-hospital death was 2 versus 5%. The initial in-hospital and total 1 year medical costs for PTCA were 56 and 47%, respectively, less than for CABG (including patients who later required either CABG or repeat PTCA). A subsequent procedure was required in 24% of PTCA patients versus 3% of CABG patients. Although the PTCA procedural mortality was lower in this study, the 1 year survival was similar, possibly reflecting that revascularization was more complete with CABG. However, the level of patient satisfaction at the time of follow-up and the activity level were similar between the two groups (57).

Comparisons of survival in nonmatched groups of patients of all ages with follow-up to 5 years have shown no significant differences between CABG and coronary angioplasty, although many tend to favor CABG (58). One study suggested that elderly patients with three-vessel coronary disease have a considerable comparative survival benefit from coronary bypass surgery compared to coronary angioplasty (58); that some patients with two-vessel disease may derive considerable benefit from the bypass operation compared to angioplasty; and that there may be no benefit in terms of survival in patients with single-vessel disease (59). The duration of freedom from angina appears to be less after initial coronary angioplasty than after initial coronary bypass surgery. There appears to be no definite difference in the incidence of late myocardial infarction between patients treated with CABG and PTCA (57,59,60).

McCallister et al. (57), Reeder et al. (61), and Alexander et al. (62), in studies from three different institutions, confirmed that in-hospital as well as total 1 year costs are less in patients of all ages undergoing PTCA versus CABG and that the hospital stay was shorter in PTCA patients. The incidence of restenosis from PTCA (±35% per lesion dilated) must be compared with more favorable 1 year SVG and LIMA patency rates (90 and 95%, respectively) after CABG. A significant consideration is that eventually ±40% of patients undergoing PTCA require a repeat revascularization procedure versus 3–6% of CABG patients.

An early study by McCallister et al. at our institution reviewed 68 consecutive patients undergoing PTCA and 107 consecutive patients treated with CABG, both over 70 years of age (47). Patients treated with PTCA versus CABG were more symptomatic before treatment (78% versus 46% were functional class IV, respectively); however, early mortality was quite similar (4.7%) for PTCA and CABG. Patients treated with CABG appeared to be less symptomatic at follow-up (47).

In 1986, Jones et al. reported a nonrandomized comparison of CABG versus PTCA in patients greater than 65 years of age (63). The in-hospital mortality for PTCA was zero versus 2.6% for surgery and the incidence of CVA was 0 and 2.6% for PTCA and CABG, respectively (63).

McCallister and Webb at our institution reviewed the early and late results of PTCA and CABG in 100 consecutive patients over the age of 70 in both: our early and late experience with patients undergoing PTCA (1980–1983 and 1986) and CABG (1972–1979 and 1986; Table 4) (64). In the early experience with PTCA and CABG, the in-hospital mortality rate and early complication rate were higher in patients undergoing PTCA. The survival at approximately 10 years in the CABG group versus 8 years in the PTCA group was 48 and 52%, respectively, with slightly greater angina relief in the PTCA group. There were 49 subsequent revascularization procedures in the PTCA group versus 6 in the CABG group. In comparison, in the late experience, the incidence of procedural death and major complications was 12 versus 1% and 19 versus 6%, respectively, in the CABG versus PTCA groups. There were three strokes in the CABG group and none in the PTCA group. At 3 years of follow-up, more patients with PTCA had angina; 66% of CABG patients were alive versus 79% of patients who underwent PTCA. Subsequent revascularization procedures were required in 3 CABG patients versus 42 PTCA patients (64).

In a recent review from our institution, 195 consecutive patients over 70 years of age who underwent CABG in 1987–1988 were compared with a cohort of 195 consecutive PTCA patients matched for left ventricular (LV) function (24). The incidence of multivessel disease was higher in CABG patients (97%) compared with the PTCA patients (84%; $p < 0.001$); all other baseline variables were similar. Multivariate correlates of long-term survival were LV dysfunction, prior CABG, and prior myocardial infarction. In this study early morbidity and mortality were higher in patients treated with CABG versus PTCA (Table 5). Long-term survival was similar, although event-free survival (freedom from MI, CABG, death) and freedom from revascularization procedures favored CABG (24).

These comparative, although nonrandomized, studies comprising PTCA and CABG in the same single institution generally support the following conclusions: PTCA can be done at a lower cost, with a shorter hospital stay, and with an initial decrease in hospital mortality and morbidity and, in particular, a decrease in the incidence of stroke. A treatment strategy choosing PTCA results

**Table 4** Early and Late Experience with CABG and PTCA in Patients $\geqslant$ 70 Years of Age (64)

| | Date | *N* | Mean age | Procedural death | Total major complications | CVA | Duration of follow-up (years) | Late death (noncardiac) | Functional class I/II angina at follow-up (%) | Lost to follow-up | Late CABG/PTCA |
|---|---|---|---|---|---|---|---|---|---|---|---|
| Early CABG | 1972–1979 | 100 | 72.6 | 4 | 23 | 0 | 10 | 48 (13) | 85 | 12 | 3/3 |
| Early PTCA | 1980–1983 | 100 | 73.8 | 9 | 41 | 0 | 8 | 39 (11) | 77 | 0 | 22/27 |
| Late CABG | 1986 | 100 | 73.6 | 12 | 19 | 3 | 3 | 22 (8) | 89 | 0 | 0/3 |
| Late PTCA | 1986 | 100 | 74.5 | 1 | 6 | 0 | 3 | 20 (5) | 82 | 0 | 12/30 |

**Table 5** Results of CABG Versus PTCA in Patients > 70 Years of Age (24)

| | PTCA, $n = 195$ (%) | CABG, $n = 195$ (%) | $p$ Value |
|---|---|---|---|
| In-hospital death | 2 | 9 | <0.01 |
| In-hospital stroke | 0 | 5 | <0.001 |
| In-hospital infarct | 1 | 6 | <0.01 |
| Survival | | | |
| 1 Year | 84 | 86 | NS |
| 5 Years | 62 | 65 | NS |
| Event free | | | |
| 1 Year | 76 | 81 | <0.01 |
| 5 Years | 40 | 59 | <0.01 |
| Repeat PTCA or CABG | 38 | 7 | <0.001 |

in considerably more subsequent revascularization procedures. Late survival appears to favor CABG, particularly in those patients who did not receive complete revascularization at the time of the initial procedure, and CABG patients in general have a lower incidence of angina pectoris at long-term follow-up.

## CONCLUSION

CABG and PTCA are both effective in the treatment of ischemic heart disease in appropriately selected elderly patients. The decision process to advise revascularization is often difficult and reflects the increased mortality and morbidity expected with any interventional procedure with advanced age, including diagnostic cardiac catheterization (65). The challenge to the clinician caring for the older patient is to choose the appropriate therapy or combination of therapy, medical, surgical, or angioplasty, based on the available data in the literature, the experience and results at the physician's institution, and the circumstances of each individual patient.

## REFERENCES

1. Wenger NK, O'Rourke RA, Marcus FI. Care of elderly patients with cardiovascular disease. *Ann Intern Med* 1988; 109:425–428.
2. American Heart Association. Estimated cardiovascular operations and procedures by sex, age and region. Heart and Stroke Facts. 1992:17.
3. Kirklin JW, McCallister BD, et al. ACC/AHA Task Force Report. Guidelines and

indications for coronary artery bypass surgery. *J Am Coll Cardiol* 1991; 17(3):543–589.

4. Ashor GW, Meyer B, et al. Coronary artery disease: Surgery in 100 patients 65 years of age and older. *Arch Surg* 1973; 107:30–33.
5. Gersh BJ, Kronmal RA, et al. Coronary arteriography and coronary artery bypass surgery: Morbidity and mortality in patients ages 65 years or older. *Circulation* 1983; 67:483–491.
6. Gersh BJ, Kronmal RA, et al. Long-term (5 year) results of coronary bypass surgery in patients 65 years or older: A report from the coronary artery surgery study. *Circulation* 1983; 68(Suppl. II):II-190–199.
7. Rahimtoola SH, Grunkemeier GL, Starr A. Ten year survival after coronary artery bypass surgery for angina in patients aged 65 years and older. *Ther Prev Coronary Artery Surg* 1986; 74:509–517.
8. Loop FD, Lytle BW, et al. Coronary artery bypass graft surgery in the elderly—indications and outcome. *Cleve Clin J Med* 1988; 55:23–24.
9. Faro RS, Golden MD, et al. Coronary revascularization in septuagenarians. *J Thorac Cardiovasc* 1983; 86:616–620.
10. McCallister BD, Schmeidt M, et al. Coronary artery bypass in patients over the age of 70: Initial and late results (abstract). *Circulation* 1975; 52(Suppl. II):11–91.
11. Killen AD. Cardiac surgery in the elderly. In: Surgical Care for the Elderly. Baltimore: Williams & Wilkins, 1988:203–220.
12. Meyer J, Wukaysch DC, et al. Coronary artery bypass in patients over 70 years of age: Indications and results. *Am J Cardiol* 1975; 36:342–345.
13. Rose DM, Gelbfish J, et al. Analysis of morbidity and mortality in patients 70 years of age and over undergoing isolated coronary artery bypass surgery. *Am Heart J* 1985; 110:341–346.
14. Knapp WS, Douglas JS Jr, et al. Efficacy of coronary artery bypass grafting in elderly patients with coronary artery disease. *Am J Cardiol* 1981; 47:923–930.
15. Edwards FH, Taylor AJ, et al. Current status of coronary artery operation in septuagenarians. *Ann Thorac Surg* 1991; *J Cardiol* 1983; 52(2):265–269.
16. Horneffer PJ, Gardner TJ, et al. The effects of age on outcome after coronary bypass surgery. *Circulation* 1987; 76(Suppl.5):6–12.
17. Hochberg MS, Levine FH, et al. Isolated coronary artery bypass grafting in patients seventy years of age and older—early and late results. *J Thorac Cardiovasc Surg* 1982; 84:219–223.
18. Pelletier LC, Castonguay YR, et al. Open-heart surgery in elderly patients. *Can Med Assoc J* 1983; 128:409–412.
19. Dorros G, Lewin RF, et al. Coronary artery bypass surgery in patients over age 70: Report from the Milwaukee Cardiovascular Data Registry. *Clin Cardiol* 1987; 10:377–382.
20. Elayda MA, Hall RJ, et al. Coronary revascularization in the elderly patient. *J Am Coll Cardiol* 1984; 3:1398–1403.
21. Berry BE, Acree PW, et al. Coronary artery bypass operations in septuagenarians. *Ann Thorac Surg* 1981; 31:310–313.

22. Bhattacharya SK, Teskey JM, et al. Risks and benefits of open-heart surgery in patients 70 years of age and older. *Can J Surg* 1984; 27:150–152.
23. Montague NT, Kouchoukos NT, et al. Morbidity and mortality of coronary bypass grafting in patients 70 years of age and older. *Ann Thorac Surg* 1985; 39:552–557.
24. Sutton MB, O'Keefe JH, McCallister BD, Vacek JL, Piehler JM, Ligon RW, Hartzler CO. Coronary bypass versus angioplasty in the elderly. (Abstr.) J Am Coll Cardiol 1993; 21(2):72A.
25. Salomon NW, Page US, et al. Coronary artery bypass grafting in elderly patients—comparative results in a consecutive series of 469 patients older than 75 years. *J Thorac Cardiovasc Surg* 1991; 101:209–218.
26. Horvath KA, DiSesa VJ, et al. Favorable results of coronary artery bypass grafting in patients older than 75 years. *J Thorac Cardiovasc Surg* 1990; 99:92–96.
27. Rich MW, Keller AJ, et al. Morbidity and mortality of coronary bypass surgery in patients 75 years of age or older. *Ann Thorac Surg* 1988; 46:638–644.
28. Naunheim KS, Kern MJ, et al. Coronary artery bypass surgery in patients aged 80 years or older. *Am J Cardiol* 1987; 59:804–807.
29. Edmunds LH Jr, Stephenson LW, et al. Open-heart surgery in octogenarians. *N Engl J Med* 1988; 319:131–136.
30. Mullany CJ, Darling GE, et al. Early and late results after isolated coronary artery bypass surgery in 159 patients aged 80 years and older. *Circulation* 1990; 82(Suppl. IV): IV-229–236.
31. Ko W, Krieger KH, et al. Isolated coronary artery bypass grafting in one hundred consecutive octogenarian patients—a multivariate analysis. *J Thorac Cardiovasc Surg* 1991; 102:532–538.
32. Gersh BJ, Kronmal RA, et al. Comparison of coronary artery bypass surgery and medical therapy in patients 65 years of age or older. *N Engl J Med* 1985; 313:217–224.
33. Bedotto JB, Rutherford BD, McConahay DR, Johnson WL, Giorgi LV, Shimshak TM, O'Keefe Jr, Ligon RW, Hartzler GO. Results of multivessel percutaneous transluminal coronary angioplasty in persons aged 65 years and older. *Am J Cardiol* 1991; 67:1051–1055.
34. Mock MB, Holmes DR, Vliestra RE, Gersh BJ, Detre KM, Kelsey SF, Orszulak TA, Schaff HV, Piehler JM, Van Raden MUJ, Passamani ER, Kent KM, Gruetzig AR. Percutaneous transluminal coronary angioplasty (PTCA) in the elderly patient: Experience in the National Heart, Lung and Blood Institute PTCA Registry. *Am J Cardiol* 1984; 534:89C–91C.
35. Dorros G, Janke L. Percutaneous transluminal coronary angioplasty in patients over the age of 70 years. *Cathet Cardiovasc Diagn* 1986; 12:223–229.
36. Raizner AE, Hust RG, Lewis JM, Winters WL, Batty JW, Roberts R. Transluminal coronary angioplasty in the elderly. *Am J Cardiol* 1986; 57:29–32.
37. Holt GW, Sugrue DD, Bresnahan JF, Vliestra RE, Bresnahan DR, Reeder GS, Holmes DR. Results of percutaneous transluminal coronary angioplasty for unstable angina pectoris in patients 70 years of age and older. *Am J Cardiol* 1988; 61:994–997.
38. Simpfendorfer C, et al. Early and long-term results of percutaneous transluminal

coronary angioplasty in patients 70 years of age and older with angina pectoris. *Am J Cardiol* 1988; 62:959.
39. Urban P, Fox K, Crean P, Shapiro L, Rickards. Coronary balloon angioplasty for elderly patients with severe angina. *Br Heart J* 1987; 58:465–468.
40. Mills TJ, Smith HC, Vliestra RE. PTCA in the elderly: Results and expectations. *Geriatrics* 1989; 44:71–79.
41. Jeroudi MO, et al. Percutaneous transluminal coronary angioplasty in octogenarians. *Ann Intern Med* 1990; 113:423.
42. Hartzler GO, Rutherford B, McConahay DR, Johnson WL, Giorgi LV. "High-risk" percutaneous transluminal coronary angioplasty. *Am J Cardiol* 1988; 61:33G–37G.
43. Good TH, Calkins M, Ligon R, McCallister BD, Hartzler CO. PTCA in the ultra-elderly. *Circulation* 1987; 76:4.
44. Shimshak TM, Giorgi LV, Johnson WL, McConahay DR, Rutherford BD, Ligon RW, Hartzler GO. Procedural results of 10,000 PTCAs—a 10-year experience. *Circulation* 1990; 82:(Suppl. III):III–652.
45. Giorgi LV, Rutherford BD, McConahay DR, Johnson WL, Shimshak TM, Hartzler GO. Is age an independent risk factor for PTCA-related mortality? *Circulation* 1990; 82(Suppl.III):III–627.
46. Hartzler GO, Rutherford BD, McConahay DB, Johnson WL, Ligon B, Calkins MM. Late results of multiple lesion coronary angioplasty in the aged population. *J Am Coll Cardiol* 1986; 7:21A.
47. McCallister BD, Hartzler GO, Reed WA, et al. Percutaneous transluminal coronary angioplasty in elderly patients: A comparison with coronary artery bypass surgery. *J Am Coll Cardiol* 1983; 1(2):656.
48. Topol EJ, Califf RM, George BS, et al. A randomized trial of immediate versus delayed elective angioplasty after intravenous tissue plasminogen activator in acute myocardial infarction. *N Engl J Med* 1987; 317:581–588.
49. Topol EJ, Califf RM, Kereiakes DJ, et al. Thrombolysis and angioplasty in myocardial infarction (TAMI) trial. *J Am Coll Cardiol* 1987; 10:65B–74B.
50. Simons ML, Arnold AE, Betriu A, et al. Thrombolysis with tissue plasminogen activator in acute myocardial infarction: No additional benefit from immediate percutaneous transluminal coronary angioplasty. *Lancet* 1988; 1:1907–203.
51. Allan JJ, O'Keefe JH, Vacek JL, Piehler JM, McCallister BD, Hartzler GO. Relative merits of coronary bypass surgery and coronary angioplasty in multivessel disease and impaired left ventricular function (abstract). *Circulation* 1991; 84(4):II–465.
52. O'Keefe JH, Rutherford BD, Ligon RW, McConahay DR, Johnson WL, Giorgi LV, Crockett JE, McCallister BD, Conn RD, Gura GM, Good TH, Steinhaus DM, Bateman TM, Shimshak TM, Hartzler GO. Early results and long-term outcome of coronary angioplasty for acute myocardial infarction. *Am J Cardiol* 1989; 64:1221–1230.
53. Holland KH, O'Neill WW, Bates ER, Pitt B, Topol EJ. Emergency percutaneous transluminal coronary angioplasty during acute myocardial infarction for patients more than 70 years of age. *Am J Cardiol* 1989; 63:399–403.

54. Lee TC, Laramee LA, Rutherford BD, McConahay DR, Johnson WL, Giorgi LV, Ligon RW, Hartzler GO. Emergency percutaneous transluminal coronary angioplasty for acute myocardial infarction in patients 70 years of age and older. *Am J Cardiol* 1990; 66:663–667.
55. McCallister BD, Ligon RW, O'Keefe JH, Hartzler GO. Late outcome following coronary angioplasty: A multivariate and univariate analysis of the risk of patient-related clinical variables. *J Am Coll Cardiol* 1992; 19(3):23A.
56. TIMI Research Group. Immediate vs. delayed catheterization and angioplasty following thrombolytic therapy for acute myocardial infarction. *JAMA* 1988; 260:2849–2858.
57. McCallister BD, Ligon R, Stack M, Borkon M, Hartzler GO. A comparison of socioeconomics and outcome after multivessel coronary angioplasty or bypass surgery. *J Am Coll Cardiol* 1989; 13(2):230A.
58. Akins CW, Block PC, Palacios IF, et al. Comparison of coronary artery bypass grafting of percutaneous transluminal coronary angioplasty as initial treatment strategies. *Ann Thorac Surg* 1989; 47:507–516.
59. Garrahi HY, Cox DA, Cavender B, et al. Survival following coronary angioplasty in elderly patients. Comparison with bypass surgery (abstract). *Circulation* 1990; 82(Suppl. III):III–618.
60. Acinapura AJ, Cunningham JN, Jacobowitz IJ, et al. Efficacy of percutaneous transluminal coronary angioplasty compared with single vessel bypass. *J Thorac Cardiovasc Surg* 1985; 89:34–41.
61. Reeder GS, Krishan I, Nobrega FT, et al. Is percutaneous coronary angioplasty less expensive than bypass surgery? *N Engl J Med* 1984; 311:1157–1162.
62. Alexander JR, Black MB, Ruben GS, et al. Comparative costs of percutaneous transluminal coronary angioplasty and coronary artery bypass grafting and multivessel coronary artery disease. *Am J Cardiol* 1988; 62:809–811.
63. Jones EL, Abi-Mansour P, Gruntzig AR. Coronary artery bypass surgery and percutaneous transluminal coronary angioplasty in the elderly patient. *Cardiology* 1986; 73:223–234.
64. McCallister BD, Webb D. A comparison of early and late results in patients over the age of 70 having PTCA and coronary bypass surgery. Personal communication.
65. Kennedy JW, Baxley WA, Bunnell IL, et al. Mortality related to cardiac catheterization and angiography. *Cathet Cardiovasc Diagn* 1982; 8:323–340.
66. Grines CL, Browne KF, Marco J, et al. A comparison of immediate angioplasty with thrombolytic therapy for acute myocardial infarction. N Engl J Med 1993; 328:673–679.
67. Stone GW, Grines CL, Vliestra R, et al. Primary angioplasty is the preferred therapy for women and the elderly with acute myocardial infarction—results of the Primary Angioplasty in Myocardial Infarction (PAMI) trial. (Abstr.) J Am Coll Cardiol 1993; 21(2):330A.
68. Stone GW, Grines CL, Browne KF, et al. Primary angioplasty reduces in-hospital mortality and morbidity in acute anterior myocardial infarction—results of the Primary Angioplasty in Myocardial Infarction (PAMI) trial. J Am Coll Cardiol 1993; 21(2):331A.

# 14

# Aortic Valve Disease in the Elderly

**Wilbert S. Aronow**
*Mount Sinai School of Medicine, New York, New York and Hebrew Hospital Home, Bronx, New York*

**Donald D. Tresch**
*Medical College of Wisconsin and University of Wisconsin, Milwaukee, Wisconsin*

**Michele Nanna**
*Albert Einstein College of Medicine, Bronx, New York*

## INTRODUCTION

### Etiology and Prevalence

Aortic stenosis in the elderly is usually due to stiffening, scarring, and calcification of the valve leaflets. The commissures are not fused as in rheumatic aortic stenosis. Calcific deposits in the aortic valve are common in elderly perons and may lead to valvular aortic stenosis (1–4). Calcific deposits in the aortic valve were present in 22 of 40 necropsy patients (55%) aged 90–103 years (2). Calcium of the aortic valve and mitral annulus may coexist (1–3,5,6).

In a prospective study in a long-term health care facility of unselected elderly patients older than 62 years (mean age 82 ± 8 years) with technically adequate M-mode and two-dimensional echocardiograms of the aortic and mitral valves, a calcified aortic valve occurred in 28 of 119 men (24%) and in 67 of 354 women (19%) (3). Calcified or thickened aortic cusps or root occurred in 65 of 119 men (55%) and in 176 of 354 women (50%) (3). Mitral annular calcium was present in 84% of 95 patients with calcified aortic cusps, in 70% of 146 patients with thickened aortic cusps or root, and in 33% of 232 patients with normal aortic cusps and root (3). Aortic valve calcification, aortic sclerosis, and mitral annular calcium are degenerative processes (1,2,7), accounting for their high prevalence in this elderly population.

In a prospective study in a long-term health care facility of 571 unselected elderly patients older than 62 years (mean age 82 ± 8 years) with technically adequate M-mode and two-dimensional echocardiograms of the aortic valve, 292 patients (51%) had calcified or thickened aortic cusps or root (8). A serum total cholesterol $\geqslant$ 200 mg/dl, a history of systemic hypertension, diabetes mellitus, and a serum high-density lipoprotein cholesterol $<$ 35 mg/dl were more prevalent in elderly patients with calcified or thickened aortic cusps or root than in elderly patients with normal aortic cusps and root (8). These and other data suggest that aortic valve calcium, mitral annular calcium, and coronary atherosclerosis in the elderly have similar predisposing factors (8–10).

The frequency of aortic stenosis increases with age. In a prospective study in a long-term health care facility of unselected elderly patients older than 62 years (mean age 82 ± 8 years) with technically adequate M-mode and two-dimensional echocardiograms and continuous wave Doppler recordings for determining the prevalence and severity of valvular aortic stenosis, valvular aortic stenosis was diagnosed in 142 of 781 elderly patients (18%) (4). Severe aortic stenosis (peak gradient across the aortic valve $\geqslant$ 50 mm Hg) occurred in 19 of 781 elderly patients (2%). Moderate aortic stenosis (peak gradient across the aortic valve 26–49 mm Hg) was present in 49 of 781 elderly patients (6%). Mild aortic stenosis (peak gradient across the aortic valve 10–25 mm Hg) occurred in 74 of 781 elderly patients (10%).

## Symptoms

Angina pectoris, syncope, and congestive heart failure are the three classic manifestations of severe aortic stenosis. Angina pectoris is the most common symptom associated with aortic stenosis in the elderly. Coexistent coronary artery disease is frequently present in these patients. However, angina pectoris may occur in the absence of coronary artery disease as a result of an increase in myocardial oxygen demand with a reduction in myocardial oxygen supply at the subendocardial level. Ross and Braunwald (11) found that the average survival rate was 3 years after the onset of angina pectoris in patients with severe aortic stenosis.

Syncope in patients with aortic stenosis may be due to decreased cerebral perfusion following exertion, when arterial pressure drops because of systemic vasodilatation in the presence of a fixed cardiac output. Left ventricular failure with a decrease in cardiac output may also cause syncope. Syncope at rest may also be caused by transient ventricular fibrillation, transient atrial fibrillation with a marked reduction in cardiac output, or transient atrioventricular block caused by extension of the valve calcification into the conduction system. Coexistent cerebrovascular disease with transient cerebral ischemia may contribute to syncope in elderly patients with aortic stenosis. Ross and Braunwald (11) reported that the average survival rate after the onset of syncope in patients with severe aortic stenosis was 3 years.

Exertional dyspnea, paroxysmal nocturnal dyspnea, orthopnea, and pulmonary edema may be caused by pulmonary venous hypertension associated with aortic stenosis. Coexistent coronary artery disease and systemic hypertension may contribute to congestive heart failure in elderly patients with aortic stenosis. Atrial fibrillation may also precipitate congestive heart failure in these patients. Ross and Braunwald (11) found that the average survival rate after the onset of congestive heart failure in patients with severe aortic stenosis was 1.5–2 years. In our elderly population, congestive heart failure, syncope, or angina pectoris was present in 18 of 74 patients (24%) with mild aortic stenosis, in 30 of 49 patients (61%) with moderate aortic stenosis, and in 17 of 19 patients (89%) with severe aortic stenosis (4).

Sudden death occurs mainly in symptomatic aortic stenosis patients (11–13). Sudden death may also occur in 3–5% of asymptomatic patients with aortic stenosis (11,13) Marked fatigue and peripheral cyanosis in patients with aortic stenosis may be caused by a low cardiac output. Cerebral emboli causing stroke or transient cerebral ischemic attack, bacterial endocarditis, and gastrointestinal bleeding may also occur in elderly patients with aortic stenosis.

## Signs

A systolic ejection murmur heard in the second right intercostal space, down the left sternal border toward the apex, or at the apex is classified as an aortic stenosis ejection murmur (ASEM) (3,4,14,15). An ASEM is commonly heard in elderly patients (1,3,14), occurring in 265 of 565 unselected elderly patients (47%) in a long-term health care facility (3). Of 220 elderly patients with an ASEM and technically adequate M-mode and two-dimensional echocardiograms of the aortic valve, 207 (94%) had aortic cuspal or root calcification or thickening (3). Of 75 elderly patients with an ASEM, valvular aortic stenosis was diagnosed by continuous wave Doppler echocardiography in 42 patients (56%) (15).

Table 1 shows that an ASEM was heard in 100% of 19 elderly patients with severe aortic stenosis, in 100% of 49 elderly patients with moderate aortic stenosis, and in 95% of 74 elderly patients with mild aortic stenosis (4). However, the ASEM may become softer or absent in patients with congestive heart failure associated with severe aortic stenosis because of a low cardiac output. The intensity and maximal location of the ASEM and transmission of the ASEM to the right carotid artery do not differentiate among mild, moderate, and severe aortic stenosis (3,4,15). The ASEM may be heard only at the apex in some elderly patients with aortic stenosis. The apical systolic ejection murmur may also be louder and more musical than the basal systolic ejection murmur in some elderly patients with aortic stenosis. The intensity of the ASEM in aortic stenosis

**Table 1** Correlation of Physical Signs of Valvular Aortic Stenosis with the Severity of Aortic Stenosis in Elderly Patients

| | Severity of aortic stenosis (%) | | |
|---|---|---|---|
| Physical sign | Mild ($n = 74$) | Moderate ($n = 49$) | Severe ($n = 19$) |
| ASEM | 95 | 100 | 100 |
| Prolonged duration ASEM | 3 | 63 | 84 |
| Late-peaking ASEM | 3 | 63 | 84 |
| Prolonged carotid upstroke time | 3 | 33 | 53 |
| $A_2$ absent | 0 | 10 | 16 |
| $A_2$ decreased or absent | 5 | 49 | 74 |

ASEM = aortic systolic ejection murmur; $A_2$ = aortic second sound.
*Source*: Adapted from Aronow and Kronzon (4).

increases with squatting and by inhalation of amyl nitrite and decreases during the Valsalva maneuver.

Prolonged duration of the ASEM and late peaking of the ASEM best differentiate severe aortic stenosis from mild aortic stenosis (3,4,15). However, these physical signs do not distinguish between severe and moderate aortic stenosis (Table 1) (4,15).

A prolonged carotid upstroke time does not differentiate between severe and moderate aortic stenosis (4,15). A prolonged carotid upstroke time was palpable in 3% of elderly patients with mild aortic stenosis, in 33% of elderly patients with moderate aortic stenosis, and in 53% of elderly patients with severe aortic stenosis (Table 1) (4). Stiff noncompliant arteries may mask a prolonged carotid upstroke time in elderly patients with severe aortic stenosis. The pulse pressure may also be normal or wide rather than narrow in elderly patients with severe aortic stenosis because of loss of vascular elasticity. An aortic ejection click is rare in elderly patients with aortic stenosis because the valve cusps are immobile (4,15).

An absent or decreased $A_2$ occurs more frequently in elderly patients with severe or moderate aortic stenosis than in patients with mild aortic stenosis (Table 1) (4,15). However, an absent or reduced $A_2$ does not differentiate between severe and moderate aortic stenosis (4,15). The presence of atrial fibrillation, reversed splitting of $S_2$, or an audible fourth heart sound at the apex also does not differentiate between severe and moderate aortic stenosis in elderly patients (15).

Table 2 compares clinical manifestations of valvular aortic stenosis in elderly and younger patients (16). The rigid calcified valve with commissural fusion

**Table 2** Clinical Manifestations of Elderly and Younger Patients with Valvular Aortic Stenosis

| | Elderly | Younger |
|---|---|---|
| Sex | M = F | 3 M, 1 F |
| Etiology | Degenerative | Congenital, rheumatic |
| Valve deformity | Tricuspid<br>No commissural fusion | Bicuspid<br>Commissural fusion |
| Systemic blood pressure | Elevated or normal | Usually low |
| Pulse pressure | Frequently wide | Narrow |
| Carotid upstroke | Normal | Diminished, slow |
| Left ventricular hypertrophy by palpation | Uncommon | Common |
| Thrill by palpation | Uncommon | Common |
| Ejection sound | Uncommon | Common |
| $S_4$ | Common | Common |
| Systolic murmur | Musical, apical | Harsh, rough, upper sternum |
| Atrial fibrillation | 25% | Rare |
| Aortic valve calcium | Common | Variable |
| Mitral annular calcium | Common | Uncommon |

*Source*: Modified from Tresch (16).

usually found in younger patients is responsible for the ejection sound so commonly audible in younger patients with aortic stenosis. Moreover, such a valve is a suitable mechanism to produce the classic harsh, rough, grunting murmur, which is usually loudest at the right base and with radiation upward to the right carotid. In certain elderly patients, by contrast, a calcified stenotic trileaflet aortic valve without commissural fusion may produce a "spray" of the blood flow instead of a "jet" into the ascending aorta. Thus, the harsh murmur at the right base may be appreciably less intense and comparatively inconspicuous. Because of the lack of commissural fusion, an ejection sound is usually not present. Since the cusps are not fused, the murmur may be a higher frequency, musical systolic murmur that is heard all over the precordium. The murmur may be heard well at or near the cardiac apex and may be confused with mitral regurgitation.

## Pathophysiology

In valvular aortic stenosis, there is resistance to ejection of blood from the left ventricle into the aorta, with a pressure gradient across the aortic valve during systole and an increase in left ventricular systolic pressure. The pressure overload on the left ventricle leads to concentric left ventricular hypertrophy, with an increase in left ventricular wall thickness and mass, normalizing systolic wall stress, and maintenance of normal left ventricular ejection fraction and cardiac output (17,18). A compensated hyperdynamic response is common in elderly women (19).

The compensatory concentric left ventricular hypertrophy leads to abnormal left ventricular compliance, left ventricular diastolic dysfunction with reduced left ventricular diastolic filling, and increased left ventricular end-diastolic pressure, further increased by left atrial systole. Left atrial enlargement develops. Atrial systole plays an important rôle in diastolic filling of the left ventricle in patients with aortic stenosis (20). Loss of effective atrial contraction may cause immediate clinical deterioration in patients with severe aortic stenosis.

Sustained left ventricular hypertrophy eventually leads to left ventricular chamber dilatation with decreased left ventricular ejection fraction and, ultimately, congestive heart failure. The stroke volume and cardiac output decrease, the mean left atrial and pulmonary capillary pressures increase, and pulmonary hypertension develops. Elderly patients with both obstructive and nonobstructive coronary artery disease have an increased incidence of left ventricular enlargement and left ventricular systolic dysfunction (21).

## Laboratory Examination

Table 3 shows that echocardiography is more sensitive than electrocardiography in detecting left ventricular hypertrophy in elderly patients with valvular aortic stenosis (4). The heart size is usually normal on the chest x-ray in patients with aortic stenosis. Rounding of the left ventricular border and apex may occur as a result of concentric left ventricular hypertrophy. Poststenotic dilatation of the ascending aorta is commonly seen. Calcification of the aortic valve is best seen by echocardiography or fluoroscopy.

Involvement of the conduction system by calcific deposits may occur in patients with aortic stenosis. Of 51 elderly patients with aortic stenosis who underwent aortic valve replacement, conduction defects occurred in 58% of 31 patients with mitral annular calcium and in 25% of 20 patients without mitral annular calcium (6). Of 77 elderly patients with aortic stenosis, first-degree atrioventricular block occurred in 18% of patients, left bundle branch block in 10% of patients, intraventricular conduction defect in 6% of patients, right bundle branch block in 4% of patients, and left axis deviation in 17% of patients (22).

Complex ventricular arrhythmias may be detected by 24 h ambulatory electrocardiography in patients with aortic stenosis. Elderly patients with complex ventricular arrhythmias associated with valvular aortic stenosis have a higher incidence of new coronary events than elderly patients with aortic stenosis and no complex ventricular arrhythmias (23).

**Table 3** Prevalence of Electrocardiographic and Echocardiographic Left Ventricular Hypertrophy (LVH) in Elderly Patients with Mild, Moderate, and Severe Valvular Aortic Stenosis

| | Severity of aortic stenosis (%) | | |
|---|---|---|---|
| | Mild ($n = 74$) | Moderate ($n = 49$) | Severe ($n = 19$) |
| Electrocardiographic LVH | 11 | 31 | 58 |
| Echocardiographic LVH | 74 | 96 | 100 |

*Source*: Adapted from Aronow and Kronzon (4).

## Echocardiography and Doppler Echocardiography

M-mode and two-dimensional echocardiography and Doppler echocardiography are very useful in the diagnosis of aortic stenosis. Echocardiography can detect thickening, calcification, and decreased excursion of aortic valve leaflets (3). Left ventricular hypertrophy is best diagnosed by echocardiography (4). Chamber dimensions and measurements of left ventricular end-systolic and end-diastolic volumes, left ventricular ejection fraction, and assessment of global and regional left ventricular wall motion give important information on left ventricular systolic function.

Doppler echocardiography is used to measure peak and mean transvalvular gradients across the aortic valve and to identify associated valve lesions. Aortic valve area can be calculated by the continuity equation using pulsed Doppler echocardiography to measure left ventricular outflow tract velocity, continuous wave Doppler echocardiography to measure transvalvular flow velocity, and two-dimensional long-axis view to measure left ventricular outflow tract area (24,25). Aortic valve area can be detected reliably by the continuity equation in elderly persons with valvular aortic stenosis (25). Figures 1 through 5 illustrate two-dimensional echocardiographic findings (Figs. 1 and 3), continuous wave Doppler echocardiographic findings (Figs. 2 and 4), and simultaneous left ventricular and femoral arterial pressure tracings (Fig. 5) in elderly patients with severe valvular aortic stenosis.

Shah and Graham (26) found that the agreement in quantitation of the severity of aortic stenosis between Doppler echocardiography and cardiac catheterization was greater than 95%. Patients with a peak jet velocity $\geqslant$ 4.5 m/s had critical aortic stenosis, and those with a peak jet velocity $<$ 3.0 m/s had noncritical aortic stenosis. Slater et al. (27) demonstrated a concordance between

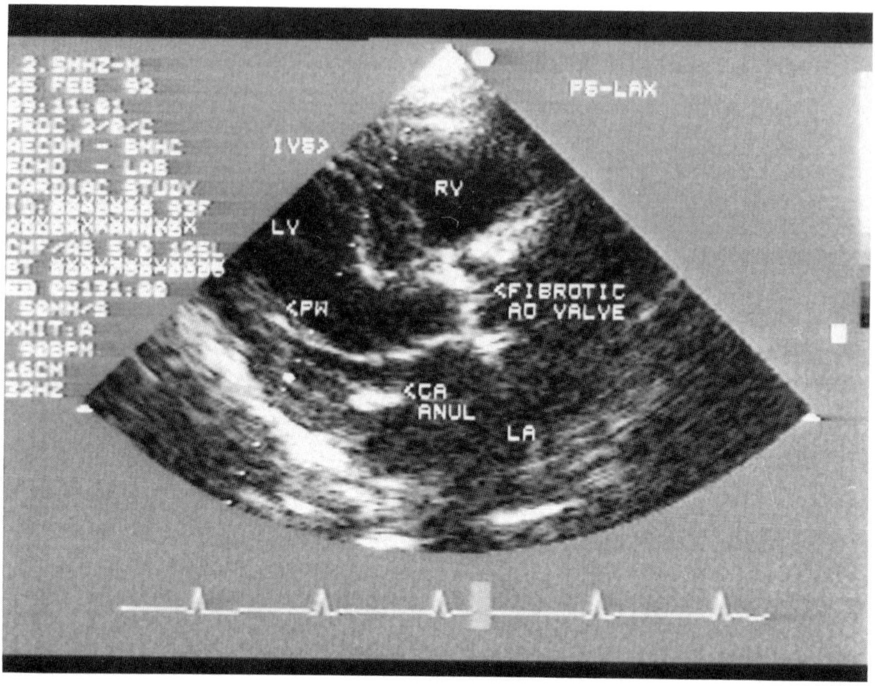


**Figure 1** Two-dimensional echocardiographic image from a parasternal long-axis view of a 93-year-old female with aortic stenosis and moderately depressed left ventricular function showing a fibrotic aortic valve and mitral anular calcification. PS-LAX = parasternal long-axis view; RV = right ventricular cavity; LV = left ventricular cavity; IVS = interventricular septum; PW = posterior wall; CA Annul = mitral annulus calcification; LA = left atrium; AO = aorta.

Doppler echocardiography and cardiac catheterization in the decision to operate or not to operate in 61 of 73 patients (84%) with valvular aortic stenosis.

Cardiac catheterization was performed in 105 patients in whom Doppler echocardiography demonstrated an aortic valve area $\leqslant 0.75$ cm$^2$ or a peak jet velocity $\geqslant 4.5$ m/s, consistent with critical aortic stenosis (28). Doppler echocardiography was 97% accurate in this subgroup. Cardiac catheterization was performed in this study in 133 patients with noncritical aortic stenosis. Doppler echocardiography was 95% accurate in this subgroup. Although most elderly persons do not require cardiac catheterization before aortic valve surgery, they require selective coronary arteriography before aortic valve surgery. Patients in whom Doppler echocardiography shows a peak jet velocity between 3.6 and 4.4 m/s and an aortic valve area $> 0.8$ cm$^2$ should undergo cardiac catheterization

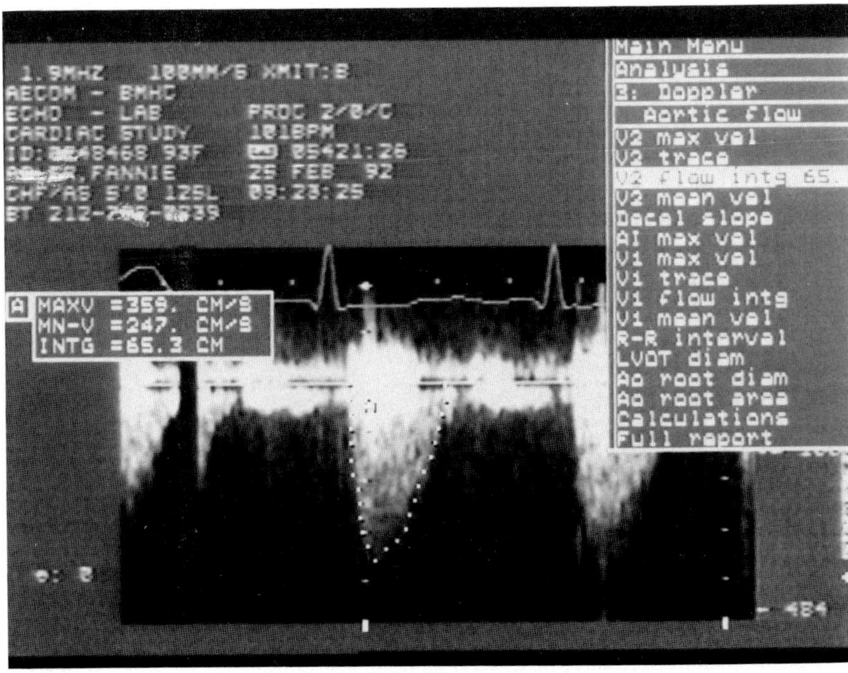


**Figure 2** Continuous wave Doppler recording of the velocity profile across the aortic valve in the same patient shown in Figure 1. A 52 mm Hg gradient across the aortic valve is measured using the Bernoulli equation. Indexed aortic valve area measured by the continuity equation using Doppler data = 0.5 $cm^2/m^2$.

if they have cardiac symptoms attributable to aortic stenosis (26). Patients with a peak jet velocity between 3.0 and 3.5 m/s and a left ventricular ejection fraction < 50% may have severe aortic stenosis, requiring aortic valve replacement, and should undergo cardiac catheterization (26). Patients with a peak jet velocity between 3.0 and 3.5 m/s and a left ventricular ejection fraction > 50% probably do not need aortic valve replacement but should undergo cardiac catheterization if they have symptoms of severe aortic stenosis (26).

## Natural History

Patients with symptomatic severe valvular aortic stenosis have a poor prognosis (11–13,29). At the National Institutes of Health, 52% of patients with symptomatic severe valvular aortic stenosis not operated on were dead at 5 years (12,13). At 10 years follow-up, 90% of these patients were dead.

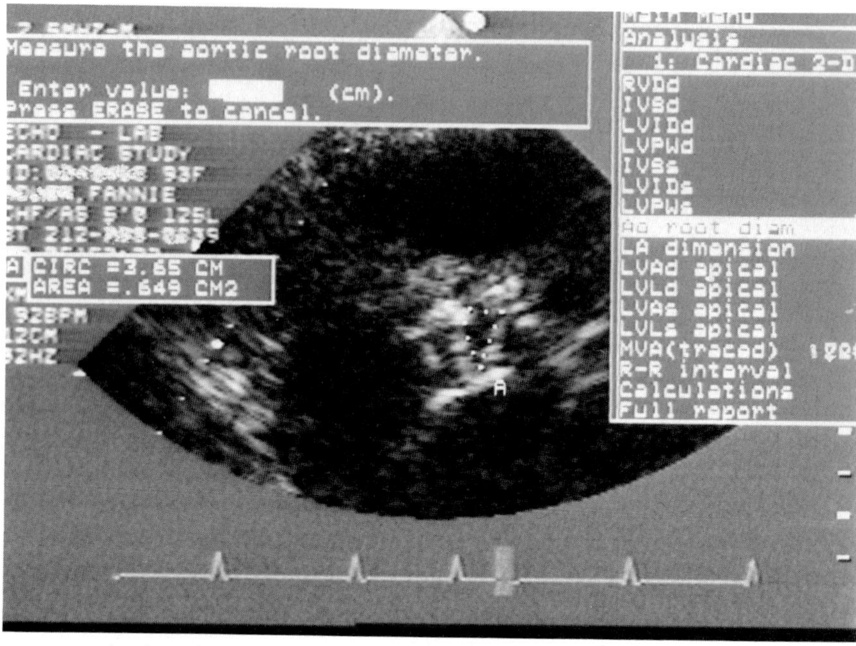


**Figure 3** Two-dimensional echocardiographic image obtained in the same patient in Figures 1 and 2 from a short-axis parasternal view in which the aortic valve orifice is mapped, yielding an indexed area of 0.4 $cm^2/m^2$.

Kennedy et al. (30) followed 66 patients with moderate valvular aortic stenosis diagnosed by cardiac catheterization (aortic valve area 0.7–1.2 $cm^2$). In 38 patients with symptomatic moderate valvular aortic stenosis and 28 patients with minimally symptomatic moderate valvular aortic stenosis, the probabilities of avoiding death from aortic stenosis were 0.86 for patients with symptomatic aortic stenosis and 1.0 for patients with minimally symptomatic aortic stenosis at 1 year follow-up, 0.77 for patients with symptomatic aortic stenosis and 1.0 for patients with minimally symptomatic aortic stenosis at 2 years, 0.77 for patients with symptomatic aortic stenosis and 0.96 for patients with minimally symptomatic aortic stenosis at 3 years, and 0.70 for patients with symptomatic aortic stenosis and 0.90 for patients with minimally symptomatic aortic stenosis at 4 years (30). During 35 months mean follow-up in this study, 21 patients underwent aortic valve replacement.

Three studies have demonstrated that patients with asymptomatic severe valvular aortic stenosis are at low risk for death and can be followed until symptoms develop (31–33). Turina et al. (31) followed 17 patients with asymptomatic

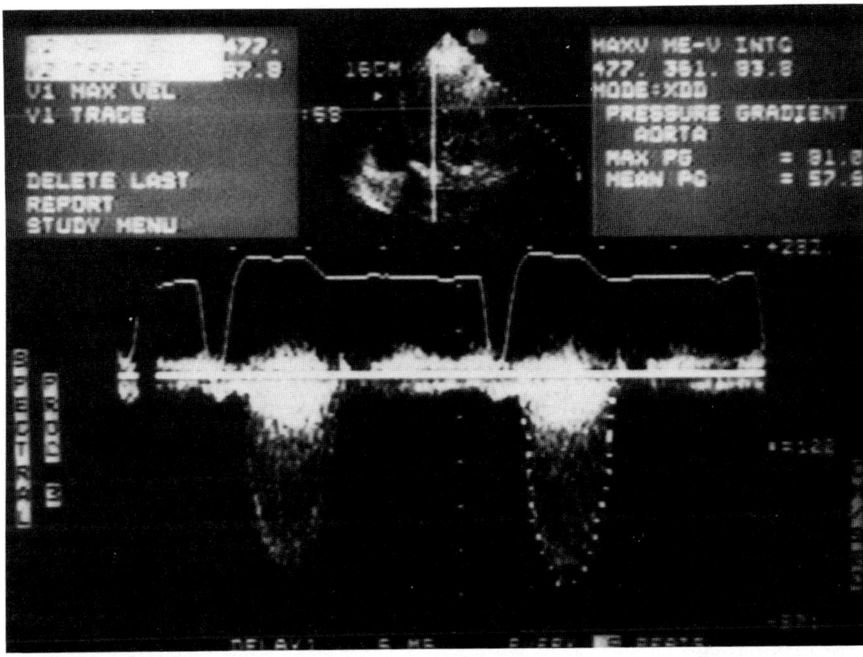


**Figure 4** Continuous wave Doppler recording of the velocity profile across the aortic valve in an elderly patient with aortic stenosis and normal left ventricular systolic function. The indexed aortic valve area is 0.5 $cm^2/m^2$ by both Gorlin's formula and the Doppler continuity equation. The peak gradient across the aortic valve by Bernouilli's equation is 81 mm Hg, a value higher than that recorded in Figure 2 for the same indexed aortic valve area.

or mildly symptomatic aortic stenosis. During the first 2 years, none died or had aortic valve surgery. At 5 years follow-up, 94% were alive and 75% were free of cardiac events. Kelly et al. (32) followed 51 asymptomatic patients with severe valvular aortic stenosis. During 17 months mean follow-up, 21 (41%) of the patients became symptomatic. Only 2 of the 51 patients (4%) died of cardiac causes. In both patients, death was preceded by the development of angina pectoris or congestive heart failure. Pellikka et al. (33) observed that 113 of 143 patients (79%), mean age 72 years, with asymptomatic severe aortic stenosis were not initially referred for aortic valve replacement or percutaneous aortic balloon valvuloplasty. During 20 months mean follow-up, 37 of 113 patients (33%) became symptomatic. The actuarial probability of remaining free of cardiac events associated with aortic stenosis, including cardiac death and aortic valve surgery, was 95% at 6 months, 93% at 1 year, and 74% at 2 years. No

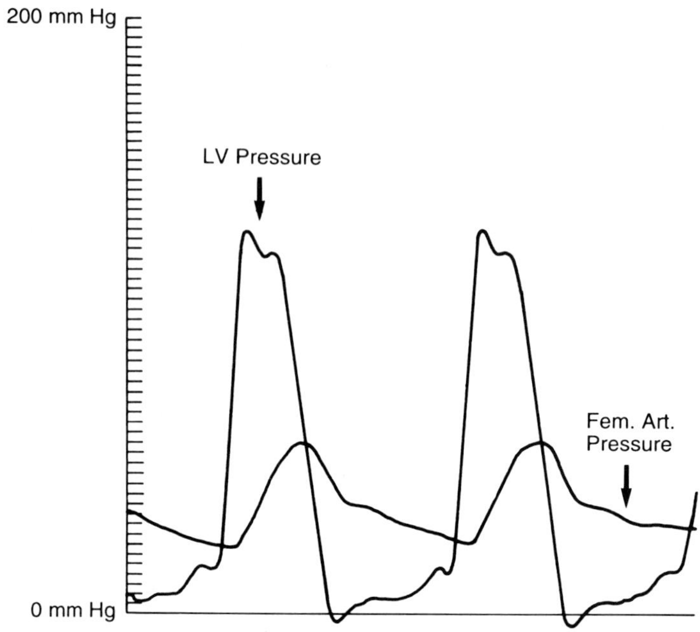


**Figure 5** Simultaneous left ventricular and femoral artery pressure recordings obtained in the same patient in Figure 4 confirming a large gradient across the aortic valve with a maximum value of 81 mm Hg (instantaneous pressure). Fem. Art. = femoral artery pressure tracing; LV = left ventricular pressure tracing.

asymptomatic patient with severe aortic stenosis developed sudden cardiac death while asymptomatic.

Hammermeister et al. (34) followed 106 patients with unoperated valvular aortic stenosis in the Veterans Administration Cooperative Study on Valvular Heart Disease for a mean duration of 5 years. During follow-up, 60 of 106 patients (57%) died. Multivariate analysis demonstrated that measures of the severity of the valvular aortic stenosis, the presence of coronary artery disease, and the presence of congestive heart failure were the important predictors of survival in unoperated patients.

## Medical Management

Prophylactic antibiotics should be used to prevent bacterial endocarditis in patients with valvular aortic stenosis, according to American Heart Association guidelines (35). Patients with congestive heart failure, exertional syncope, or angina pectoris associated with moderate or severe valvular aortic stenosis should undergo aortic valve replacement promptly. Patients with asymptomatic aortic stenosis should report the development of symptoms possibly related to aortic stenosis immediately to the physician. If significant valvular aortic stenosis is present in asymptomatic elderly patients, clinical examination and an electrocardiogram and Doppler echocardiogram should be performed at 6 month intervals. Nitrates should be used with caution in patients with angina pectoris and aortic stenosis to prevent the occurrence of orthostatic hypotension and syncope. In patients with congestive heart failure due to aortic stenosis, medical therapy does not relieve the mechanical obstruction to left ventricular outflow. Diuretics should be used with caution to prevent a decrease in cardiac output and hypotension. Vasodilators should be avoided. We observed that 30 of 48 elderly patients (63%) with congestive heart failure associated with aortic stenosis had a normal left ventricular ejection fraction. Digitalis should not be used in these patients unless needed to control a rapid ventricular rate associated with atrial fibrillation.

## Balloon Aortic Valvuloplasty

Aortic valve replacement is the procedure of choice for symptomatic elderly patients with severe valvular aortic stenosis. In a Mayo Clinic study, the actuarial survival of 50 elderly patients, mean age 77 years, with symptomatic severe aortic stenosis in whom aortic valve replacement was refused (45 patients) or deferred (5 patients) was 57% at 1 year, 37% at 2 years, and 25% at 3 years (36). Because of the poor survival in this group of patients, balloon aortic valvuloplasty should be considered when operative intervention is refused or deferred.

Balloon aortic valvuloplasty is effective palliative therapy for some elderly patients with symptomatic valvular aortic stenosis (37–45). Rodriguez et al. (43) demonstrated in 42 elderly patients, mean age 78 years, undergoing aortic valvuloplasty that the 2 year survival was 36% in patients with left ventricular ejection fraction $< 40\%$ and 80% in patients with left ventricular ejection fraction $\geqslant 40\%$. The 2 year event-free survival (freedom from aortic valve surgery or severe congestive heart failure) was 0% in patients with left ventricular ejection fraction $< 40\%$ and 34% in patients with left ventricular ejection fraction $\geqslant 40\%$ (43). Block and Palacios (38) observed recurrence of symptoms, death, or hemodynamic evidence of restenosis in 56% of 90 elderly patients, mean age 79 years, an average of 5.5 months after aortic valvuloplasty. Kuntz et al. (44) observed immediate clinical improvement after successful aortic valvuloplasty in the majority of 205 elderly patients, mean age 78 years, but restenosis in more than 50% of the patients within 1–2 years. On the basis of the available data, balloon aortic valvuloplasty should be considered for elderly patients with symptomatic severe valvular aortic stenosis who are not candidates for aortic valve surgery and possibly for patients with severe left ventricular dysfunction as a bridge to subsequent aortic valve surgery (44,45).

## Aortic Valve Replacement

Aortic valve replacement is the procedure of choice for symptomatic elderly patients with severe aortic stenosis. The bioprosthesis has less structural failure in elderly patients than in younger patients and is preferable to the mechanical prosthetic valve for aortic valve replacement in the elderly (46). Patients with mechanical prostheses need anticoagulant therapy indefinitely. Patients with porcine bioprostheses require anticoagulant therapy for 3 months after hospital discharge and then may be treated with antiplatelet therapy alone (47).

Arom et al. (48) performed aortic valve replacement in 273 patients aged 70–89 years (mean age 75 years), 162 with aortic valve replacement alone, and 111 with aortic valve replacement plus coronary artery bypass. Operative mortality was 5%. Late mortality at 33 months mean follow-up was 18%. Actuarial analysis showed at 5 years follow-up that overall survival was 66% for patients with aortic valve replacement alone, 76% for patients with aortic valve replacement plus coronary artery bypass, and 74% for a similar age group in the general population.

Culliford et al. (47) performed aortic valve replacement in 71 patients aged ⩾ 80 years, 35 with aortic valve replacement alone and 36 with aortic valve replacement plus coronary artery bypass. Hospital mortality was 6% for patients with aortic valve replacement alone and 19% for patients with both aortic valve replacement plus coronary artery bypass. At 1 year follow-up, survival from late cardiac death was 100% for patients who had aortic valve replacement alone and 96% for patients who had aortic valve replacement plus coronary artery bypass. At 3 years follow-up, survival from late cardiac death was 100% for patients who had aortic valve replacement alone and 91% for patients who had aortic valve replacement plus coronary artery bypass. Freedom from all valve-related complications (thromboembolism, anticoagulant-related complications, endocarditis, and reoperation or prosthetic failure) was 93% at 1 year follow-up and 80% at 3 years follow-up. At follow-up, 65% of survivors were in New York Heart Association functional class I or II, 31% in New York Association functional class III, and 4% in New York Heart Association functional class IIII.

Levinson et al. (49) performed aortic valve replacement in 71 octogenarians, mean age 82 years. The operative mortality was 9% in these elderly patients. At 28 months mean follow-up, 100% of the survivors were in New York Heart Association functional class I or II. Actuarial 1, 5, and 10 year survival rates were 83, 67, and 49%, respectively.

Aortic valve replacement is associated with a reduction in left ventricular mass and in improvement of left ventricular diastolic filling (50). Hoffmann and Burckhardt (51) performed a prospective study in 100 patients who had aortic valve replacement. At 41 months mean follow-up, the yearly cardiac mortality rate was 8% in patients with electrocardiographic left ventricular hypertrophy and repetitive ventricular premature complexes ≥ two couplets per 24 h during 24 h ambulatory electrocardiographic monitoring and 0.6% in patients without either of these findings.

## AORTIC REGURGITATION

### Etiology and Prevalence

Acute aortic regurgitation in the elderly may be due to infective endocarditis, rheumatic fever, aortic dissection, trauma, following prosthetic valve surgery, or rupture of the sinus of Valsalva and causes sudden severe left ventricular failure. Chronic aortic regurgitation in the elderly may be caused by valve leaflet disease (secondary to any cause of aortic stenosis, infective endocarditis, rheumatic fever, congenital heart disease, rheumatoid arthritis, ankylosing spondylitis, following prosthetic valve surgery, or myxomatous degeneration of the valve) or by aortic root disease. Examples of aortic root disease causing chronic aortic regurgitation in the elderly include association with systemic hypertension, syphilitic aortitis, cystic medial necrosis of the aorta, ankylosing spondylitis, rheumatoid arthritis, Reiter's disease, systemic lupus erythematosus, Ehlers-Danlos syndrome, and pseudoxanthoma elasticum. Mild or moderate aortic regurgitation was also diagnosed by Doppler echocardiography in 9 of 29 patients (31%) with hypertrophic cardiomyopathy (52). Margonato et al. (53) linked the increased prevalence of aortic regurgitation with age to aortic valve thickening.

The prevalence of aortic regurgitation increases with age (53–55). In a prospective study in a long-term health care facility of 450 unselected elderly patients older than 62 years (range 82 ± 8 years) with technically adequate M-mode and two-dimensional echocardiograms and pulsed Doppler recordings of the aortic valve, aortic regurgitation was diagnosed in 39 of 114 men (34%) and in 92 of 336 women (27%) (55). Severe or moderate aortic regurgitation was diagnosed in 74 of 450 patients (16%). Mild aortic regurgitation was diagnosed in 57 of 450 patients (13%).

### Symptoms

Patients with acute aortic regurgitation develop symptoms due to the sudden onset of congestive heart failure, with marked dyspnea and weakness. Patients with chronic aortic regurgitation may remain asymptomatic for many years. Mild dyspnea on exertion and palpitations, especially on lying down, may occur. Exertional dyspnea, orthopnea, paroxysmal noctural dyspnea, fatigue, and edema are common clinical symptoms when left ventricular failure develops. Syncope is rare. Angina pectoris occurs less often in patients with aortic regurgitation than in patients with aortic stenosis and may be due to coexistent coronary artery disease. However, nocturnal angina pectoris, often accompanied by flushing, diaphoresis, and palpitations, may occur when the heart rate slows and the arterial diastolic pressure falls to very low levels. Most patients with severe aortic regurgitation who do not have surgery die within 2 years after congestive heart failure develops (56).

## Signs

The aortic regurgitation murmur is typically a high-pitched blowing diastolic murmur that begins immediately after $A_2$. The diastolic murmur is best heard along the left sternal border in the third and fourth intercostal spaces when aortic regurgitation is due to valvular disease. The murmur is best heard along the right sternal border when aortic regurgitation is due to dilatation of the ascending aorta. The diastolic murmur is best heard with the diaphragm of the stethoscope with the patient sitting up, leaning forward, and holding the breath in deep expiration. The severity of aortic regurgitation correlates with the duration of the diastolic murmur, not with the intensity of the murmur.

Grayburn et al. (57) heard an aortic regurgitation murmur in 73% of 82 patients with aortic regurgitation and in 8% of 24 patients without aortic regurgitation. Saal et al. (58) heard an aortic regurgitation murmur in 80% of 35 patients with aortic regurgitation and in 10% of 10 patients without aortic regurgitation. Meyers et al. (59) heard an aortic regurgitation murmur in 73% of 66 patients with aortic regurgitation and in 22% of 9 patients without aortic regurgitation. Table 4 shows that an aortic regurgitation murmur was heard in 95% of 74 elderly patients with severe or moderate aortic regurgitation diagnosed by pulsed Doppler echocardiography, in 61% of 57 elderly patients with mild aortic regurgitation, and in 3% of 319 elderly patients with no aortic regurgitation (55).

In patients with chronic severe aortic regurgitation, the left ventricular apical impulse is diffuse, hyperdynamic, and displaced laterally and inferiorly. A rumbling diastolic murmur (Austin Flint) may be heard at the apex, with its intensity reduced by inhalation of amyl nitrite. A short basal systolic ejection murmur is heard. A palpable left ventricular rapid filling wave and an audible $S_3$ at the apex are usually found. Physical findings due to a large left ventricular stroke volume and a rapid diastolic runoff in patients with severe aortic regurgitation include a wide pulse pressure with an increased systolic arterial pressure and an

**Table 4** Correlation of Aortic Regurgitation Murmur with Severity of Aortic Regurgitation (AR) in Elderly Patients with Chronic Aortic Regurgitation

| | AR murmur (%) |
|---|---|
| Severe or moderate AR (74) | 95 |
| Mild AR (57) | 61 |
| No AR (319) | 3 |

*Source*: Adapted from Aronow and Kronzon (55).

abnormally low diastolic arterial pressure, an arterial pulse that abruptly rises and collapses, a bisferiens pulse, bobbing of the head with each heart beat, booming systolic and diastolic sounds heard over the femoral artery, capillary pulsations, and systolic and diastolic murmurs over the femoral artery when compressing it proximally and distally.

## Pathophysiology

Chronic aortic regurgitation increases left ventricular end-diastolic volume. The largest left ventricular end-diastolic volumes are seen in patients with chronic severe aortic regurgitation. Left ventricular stroke volume increases to maintain the forward stroke volume. The increased preload causes an increase in left ventricular diastolic stress and the addition of sarcomeres in series. This results in an increase in the ratio of the left ventricular chamber size to wall thickness. This pattern of left ventricular hypertrophy is called eccentric left ventricular hypertrophy.

Primary myocardial abnormalities or ischemia due to coexistent coronary artery disease depress the contractile state. Left ventricular diastolic compliance decreases, left ventricular end-systolic volume increases, left ventricular end-diastolic pressure rises, left atrial pressure increases, and pulmonary venous hypertension results. When the left ventricular end-diastolic radius to wall thickness ratio rises, left ventricular systolic wall stress increases abnormally because of the preload and afterload mismatch (18,60). Additional stress then reduces the left ventricular ejection fraction response to exercise (61). Eventually, the left ventricular ejection fraction, forward stroke volume, and effective cardiac output are reduced at rest. We observed that an abnormal resting left ventricular ejection fraction occurred in 8 of 25 elderly patients (32%) with congestive heart failure associated with chronic severe aortic regurgitation.

In patients with acute severe aortic regurgitation, the left ventricle cannot adapt to the increased volume overload. Forward stroke volume falls, left ventricular end-diastolic pressure increases rapidly to high levels (62), and pulmonary hypertension and pulmonary edema result. The rapid rise of the left ventricular end-diastolic pressure to exceed the left atrial pressure in early diastole causes premature closure of the mitral valve (63). This prevents backward transmission of the elevated left ventricular end-diastolic pressure to the pulmonary venous bed.

## Laboratory Examination

The electrocardiogram may initially be normal in patients with acute severe aortic regurgitation. Roberts and Day (64) showed in 30 necropsy patients with chronic severe aortic regurgitation that the electrocardiogram did not accurately predict the severity of aortic regurgitation or cardiac weight. Using various electrocardiographic criteria, the prevalence of left ventricular hypertrophy varied from 30% ($RV_6 > RV_5$) to 90% (total 12-lead QRS voltage > 175 mm). The P-R interval was prolonged in 28% of patients, and the QRS duration was $\geqslant 0.12$ s in 20% of patients (64).

The chest x-ray in patients with acute severe aortic regurgitation may show a normal heart size and pulmonary edema. The chest x-ray in patients with chronic severe aortic regurgitation usually shows a dilated left ventricle, with elongation of the apex inferiorly and posteriorly and a dilated aorta. Aneurysmal dilatation of the aorta suggests that aortic root disease is causing the aortic regurgitation. Linear calcifications in the wall of the ascending aorta are observed in syphilitic aortic regurgitation and in degenerative disease.

## Echocardiography and Doppler Echocardiography

M-mode and two-dimensional echocardiography and Doppler echocardiography are very useful in the diagnosis of aortic regurgitation. Two-dimensional echocardiography can provide information establishing the etiology of the aortic regurgitation and measurements of left ventricular function. Eccentric left ventricular hypertrophy is diagnosed by echocardiography if the left ventricular mass index is increased with a relative wall thickness < 0.45 (65–67). Echocardiographic measurements reported to predict an unfavorable response to aortic valve replacement in patients with chronic aortic regurgitation include a left ventricular end-systolic dimension > 55 mm (68), a left ventricular shortening fraction < 25% (68), a left ventricular diastolic radius to wall thickness ratio > 3.8 (69), a left ventricular end-diastolic dimension index > 38 $mm/m^2$ (69), and a left ventricular end-systolic dimension index > 26 $mm/m^2$ (69).

Grayburn et al. (57) showed that pulsed Doppler echocardiography correctly identified the presence of aortic regurgitation in 57 of 57 patients (100%) with $\geqslant 2^+$ aortic regurgitation and in 22 of 25 patients (88%) with $1^+$ aortic regurgitation. Saal et al. (58) demonstrated that pulsed Doppler echocardiography identified the presence of aortic regurgitation in 34 of 35 patients (97%) with documented aortic regurgitation. Continuous wave Doppler echocardiography has also been shown to be very useful in diagnosing and quantitating aortic regurgitation (70,71). Aortic regurgitation is best assessed by color flow Doppler imaging (72). Figure 6 illustrates two-dimensional echocardiographic and color Doppler findings in an elderly patient with chronic severe aortic regurgitation. Figure 7 illustrates continuous wave Doppler findings in the elderly patient with chronic severe aortic regurgitation shown in Figure 6.

## Natural History

Patients with acute aortic regurgitation should have immediate aortic valve replacement because death may occur within hours to days. Of patients with hemodynamically significant chronic aortic regurgitation treated medically, 75% are alive at 5 years after diagnosis (29). Of patients with moderate to severe chronic aortic regurgitation, 50% are alive at 10 years after diagnosis (29,73). The 10 year survival rate for patients with mild to moderate chronic aortic regurgitation is 85–95% (29,74).

Of 14 patients with chronic severe aortic regurgitation who did not have surgery, 13 (93%) died within 2 years of developing congestive heart failure (56). The mean survival time after the onset of angina pectoris is 5 years (73).

During 8 years mean follow-up of 104 asymptomatic patients with chronic severe aortic regurgitation and normal left ventricular ejection fraction, 2 patients (2%) died suddenly, and 23 patients (22%) had aortic valve replacement (75). Of the 104 patients, 19 (18%) had aortic valve replacement because of cardiac symptoms and 4 patients (4%) had aortic valve replacement because of the development of left ventricular systolic dysfunction in the absence of cardiac symptoms. Multivariate analysis showed that age, initial end-systolic dimension, and rate of change in end-systolic dimension and resting left ventricular ejection fraction during serial studies predicted the outcome.

## Medical and Surgical Management

Asymptomatic patients with mild or moderate aortic regurgitation do not require therapy. However, prophylactic antibiotics should be used to prevent bacterial endocarditis in patients with aortic regurgitation, according to American Heart Association guidelines (35). Echocardiographic evaluation of left ventricular end-systolic dimension should be performed yearly if the measurement is less than 50 mm but every 3–6 months if the left ventricular end-systolic dimension is 50–54 mm. Aortic valve replacement should be considered when the left ventricular end-systolic dimension exceeds 55 mm, even in the absence of cardiac symptoms (68).

Patients with asymptomatic chronic severe aortic regurgitation should be treated with hydralazine (76) or nifedipine (77) therapy to reduce the left ventricular volume overload. Infections should be treated promptly. Systemic hypertension increases the regurgitant flow and should be treated. Drugs that depress left ventricular function, such as $\beta$-adrenergic blockers, should not be used. Arrhythmias should be treated. Patients with aortic regurgitation due to syphilitic aortitis should receive a course of penicillin therapy. Prophylactic resection should be considered in patients with Marfan's syndrome when the aortic root diameter exceeds 55 mm (78).

Bacterial endocarditis should be treated with intravenous antibiotics. Indications for aortic valve replacement in patients with aortic regurgitation due to bacterial endocarditis are congestive heart failure, uncontrolled infection, myocardial or valvular ring abscess, prosthetic valve dysfunction or dehiscence, and multiple embolic episodes (79–81).

Congestive heart failure should be treated with sodium restriction, diuretics, digitalis, vasodilator therapy, and aortic valve replacement. Angina pectoris should be treated with nitrates.

Patients with acute severe aortic regurgitation should undergo valve replacement immediately. Patients with chronic severe aortic regurgitation should have aortic valve replacement if they develop symptoms of congestive heart failure, such as paroxysmal nocturnal dyspnea, orthopnea, or dyspnea at rest; angina pectoris; syncope; or exertional dyspnea severe enough to interfere with the quality of life (75). Aortic valve replacement should also be performed in asymptomatic patients with chronic severe aortic regurgitation if they develop left ventricular systolic dysfunction (75).

Patients undergoing aortic valve replacement for severe aortic regurgitation have an excellent postoperative survival if the preoperative left ventricular ejection fraction is normal (82,83). If left ventricular systolic dysfunction was present for less than 1 year, patients also did well postoperatively. However, if the patient with severe aortic regurgitation has an abnormal left ventricular ejection fraction and impaired exercise tolerance and/or prolonged left ventricular systolic dysfunction, the postoperative survival is poor (82,83).

The operative mortality for aortic valve replacement in patients with severe aortic regurgitation is similar to that in patients with aortic valve replacement for aortic stenosis. The mortality rate is slightly increased in patients with infective endocarditis and in those also requiring replacement of the ascending aorta. The bioprosthesis is preferable to the mechanical prosthetic valve for aortic valve replacement in the elderly (46). Patients with porcine bioprostheses require anticoagulant therapy for 3 months after hospital discharge and then may be treated with antiplatelet therapy alone (46).

In a prospective study, aortic valve replacement in 38 patients with severe aortic regurgitation normalized left ventricular chamber size and mass in two-

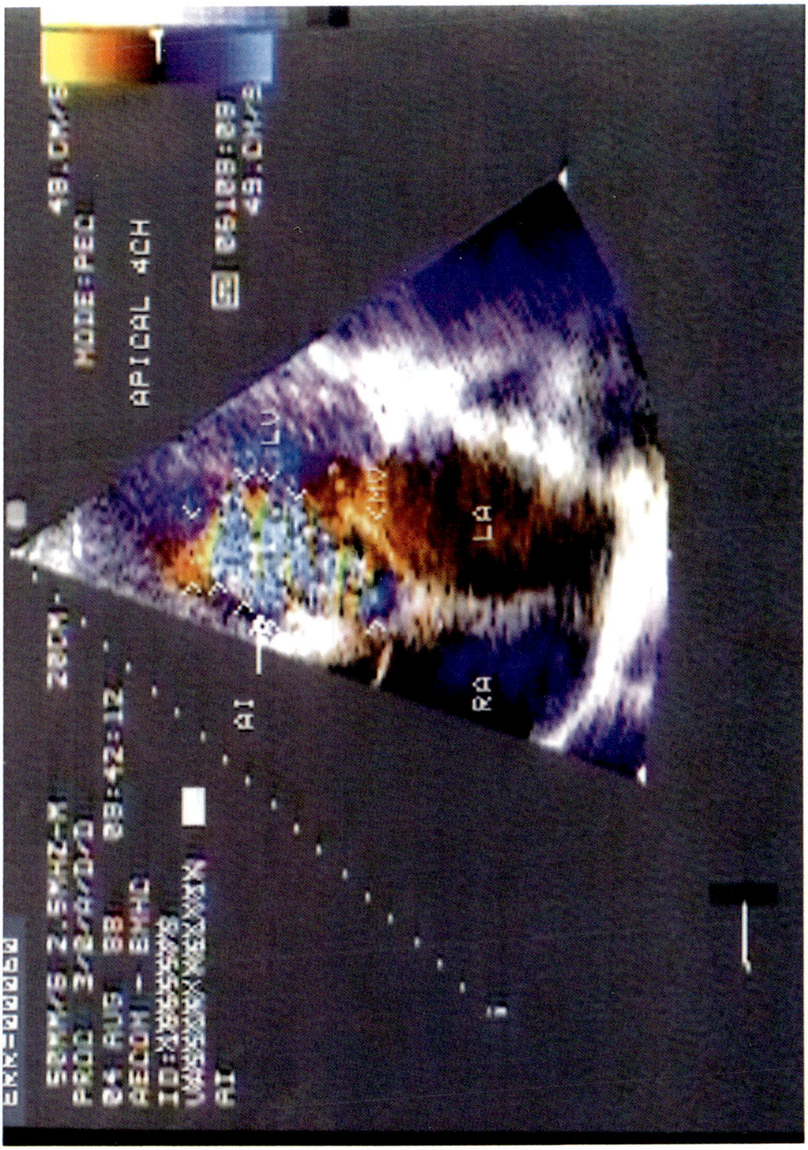


**Figure 6** Two-dimensional echocardiographic image from an apical four-chamber view in an elderly patient with severe aortic insufficiency, showing a large diastolic aliasing color Doppler jet in the left ventricular outflow tract. AI = aortic insufficiency; LV = left ventricular cavity; MV = mitral valve leaflets; LA = left atrium; RA = right atrium.

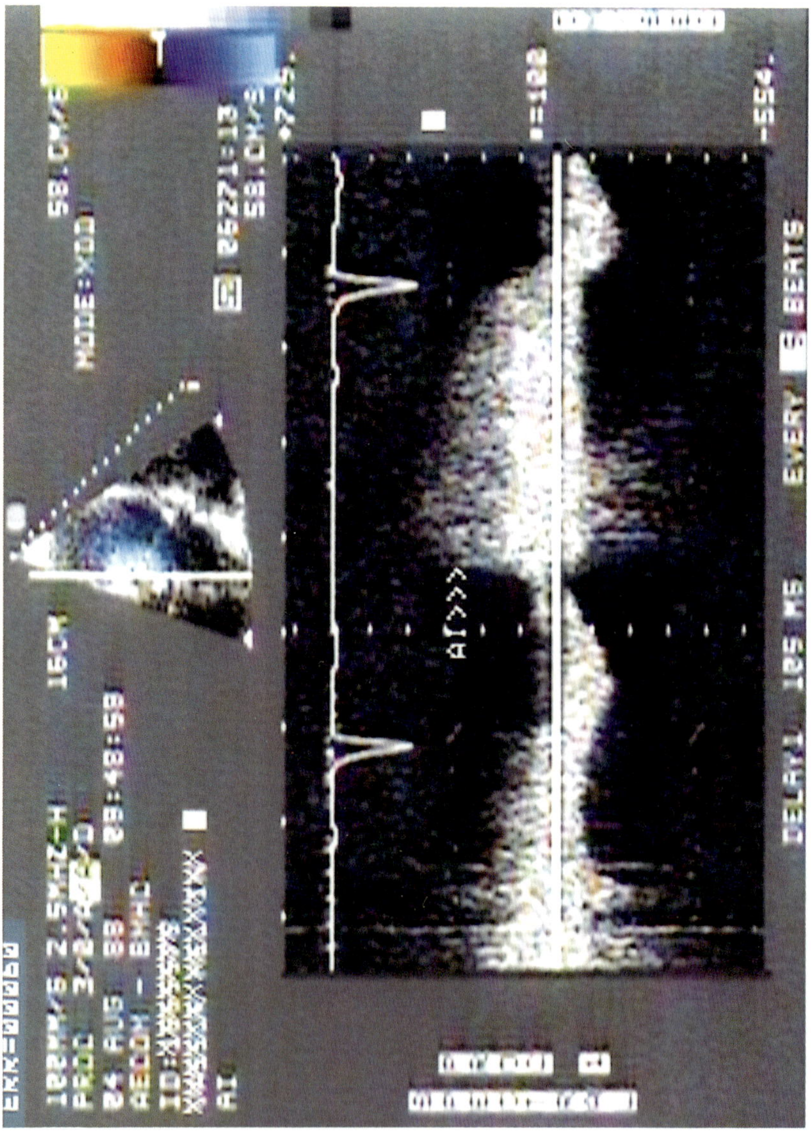


**Figure 7** Continuous wave Doppler recording of the velocity profile across the aortic valve in the same patient shown in Figure 6. A holosystolic decrescendo high-velocity profile is recorded from the left ventricular outflow tract, characteristic of aortic insufficiency. AI = aortic insufficiency.

thirds of patients undergoing surgery (84). At 9 months follow-up after aortic valve replacement, 58% of patients had a normal left ventricular end-diastolic dimension and 50% of patients had a normal left ventricular mass. During further follow-up (18–56 months postoperatively), 66% of patients had a normal left ventricular end-diastolic dimension and 68% of patients had a normal left ventricular mass. The left ventricular end-diastolic dimension normalized in 86% of patients with a preoperative left ventricular end-systolic dimension $\leqslant$ 55 mm. A preoperative left ventricular end-systolic dimension $>$ 55 mm occurred in 81% of patients with postoperative persistent left ventricular dilatation.

## REFERENCES

1. Roberts WC, Perloff JK, Costantino T. Severe valvular aortic stenosis in patients over 65 years of age. *Am J Cardiol* 1971; 27:497–506.
2. Waller BF, Roberts WC. Cardiovascular disease in the very elderly. An analysis of 40 necropsy patients aged 90 years or over. *Am J Cardiol* 1983; 51:403–421.
3. Aronow WS, Schwartz KS, Koenigsberg M. Correlation of aortic cuspal and aortic root disease with aortic systolic ejection murmurs and with mitral anular calcium in persons older than 62 years in a long-term health care facility. *Am J Cardiol* 1986; 58:651–652.
4. Aronow WS, Kronzon I. Prevalence and severity of valvular aortic stenosis determined by Doppler echocardiography and its association with echocardiographic and electrocardiographic left ventricular hypertrophy and physical signs of aortic stenosis in elderly patients. *Am J Cardiol* 1991; 67:776–777.
5. Roberts WC, Perloff JK. Mitral valvular disease: A clinicopathological survey of the conditions causing the mitral valve to function abnormally. *Ann Intern Med* 1972; 77:939–975.
6. Nair CK, Aronow WS, Stokke K, Mohiuddin SM, Thomson W, Sketch MH. Cardiac conduction defects in patients older than 60 years with aortic stenosis with and without mitral anular calcium. *Am J Cardiol* 1984; 53:169–172.
7. Sell S, Scully RE. Aging changes in the aortic and mitral valves. *Am J Patholol* 1965; 46:345–365.
8. Aronow WS, Schwartz KS, Koenigsberg M. Correlation of serum lipids, calcium, and phosphorus, diabetes mellitus and history of systemic hypertension with presence or absence of calcified or thickened aortic cusps or root in elderly patients. *Am J Cardiol* 1987; 59:998–999.
9. Roberts WC. The senile cardiac calcification syndrome. *Am J Cardiol* 1986; 58:572–574.
10. Aronow WS, Schwartz KS, Koenigsberg M. Correlation of serum lipids, calcium, and phosphorus, diabetes mellitus, aortic valve stenosis, and history of hypertension with presence or absence of mtral anular calcium in persons older than age 62 years in a long-term health care facility. *Am J Cardiol* 1987; 59:381–382.
11. Ross J Jr, Braunwald E. Aortic stenosis. *Circulation* 1968; 37(Suppl. V):V-61–67.

12. Frank S, Johnson A, Ross J Jr. Natural history of valvular aortic stenosis. *Br Heart J* 1973; 35:41–46.
13. Braunwald E. On the natural history of severe aortic stenosis. *J Am Coll Cardiol* 1990; 15:1018–1020.
14. Bruns DL, Van Der Hauwaert LG. The aortic systolic murmur developing with increased age. *Br Heart J* 1958; 20:370–378.
15. Aronow WS, Kronzon I. Correlation of prevalence and severity of valvular aortic stenosis determined by continuous-wave Doppler echocardiography with physical signs of aortic stenosis in patients aged 62 to 100 years with aortic systolic ejection murmurs. *Am J Cardiol* 1987; 60:399–401.
16. Tresch DD. Atypical presentations of cardiovascular disorders in the elderly. *Geriatrics* 1987; 42(10):31–46.
17. Kennedy JW, Twiss RD, Blackmon JR, Dodge HT. Quantitative angiocardiography. III. Relationships of left ventricular pressure, volume and mass in aortic valve disease. *Circulation* 1968; 38:838–845.
18. Hood WP Jr, Rackley CE, Rolett EL. Wall stress in the normal and hypertrophied human left ventricle. *Am J Cardiol* 1968; 22:550–558.
19. Carroll JD, Carroll EP, Feldman T, Ward DM, Karp RB. Differential response of the left ventricle to aortic stenosis in elderly women versus men (abstract). *Circulation* 1991; 84(Suppl. II):II–2.
20. Stott DK, Marpole DG, Bristow JD, Kloster FE, Griswold HE. The role of left atrial transport in aortic and mitral stenosis. *Circulation* 1970; 41:1031–1041.
21. Vekshtein VI, Alexander RW, Yeung AC, Plappert T, St John Sutton MG, Ganz P, Selwyn AP, Bittl JA. Coronary atherosclerosis is associated with left ventricular dysfunction and dilatation in aortic stenosis. *Circulation* 1990; 82:2068–2074.
22. Finegan RE, Gianelly RE, Harrison DC. Aortic stenosis in the elderly. Relevance of age to diagnosis and treatment. *N Engl J Med* 1969; 281:1261–1264.
23. Aronow WS, Epstein S, Koenigsberg M, Schwartz KS. Usefulness of echocardiographic abnormal left ventricular ejection fraction, paroxysmal ventricular tachycardia and complex ventricular arrhythmias in predicting new coronary events in patients over 62 years of age. *Am J Cardiol* 1988; 61:1349–1351.
24. Teirstein P, Yeager M, Yock PG, Popp RL. Doppler echocardiographic measurement of aortic valve area in aortic stenosis: A noninvasive application of the Gorlin formula. *J Am Coll Cardiol* 1986; 8:1059–1065.
25. Come PC, Riley MF, McKay RG, Safian R. Echocardiographic assessment of aortic valve area in elderly patients with aortic stenosis and of changes in valve area after percutaneous balloon valvuloplasty. *J Am Coll Cardiol* 1987; 10:115–124.
26. Shah PM, Graham BM. Management of aortic stenosis: Is cardiac catheterization necessary? *Am J Cardiol* 1991; 67:1031–1032.
27. Slater J, Gindea AJ, Freedberg RS, Chinitz LA, Tunick PA, Rosenzweig BP, Winer HE, Goldfarb A, Perez JL, Glassman E, Kronzon I. Comparison of cardiac catheterization and Doppler echocardiography in the decision to operate in aortic and mitral valve disease. *J Am Coll Cardiol* 1991; 17:1026–1036.
28. Galan A, Zoghbi WA, Quinones MA. Determination of severity of valvular aortic stenosis by Doppler echocardiography and relation of findings to clinical outcome

and agreement with hemodynamic measurements determined at cardiac catheterization. *Am J Cardiol* 1991; 67:1007–1012.
29. Rapaport E. Natural history of aortic and mitral valve disease. *Am J Cardiol* 1975; 35:221-227.
30. Kennedy KD, Nishimura RA, Holmes DR Jr, Bailey KR. Natural history of moderate aortic stenosis. *J Am Coll Cardiol* 1991; 17:313–319.
31. Turina J, Hess O, Sepulcri F, Krayenbuehl HP. Spontaneous course of aortic valve disease. *Eur Heart J* 1987; 8:471–483.
32. Kelly TA, Rothbart RM, Cooper CM, Kaiser DL, Smucker ML, Gibson RS. Comparison of outcome of asymptomatic to symptomatic patients older than 20 years of age with valvular aortic stenosis. *Am J Cardiol* 1988; 61:123–130.
33. Pellikka PA, Nishimura RA, Bailey KR, Tajik AJ. The natural history of adults with asymptomatic, hemodynamically significant aortic stenosis. *J Am Coll Cardiol* 1990; 15:1012–1017.
34. Hammermeister KE, Cantor AB, Burchfiel CM, Sethi GK, Hong DM, VA Cooperative Study on Valvular Heart Disease. Clinical, haemodynamic and angiographic predictors of survival in unoperated patients with aortic stenosis. *Eur Heart J* 1988; 9(Suppl. E):65–69.
35. Dajani AS, Bisno AL, Chung KJ, Durack DT, Freed M, Gerber MA, Karchmer AW, Millard HD, Rahimtoola S, Shulman ST, Watanakunakorn C, Taubert KA. Prevention of bacterial endocarditis. Recommendations by the American Heart Association. *JAMA* 1990; 264:2919–2922.
36. O'Keefe JH Jr, Vlietstra RE, Bailey KR, Holmes DR Jr. Natural history of candidates for balloon aortic valvuloplasty. *Mayo Clin Proc* 1987; 62:986–991.
37. Litvack F, Jakubowski AT, Buchbinder NA, Eigler N. Lack of sustained clinical improvement in an elderly population after percutaneous aortic valvuloplasty. *Am J Cardiol* 1988; 62:270–275.
38. Block PC, Palacios IF. Clinical and hemodynamic follow-up after percutaneous aortic valvuloplasty in the elderly. *Am J Cardiol* 1988; 62:760–763.
39. Safian RD, Berman AD, Diver DJ, McKay LL, Come PC, Riley MF, Warren SE, Cunningham MJ, Wyman RM, Weinstein JS, Grossman W, McKay RG. Balloon aortic valvuloplasty in 170 consecutive patients. *N Engl J Med* 1988; 319:125–130.
40. Lewin RF, Dorros G, King JF, Mathiak L. Percutaneous transluminal aortic valvuloplasty: Acute outcome and follow-up of 125 patients. *J Am Coll Cardiol* 1989; 14:1210–1217.
41. Brady ST, Davis CA, Kussmaul WG, Laskey WK, Hirshfeld JW, Herrmann HC. Percutaneous aortic balloon valvuloplasty in octogenarians: Morbidity and mortality. *Ann Intern Med* 1989; 110:761–766.
42. Letac B, Cribier A, Koning R, Lefebvre E. Aortic stenosis in elderly patients aged 80 or older. Treatment by percutaneous balloon valvuloplasty in a series of 92 cases. *Circulation* 1989; 80:1514–1520.
43. Rodriguez AR, Kleiman NS, Minor ST, Zoghbi WA, West MS, DeFelice CA, Samuels DA, Cashion R, Pickett JD, Lewis JM, Raizner AE. Factors influencing the outcome of balloon aortic valvuloplasty in the elderly. *Am Heart J* 1990; 120:373–380.

44. Kuntz RE, Tosteson ANA, Berman AD, Goldman L, Gordon PC, Leonard BM, McKay RG, Diver DJ, Safian RD. Predictors of event-free survival after balloon aortic valvuloplasty. *N Engl J Med* 1991; 325:17–23.
45. Cheitlin MD. Severe aortic stenosis in the sick octogenarian. A clear indicator for balloon valvuloplasty as the initial procedure. *Circulation* 1989; 80:1906–1908.
46. Borkon AM, Soule LM, Baughman KL, Baumgartner WA, Gardner TJ, Watkins L, Gott VL, Hall KA, Reitz BA. Aortic valve selection in the elderly patient. *Ann Thorac Surg* 1988; 46:270–277.
47. Culliford AT, Galloway AC, Colvin SB, Grossi EA, Baumann FG, Esposito R, Ribakove GH, Spencer FC. Aortic valve replacement for aortic stenosis in persons aged 80 years and over. *Am J Cardiol* 1991; 67:1256–1260.
48. Arom K, Nicoloff D, Lindsay W, Northrup W, Kersten T, Emery R. Aortic valve replacement in the elderly: operative risks and long-term results (abstract). *J Am Coll Cardiol* 1990; 15:96A.
49. Levinson JR, Akins CW, Buckley MJ, Newell JB, Palacios IF, Block PC, Fifer MA. Octogenarians with aortic stenosis. Outcome after aortic valve replacement. *Circulation* 1989; 80(Suppl. I):I-49–56.
50. Gilchrist IC, Waxman HL, Kurnik PB. Improvement in early diastolic filling dynamics after aortic valve replacement. *Am J Cardiol* 1990; 66:1124–1129.
51. Hoffmann A, Burckhardt D. Patients at risk for cardiac death late after aortic valve replacement. *Am Heart J* 1990; 120:1142–1147.
52. Theard MA, Bhatia SJS, Plappert T, St John Sutton MG. Doppler echocardiographic study of the frequency and severity of aortic regurgitation in hypertrophic cardiomyopathy. *Am J Cardiol* 1987; 60:1143–1147.
53. Margonato A, Cianflone D, Carlino M, Conversano A, Nitti C, Chierchia S. Frequence and significance of aortic valve thickening in older asymptomatic patients and its relation to aortic regurgitation. *Am J Cardiol* 1989; 64:1061–1062.
54. Akasaka T, Yoshikawa J, Yoshida K, Okumachi F, Koizumi K, Shiratori K, Takao S, Shakudo M, Kato H. Age-related valvular regurgitation: A study by pulsed Doppler echocardiography. *Circulation* 1987; 76:262–265.
55. Aronow WS, Kronzon I. Correlation of prevalence and severity of aortic regurgitation detected by pulsed Doppler echocardiography with the murmur of aortic regurgitation in elderly patients in a long-term health care facility. *Am J Cardiol* 1989; 63:128–129.
56. Massell BF, Amezcua FJ, Czoniczer G. Prognosis of patients with pure or predominant aortic regurgitation in the absence of surgery (abstract). *Circulation* 1966; 34(Suppl. III):III–164.
57. Grayburn PA, Smith MD, Handshoe R, Friedman BJ, DeMaria AN. Detection of aortic insufficiency by standard echocardiography, pulsed Doppler echocardiography, and auscultation. A comparison of accuracies. *Ann Intern Med* 1986; 104:599–605.
58. Saal AK, Gross BW, Franklin DW, Pearlman AS. Noninvasive detection of aortic insufficiency in patients with mitral stenosis by pulsed Doppler echocardiography. *J Am Coll Cardiol* 1985; 5:176–181.
59. Meyers DG, Sagar KB, Ingram RF, Paulsen WJH, Romhilt DW. Diagnosis of aor-

tic insufficiency: Comparison of auscultation and M-mode echocardiography to angiography. *South Med J* 1982; 75:1192–1194.
60. Ross J Jr. Afterload mismatch and preload reserve: A conceptual framework for the analysis of ventricular function. *Prog Cardiovasc Dis* 1976; 18:256–264.
61. Greenberg B, Massie B, Thomas D, Bristow JD, Cheitlin M, Broudy D, Szlachcic J, Krishnamurthy G. Association between the exercise ejection fraction response and systolic wall stress in patients with chronic aortic insufficiency. *Circulation* 1985; 71:458–465.
62. Welch GH Jr, Braunwald E, Sarnoff SJ. Hemodynamic effects of quantitatively varied experimental aortic regurgitation. *Circ Res* 1957; 5:546–551.
63. Mann T, McLaurin LP, Grossman W, Craige E. Assessing the hemodynamic severity of acute aortic regurgitation due to infective endocarditis. *N Engl J Med* 1975; 293:108–113.
64. Roberts WC, Day PJ. Electrocardiographic observations in clinically isolated, pure, chronic, severe aortic regurgitation: Analysis of 30 necropsy patients aged 19 to 65 years. *Am J Cardiol* 1985; 55:431–438.
65. Savage DD, Garrison RJ, Kannel WB, Levy D, Anderson SJ, Stokes J III, Feinleib M, Castelli WP. The spectrum of left ventricular hypertrophy in a general population sample: The Framingham Study. *Circulation* 1987; 75(Suppl. I):I-26–33.
66. Aronow WS, Ahn C, Kronzon I, Koenigsberg M. Congestive heart failure, coronary events, and atherothrombotic brain infarction in elderly blacks and whites with systemic hypertension and with and without echocardiographic and electrocardiographic evidence of left ventricular hypertrophy. *Am J Cardiol* 1991; 67:295–299.
67. Koren MJ, Devereux RB, Casale PN, Savage DD, Laragh JH. Relation of left ventricular mass and geometry to morbidity and mortality in uncomplicated essential hypertension. *Ann Intern Med* 1991; 114:345–352.
68. Henry WL, Bonow RO, Borer JS, Ware JH, Kent KM, Redwood DR, McIntosh CL, Morrow AG, Epstein SE. Observations on the optimum time for operative intervention for aortic regurgitation. I. Evaluation of the results of aortic valve replacement in symptomatic patients. *Circulation* 1980; 61:471–483.
69. Gaasch WH, Carroll JD, Levine HJ, Criscitiello MG. Chronic aortic regurgitation: Prognostic value of left ventricular end-systolic dimension and end-diastolic radius/thickness ratio. *J Am Coll Cardiol* 1983; 1:775–782.
70. Grayburn PA, Handshoe R, Smith MD, Harrison MR, DeMaria AN. Quantitative assessment of the hemodynamic consequences of aortic regurgitation by means of continuous wave Doppler recordings. *J Am Coll Cardiol* 1987; 10:135–141.
71. Beyer RW, Ramirez M, Josephson MA, Shah PM. Correlation of continuous-wave assessment of chronic aortic regurgitation with hemodynamics and angiography. *Am J Cardiol* 1987; 60:852–856.
72. Perry GJ, Helmcke F, Nanda NC, Byard C, Soto B. Evaluation of aortic insufficiency by Doppler color flow mapping. *J Am Coll Cardiol* 1987; 9:952–959.
73. Dexter L. Evaluation of the results of cardiac surgery. In: Jones AM, ed. Modern Trends in Cardiology, Vol. 2. New York: Appleton-Century-Crofts, 1969:311-333.

74. Hegglin R, Scheu H, Rothlin M. Aortic insufficiency. *Circulation* 1968; 38 (Suppl. V):V-77–92.
75. Bonow RO, Lakatos E, Maron BJ, Epstein SE. Serial long-term assessment of the natural history of asymptomatic patients with chronic aortic regurgitation and normal left ventricular systolic function. *Circulation* 1991; 84:1625–1635.
76. Greenberg B, Massie B, Bristow JD, Cheitlin M, Siemienczuk D, Topic N, Wilson RA, Szlachcic J, Thomas D. Long-term vasodilator therapy of chronic aortic insufficiency: A randomized double-blind, placebo-controlled clinical trial. *Circulation* 1988; 78:92–103.
77. Scognamiglio R, Fasoli G, Ponchia A, Dalla-Volta S. Long-term nifedipine unloading therapy in asymptomatic patients with chronic severe aortic regurgitation. *J Am Coll Cardiol* 1990; 16:424–429.
78. McDonald GR, Schaff HV, Pyeritz RE, McKusick VA, Gott VL. Surgical management of patients with the Marfan syndrome and dilatation of the ascending aorta. *J Thorac Cardiovasc Surg* 1981; 81:180–186.
79. Alsip SG, Blackstone EH, Kirklin JW, Cobbs CG. Indications for cardiac surgery in patients with active infective endocarditis. *Am J Med* 1985; 78(Suppl. 6B):138–148.
80. Karp RB. Role of surgery in infective endocarditis. *Cardiovasc Clin* 1987; 17(3):141–162.
81. Cobbs CG, Gnann JW. Indications for surgery. In: Sande MA, Kaye D, Root RK, eds. Endocarditis. New York: Churchill Livingstone, 1984:201–212.
82. Bonow RO, Picone AL, McIntosh CL, Jones M, Rosing DR, Maron BJ, Lakatos E, Clark RE, Epstein SE. Survival and functional results after valve replacement for aortic regurgitation from 1976 to 1983: Impact of preoperative left ventricular function. *Circulation* 1985; 72:1244–1256.
83. Bonow RO. Noninvasive evaluation: prognosis and timing of operation in symptomatic and asymptomatic patients with chronic aortic regurgitation. In: Cohn LH, DiSesa VJ, eds. Aortic Regurgitation: Medical and Surgical Management. New York: Marcel Dekker, 1986:55–86.
84. Roman MJ, Klein L, Devereux RB, Kligfield P, Niles NW, Hochreiter C, Isom OW, Borer JS. Reversal of left ventricular dilatation, hypertrophy, and dysfunction by valve replacement in aortic regurgitation. *Am Heart J* 1989; 118:553–563.

# 15

# Mitral Valvular Disease in the Elderly

**Donald D. Tresch**
*Medical College of Wisconsin and University of Wisconsin, Milwaukee, Wisconsin*

## INTRODUCTION

It has been shown that the mitral valve undergoes structural changes related to aging (1–3). The anterior leaflet demonstrates lipid disposition, nodular thickening at the free edges, and atheromatosis of the ventricular surface. This atheromatosis differs from vascular atheromatosis in that thrombosis, hemorrhage, and calcification are not present. The posterior leaflet demonstrates small puckered scars and diffuse opacification of the leaflet. Microscopically, collagen fibers become disorganized, the posterior leaflet demonstrates fibroelastic hyperplasia, and there is microscopic calcification of both valve leaflets.

Most of these changes are thought to be secondary to years of stress and adaptive processes secondary to the stress. Usually such changes do not produce significant valvular dysfunction, and clinically the process is silent. Two degenerative aging processes, mitral annulus calcification and mucoid (or myxomatous) degeneration of the valve leaflets and chordae tendineae, however, can produce significant valvular dysfunction (4,5).

In certain elderly patients these degenerative aging changes may be so severe that significant valvular dysfunction occurs with clinical manifestations. In other elderly patients the aging changes may be superimposed on inherited or acquired valvular disorders, with clinical manifestations resulting from significant valvular dysfunction secondary to the combined disorders. Some diseases, such as coronary artery disease, may not cause any mitral valvular dysfunction until the patient is elderly, when the general cardiac disease is clinically manifested. Rheumatic mitral valve disease, even though acquired early in life, may become clinically symptomatic only when the patient reaches his or her seventh or eighth decade, at which time the heart decompensates secondary to the years of accumulated stress from the valvular dysfunction. Other elderly patients can have an inherited, acquired, or aging mitral valvular disorder, which is clinically silent until a systemic illness, such as an infection, affects the abnormal valve with the development of clinical symptoms (endocarditis).

Specific mitral valvular disorders in the elderly may produce clinical symptoms, which are similar to those in younger patients who have the same valvular disorders. In some elderly persons, however, the clinical manifestations are different from those usually seen in younger patients with the disease. Because of this different presentation, the valvular disorder may be clinically missed or the patient's symptoms are misdiagnosed as related to another abnormality. Furthermore, valvular disorders in the elderly can have more severe clinical manifestations than are usually seen in younger patients with the disorder and management will have to be modified.

## MITRAL VALVULAR INCOMPETENCE

### Mitral Valve Prolapse

Mitral valve prolapse (MVP) is a common valvular abnormality with distinct anatomical findings. The disorder occurs in all ages, with reported prevalence varying from 5 to 21% depending on the diagnostic technique and the population tested (6–9). Gross pathology typically reveals the mitral leaflets, both anterior and posterior, to be enlarged, redundant, and voluminous and appear deformed, giving the appearance of a parachute, or what has been referred to as "ballooning" (Fig. 1). The posterior leaflet is more commonly involved or may be more severely affected than the anterior leaflet. Because of this involvement, the posterior leaflet may be twice the depth of the anterior leaflet, instead of the normal one-third to one-half. The annular circumference of the valve is increased, and the chordae tendineae are often elongated and generally thin. The commissures of the leaflets do not demonstrate fusion, a finding that distinguishes MVP from a rheumatic valve.

Microscopically, abnormal collagen tissue replaces the normal homogenous collagen of the fibrosa of the leaflets; the abnormal tissue demonstrates thinning, fragmentation, and loss of fiber orientation. The increase in this abnormal collagen tissue is mainly due to excessive mucopolysaccarides, which may be secondary to a fundamental abnormality in collagen metabolism (myxomatous degeneration) (10). This myxomatous degeneration leads to softening of the

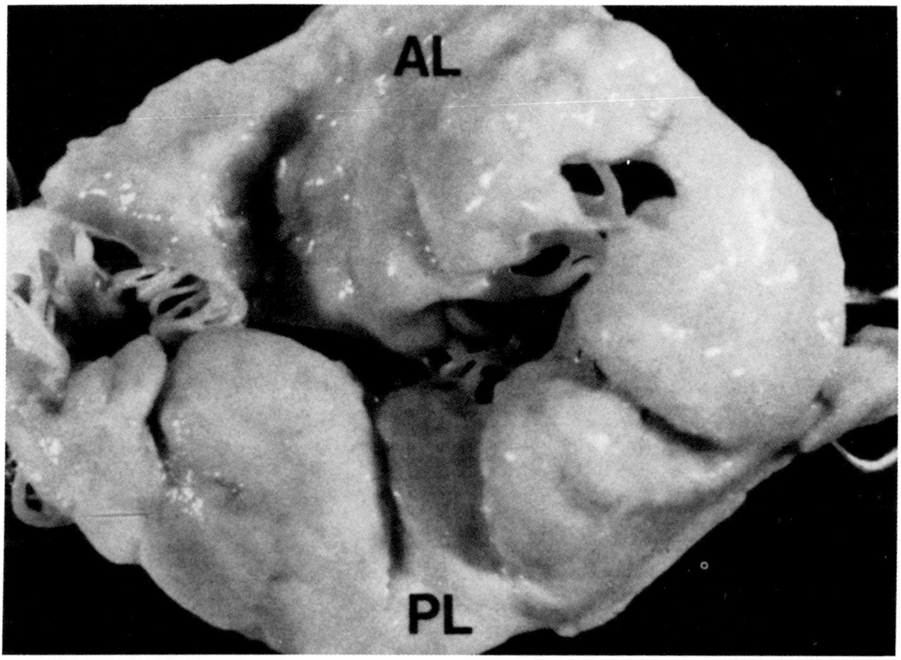


**Figure 1** Excised mitral valve displaying gross changes of mitral valve prolapse. Leaflets are enlarged and redundant, giving the appearance of a parachute—"ballooning." (Reprinted with permission from Ref. 101.)

fibrosa with stretching of the affected leaflet, which causes prolapse of the leaflet into the left atrium. The annulus and chordae tendineae are also usually affected with degenerative changes similar to those in the fibrosa of the valve leaflets, and the elongated redundant chordae tendineae may also be responsible for producing prolapse of the leaflets.

Anatomically, the final structural abnormality of mitral valve prolapse is disproportion between the left ventricular size and the mitral valve (Fig. 2). The valve is "too big" for the ventricle, or the ventricle is "too small" for the valve. In certain cases this disproportion between the ventricle and the valve may not be presented at the beginning of systole and only becomes evident during systole, as the ventricular volume dynamically changes.

Numerous conditions, including Marfan's syndrome (11), Ehlers-Danlos syndrome (11,12), muscular dystrophy (13), congenital abnormalities, particularly atrial septal defect (14), and rheumatic heart disease (15), have all been associated with MVP. The specific pathogenesis of mucoid degeneration that

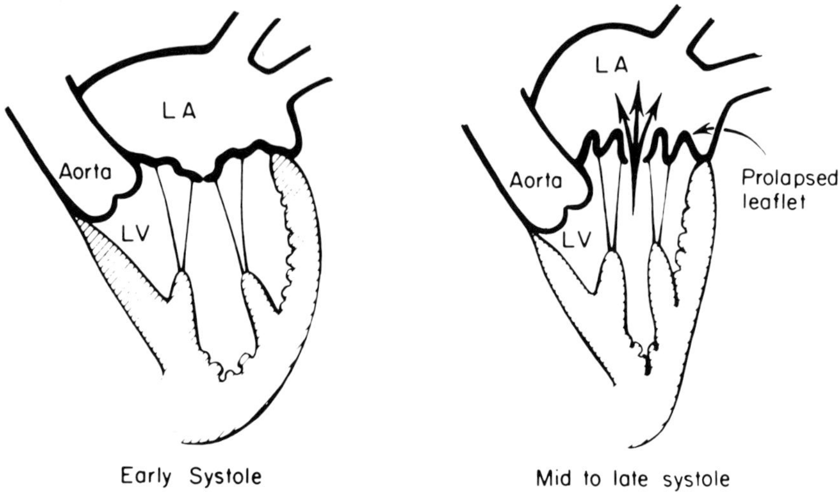


**Figure 2** The mitral valve is noted to be large and redundant, but competent, at the beginning of systole. In mid- to late systole, with changes in left ventricular volume, the valve is "too large," and prolapse occurs with mitral insufficiency. (Reprinted with permission from Ref. 102.)

results in MVP, however, remains unknown. Most likely it is a nonspecific change that results from a number of factors, with a genetic etiology playing a major role.

Pomerance (5) reported findings of severe mucoid degeneration of the mitral valve in approximately 1% of autopsies in patients over 50 years of age. Whether this mucoid degeneration related to aging is the major cause of the clinical entity, mitral valve prolapse syndrome, seen in elderly patients remains unclear.

## Diagnosis of Mitral Valve Prolapse

The diagnosis of MVP is usually made from the physical examination and confirmed by the echocardiographic findings. On occasion, however, the physical examination, including the cardiac auscultatory findings, is completely normal, and the echocardiogram demonstrates findings of MVP (16,17). The general appearance of the person with MVP may be entirely normal, although one may be struck by the asthenic body habitus and thoracic bony abnormalities. Pectus excavatum, "straight back," and scoliosis are so common that they may in some cases be considered part of the syndrome. Ansari (18) found in a series of 50 patients with straight back syndrome that 64% had MVP, whereas only

17.5% of age- and sex-matched controls demonstrated echocardiographic findings of MVP.

The typical auscultatory findings produced by MVP are a midsystolic click followed by a mid- to late systolic murmur. The click, or "snapping sound," however, can be quite variable in location and intensity. These sounds are thought to originate from the redundant valve leaflets or tensing of the chordae. A single systolic click may be heard, or multiple clicks may be present. The click may vary in timing and also be transient, disappearing from one examination to the next.

As with the click, the murmur is also variable in timing and intensity. The typical murmur occurs in mid- to late systole and is "blowing" in quality. In some persons the murmur may be holosystolic, with radiation into the axilla, displaying all the qualities of a murmur of typical mitral regurgitation. In contrast, occasionally the murmur may have an "ejection" quality and be heard extremely well at the base. The "honking" and "whooping" murmurs associated with mitral incompetence have also been reported.

Variability of the systolic click and murmur appears to be the hallmark of the auscultatory findings in MVP. This variability may be modified by bedside maneuvers (both physical and pharmacological), and it should be emphasized that the findings may be completely missed unless a specific effort is made to bring them out.

Maneuvers that decrease left ventricular volume, resulting in a smaller chamber size and accentuating leaflet or chordae redundancy, produce earlier and more pronounced systolic prolapse of the mitral leaflet, and the murmur and click occur earlier in systole, plus the murmur is louder (Fig. 3). In contrast, maneuvers that increase left ventricular size delay the onset of the click and murmur in systole, and in certain cases, the murmur is softer or may even disappear.

These maneuvers are quite helpful and are mandatory in attempting to elicit the typical auscultatory findings of MVP. Nevertheless, some investigators (16,17) have reported that 10–20% of persons with MVP remain "silent" to auscultation, even when maneuvers are performed.

The chest x-ray may confirm the thoracic bony abnormalities of a straight back, pectus excavatum, and scoliosis or may be entirely normal. In uncomplicated MVP, the cardiac silhouette is rarely enlarged.

The electrocardiographic abnormalities seen in patients with MVP are usually nonspecific ST-T wave changes with partial or total T wave inversion with and without ST depression in leads II, III, and AVF and occasionally involving left precordial leads (19,20). Almost all types of arrhythmias have been reported in patients with MVP, although the most common are supraventricular and ventricular premature contractions and ventricular tachycardia. Prolonged Q-T

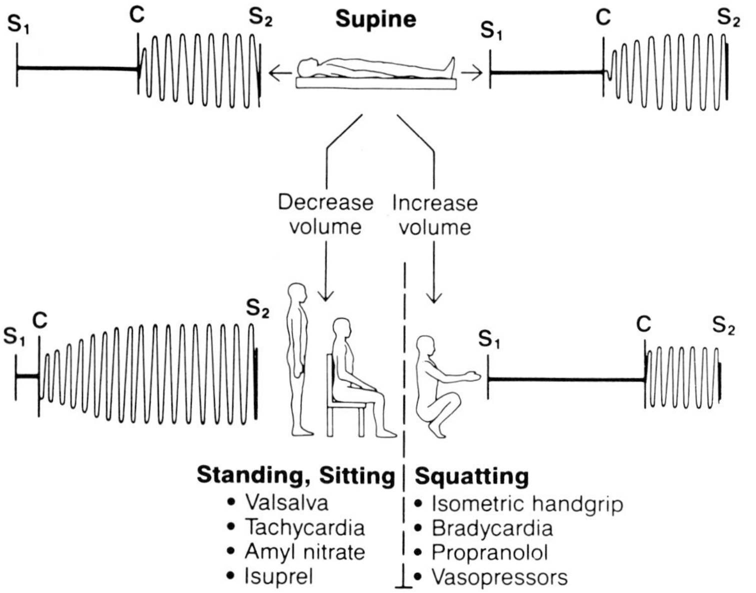


**Figure 3** Typical auscultatory findings in mitral valve prolapse and change in intensity and timing of murmur and click with maneuvers. The variability of the timing and intensity of the murmurs depends on the position of the patient. (Reprinted with permission from Ref. 103.)

interval has been reported, as have bradyarrhythmias and Wolfe-Parkinson-White syndrome, in patients with MVP.

The echocardiogram is usually considered the most definitive laboratory test for confirming the diagnosis of MVP (21,22). Two distinctive M-mode echocardiographic patterns have been reported: the classic and most definitive is the abrupt late posterior displacement (prolapse) of either or both leaflets in mid- and late systole, and the other finding is the "hammocklike" parasystolic displacement of the leaflets (Fig. 4). Most authorities state that the posterior displacement must exceed 2–3 mm below the mitral closure to be able to make a definitive diagnosis of MVP by M-mode echocardiography. Two-dimensional echocardiography has been beneficial in determining echocardiographic criteria for diagnosing MVP. With two-dimensional echocardiography the mitral annulus is clearly visible as a reference point, and systolic displacement of either the anterior or posterior leaflets into the left atrium can be readily appreciated (Fig. 5). Other two-dimensional echocardiographic findings of MVP are thickening of the mitral valve leaflets as a result of redundancy, dilatation of the mitral annulus, and coexistence of prolapse of other cardiac valves. Transeso-

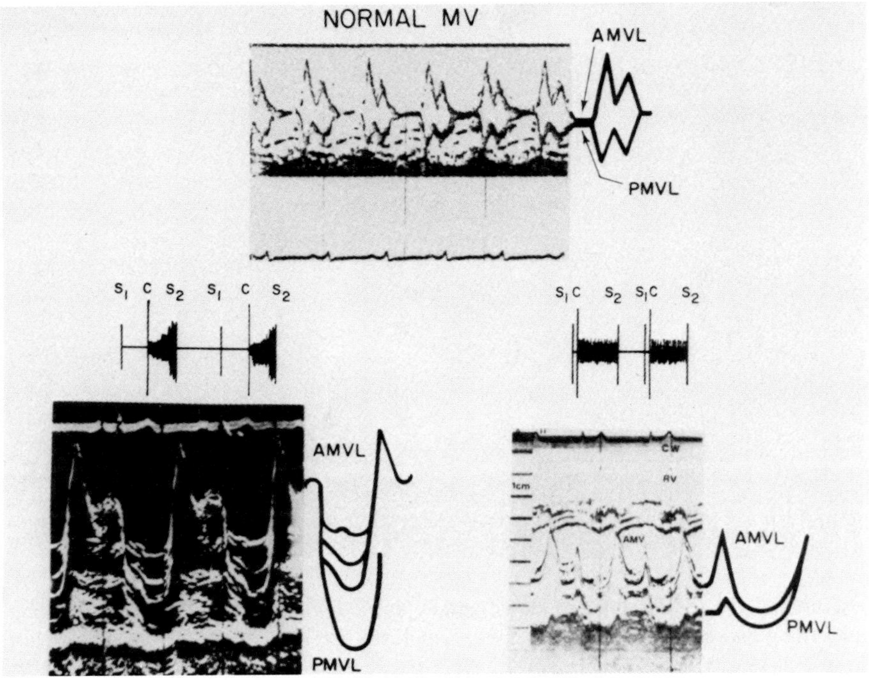


**Figure 4** Normal M-mode echocardiogram; echocardiograms showing two types of mitral valve prolapse and simultaneous echocardiograms and phonocardiograms. AMVL = anterior mitral valve leaflet; PMVL = posterior mitral valve leaflet; MV = mitral valve. (Reprinted with permission from Ref. 102.)

phageal echocardiography has recently been developed and can also be useful in diagnosing MVP (see Chap. 3).

Left ventricular angiography is usually not necessary to make the diagnosis of MVP but can confirm the abnormality. In the right anterior oblique projection, the bulging of the leaflets (one or both) into the left atrium is considered diagnostic of MVP (Fig. 6). Care should be taken not to overdiagnose MVP in the presence of normal radiographic variants, since normal "pouches" or fornices of the normal valve may be misinterpreted as abnormal prolapse.

## Mitral Valve Prolapse Syndrome

Mitral valve prolapse syndrome (MVPS) is the presence of anatomical MVP accompanied by a set of clinical symptoms and features. The syndrome is considered the most common cardiac disorder seen by the practicing physician (23), and it has now been shown that MVP is the most common etiology of mitral valvular incompetence for which mitral valve surgery is necessary (24).

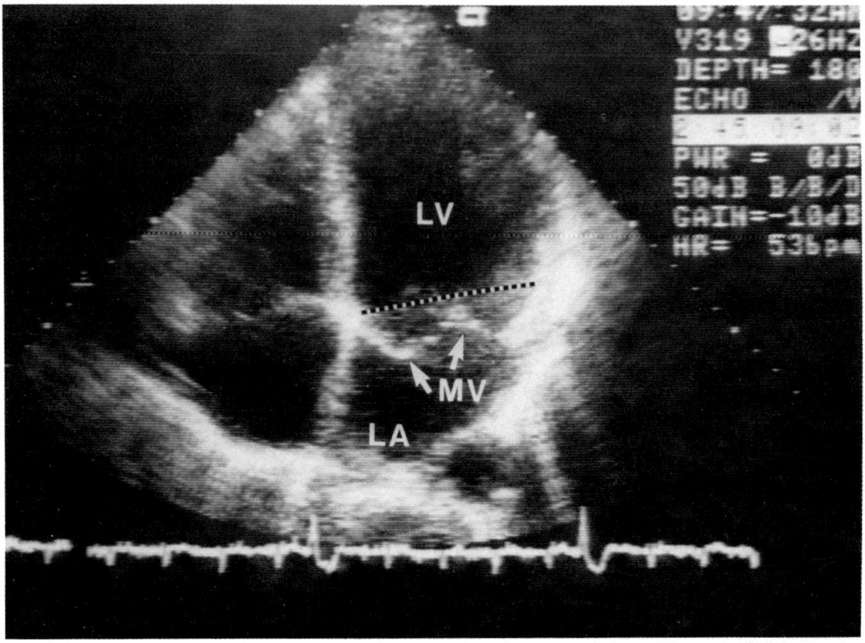


**Figure 5** Two-dimensional echocardiogram (apical four-chamber view) demonstrating thickening and prolapse of leaflets above annulus plane. LA = left atrium; LV = left ventricle; MV = mitral valve.

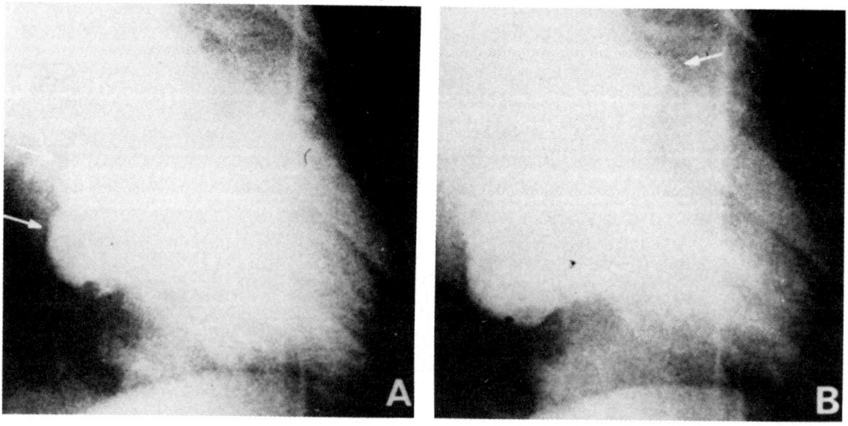


**Figure 6** Early (A) and late (B) systolic frames of a left ventriculogram in right anterior oblique projection showing a triscallop prolapse of the posterior mitral leaflet. Specific scallops are defined by arrows. Mitral incompetence is present. (Reprinted with permission from Ref. 104.)

Patients with MVP may be asymptomatic, although it has been shown that approximately 80% of patients with MVP have symptoms (25). Symptoms are often nonspecific and include chest pain, palpitations, dyspnea, dizziness, easy fatigability, and anxiety attacks. On occasion patients with MVP present with supraventricular tachycardia and, infrequently, ventricular tachycardia or ventricular fibrillation. There is a good deal of controversy concerning the actual prevalence of symptoms in persons with MVP compared to a matched control population. Deveraux et al. (26) found no difference in prevalence of chest pain, dyspnea, or anxiety between persons with MVP and a control group of subjects without MVP, whereas palpitations were more common in persons with MVP. The Framingham Heart Study (27) reported that chest pain, dyspnea, or syncope was not specifically associated with MVP.

Heart failure may develop in persons with MVP when mitral incompetence is severe. The heart failure can be insidious and progressive or may be abrupt, with development of acute pulmonary edema when the severe mitral incompetence is related to an acute spontaneous rupture of the chordae tendineae.

## Comparison of Elderly Patients and Younger Patients with MVP and MVPS

Mitral valve prolapse syndrome usually becomes clinically manifested in the third through fifth decades and is more common in women than men in this age group (28,29). This gender difference has been reported by some investigators to decrease with age, although studies by Levy and Savage (30) demonstrated that irrespective of the diagnostic criteria used to define MVP, there is a 2.1 female-to-male ratio, regardless of the patient's age.

Recently, mitral valve prolapse has become increasingly recognized in the population 60 years of age or older. The natural history of the disorder remains unclear, and it is not known if the condition in the elderly represents a sudden onset of the entity or the disease has progressed to the point at which it becomes clinically recognizable.

The majority of elderly patients with MVP and MVPS have features similar to those in younger patients with the mitral valve disorder (Table 1). The older patient, like the younger patient, may be entirely asymptomatic, and MVP is diagnosed by the auscultatory findings. Tresch and associates (31) reported 40 patients over the age of 60 years who were found to have MVP on echocardiography; approximately one-fourth of the patients were asymptomatic, and the echocardiogram was obtained because of a heart murmur. Higgins and associates (32) reported similar findings when studying 40 elderly patients (mean age 66 years) with echocardiographic findings of MVP; 15 of the 40 patients with MVP were without symptoms.

As in younger patients with MVPS, most elderly patients' symptoms are nonspecific, with palpitations and atypical chest pain not unusual. Some investi-

**Table 1** Clinical Findings in Elderly Patients with Mitral Valve Prolapse

| Study | Number of patients | Ages (years) | Asymptomatic | Absence of murmur | AF | Chest pain | Palpitations | Syncope | Endocarditis | CHF |
|---|---|---|---|---|---|---|---|---|---|---|
| Kolibash et al. (33) | 62 | 60–81 (67)[a] | 0 | 1 (2%) | 3 (5%) | 20 (32%) | 11 (18%) | 5 (8%) | — | 26 (42%) |
| Higgins et al. (32) | 40 | 50–90 (66)[a] | 15 (38%) | 11 (28%) | 14 (35%) | 6 (15%) | 15 (38%) | —[b] | 3 (8%) | —[b] |
| Tresch et al. (31) | 40 | 61–86 (67)[a] | 11 (28%) | 5 (13%) | 4 (10%) | 9 (22%) | 20 (25%) | 4 (10%) | 4 (10%) | 10 (25%) |

AF = atrial fibrillation; CHF = congestive heart failure.
[a] Mean age in parentheses.
[b] Not mentioned.

gators (31,33), however, have found elderly patients to be more disabled by the disorder than younger patients. Kolibash and associates (33), in a study of patients over 60 years of age (mean age 67) with MVPS, found approximately 30% presented with disabling chest pain, which had characteristics suggestive of ischemic pain in most cases. Of the 62 patients in Kolibash's study, 16 presented with symptoms (syncope and palpitations) related to arrhythmias; 2 patients with syncope had prehospital cardiac arrests and required cardiopulmonary resuscitation. Approximately 35% of the patients in the Tresch (31) and Higgins (32) groups' studies complained of symptoms thought to be related to arrhythmias, although none of the patients in those two studies had sustained cardiac arrest.

The main clinical feature that appears different between elderly patients and younger patients with MVPS is the occurrence of heart failure. In younger patients with MVPS, severe mitral incompetence producing left ventricular failure appears to be rare. This may not be the case in elderly patients, and studies (31,33–35) have demonstrated heart failure to be a presenting symptom in the elderly patient with MVPS. In 1976, Collins et al. (35) reported 4 patients, all over 65, range 65–76, who presented with heart failure; in 2 of the 4 patients the heart failure was of acute onset, 1 week or less. All 4 patients died, and at autopsy all 4 patients demonstrated severe myxomatous changes of the mitral valve and findings consistent with MVP; 2 of the 4 patients demonstrated ruptured chordae. More recently, both the Tresch (31) and Kolibash (33) groups reported elderly patients with MVPS who presented with heart failure. Tresch et al. (31) found 25% of patients over 60 years with MVPS presented with heart failure. The percentage of elderly patients with heart failure in the Kolibash group's study (33) was even higher: 26 of 66 patients (43%) with MVP presented with heart failure. Of the 10 patients with heart failure in Tresch's study, 5, and 16 of 26 patients with heart failure in Kalibash's study required valvular surgery.

In another study, Tresch and associates (34) analyzed clinical features of 30 patients who required valvular surgery (mitral valve replacement or repair) for severe mitral incompetence secondary to MVP. The mean age of the patients was 59.5 years, range 25–72, and the majority (20) of the patients were male. The patients were usually aware of having a heart murmur for many years (mean duration 15.3 years), although symptoms of heart failure were of recent onset; 24 of the 30 patients had symptoms for less than 1 month, and many of the patients presented with acute pulmonary edema. At the time of the presentation with heart failure, the patients' auscultatory findings were usually a loud holosystolic murmur characteristic of severe mitral incompetence. A systolic click was not detected, even though auscultatory findings before the onset of heart failure were commonly the typical mid- to late systolic murmur preceded by a nonejection systolic click. In 2 of the 30 patients, instead of the typical holosystolic blowing murmur of mitral incompetence, an ejection type of murmur heard best at the upper left sternal border, mimmicking the murmur of aortic valvular stenosis, was detected. At the time of their presentation with heart failure, 13 of the patients (43%) demonstrated atrial fibrillation. Chest x-ray revealed significant pulmonary congestion in all patients, although only moderate to mild cardiomegaly was noted. Cardiac catheterization in all patients revealed findings of severe mitral incompetence, and angiographic studies demonstrated prolapsing mitral valve leaflets with "wide-open" regurgitation. At the time of surgery all patients demonstrated a myxomatous mitral valve with a dilated mitral annulus and redundant leaflets. Of the 30 patients 17 also demonstrated ruptured chordae tendineae; the posterior chorda was ruptured in 11 patients, the anterior chorda in 4 patients, and in 2 patients both chordae were ruptured (Fig. 7).

Other investigators (33,35–40) reported similar findings in elderly patients with MVPS who required mitral valve surgery for heart failure. Even though the syndrome of MVPS is more common in young women than men, patients requiring valvular surgery are more commonly men and usually older than 50 years, with many patients older than 70 years. Usually the patient is aware of having a heart murmur for many years (>20 or 30 years), with typical auscultatory findings of a mid- to late systolic murmur preceded by a midsystolic click. The onset of heart failure is abrupt, however, at which time the patient usually demonstrates a loud holosystolic murmur, a systolic click is not detected, and commonly atrial fibrillation is present. At the time of surgery the typical findings of MVP are noted, and not uncommonly, ruptured chordae are found. This clinical presentation is compatible with acute mitral valvular incompetence superimposed on chronic mild valvular incompetence. In other cases, the onset of heart failure may not be as abrupt and may have a more chronic, progressive presentation. The specific reason for the increased incidence of this chronic failure in this subset of elderly patients with MVP is unclear. The possibility of mild valvular incompetence progressing over the years to severe incompetence (mitral incompetency begets more mitral incompetence) should be considered.

Other complications that must be considered in elderly patients with MVPS are infectious endocarditis and cerebral thromboembolism. Clemens and associates (41), in a case-controlled study of hospitalized patients who had echocardiographic findings of MVP and who lacked any other known cardiovascular risk factors for endocarditis, found a significantly higher risk for endocarditis in patients with MVP than for those without MVP. Similar conclusions have been reached in other recent studies (42–44). McMahon and associates (44), in a review of the literature, reported that the risk of endocarditis in patients with MVPS is two to three times greater in men than women, with the risk most marked in patients over age 45 when the MVP is associated with mitral incompetence. The absolute risk of endocarditis in patients with MVP without clinical

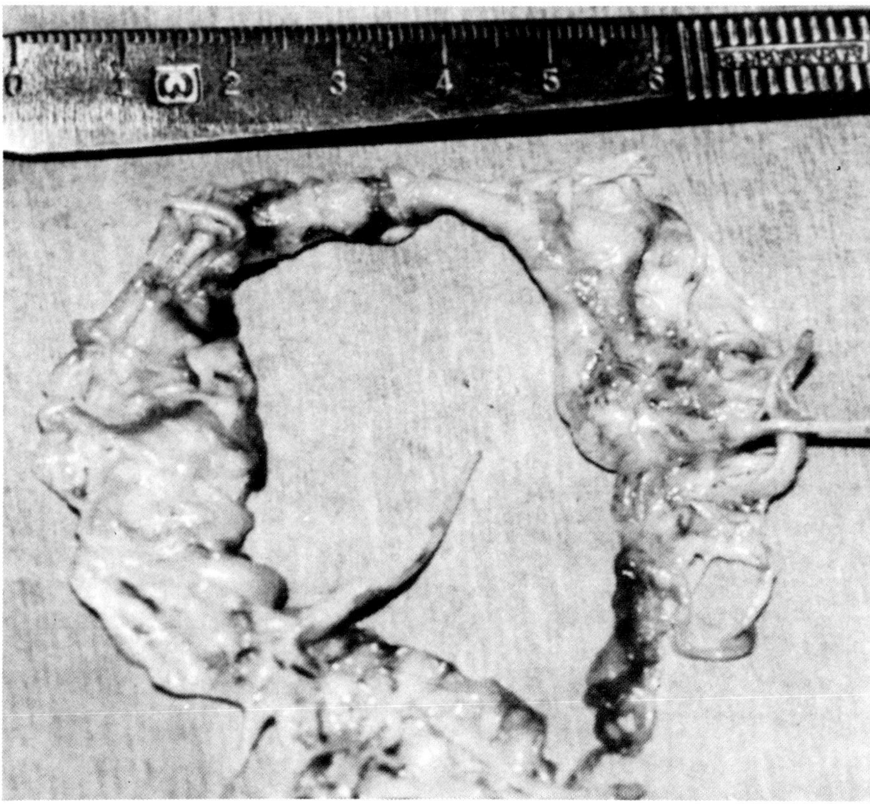

**Figure 7** Mitral valve excised during surgery in 67-year-old male with mitral valve prolapse. Note dilated annular circumference with ruptured chordae. (Reprinted with permission from Ref. 34.)

or Doppler findings of mitral valvular incompetence is considered by some authorities to be so low that prophylactic antibiotics are not considered necessary in this subset of patients with MVP (44–46).

Patients with MVP have been found by some investigators (47–52) at increased risk for cerebral ischemic events. Sandok and Guiliani (47), in a study of 1138 persons with MVP (mean age 48 years), found a 3.5% incidence of cerebral ischemic events and suggested that the prevalence of such events in persons with MVP was four times greater than the rate expected in the normal population. Interestingly, as in patients with MVPS who require valvular surgery and develop endocarditis, the association of MVP with ischemic cerebral events has been found to be more common in men than women (48,49). When comparing younger (mean age 34 years) and older (mean age 65 years) persons with MVP and occurrence of cerebral ischemic events, Barnett and associates (49) concluded that MVP played a role in cerebral ischemia and/or cerebral infarction in younger persons with the disorder but most likely not in older persons. Other studies (48,50,51) have reported similar findings, although in the Sandok and Guiliani study (47) the incidence of MVP-associated cerebral ischemia did not vary with patient age. Hart and Easton (52), when reviewing the literature, suggested that the so-called difference in MVP-associated cerebral ischemia events between younger and older adults is merely related to the difficulty of demonstrating the MVP stroke relationship in older adults in whom atheroemboli mechanisms predominate. They estimated that the incidence of MVP-related strokes in young adults is only 1 per 100,000 per year, whereas in older adults who have a stroke incidence of 80 per 100,000 per year, the contribution of MPV (estimated to be 1.25%) could easily be overlooked.

Despite the increased prevalence of cerebral ischemic events in patients with MVP, most authorities (47,49,50) do not recommend preventive treatment in patients with MVP who have not had a cerebral ischemic event. In elderly patients with MVP who experience a cerebral ischemic event, a thorough evaluation should be performed to rule out other potentially responsible etiologies before attributing the event to MVP. When no other mechanism is recognized, MVP may be presumed to be the etiology and antiplatelet drugs are recommended. In patients with recurrent cerebral events thought to be related to MVP, anticoagulation is suggested.

## Rheumatic and Other Etiologies of Chronic Mitral Valve Incompetence

In addition to MVP, the other common disorders producing mitral valvular incompetence in the elderly include rheumatic heart disease, coronary artery disease, and calcified mitral annulus. The disorder of calcified mitral annulus with resultant mitral incompetence is discussed in Chapter 16.

Residual rheumatic heart disease is found in the elderly. Although the disorder is less common than in the general population, the incidence of rheumatic mitral valvular disease in the elderly is higher than commonly realized. Hargreaves (53), in an autopsy study, found rheumatic mitral incompetence or stenosis or both in 3.1% of autopsies in patients over the age of 50. Most investigators (54) have reported mitral incompetence to be the predominant valvular lesion in elderly patients with rheumatic mitral valve disease. As in MVP, echocardiography with Doppler examination is very useful in diagnosing and assessing the severity of rheumatic mitral valvular incompetence.

One of the main problems when approaching elderly patients with chronic mitral valvular incompetence, regardless of the etiology, is the timing of surgical intervention. (Management of heart failure, arrhythmias, and endocarditis is discussed in Chapters 20–23 and 17, respectively.) The problem of proper timing of mitral valve surgery may be even more difficult in elderly patients than in younger patients with mitral incompetence. The more severe left ventricular dysfunction usually present in elderly patients and the high association of concomitant serious illnesses in this age group, both of which are associated with a high surgical risk, make most physicians hesitant when considering mitral valve surgery in the elderly patient (55,56). Also, some investigators have reported advanced age to be an independent predictor of operative mortality in valvular surgery (57–60). In the last two decades, however, with advances in intraoperative techniques and the design of better valvular prostheses, postoperative mortality in elderly patients has significantly improved. Instead of valve replacement, mitral valve repair has now become another option in the elderly patient, and in some studies (61–63) valvular repair has been associated with a significantly lower operative mortality and better long-term survival than valve replacement. The other added advantage of valve repair that is an important consideration in the elderly patient is the lack of the necessity of long-term anticoagulation.

Despite remarkable improvements in heart surgery, it is estimated that the results will be suboptimal in approximately 30% of patients undergoing valvular surgery (64,65). Most investigators relate these poor postoperative results directly to the timing of surgery, with valvular surgery performed too late in the course of the disease, after irreversible left ventricular dysfunction has developed.

During the development of chronic systolic volume overload secondary to the valvular incompetence, the cardiovascular system compensates to limit the deleterious effect of the disease on left ventricular function and clinical symptoms. As a consequence, many patients with chronic mitral incompetence are without symptoms until the seventh or eighth decade. As the volume overload progressed, however, the left ventricle is no longer able to compensate and deterioration of ventricular function occurs. Commonly, at this stage of progressive volume overload ventricular decompensation occurs and the patient becomes symptomatic before irreversible damage occurs to the left ventricle. Unfortunately, this deterioration is not always associated with symptoms, and valvular surgery may be delayed until irreversible ventricular damage is present. In such cases, surgery produces suboptimal results, with high operative mortality and inadequate relief of the patient's symptoms.

Retrospective studies (61–68) have been used to identify preoperative markers of significant progressive left ventricular dysfunction, and such markers may be used to determine optimum timing of valvular surgery. Depending on the study, indices vary to a degree, although increasing left ventricular dimension in range of 45–50 mm in end systole or a resting left ventricular ejection fraction of less than 50% are two markers that are commonly used (66–68). Such markers may be determined by periodic echocardiography and/or radionuclide angiography. Some authorities recommend obtaining the examinations every 6–12 months in patients with chronic mitral incompetence.

In summary, valvular surgery should be considered in elderly patients with chronic mitral valvular incompetence whose symptoms have progressed to New York Heart Association (NYHA) functional class III or IV and are not functionally incapacitated from other illnesses. In addition, mitral valve surgery should be considered when indicators of left ventricular dysfunction are present even in the absence of severe or limiting symptoms.

## MITRAL VALVULAR STENOSIS

Mitral valvular stenosis in the adult is usually always rheumatic in origin. Mitral "stenosis" has been reported to occur secondary to severe annular calcification in patients with small hypertrophied ventricles (see Chap. 16) (69). Mitral valvular stenosis commonly manifests clinically in the third to fourth decade, and studies have reported that the average age of death in patients with mitral stenosis is between 40 and 45 years (70). However, certain patients with mitral stenosis survive into their seventh and eighth decades, with the patient unaware of having the valvular disorder. Limas (71), in an autopsy study, found the incidence of mitral valvular stenosis to be 2.5% in patients older than 65 years; the mean age of the patients was 77 years, and the oldest patient was aged 86 years. Only 35% of the 39 patients with mitral stenosis had a history of rheumatic fever. In 65% of the cases mitral stenosis was the only valvular abnormality. Review of the patients' clinical findings revealed that the typical diastolic murmur of mitral stenosis was detected in only 40% of the patients, although 50% had atrial fibrillation and heart failure was the major clinical manifestation. The average duration of atrial fibrillation before death in these patients was 8 years. Clinical evidence of embolization was noted in 35% of the patients with embolization resulting in a cerebral event in the majority of patients.

Recently, Sherrid and associates (72) reported 18 patients with mitral stenosis in whom the diagnosis was unsuspected until an echocardiogram was performed. The median age of these patients was 72 years; only 1 patient was less than 50 years of age. Of the 18 patients 8 were referred for echocardiogram because of evaluation of heart failure, 3 patients were referred because of cerebral vascular accidents and atrial fibrillation, and 5 patients were referred for aortic valve disease. Before the echocardiogram, a diastolic murmur was not noted in any of the 18 patients. The authors speculated that 7 patients had coexisting conditions besides mitral stenosis that may have obscured the auscultation findings of mitral stenosis, although after the echocardiogram was performed, a diastolic murmur was detected in 8 of the 13 patients examined. The degree of stenosis varied from mild to severe, with a valve area less than or equal to 1.5

$cm^2$ in 8 patients. After evaluation 2 patients underwent mitral valve surgery, with improvement of heart failure, and 3 patients were begun on anticoagulation therapy. An additional 2 patients were offered surgery and balloon valvuloplasty, respectively, but declined.

As noted in these two studies, the diagnosis of mitral stenosis in elderly patients is frequently missed. Occasionally, truly silent mitral stenosis occurs, that is, mitral stenosis without an appreciative apical murmur (73,74). More often, the murmur may be overlooked on examination, especially if there is a low index of suspicion or if other medical conditions are present that complicate the physical examination. If the suspicion is high, even if a diastolic murmur is not detected, echocardiography should be performed, which makes the definitive diagnosis (75,76). In addition, echocardiography and Doppler echocardiography should be able to assess the severity of the stenosis. The elderly patient, especially if the patient is a woman, who presents with atrial fibrillation and demonstrates findings of embolization should arouse suspicions that underlying mitral stenosis may be the etiology of the patient's symptoms. Also, the clinical picture of an elderly patient presenting with pulmonary congestion with radiographic findings of an isolated enlarged left atrium and pulmonary hypertension should alert the physician that mitral stenosis may be present.

As in the younger patient with mitral stenosis, many elderly patients with this valvular disorder can be treated medically. Digitalization usually slows the ventricular heart rate if atrial fibrillation is present, and diuretics control the congestive symptoms. In certain cases, verapamil, diltiazem, or a $\beta$-blocker, in combination with digitalis, may be necessary to slow the heart rate. "Unloading therapy" with vasodilators is not usually considered beneficial in patients with mitral stenosis and may result in a significant decrease in cardiac output (77). Anticoagulation to prevent embolization is considered mandatory in all patients with mitral stenosis who demonstrate atrial fibrillation, and some authorities consider anticoagulation mandatory in all patients with mitral stenosis regardless of the patient's heart rhythm (78). The role of interventional therapy to prevent recurrent embolization in patients with mitral stenosis is controversial. Some authorities recommend valvular surgery or valvuloplasty in all patients with mitral stenosis who have experienced embolization regardless of the severity of the stenosis (79,80). Other authorities favor medical therapy with anticoagulation unless the stenosis is significant or the patient has recurrent embolization while taking anticoagulants (81,82).

## MITRAL VALVE SURGERY AND MITRAL VALVULOPLASTY IN THE ELDERLY

With the significant advances in surgical technology, the improvement in anesthetic agents and techniques, and the improved design of valvular prostheses, valvular surgery is increasingly used in elderly patients with severe mitral valve disease (83,84). Hochberg et al. (85), reporting the National Institute of Health (NIH) experience with mitral valve replacement between 1968 and 1977, found a hospital mortality of 14% in patients aged 60 years or older, compared to a 10% mortality in patients under the age of 60 years. The valvular surgery was classified as performed for pure or predominant mitral stenosis or pure or predominant mitral regurgitation. None of the patients had coronary artery bypass surgery, and the presence of coronary artery disease was not discussed. Indicators for surgery did not differ between the age groups; patients with symptoms of mitral valve disease were considered for operation if they were unable to maintain an acceptable life-style despite optimal medical therapy. Late cardiac death at a mean follow-up of 54 months occurred in 14% of older patients and 17% of younger patients. These early and late deaths were not significantly different between the age groups, although the hospital mortality rate for elderly patients in the predominantly mitral regurgitation subgroup was considerably higher than that of younger patients (22 versus 6%). Also, approximately 25% of the total elderly patients sustained postoperative strokes, and two elderly patients had pulmonary embolism. The authors concluded that mitral valve surgery could be performed in selective elderly patients, as well as younger patients, and the results were encouraging.

The results of the NIH study are comparable to the results of earlier studies of cardiac surgery in the elderly, which have demonstrated operative mortality in mitral valve surgery to range from 0 to 20%, with late deaths from 0 to 16% (Table 2) (86,89). A more recent study from the University of Toronto (90) reported an operative mortality of 15.1% in patients 70 years or older having mitral valve surgery (both replacement and repair), compared to a mortality of 4.5% in patients under the age of 70 years; the results were significantly different. Significant predictors of increased operative mortality for the older patients were urgent surgery, presence of coronary artery disease, whether grafted or nongrafted, female gender, and depressed left ventricular function. Coronary artery bypass surgery was associated with improved results, as opposed to nongrafting. In this study there was no significant difference in operative mortality between mitral valve replacement or repair in the elderly patients. This finding was unexpected: most studies have demonstrated reduced mortality with mitral valve repair compared to valve replacement whether the etiology of the valvular lesion is rheumatic (61), myxomatous (62), or ischemic (63).

In the last few years a number of studies (91–94) of valvular heart surgery in octogenarians have been reported (Table 3). In most of the studies the mitral valve surgery was performed in conjunction with coronary bypass surgery, and in some cases, emergency surgery was necessary. The number of patients having mitral valve surgery was small, and the operative mortality was variable, ranging from 16 to 35%, with a 66% operative mortality reported in certain

**Table 2** Mitral Valve Surgery in the Elderly

| Study | Year | Number of patients | Age (years) | Early deaths (%)[a] | Late deaths (%)[b] |
|---|---|---|---|---|---|
| Hochberg et al. (85) | 1979 | 43 | ≥60 | 14 | 14 |
| Bessone et al. (88) | 1977 | 14 | ≥70 | 0 | 0 |
| Shanahan et al. (86) | 1975 | 31 | ≥60 | 23 | 16 |
| Barnhorst et al. (89) | 1974 | 60 | >65 | 20 | — |
| Oh et al. (87) | 1973 | 22 | ≥60 | 18 | 14 |

[a] Death occurring during hospitalization.
[b] All deaths occurring during follow-up, which varied from 1 to 72 months.
*Source*: Adapted from Hochberg et al. (85).

cases (91) when emergency operation with mitral valve replacement or repair plus coronary bypass grafting was necessary. Mortality from mitral valve surgery was higher than the mortality associated with aortic valve surgery or isolated coronary artery bypass surgery. Even though operative mortality was high in these very old patients compared to younger patients, most of the very old patients had improvement in functional class following surgery and were assessed to benefit from the surgery. The conclusion of the investigators was that operative intervention can be a reasonable therapeutic option in very old patients with advanced valvular disease in whom medical therapy had failed.

**Table 3** Mitral Valve Surgery in Octogenarians

| Study | Intervention | Number of patients | Early deaths | Late deaths |
|---|---|---|---|---|
| Rich et al. (92) | MVR + CAB[a] | 4 | 1 | 0 |
| Freeman et al. (91) | MVR + CAB | 21 | 6 | — |
| Edmunds et al. (94) | MVR | 3 | 0 | 2 |
| Edmunds et al. (94) | MVR + CAB | 1 | 1 | — |
| Tsai et al. (93) | MVR | 2 | 1 | 0 |
| Tsai et al. (93) | MVR + CAB[a] | 8 | 3 | 3 |
| Tsai et al. (93) | MV repair + CAB | 2 | 0 | 0 |
| Freeman et al. (91) | MVR + CAB[b] | 6 | 4 | — |

CAB = coronary artery bypass; MVR = mitral valve replacement.
[a] Surgery included both urgent and elective procedures.
[b] All surgery was emergency.

In elderly patients with pure mitral stenosis and a critical valve area of 1.0 $cm^2$, interventional therapy is necessary. Rather than mitral valve replacement, open mitral commissurotomy may be an option in certain elderly patients with mitral stenosis. Open commissurotomy in this age is usually quite low, less than 5% (95). Unfortunately, the majority of stenotic valves in this age group are usually calcified and severely deformed, with associated significant mitral incompetence; thus valve replacement is the surgery of choice.

Recently, percutaneous balloon valvotomy has become another interventional therapy in treating patients with critical mitral valve stenosis. Since the first balloon dilatation for mitral stenosis was described in 1984 by Inoue et al. (96), the technique has become increasing popular. Initially, the intervention was used in young patients with pliant valves and then used successfully in middle-aged patients. As expected with an intervention that does not require general anesthesia or thoracotomy and may be performed in patients with general debilitating conditions, percutaneous mitral balloon valvotomy has been used in elderly patients with critical mitral valve stenosis. Unfortunately, many elderly patients demonstrate clinical and mitral valvular characteristics (atrial fibrillation and calcified leaflets), which are not conducive to good results with valvotomy; however, it has been shown that mitral balloon valvotomy can be an attractive alternative to surgical therapy in certain elderly patients with critical mitral valve stenosis.

Shaw and associates (97) reported 20 patients, all over 70 years of age (mean age 74.2), who underwent mitral valvotomy. In addition to their mitral valve disorder, all patients had at least one additional cardiac, respiratory, or general medical problem; 10 of the 20 patients had been judged unsuitable for an operation by a cardiac surgeon. Valvular dilatation was achieved in 17 of the 20 patients, and no procedure-related morbidity occurred. Of the 17 patients in whom dilatation was achieved, 15 showed syptomatic improvement at 1 month postvalvuloplasty, and at 1 year, 10 patients maintained this improvement.

More recently, three other studies (98–100) have reported percutaneous mitral valvotomy in elderly patients. Goicolea and associates (98), when comparing 39 patients 65 years or older to 196 patients younger than 65 years, found elderly patients were more functionally impaired before the valvotomy and had more severe valve deformities. There was no difference in procedure complications, however, and improvement was comparable in the two age groups; at 6 months follow-up 92% of the younger patients and 91% of the elderly patients demonstrated improvement in cardiac functional state compared to the prevalvotomy state. In a multicenter study, Feldman and associates (99) found, as in the Goicolea group's study, that patients aged 75 years or older (mean age 81 years) who had mitral valvotomy demonstrated more functional impairment before the procedure compared to younger patients, and their valves were more seriously deformed. In this study failed procedures were more common in the elderly patients, although the mitral valve area increased 50% or more in 68% of the elderly patients.

In one of the largest series of elderly patients (65 years or older, mean age 72) who have had mitral valvotomy, Tuzcu and associates (100) found that a successful outcome (defined as mitral valve area of 1.5 $cm^2$ or greater without a two-grade increase in mitral regurgitation and without left-to-right shunt, with a pulmonary-to-system flow ratio of 1.5:1 or greater) was achieved in 46 (46%) of 99 patients. As in the other studies, before the valvotomy the majority of elderly patients were severely functionally impaired, with approximately 85% of the patients in NYHA functional class III or IV, and 37 patients had at least two or more comorbidities; 15 patients had four or more comorbidities. In the majority of patients the mitral valve was severely deformed, with significant valvular calcification, before the valvotomy. Of the 99 patients 3 died of causes related to the procedure; all deaths occurred early in the authors' experience with percutaneous valvotomy. During the follow-up period 14 patients underwent mitral valve replacement. The operative mortality of these 14 patients was 14%. The majority of patients were functionally improved compared to their prevalvotomy state, with 66% of the patients in NYHA functional class I or II. The actuarial survivals with freedom from mitral valve replacement and with freedom from NYHA functional class III or IV of the patients at 1, 2, and 3 years were 72, 53, and 46%, respectively. The authors concluded that because of the severely deformed mitral valve morphology commonly seen in elderly patients with mitral stenosis, valvotomy may be less anatomically successful than in younger patients undergoing valvotomy. The majority of elderly patients will be clinically improved, however, and mitral valvotomy appears to be an excellent therapy for certain elderly patients with symptomatic mitral stenosis. Selection of therapy must be made on an individual basis.

## REFERENCES

1. Pomerance A. Aging changes in human heart valves. *Br Heart J* 1967; 29:222–226.
2. McMillan JB, Lev M. The aging heart. I. Endocardium. *J Gerontol* 1959; 14:268–283.
3. Bloor CM. Valvular heart disease in the elderly. *J Am Geriatr Soc* 1982; 30:466–472.
4. Robert WC. The senile cardiac calcification syndrome. *Am J Cardiol* 1986; 58:572–574.
5. Pomerance A. Ballooning deformity (mucoid degeneration) of the atrioventricular valves. *Br Heart J* 1969; 31:343–348.
6. Procacci PM, Savran SV, Schreiter SL, Bryson AL. Prevalence of clinical mitral valve prolapse in 1169 young women. *N Engl J Med* 1976; 294:1086–1088.
7. Hickey AJ, Wolfers J, Wilcken DEL. Mitral valve prolapse: Prevalence in an Australian population. *Med J Aust* 1981; 1:31–33.
8. Bloch A, Vignola PA, Walker H, et al. Echocardiographic spectrum of posterior systolic motion of the mitral valve in the general population. *J Clin Ultrasound* 1977; 5:243–247.

9. Markiewicz W, Stoner J, London E, et al. Mitral valve prolapse in 100 presumably health young females. *Circulation* 1976; 53:464–473.
10. Davies MJ, Moore BP, Braimbridge MV. The floppy mitral valve. Study of incidence, pathology and complications in surgical, necropsy and forensic material. *Br Heart J* 1978; 40:468–481.
11. O'Rourke RA, Crawford MH. The systolic click-murmur syndrome: Clinical recognition and management. *Curr Probl Cardiol* 1976; 1:1–60.
12. Cabeen WR Jr, Reza MJ, Kovick RB, Stern MS. Mitral valve prolapse and conduction defects in Ehlers-Danlos syndrome. *Arch Intern Med* 1977; 137:1227–1231.
13. Sanyal SK, Johnson WW, Dische MR, Pitner ES, Beard C. Dystrophic degeneration of papillary muscle and ventricular myocardium. A basic for mitral valve prolapse in Duchenne's muscular dystrophy. *Circulation* 1980; 62:430–431.
14. Rippe JM, Sloss LJ, Angoff G, Alpert JS. Mitral valve prolapse in adults with congenital heart disease. *Am Heart J* 1979; 97:561–573.
15. Weinrauch LA, McDonald DC, DeSilva RA, Hawkins ET, Leland OS, Shubrooks SJ. Mitral prolapse in rheumatic mitral stenosis. *Chest* 1977; 72:752–756.
16. Devereux RB, Perloff JK, Reichek N, Josephson MD. Mitral valve prolapse. *Circulation* 1976; 54:3–14.
17. Hickey AJ, Wilcken DEL. Age and the clinical profile of idiopathic mitral valve prolapse. *Br Heart J* 1986; 55:582–586.
18. Ansari A. The straight back syndrome, current perspective: More often associated with valvular heart disease than pseudoheart disease. *Clin Cardiol* 1985; 8:290–305.
19. Lobstein HP, Horwitz LD, Curry GC, Mullins CB. Electrocardiographic abnormalities and coronary arteriograms in the mitral click-murmur syndrome. *N Engl J Med* 1973; 289:127–131.
20. Pocock WA, Barlow JB. Etiology and electrocardiographic features of the billowing posterior mitral leaflet syndrome. *Am J Med* 1971; 51:731–739.
21. Popp RL, Brown OR, Silverman JF, Harrison DC. Echocardiographic abnormalities in the mitral valve prolapse syndrome. *Circulation* 1974; 49:428–433.
22. DeMaria AN, King JF, Bogren HG, Lies JE, Mason DT. The variable spectrum of echocardiographic manifestations of the mitral prolapse syndrome. *Circulation* 1974; 50:33–41.
23. Savage DD, Garrison RJ, Devereaux RB, et al. Mitral valve prolapse in the general population. I. Epidemiologic features: The Framingham Study. *Am Heart J* 1983; 106:571–576.
24. Waller BF, Morrow AG, Maron BJ, et al. Etiology of clinically isolated, severe, chronic, pure mitral regurgitation: Analysis of 97 patients over 30 years of age having mitral valve replacement. *Am Heart J* 1982; 104:276–288.
25. Jeresaty RM. Mitral valve prolapse-click syndrome. *Prog Cardiovasc Dis* 1973; 15:623–652.
26. Devereaux RB, Kramer-Fox R, Browne T. Relation between clinical features of the mitral valve prolapse syndrome and echocardiographically documented mitral valve prolapse. *J Am Coll Cardiol* 1986; 8:763–772.

27. Savage DD, Devereaux RB, Garrison RJ, et al. Mitral valve prolapse in the general population. II. Clinical features: The Framingham Study. *Am Heart J* 1983; 106:577–581.
28. Fontana ME, Pence HL, Leighton RF, Wooley CF. The varying clinical spectrum of the systolic click-late systolic murmur. *Circulation* 1970; 41:807–816.
29. Barlow JB, Bosman CK, Pocock WA, Merchand P. Late systolic murmur and nonejection (mid-late) systolic clicks: An analysis of 90 patients. *Br Heart J* 1968; 30:203–218.
30. Levy D, Savage DD. Prevalence and clinical features of mitral valve prolapse. *Am Heart J* 1987; 113:1281–1290.
31. Tresch DD, Siegel R, Keelan MH Jr, Gross CM, Brooks HL. Mitral valve prolapse in the elderly. *J Am Geriatr Soc* 1979; 27:421–424.
32. Higgins CB, Reinke RT, Gosink BB, Leopold GR. The significance of mitral valve prolapse in middle-aged and elderly men. *Am Heart J* 1976; 91:292–296.
33. Kolibash AJ, Bush CA, Fontana MB, Ryan JM, Kilman J, Wooley CF. Mitral valve prolapse syndrome: Analysis of 62 patients aged 60 years and older. *Am J Cardiol* 1983; 52:534–539.
34. Tresch DD, Doyle TP, Boncheck LI, Siegel R, Keelan MH Jr, Olinger GN, Brooks HL. Mitral valve prolapse requiring surgery. *Am J Med* 1985; 78:245–250.
35. Collins R, Cotton RE, Duff RS. Symptomatic mitral myxomatous transformation in the elderly. *Thorax* 1976; 31:765–770.
36. Jeresaty RM, Edwards JE, Chawla SK. Mitral valve prolapse and ruptured chordae tendineae. *Am J Cardiol* 1985; 55:138–142.
37. Cooley DA, Gerami S, Hallman GL, Wukasch DC, Hall RJ. Mitral insufficiency due to myxomatous transformation: "Floppy valve syndrome." *J Cardiovasc Surg* 1972; 13:346–349.
38. Salomon NW, Stinson EB, Griepp RB, Shumway NE. Surgical treatment of degenerative mitral regurgitation. *Am J Cardiol* 1976; 38:463–468.
39. Wilcken DEL, Hickey AJ. Lifetime risk for patients with mitral valve prolapse of developing severe valve regurgitation requiring surgery. *Circulation* 1988; 78:10–14.
40. Singh R, Schrank JP, Nolan SP, McQuire LB. Spontaneous rupture of mitral chordae tendinae. *JAMA* 1972; 219:189–193.
41. Clemens JD, Horwitz RI, Jaffe CC, et al. A controlled evaluation of the risk of bacterial endocarditis in persons with mitral valve prolapse. *N Engl J Med* 1982; 307:776–781.
42. Lachman AS, Bramnell-Jones DM, Lakier JB, Pocock WA, Barlow JB. Infective endocarditis in the billowing mitral leaflet. *Br Heart J* 1975; 37:326–330.
43. Danchin N, Voiriot P, Bariancon S, Bairati I, Mathieu P, Deschamps JP, Dureux JB, Cherrier F. Mitral valve prolapse as a risk factor for infective endocarditis. *Lancet* 1989; 1:743–745.
44. McMahon SW, Roberts JK, Kramer-Fox R, Zucker DM, Roberts RG, Devereux RB. Mitral valve prolapse and infective endocarditis. *Am Heart J* 1987; 113:1291–1298.

45. McMahon SW, Hickey AJ, Wilcken DEL, Wittes JT, Feneley MP, Hickie JB. Risk of infective endocarditis in mitral valve prolapse with and without precordial systolic murmurs. *Am J Cardiol* 1987; 58:105–108.
46. Dajani AS, Bisno AL, Chung KJ, Durack DT, et al. Prevention of bacterial endocarditis. *JAMA* 1990; 264:2919–2922.
47. Sandok BA, Guiliani ER. Cerebral ischemic events in patients with mitral valve prolapse. *Stroke* 1982; 13:448–450.
48. Watson RT. TIA, stroke, and mitral valve prolapse. *Neurology* 1979; 29:886–889.
49. Barnett HJM, Boughner DR, Taylor DW, Cooper RE, Kostuk WJ, Nichol PM. Further evidence relating mitral valve prolapse to cerebral ischemic events. *N Engl J Med* 1980; 302:139–144.
50. Kostuk WJ, Boughner DR, Barnett HJM, Silver MD. Strokes: A complication of mitral-leaflet prolapse? *Lancet* 1977; 1:313–316.
51. Scharf RE, Hennerici M, Bluschice V, Lueck J, Kladetzky RG. Cerebral ischemia in young patients—is it associated with mitral valve prolapse and abnormal platelet activity in vitro? *Stroke* 1982 13:454–458.
52. Hart RG, Easton JD. Mitral valve prolapse and cerebral infarction. *Stroke* 1982; 13:429–430.
53. Hargreaves I. Rheumatic mitral valve disease in the elderly: Incidence found at autopsy. *Br Med J* 1961; 2:342.
54. Bedford PD, Caird FI. Valvular Disease of the Heart in Old Age. Churchill Livingstone, Edinburgh, 1960.
55. Gersh BJ, Kronmal RA, Frye RL, et al. Coronary arteriography and coronary artery bypass surgery: Morbidity and mortality in patients ages 65 years or older. A report from the Coronary Artery Surgery Study. *Circulation* 1983; 67:483–491.
56. Czer LS, Gray RJ, DeRobertis MA, et al. Mitral valve replacement: Impact of coronary artery disease and determinants of prognosis after revascularization. *Circulation* 1984; 70(Suppl. I):198–207.
57. Stephenson LW, McVaugh MH III, Edmunds LH Jr. Surgery using cardiopulmonary bypass in the elderly. *Circulation* 1978; 58:250–254.
58. Sethi GK, Miller CD, Souchek J, Oprian C, Henderson WG, Hassal Z, Folland E, Khuri S, Stewart SM, Burchfield C, Hammermeister KE. Clinical, hemodynamic and angiographic predictors of operative mortality in patients undergoing single valve replacement. *J Thorac Cardiovasc Surg* 1987; 93:884–897.
59. Loop FD, Lytle BW, Cosgrove DM, et al. Coronary artery bypass graft surgery in the elderly: Indications and outcome. *Cleve Clin J Med* 1988; 55:23–24.
60. Scott WC, Miller DC, Haverich A, Mitchell RS, Oyer PE, Stinson EB, Jamieson SW, Baldwin JC, Shumway NE. Operative risk of mitral valve replacement: Discriminant analysis of 1,329 procedures. *Circulation* 1985; 72(Suppl. II):108–119.
61. Duran CG, Pomar JL, Reveuelta JM, Gallo I, Poveda J, Ochoteco A, Ubago JL. Conservative operation for mitral insufficiency. *J Thorac Cardiovasc Surg* 1980; 79:326–337.

62. Reed GE, Pooley RW, Moggio RA. Durability of measured mitral annuloplasty, seventeen year study. *J Thorac Cardiovasc Surg* 1980; 79:321–325.
63. Kay GL, Kay JH, Zubiate P, Yokoyama T, Mendez M. Mitral valve repair for mitral regurgitation secondary to coronary artery disease. *Circulation* 1986; 74(Suppl. I):88–98.
64. Crawford MH, Souchek J, Oprian CA, et al. Determinants of survival and left ventricular performance after mitral valve replacement. *Circulation* 1990; 81:1173–1181.
65. Hwang MH, Hammermeister KE, Oprian C, et al. Preoperative identification of patients likely to have left ventricular dysfunction after aortic valve replacement. *Circulation* 80(Suppl. I):65–76.
66. Breisblatt W, Goodyer AVN, Zaret BL, et al. An improved index of left ventricular function in chronic mitral regurgitation. *Am J Cardiol* 1986; 57:1105–1108.
67. Waggoner AD, Kumpuris AG, Shah AA, et al. Determinants of post-operative regression of left ventricular dilatation in chronic mitral regurgitation. *Circulation* 1979; 60(Suppl. II):38.
68. Phillips HR, Levine FH, Carter JE, et al. Mitral valve replacement for isolated mitral regurgitation: Analysis of clinical course and late postoperative left ventricular ejection fraction. *Am J Cardiol* 1981; 48:647–654.
69. Hammer WJ, Roberts WC, deLeon AC. "Mitral stenosis" secondary to combined "massive" mitral annular calcific deposits and small, hypertrophied left ventricles. *Am J Med* 1978; 64:371–376.
70. Kaufman P, Poliakoff H. Studies on aging heart. Pattern of rheumatic heart disease in old age (clinical pathological study). *Ann Intern Med* 1950; 32:889–904.
71. Limas CJ. Mitral stenosis in the elderly. *Geriatrics* 1971; 26:75–79.
72. Sherrid M, Goyal A, Delia E, Khoo G, Heropoulos M, McCabe JB, Dwyer EM Jr. Unsuspected mitral stenosis. *Am J Med* 1991; 90:189–192.
73. Likoff W, Segal B, Kaspar A, Kasparian H, Novack P. Silent rheumatic valvular heart disease. *Dis Chest* 1966; 49:362–364.
74. Proctor HW. Silent valvular heart disease. In: Cardiovascular Clinics, vol. 5. Philadelphia: FA Davis, 1973; 5:77–83.
75. Weyman AE. Cross-Sectional Echocardiography. Philadelphia: Lea & Febiger, 1982:139–174.
76. Feigenbaum H. Echocardiography, 4th ed. Philadelphia: Lea & Febiger, 1986:249–262.
77. Cohn JN. Drug Treatment of Heart Failure, 2nd ed. Secaucus, NJ: Advanced Therapeutics Communications International, 1988:209.
78. Braunwald E. Valvular heart disease. In: Heart Disease: A Textbook of Cardiovascular Medicine, 3rd ed. Philadelphia: W. B. Saunders, 1983:1031.
79. McHenry MM. Systemic arterial embolism in patients with mitral stenosis and minimal dyspnea. *Am J Cardiol* 1966; 18:169–174.
80. Braunwald E. Valvular heart disease. In: Braunwald E, ed. Heart Disease: A Textbook of Cardiovascular Medicine, 3rd ed. Philadelphia: W. B. Saunders, 1988:1032.

81. Siegel R, Tresch DD, Keelan MH Jr, Brooks HL. Effects of anticoagulation on recurrent systemic emboli in mitral stenosis. *Am J Cardiol* 1987; 60:1191–1192.
82. Abernathy WS, Willis PW. Thromboembolic complications of rheumatic heart disease. In: Breast AN, Likoff W, eds. Valvular Heart Disease: Cardiovascular Clinics. Philadelphia: F. A. Davis, 1973:131–176.
83. Levinson JR, Akins CW, Buckley MJ, et al. Octogenarians with aortic stenosis: Outcome after aortic valve replacement. *Circulation* 1989; 80(Suppl. I):49–56.
84. Canepa-Anson R, Emanual RW. Elective aortic and mitral valve surgery in patients over 70 years of age. *Br Heart J* 1979; 41:493–497.
85. Hochberg MS, Derkac WM, Conkle DM, McIntosh CL, Epstein SE, Morrow AG. Mitral valve replacement in elderly patients. Encouraging postoperative clinical and hemodynamic results. *J Thorac Cardiovasc Surg* 1979; 77:422–426.
86. Shanahan MY, Windsor HM, Golding L. Open heart surgery in the elderly. *Aust N Z J Surg* 1972; 42:107–112.
87. Oh W, Hickman R, Emanual R, McDonald L, Somerville J, Ross D, Ross K, Gonzalez-Lavin L. Heart valve surgery in 114 patients over the age of 60. *Br Heart J* 1973; 35:174–180.
88. Bessone LN, Pupello DF, Blank RH, Harrison EE, Sbar S. Valve replacement in patients over 70 years. *Ann Thorac Surg* 1977; 24:417–421.
89. Barnhorst DA, Giuliani ER, Pluth JR, Danielson GK, Wallace RB, McGoon DC. Open heart surgery in patients more than 65 years old. *Ann Thorac Surg* 1974; 18:81–90.
90. Fremes SE, Goldman BS, Ivanov J, Weisel RD, David TE, Salerno T. Valvular surgery in the elderly. *Circulation* 1989; 80(Suppl. I):77–90.
91. Freeman WK, Schaff HV, O'Brien PC, Orszulak TA, Naessens JM, Tajik AJ. Cardiac surgery in the octogenarian: Perioperative outcome and clinical follow-up. *J Am Coll Cardiol* 1991; 18:29–35.
92. Rich MW, Sandza JG, Kleiger RE, Connors JP. Cardiac operations in patients over 80 years of age. *J Thorac Cardiovasc Surg* 1985; 90:56–60.
93. Tsai TP, Matloff JM, Gray RJ, Chaux A, Kass RM, Lee ME, Czer LSC. Cardiac surgery in the octogenarian. *J Thorac Cardiovasc Surg* 1986; 91:924–928.
94. Edmunds LH Jr, Stephenson LW, Edie RN, Ratcliffe MB. Open-heart surgery in octogenarians. *N Engl J Med* 1988; 319:131–136.
95. Jamieson WRE, Dooner J, Munro AI, Janusz MT, Burgess JJ, Miyagishima RR, Gerein AN, Allen P. Cardiac valve replacement in the elderly: A review of 320 consecutive cases. *Circulation* 1981; 64(Suppl. II):177–183.
96. Inoue K, Owaki T, Nakamura T, Kitamura F, Miyamoto N. Clinical application of transvenous mitral commissurotomy by a new balloon catheter. *J Thorac Cardiovasc Surg* 1984; 87:394–402.
97. Shaw TRD, Elder AT, Flapan AD, Essop AR. Mitral balloon valvotomy for patients aged over 70 years: An alternative to surgical treatment. *Age Aging* 1991; 20:299–303.
98. Goicolea J, Macaya C, Hernandez R, et al. Immediate results and clinical follow-up of percutaneous mitral valvotomy in elderly patients. *J Am Coll Cardiol* 1992; 19:378A.

99. Feldman T, Carroll JD, Bashore TM, et al. Inoue balloon mitral valvotomy on patients age 75 or older. *J Am Coll Cardiol* 1992; 19:363A.
100. Tuzcu EM, Block PC, Griffin BP, Newell JB, Palacios IF. Immediate and long-term outcome of percutaneous mitral valvotomy in patients 65 years and older. *Circulation* 1992; 85:963–971.
101. Boudoulash, Wolley CF. Mitral valve prolapse. In: Liu PN, Goodwin JF, eds. Progress in Cardiology, No. 14. Philadelphia: Lea & Febiger, 1986; 275–304.
102. Tresch DD, Siegel R. Mitral valve prolapse: How to recognize this common disorder. *Prim Cardiol* 1976; 2:8–12.
103. Tresch DD. Atypical presentations of cardiovascular disorders in the elderly. *Geriatrics* 1987; 42:31–44.
104. Ranganathan N, Silver MD, Robinson TI, Kostuk WJ, Felderhof CH, Patt NL, Wilson JK, Wigle ED. Angiographic–morphologic correlation in patients with severe mitral regurgitation due to prolapse of the posterior mitral valve leaflet. *Circulation* 1973; 48:514–518.

# 16

# Mitral Annular Calcium in the Elderly

**Wilbert S. Aronow**
*Mount Sinai School of Medicine, New York, New York and Hebrew Hospital Home, Bronx, New York*

**Chandra K. Nair**
*Creighton University School of Medicine, Omaha, Nebraska*

## INTRODUCTION

Mitral annular calcium (MAC) is a chronic degenerative process that is common in elderly persons, especially women. The amount of calcium may vary from a few spicules to a large mass behind the posterior cusp, often extending to form a ridge or ring encircling the mitral leaflets, occasionally lifting the leaflets toward the left atrium. Sphincter function loss of the mitral annulus and mechanical stretching of the mitral leaflets can cause improper coaptation of the leaflets during systole, resulting in mitral regurgitation (1). Although the calcific mass may immobilize the mitral valve, actual calcification of the leaflets is rare. In patients with severe MAC, the calcification may extend inward to involve the underside of the leaflets. Mitral stenosis may result from severe calcific deposits within the mitral annulus protruding into the orifice (2,3). Calcific deposits may extend from the mitral annulus into the membranous portions of the ventricular septum, involving the conduction system and causing rhythm and conduction disturbances (4–6). Although the annular calcium is covered with a layer of endothelium, ulceration of this lining can expose the underlying calcific deposits, which may serve as a nidus for platelet-fibrin aggregation and subsequent thromboembolic episodes (7–9). In patients with endocarditis associated with MAC, the avascular nature of the mitral annulus predisposes to periannular and myocardial abscesses (10–13).

## PREVALENCE

MAC is a degenerative process that increases with age and occurs more frequently in women than in men (7,14–23). In a prospective study of 976 unselected elderly persons in a long-term health care facility, mean age 82 ± 8 years (range 62–103 years), with technically adequate M-mode and two-dimensional echocardiograms of the mitral valve, MAC was present in 402 of 714 women (56%) and in 124 of 262 men (47%) (23). Table 1 shows the prevalence of MAC with increasing age in elderly men and elderly women (21).

## PREDISPOSING FACTORS

Because calcific deposits in the mitral annulus, in the aortic valve cusps, and in the epicardial coronary arteries are commonly associated in elderly persons and have similar predisposing factors, Roberts (17) suggested that MAC and aortic cuspal calcium are a form of atherosclerosis. MAC and aortic cuspal calcium may coexist (1,7,17–19,24–26). Breakdown of lipid deposits on the ventricular surface of the posterior mitral leaflet at or below the mitral annulus and on the aortic surfaces of the aortic valve cusps is probably responsible for the calcification (1). Increased left ventricular systolic pressure due to aortic valve stenosis increases stress on the mitral apparatus and may accelerate development of MAC (1,7,19,20,26). Tricuspid annular calcium and MAC may also coexist and have similar predisposing factors (27).

Systemic hypertension increases with age and predisposes to MAC (1,7,18,19,24,25,28). Persons with diabetes mellitus also have a higher prevalence of MAC than nondiabetic persons (1,19,24,25). MAC occurs in the teens in persons with serum total cholesterol levels > 500 mg/dl (29). Waller and Roberts (19) suggested that hypercholesterolemia predisposes to MAC. The

**Table 1** Prevalence of Mitral Annular Calcium with Increasing Age in Elderly Men and in Elderly Women

| | Mitral annular calcium | | | |
|---|---|---|---|---|
| | Men | | Women | |
| Age (years) | *n* | (%) | *n* | (%) |
| 62–70 | 4/22 | (18) | 7/35 | (20) |
| 71–80 | 13/42 | (31) | 40/116 | (34) |
| 81–90 | 44/75 | (59) | 146/226 | (65) |
| 91–100 | 19/22 | (86) | 56/63 | (89) |
| 101–103 | — | — | 3/3 | (100) |

*Source*: Adapted from Aronow et al. (21).

prevalence of hypercholesterolemia with a serum total cholesterol ⩾ 200 mg/dl was higher in elderly persons with MAC than in elderly persons without MAC (25). Roberts (8) also stated that MAC is rare in elderly persons residing in areas of the world where serum total cholesterol levels are < 150 mg/dl. However, Nair et al. (24) found no significant difference in mean serum total cholesterol level between persons younger than 60 years with MAC and a control group.

Roberts and Waller (30) found that chronic hypercalcemia predisposes to MAC. Patients undergoing dialysis for chronic renal insufficiency have an increased prevalence of MAC (30–35). Cardiac calcium in patients with chronic renal failure has been attributed to secondary hyperparathyroidism (32,35). Nair et al. (24) demonstrated a similar mean serum calcium, a higher mean serum phosphorus, and a higher mean product of serum calcium and phosphorus in patients younger than 60 years with MAC than in a control group. However, Aronow et al. (25) observed no significant difference in mean serum calcium, serum phosphorus, or product of serum calcium and phosphorus between elderly persons with and without MAC.

By accelerating left ventricular systolic pressure, hypertrophic cardiomyopathy predisposes to MAC (1). Kronzon and Glassman (36) diagnosed MAC in 12 of 18 patients (67%) older than 55 years with hypertrophic cardiomyopathy and in 4 of 28 patients (14%) younger than 55 years with hypertrophic cardiomyopathy. Nair et al. (37) found MAC in 12 of 42 patients (27%) with hypertrophic cardiomyopathy. Their patients with both MAC and hypertrophic cardiomyopathy were older than their patients with hypertrophic cardiomyopathy and no MAC. Motamed and Roberts (38) demonstrated MAC in 30 of 100 autopsy patients (30%) with hypertrophic cardiomyopathy older than 40 years and in none of 100 autopsy patients (0%) younger than 40 years with hypertrophic cardiomyopathy. Aronow and Kronzon (39) diagnosed MAC in 13 of 17 elderly persons (76%) with hypertrophic cardiomyopathy and in 176 of 362 elderly persons (49%) without hypertrophic cardiomyopathy.

## DIAGNOSIS

Calcific deposits in the mitral annulus are J, C, U, or O shaped and are visualized in the posterior third of the heart shadow (7,16,31,40–46). MAC may be diagnosed by chest x-ray films or by fluoroscopy (46). However, the procedures of choice for diagnosing MAC are M-mode and two-dimensional echocardiography.

Posterior MAC (Fig. 1) is diagnosed by M-mode echocardiography when a band of dense echoes is recorded anterior to the left ventricular posterior wall and moving parallel with it (47). These echoes end at the atrioventricular junc-

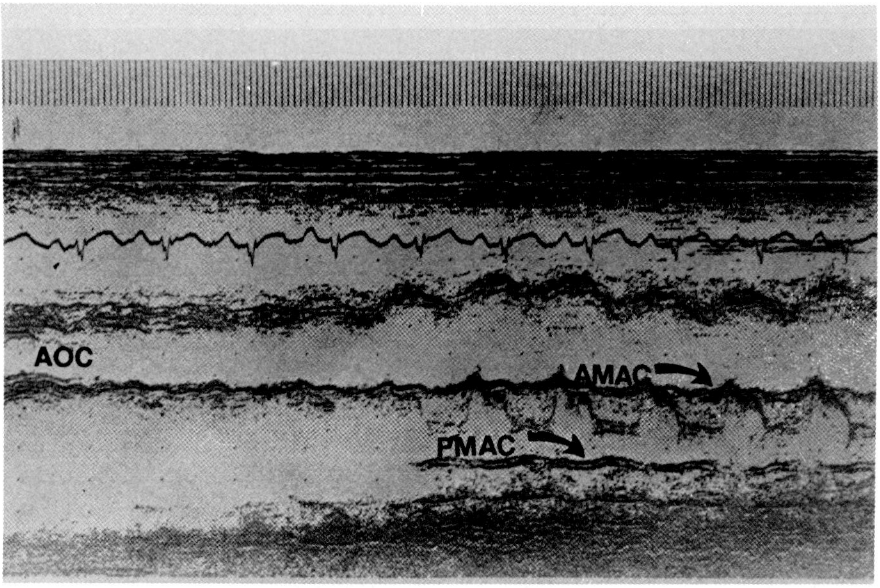


**Figure 1** M-mode echocardiogram with scan from the aortic root to the left ventricular apex in a patient with both anterior and posterior mitral annular calcium. AOC = aortic calcium; AMAC = anterior mitral annular calcium; PMAC = posterior mitral annular calcium.

tion and merge with the left ventricular posterior wall on echocardiographic sweep from the aortic root to the left ventricular apex.

Anterior MAC (Fig. 1) is diagnosed by M-mode echocardiography when a continuous band of dense echoes is observed at the level of the anterior mitral leaflet in both systole and diastole (47). These echoes are contiguous with the posterior wall of the aortic root. Calcification may extend from the mitral annulus throughout the base of the heart and into the mitral and aortic valves.

Figures 2 and 3 are two-dimensional echocardiograms showing increased echogenicity and brightness of the mitral annulus characteristic of MAC. Using multiple echocardiographic views, MAC may be classified as mild, moderate, or severe (48). The echo densities in mild MAC involve less than one-third of the annular circumference (<3 mm in width) and are usually restricted to the angle between the posterior leaflet of the mitral valve and the left ventricular posterior wall. The echo densities in moderate MAC involve less than two-thirds of the annular circumference (3–5 mm in width). The echo densities in severe MAC involve more than two-thirds of the annular circumference (>5

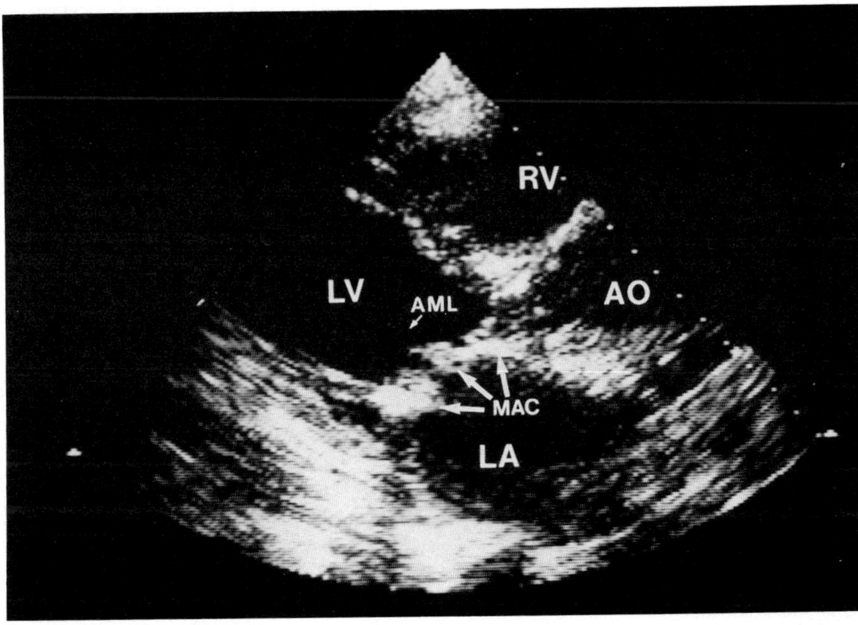


**Figure 2** Two-dimensional echocardiogram long-axis view depicting mitral annual calcium (MAC). LA = left atrium; LV = left ventricle; RV = right ventricle; AO = aorta; AML = anterior mitral leaflet.

mm in width), usually extending beneath the entire posterior mitral leaflet with or without making a complete circle.

MAC was mentioned in the original radiological report in 3 of 8 patients (38%) with MAC diagnosed at autopsy (16). Schott et al. (31) detected MAC by chest x-ray films in 2 of 41 patients (5%) with MAC diagnosed by echocardiography. Dashkoff et al. (49) detected MAC by chest x-ray films in 5 of 8 patients (63%) with MAC diagnosed by echocardiography.

In a blinded prospective study, MAC was diagnosed by M-mode and two-dimensional echocardiography in 55% of 604 unselected elderly patients in a longer-term health care facility (46). Table 2 shows that the diagnosis of MAC by chest x-ray films using a lateral chest x-ray in addition to the posterior–anterior or anterior–posterior chest x-ray had a sensitivity of 12%, a specificity of 99%, a positive predictive value of 95%, and a negative predictive value of 47%. Patients with radiographic MAC were more likely than patients without radiographic MAC to have a more severe form of the disease, with significant mitral regurgitation, functional mitral stenosis, or conduction defects. However,

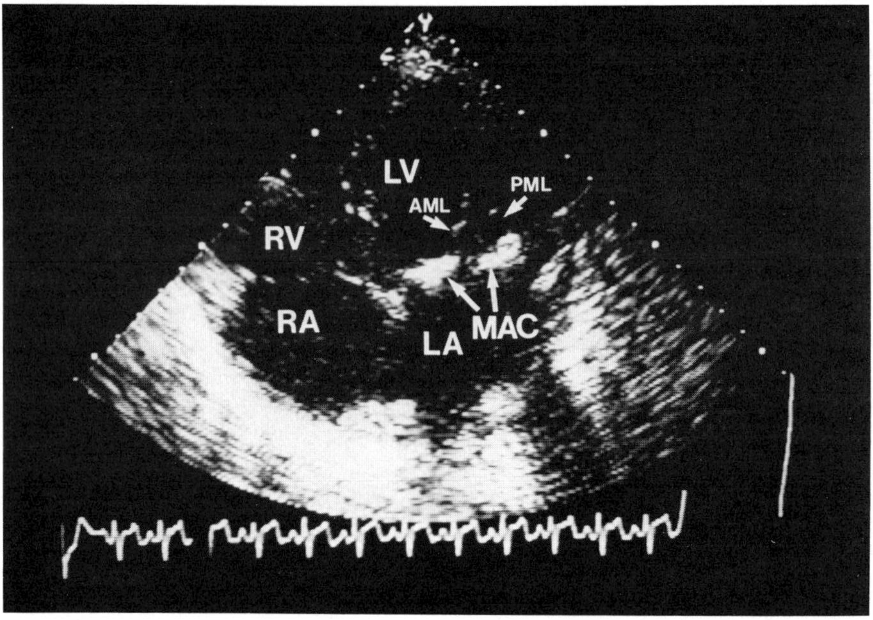


**Figure 3** Two-dimensional echocardiogram four-chamber view of a patient with mitral annular calcium (MAC). LA = left atrium; RA = right atrium; RV = right ventricle; LV = left ventricle; AML = anterior mitral leaflet; PML = posterior mitral leaflet.

patients with echocardiographically severe MAC and significant mitral regurgitation, functional mitral stenosis, or conduction defects may have no evidence of MAC on chest x-ray films. Figure 4 shows C-shaped calcification of the mitral annulus. Figure 5 illustrates J-shaped calcification of the mitral annulus.

## CHAMBER SIZE

Patients with MAC have a higher prevalence of left atrial enlargement (7,16,18,21,23,24,48,50) and left ventricular enlargement (16,18,24,48,50) than patients without MAC. In a prospective study of 976 elderly patients (526 with MAC and 450 without MAC), left atrial enlargement was 2.4 times more prevalent in patients with MAC than in the group without MAC (23).

## ATRIAL FIBRILLATION

Patients with MAC also have a higher prevalence of atrial fibrillation than patients without MAC (7,16,18,21,23,48). Table 3 shows that the prevalence of

**Table 2** Sensitivity, Specificity, Positive Predictive Value, and Negative Predictive Value of Chest X-ray Films in Detecting Mitral Annular Calcium Diagnosed by Echocardiography in Elderly Patients

| | *n* | (%) |
|---|---|---|
| Sensitivity | 39/332 | (12) |
| Specificity | 270/272 | (99) |
| Positive predictive value | 39/41 | (95) |
| Negative predictive value | 270/563 | (47) |

*Source*: Adapted from Aronow et al. (46).

atrial fibrillation was increased 12, 5, and 1.9 times in patients with MAC than in patients without MAC (18,23,48).

## CONDUCTION DEFECTS

Because of the close proximity of the mitral annulus to the atrioventricular node and the bundle of His, patients with MAC have a higher prevalence of conduction defects, such as sinoatrial disease, atrioventricular block, bundle branch block, left anterior fascicular block, and intraventricular conduction defect, than patients without MAC (4–7,26,48). The calcific deposits may also extend into the membranous portions of the interventricular septum involving the conduction system, or may even extend to the left atrium, interrupting interatrial and intraatrial conduction. In addition, MAC may be associated with a sclerodegenerative process in the conduction system. Nair et al. (48) demonstrated in their

**Table 3** Prevalence of Atrial Fibrillation in Patients With and Without Mitral Annular Calcium (MAC)

| | Atrial fibrillation | | | | |
|---|---|---|---|---|---|
| | MAC | | No MAC | | Relative |
| | *n* | (%) | *n* | (%) | risk |
| Framingham Study (18) | 20/162 | (12) | 53/5532 | (1) | 12 |
| Patients younger than 61 years (48) | 11/107 | (10) | 2/107 | (2) | 5 |
| Patients older than 62 years (mean age 82 ± 8) (23) | 90/526 | (17) | 41/450 | (9) | 1.9 |

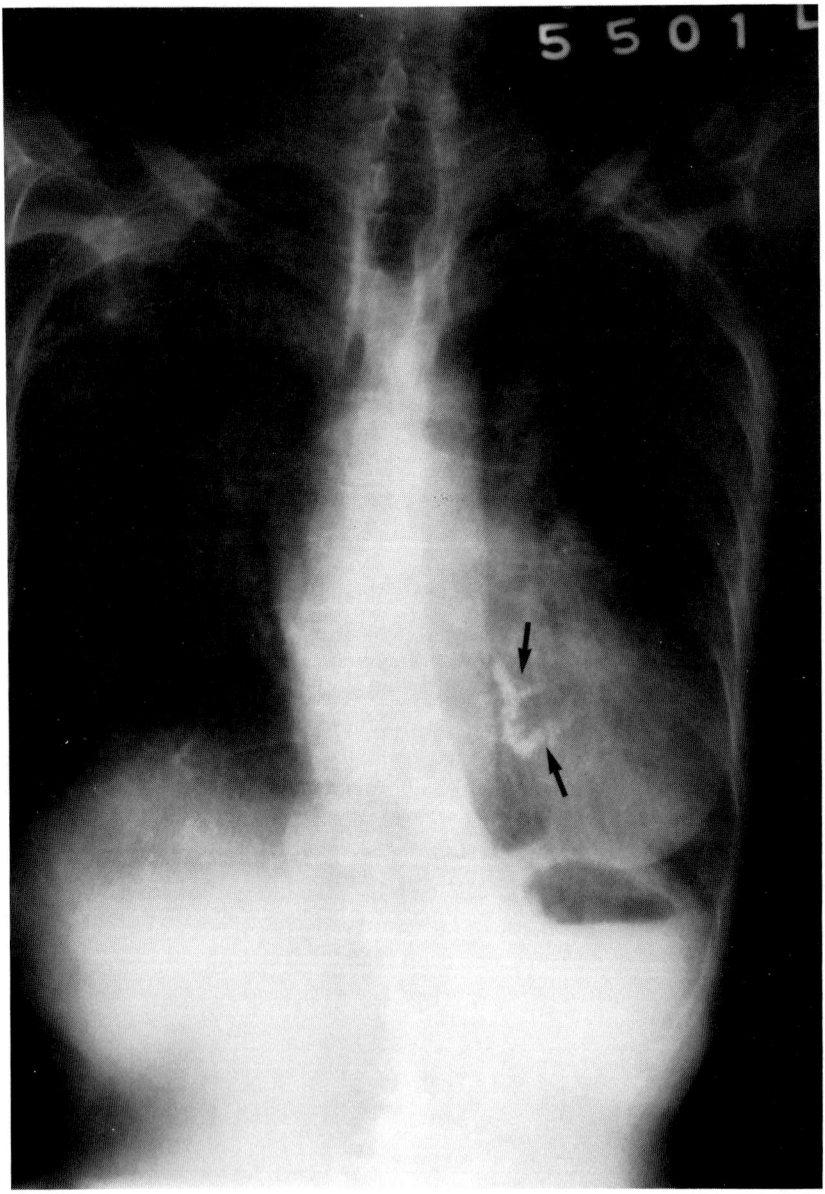


**Figure 4** Posterior–anterior chest x-ray in a patient with C-shaped calcification of the mitral annulus (arrows).

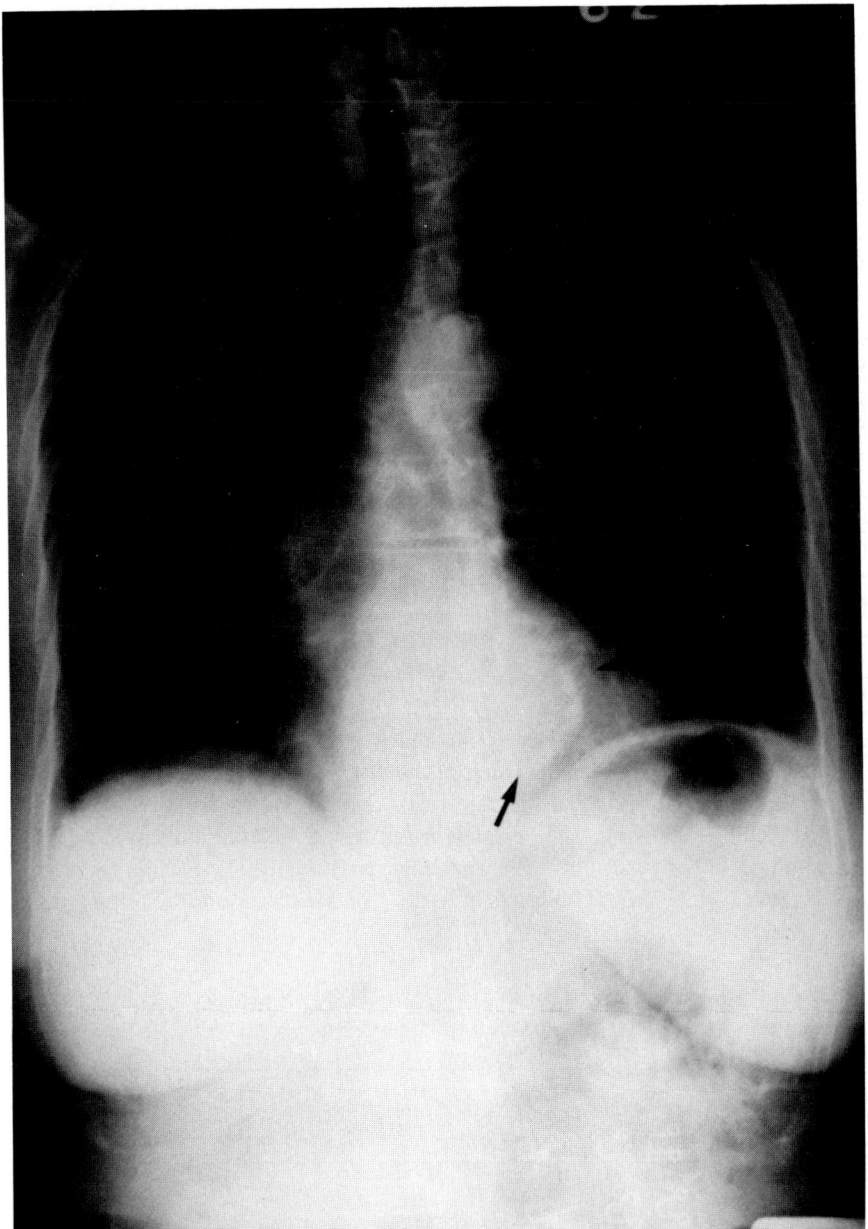

**Figure 5** Posterior–anterior chest x-ray in a patient with J-shaped calcification of the mitral annulus (arrow).

**Table 4** Prevalence of Apical Systolic Murmurs of Mitral Regurgitation (MR) in Patients with Mitral Annular Calcium

| | Prevalence of MR murmur | |
|---|---|---|
| | *n* | (%) |
| Korn et al. (16) | 14/14 | (100) |
| Schott et al. (31) | 10/14 | (71)[a] |
| Hammer et al. (2) | 2/4 | (50) |
| Fulkerson et al. (7) | 72/80 | (90) |
| Savage et al. (18) | 16/132 | (12) |
| Nair et al. (47) | 17/104 | (16) |
| Aronow et al. (22) | 129/293 | (44) |
| Aronow et al. (51) | 43/100 | (43) |

[a] MAC due to noninflammatory calcific disease.

prospective study that patients with MAC had a higher incidence of permanent pacemaker implantation because of both atrioventricular block and sinoatrial disease than patients without MAC.

## MITRAL REGURGITATION

MAC is thought to generate systolic murmurs by the sphincter action loss of the annulus and the mechanical stretching of the mitral leaflets causing mitral regurgitation and from vibration of the calcified ring or vortex formation around the annulus. Table 4 shows that the prevalence of apical systolic murmurs of mitral regurgitation in patients with MAC ranged from 12 to 100% in different studies (2,7,16,18,22,31,47,51). Table 5 states the prevalence of mitral regurgitation

**Table 5** Prevalence of Mitral Regurgitation (MR) Diagnosed by Doppler Echocardiography in Patients with Mitral Annular Calcium

| | MR | | Moderate to severe MR | |
|---|---|---|---|---|
| | *n* | (%) | *n* | (%) |
| Labovitz et al. (52) | 28/51 | (55) | 17/51 | (33) |
| Aronow et al. (51) | 54/100 | (54) | 18/100 | (18) |
| Kaul et al. (50) | 28/29 | (97)[a] | — | — |

[a] Severe mitral regurgitation in 2 of 29 patients (7%).

diagnosed by Doppler echocardiography in patients with MAC (50–52). The prevalence of mitral regurgitation associated with MAC ranged from 54 to 97% in the three Doppler echocardiographic studies (50–52). Figure 6 illustrates severe mitral regurgitation due to MAC diagnosed by color Doppler echocardiography.

The greater the severity of MAC, the greater the severity of mitral regurgitation associated with MAC. Moderate to severe mitral regurgitation was diagnosed by Doppler echocardiography in 33% of patients with MAC by Labovitz et al. (52) and in 18% of patients with MAC by Aronow and Kronzon (51). Kaul et al. (50) diagnosed severe mitral regurgitation in 7% of their patients with MAC. Kaul et al. (50) also concluded from their study that mitral regurgitation in patients with MAC is caused by a reduced sphincteric action of the mitral annulus, with MAC preventing the posterior annulus from contracting and assuming a flatter shape during systole.

## MITRAL STENOSIS

An apical diastolic murmur may be heard in patients with MAC as a result of turbulent flow across the calcified and narrowed annulus (annular stenosis). Table 6 shows that the prevalence of apical diastolic murmurs of mitral stenosis in patients with MAC ranged from 0 to 25% in different studies (2,16,18,22,31,42,47,51,52). Table 6 also indicates that mitral stenosis associated with MAC was diagnosed by Doppler echocardiography in 8% of 51 patients by Labovitz et al. (52) and in 6% of 100 patients by Aronow and Kronzon (51). Figure 7 illustrates mitral stenosis due to MAC diagnosed by Doppler echocardiography.

The reduction of mitral valve orifice in patients with MAC is due to the annular calcium and to reduced mitral excursion and mobility secondary to calcium at the base of the leaflets (51). The commissures are fused in rheumatic mitral stenosis but are not fused in mitral stenosis associated with MAC. The mitral leaflet margins in MAC may be thin and mobile, and the posterior mitral leaflet may move normally during diastole. However, Doppler echocardiographic recordings show increased transvalvular flow velocity and prolonged pressure halftime and, therefore, smaller mitral valve orifice in patients with mitral stenosis, regardless of the etiology.

## BACTERIAL ENDOCARDITIS

Bacterial endocarditis, with a high incidence of *Staphylococcus aureus* endocarditis, may complicate MAC (7,10–13,23). Patients with MAC associated with chronic renal failure are at especially increased risk for developing bacterial endocarditis (31). The calcific mass erodes the endothelium under the mitral

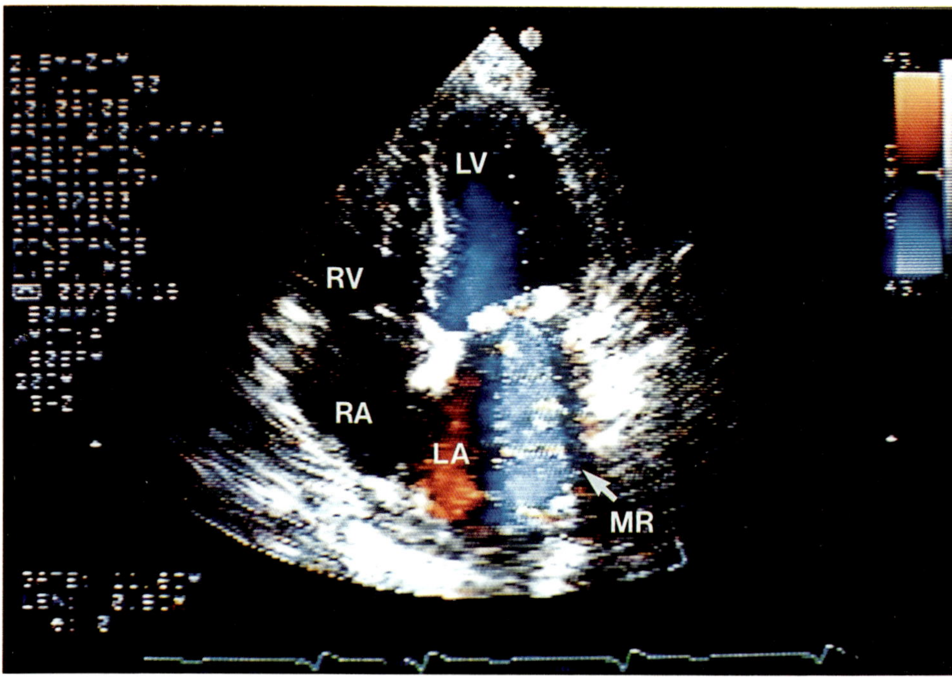


**Figure 6** Color Doppler echocardiographic findings in a patient with mitral annular calcium and severe mitral regurgitation (MR). LA = left atrium; RA = right atrium; RV = right ventricle; LV = left ventricle.

**Table 6** Prevalence of Apical Diastolic Murmurs of Mitral Stenosis (MS) and of Mitral Stenosis in Patients with Mitral Annual Calcium

| | Prevalence of MS murmur | | Prevalence of MS by Doppler echocardiography | |
|---|---|---|---|---|
| | *n* | (%) | *n* | (%) |
| Simon and Liu (42) | 5/59 | (8) | — | — |
| Korn et al. (16) | 3/14 | (21) | — | — |
| Schott et al. (31) | 2/14 | (14)[a] | — | — |
| Hammer et al. (2) | 1/4 | (25) | — | — |
| Savage et al. (18) | 2/132 | (2) | — | — |
| Nair et al. (47) | 7/104 | (7) | — | — |
| Aronow et al. (22) | 28/293 | (10) | — | — |
| Labovitz et al. (52) | 0/51 | (0) | 4/51 | (8) |
| Aronow et al. (51) | 6/100 | (6) | 6/100 | (6) |

[a] MAC due to noninflammatory calcific disease.

valve, which is exposed to transient bacteremia. The avascular nature of the mitral annulus interferes with antibiotics reaching a nidus of bacteria, predisposing to periannular and myocardial abcesses and, consequently, to a poor prognosis (10–13). Burnside and DeSanctis (10) therefore recommended prophylactic antibiotics to prevent bacterial endocarditis in patients with MAC.

Nair et al. (18) observed at 4.4 years mean follow-up no significant difference in incidence of bacterial endocarditis in 99 patients younger than 61 years with MAC compared to a control group of 101 patients. However, Aronow et al. (23) demonstrated at 39 months mean follow-up a 3% incidence of bacterial endocarditis in 526 elderly patients with MAC and a 1% incidence of bacterial endocarditis in 450 elderly patients without MAC. On the basis of these data, we recommend using prophylactic antibiotics to prevent bacterial endocarditis in patients with MAC according to American Heart Association guidelines (53).

## CARDIAC EVENTS

In a prospective study of 107 patients (8 lost to follow-up) younger than 61 years with MAC and 107 (6 lost to follow-up) age- and sex-matched control subjects, Nair et al. (48) demonstrated at 4.4 years mean follow-up that patients with MAC had a higher incidence of new cardiac events than control subjects (Table 7). In a prospective study of 526 elderly patients with MAC and 450 el-

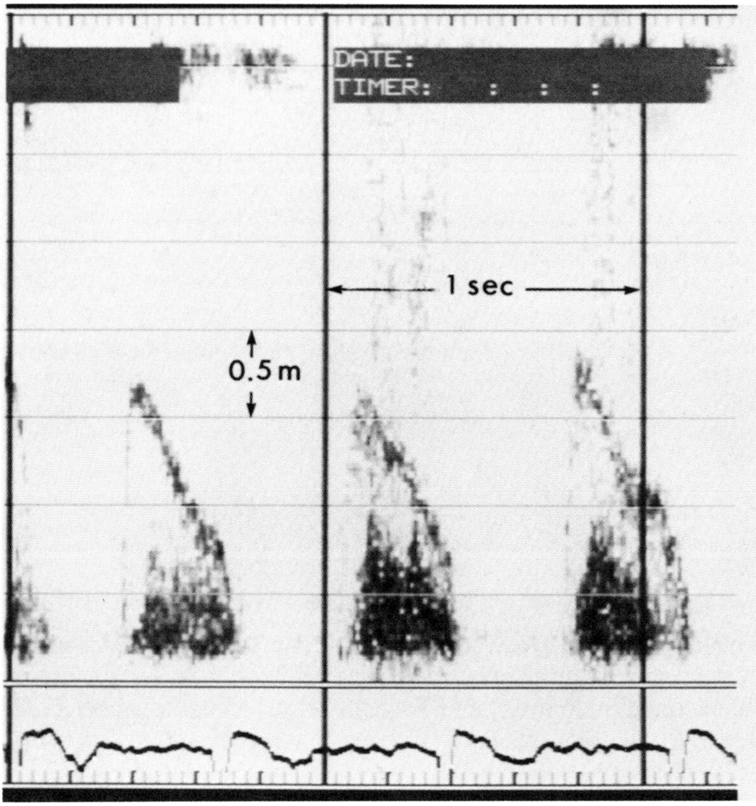


**Figure 7** Continuous wave Doppler tracing across a stenotic mitral valve orifice due to mitral annular calcium. Peak diastolic pressure gradient = 12 mm Hg. Pressure halftime = 200 ms. Mitral valve area = 1.1 cm$^2$.

derly patients without MAC, Aronow et al. (23) found at 39 months mean follow-up that the incidence of new cardiac events (myocardial infarction, primary ventricular fibrillation, or sudden cardiac death) was also higher in elderly patients with MAC than in elderly patients without MAC (Table 7).

## MITRAL VALVE REPLACEMENT

Nair et al. (54) reported that mitral valve replacement can be accomplished in patients with MAC with morbidity and mortality similar to those in patients without MAC. Following mitral valve replacement, subsequent morbidity and

**Table 7** Incidence of New Cardiac Events in Patients With and Without Mitral Annular Calcium (MAC)

| | | Cardiac events | | | | |
|---|---|---|---|---|---|---|
| | | MAC | | No MAC | | |
| | Follow-up | *n* | (%) | *n* | (%) | Relative risk |
| Nair et al. (48) | 4.4 years | | | | | |
| Total cardiac death | | 31/99 | (31) | 2/101 | (2) | 15.5 |
| Sudden cardiac death | | 12/99 | (12) | 1/101 | (1) | 12.0 |
| Congestive heart failure | | 41/99 | (41) | 6/101 | (6) | 6.8 |
| Mitral or aortic valve replacement | | 9/99 | (9) | 0/101 | (0) | — |
| Aronow et al. (23) | 39 months | | | | | |
| cardiac events,[a] if | | | | | | |
| Atrial fibrillation | | 62/90 | (69) | 22/41 | (54) | 1.3 |
| Sinus rhythm | | 157/436 | (36) | 106/409 | (26) | 1.4 |
| All patients | | 219/526 | (42) | 128/450 | (28) | 1.5 |

[a] Myocardial infarction, primary ventricular fibrillation, or sudden cardiac death.

mortality during 4.4 year mean follow-up were also similar in patients with and without MAC.

## CEREBROVASCULAR EVENTS

Although the increased prevalence of atrial fibrillation, mitral stenosis, and mitral regurgitation predisposes patients with MAC to thromboembolic stroke, some investigators consider MAC a marker of other vascular disease causing stroke rather than the primary embolic source (55). In a retrospective study of 110 elderly patients with chronic atrial fibrillation, 44 (40%) had documented thromboembolic stroke (56). In this study, the prevalence of MAC was not significantly different in elderly patients with thromboembolic stroke (80%) or without thromboembolic stroke (65%; relative risk = 1.2). However, five prospective studies have demonstrated an increased incidence of new cerebrovascular events in patients with MAC than in patients without MAC (Table 8) (23,48,57–59).

Nair et al. (48) observed at 4.4 years mean follow-up in 107 patients (8 lost to follow-up) younger than 61 years with MAC and 107 (6 lost to follow-up) age- and sex-matched control subjects that patients with MAC had a 5 times higher incidence of new thromboembolic cerebrovascular events than patients without

**Table 8** Incidence of New Cerebrovascular Events in Patients With and Without Mitral Annular Calcium (MAC)

| | | Cerebrovascular events | | | | |
|---|---|---|---|---|---|---|
| | | MAC | | No MAC | | |
| | Follow-up | *n* | (%) | *n* | (%) | risk |
| Nair et al. (48), TE cerebrovascular events | 4.4 years | 10/99 | (10) | 2/101 | (2) | 5.0 |
| Benjamin et al. (57), stroke | 8 years | 22/160 | (14) | 51/999 | (5) | 2.7 |
| Aronow et al. (23), TE stroke if | 39 months | | | | | |
| Atrial fibrillation | | 45/90 | (50) | 14/41 | (34) | 1.5 |
| Sinus rhythm | | 59/436 | (14) | 38/409 | (9) | 1.6 |
| All patients | | 104/526 | (20) | 52/450 | (12) | 1.7 |
| Boston Area Anticoagulation Trial for Atrial Fibrillation (50), ischemic stroke | 2.2 years | 10/129 | (8) | 5/291 | (2) | 4.0 |
| Aronow et al. (59), TE stroke if | 45 months | | | | | |
| 40–100% ECD | | 52/101 | (51) | 16/49 | (33) | 1.5 |
| No ECD | | 88/365 | (24) | 47/413 | (11) | 2.2 |
| TIA if | | | | | | |
| 40–100% ECD | | 8/101 | (8) | 3/49 | (6) | 1.3 |
| No ECD | | 11/365 | (3) | 3/413 | (1) | 3.0 |

TE = thromboembolic; ECD = extracranial carotid arterial disease; TIA = cerebral transient ischemic attack.

MAC (Table 8). The Framingham study demonstrated at 8 years follow-up in 160 persons with MAC and 999 persons without MAC that the incidence of stroke was increased 2.7 times in patients with MAC than in patients without MAC (Table 8) (57). At 39 months mean follow-up of 526 elderly patients with MAC and 450 elderly patients without MAC, Aronow et al. (23) found a 1.5 times higher incidence of new thromboembolic stroke in patients with MAC than in patients without MAC if atrial fibrillation was present, a 1.6 times higher incidence of new thromboembolic stroke in patients with MAC than in patients without MAC if sinus rhythm was present, and a 1.7 times higher incidence of new thromboembolic stroke in all patients with MAC than in all patients without MAC (Table 8). The Boston Area Anticoagulation Trial for Atrial Fibrillation study documented at 2.2 years mean follow-up in 129 patients with atrial fibrillation and MAC and 291 patients with atrial fibrillation without MAC a 4 times higher incidence of ischemic stroke in patients with MAC than in patients without MAC (Table 8) (58). At 45 months mean follow-up, Aronow et al. (59) observed that the incidence of thromboembolic stroke was 1.5 times higher in 101 patients with 40–100% extracranial carotid arterial disease and MAC than in 49 patients with 40–100% extracranial carotid arterial disease and no MAC and 2.2 times higher in 365 patients with MAC and no extracranial carotid arterial disease than in 413 patients with no MAC and no extracranial carotid arterial disease.

Since patients with MAC and atrial fibrillation or sinus rhythm have a higher incidence of thromboembolic stroke than patients without MAC, antithrombotic therapy should be considered in patients with MAC and no contraindications to antithrombotic therapy. In the Boston Area Anticoagulation Trial for Atrial Fibrillation study, warfarin decreased the incidence of thromboembolic stroke in patients with MAC by about 90% (60,61). The risk of major bleeding from anticoagulant therapy in elderly patients with MAC is unknown and must be investigated to determine if any decrease in risk of thromboembolic stroke will be offset by an increased risk of major bleeding from anticoagulant therapy. The Stroke Prevention in Atrial Fibrillation study will provide us with important data about the risk of major hemorrhage from warfarin therapy in patients older than 75 years (62).

Until data from prospective, randomized studies evaluating the efficacy and risk of antithrombotic therapy in patients with MAC are available, we recommend treating patients younger than 75 years of age with MAC associated with either atrial fibrillation, mitral stenosis, or moderate to severe mitral regurgitation with warfarin if they have no contraindications to anticoagulant therapy. Using clinical judgment, we would treat selected patients older than 75 years with MAC associated with either atrial fibrillation, mitral stenosis, or moderate to severe mitral regurgitation with low-dose warfarin if there is no contraindication to anticoagulant therapy.

## REFERENCES

1. Roberts WC, Perloff JK. Mitral valvular disease. A clinicopathologic survey of the conditions causing the mitral valve to function abnormally. *Ann Intern Med* 1972; 77:939–975.
2. Hammer WJ, Roberts WC, deLeon AC Jr. "Mitral stenosis" secondary to combined "massive" mitral anular calcific deposits and small, hypertrophied left ventricles. Hemodynamic documentation in four patients. *Am J Med* 1978; 64:371–376.

3. Osterberger LE, Goldstein S, Khaja F, Lakier J. Functional mitral stenosis in patients with massive annular calcification. *Circulation* 1981; 64:472–476.
4. Nair CK, Runco V, Everson GT, Boghairi A, Mooss AN, Mohiuddin SM, Sketch MH. Conduction defects and mitral annulus calcification. *Br Heart J* 1980; 44:162–167.
5. Nair CK, Sketch MH, Desai R, Mohiuddin SM, Runco V. High prevalence of symptomatic bradyarrhythmias due to atrioventricular node-fascicular and sinus node-atrial disease in patients with mitral anular calcification. *Am Heart J* 1982; 103:226–229.
6. Nair CK, Aronow WS, Stokke K, Mohiuddin SM, Thomson W, Sketch MH. Cardiac conduction defects in patients older than 60 years with aortic stenosis with and without mitral anular calcium. *Am J Cardiol* 1984; 53:169–172.
7. Fulkerson PK, Beaver BM, Auseon JC, Graber HL. Calcification of the mitral annulus: Etiology, clinical associations, complications and therapy. *Am J Med* 1979; 66:967–977.
8. Ridolfi RL, Hutchins GM. Spontaneous calcific emboli from calcific mitral annulus fibrosus. *Arch Pathol Lab Med* 1976; 100:117–120.
9. DeBono DP, Warlow CP. Mitral annulus calcification and cerebral or retinal ischaemia. *Lancet* 1979; 2:383–385.
10. Burnside JW, DeSanctis RW. Bacterial endocarditis on calcification of the mitral anulus fibrosus. *Ann Intern Med* 1972; 76:615–618.
11. Watanakunakorn C. *Staphylococcus aureus* endocarditis on the calcified mitral anulus fibrosus. *Am J Med Sci* 1973; 266:219–223.
12. Mambo NC, Silver MD, Brunsdon DFV. Bacterial endocarditis of the mitral valve associated with annular calcification. *Can Med Assoc J* 1978; 119:323–326.
13. D'Cruz IA, Collison HK, Gerrardo L, Hensel P. Two-dimensional echocardiographic detection of staphylococcal vegetation attached to calcified mitral anulus. *Am Heart J* 1982; 103:295–298.
14. Sell S, Scully RE. Aging changes in the aortic and mitral valves. *Am J Pathol* 1965; 46:345–365.
15. Pomerance A, Darby AJ, Hodkinson HM. Valvular calcification in the elderly: Possible pathogenic factors. *J Gerontol* 1978; 33:672–676.
16. Korn D, DeSanctis RW, Sell S. Massive calcification of the mitral annulus: A clinicopathologic study of fourteen cases. *N Engl J Med* 1962; 267:900–909.
17. Roberts WC. The senile cardiac calcification syndrome. *Am J Cardiol* 1986; 58:572–574.
18. Savage DD, Garrison RJ, Castelli WP, McNamara PM, Anderson SJ, Kannel WB, Feinleib M. Prevalence of submitral (anular) calcium and its correlates in a general population-based sample (the Framingham Study). *Am J Cardiol* 1983; 51:1375–1378.
19. Waller BF, Roberts WC. Cardiovascular disease in the very elderly. An analysis of 40 necropsy patients aged 90 years or over. *Am J Cardiol* 1983; 51:403–421.
20. Aronow WS, Schwartz KS, Koenigsberg M. Correlation of aortic cuspal and aortic root disease with aortic systolic ejection murmurs and with mitral anular calcium in persons older than 62 years in a long-term health care facility. *Am J Cardiol* 1986; 58:651–652.

21. Aronow WS, Schwartz KS, Koenigsberg M. Correlation of atrial fibrillation with presence or absence of mitral anular calcium in 604 persons older than 60 years. *Am J Cardiol* 1987; 59:1213–1214.
22. Aronow WS, Schwartz KS. Koenigsberg M. Correlation of murmurs of mitral stenosis and mitral regurgitation with presence or absence of mitral anular calcium in persons older than 62 years in a long-term health care facility. *Am J Cardiol* 1987; 59:181–182.
23. Aronow WS, Koenigsberg M, Kronzon I, Gutstein H. Association of mitral anular calcium with new thromboembolic stroke and cardiac events at 39-month follow-up in elderly patients. *Am J Cardiol* 1990; 65:1511–1512.
24. Nair CK, Sudhakaran C, Aronow WS, Thomson W, Woodruff MP, Sketch MH. Clinical characteristics of patients younger than 60 years with mitral anular calcium: Comparison with age- and sex-matched control subjects. *Am J Cardiol* 1984; 54:1286–1287.
25. Aronow WS, Schwartz KS, Koenigsberg M. Correlation of serum lipids, calcium and phosphorus, diabetes mellitus, aortic valve stenosis and history of systemic hypertension with presence or absence of mitral anular calcium in persons older than 62 years in a long-term health care facility. *Am J Cardiol* 1987; 59:381–382.
26. Nair CK, Sketch MH, Ahmed I, Thomson W, Ryschon K, Woodruff MP, Runco V. Calcific valvular aortic stenosis with and without mitral anular calcium. *Am J Cardiol* 1987; 60:865–870.
27. Aronow WS, Schwartz KS, Koenigsberg M. Prevalence of tricuspid anular calcium diagnosed by echocardiography in elderly patients. *Am J Noninvas Cardiol* 1987; 1:275–277.
28. Roberts WC. Morphologic features of the normal and abnormal mitral valve. *Am J Cardiol* 1983; 51:1005–1028.
29. Sprecher DL, Schaefer EJ, Kent KM, Gregg RE, Zech LA, Hoeg JM, McManus B, Roberts WC, Brewer HB Jr. Cardiovascular features of homozygous familial hypercholesterolemia: Analysis of 16 patients. *Am J Cardiol* 1984; 54:20–30.
30. Roberts WC, Waller BF. Effect of chronic hypercalcemia on the heart: An analysis of 18 necropsy patients. *Am J Med* 1981; 71:371–384.
31. Schott CR, Kotler MN, Parry WR, Segal BL. Mitral annular calcification: clinical and echocardiographic correlations. *Arch Intern Med* 1977; 137:1143–1150.
32. D'Cruz IA, Bhatt GR, Cohen HC, Glick G. Echocardiographic detection of cardiac involvement in patients with chronic renal failure. *Arch Intern Med* 1978; 138:720–724.
33. Nestico PF, DePace NL, Kotler MN, Rose LI, Brezin JH, Swartz C, Mintz GS, Schwartz AB. Calcium phosphorus metabolism in dialysis patients with and without mitral anular calcium. *Am J Cardiol* 1983; 51:497–500.
34. Forman MB, Virmani R, Robertson RM, Stone WJ. Mitral anular calcification in chronic renal failure. *Chest* 1984; 85:367–371.
35. Cohen JL, Barooah B, Segal KR, Batuman V. Two-dimensional echocardiographic findings in patients on hemodialysis for more than six months. *Am J Cardiol* 1987; 60:743–745.
36. Kronzon I, Glassman E. Mitral ring calcification in idiopathic hypertrophic subaortic stenosis. *Am J Cardiol* 1978; 42:60–66.

37. Nair CK, Kudesia V, Hansen D, Thomson W, Pagano T, Ryschon K, Sketch MH. Echocardiographic and electrocardiographic characteristics of patients with hypertrophic cardiomyopathy with and without mitral anular calcium. *Am J Cardiol* 1987; 59:1428–1430.
38. Motamed HE, Roberts WC. Frequency and significance of mitral anular calcium in hypertrophic cardiomyopathy: Analysis of 200 necropsy patients. *Am J Cardiol* 1987; 60:877–884.
39. Aronow WS, Kronzon I. Prevalence of hypertrophic cardiomyopathy and its association with mitral anular calcium in elderly patients. *Chest* 1988; 94:1295–1296.
40. Roberts WC, Waller BF. Mitral valve 'anular' calcium forming a complete circle or 'O' configuration: Clinical and necropsy observations. *Am Heart J* 1981; 101:619–621.
41. Sosman MC. The technique for locating and identifying pericardial and intracardiac calcifications. *Am J Roentgenol* 1943; 50:461–468.
42. Simon MA, Liu SF. Calcification of the mitral valve annulus and its relation to functional valvular disturbance. *Am Heart J* 1954; 48:497–505.
43. Windholz F, Grayson C. Roentgen demonstration of calcifications in the interventricular septum in cases of heart block. *Am J Roentgenol* 1947; 58:411–421.
44. Gabor GE, Mohr BD, Goel PC, Cohen B. Echocardiographic and clinical spectrum of mitral anular calcification. *Am J Cardiol* 1976; 38:836–842.
45. D'Cruz IA, Cohen HC, Prabhu R, Bisla V, Glick G. Clinical manifestations of mitral annulus calcification, with emphasis on its echocardiographic features. *Am Heart J* 1977; 94:367–377.
46. Aronow WS, Schwartz KS, Koenigsberg M. Sensitivity, specificity, positive predictive value, and negative predictive value of mitral anular calcium detected by chest roentgenograms correlated with mitral anular calcium diagnosed by echocardiography in elderly patients. *Am J Noninvas Cardiol* 1987; 1:251–253.
47. Nair CK, Aronow WS, Sketch MH, Mohiuddin SM, Pagano T, Esterbrooks DJ, Hee TT. Clinical and echocardiographic characteristics of patients with mitral anular calcification. Comparison with age- and sex-matched control subjects. *Am J Cardiol* 1983; 51:992–995.
48. Nair CK, Thomson W, Ryschon K, Cook C, Hee TT, Sketch MH Sr. Long-term follow-up of patients with echocardiographically detected mitral anular calcium and comparison with age- and sex-matched control subjects. *Am J Cardiol* 1989; 63:465–470.
49. Dashkoff N, Karakushensky M, Fortuin NJ. Echocardiographic features of mitral annulus calcification (abstract). *Circulation* 1975; 52(Suppl. II):II–34.
50. Kaul S, Pearlman JD, Touchstone DA, Esquival L. Prevalence and mechanisms of mitral regurgitation in the absence of intrinsic abnormalities of the mitral leaflets. *Am Heart J* 1989; 118:963–972.
51. Aronow WS, Kronzon I. Correlation of prevalence and severity of mitral regurgitation and mitral stenosis determined by Doppler echocardiography with physical signs of mitral regurgitation and mitral stenosis in 100 patients aged 62 to 100 years with mitral anular calcium. *Am J Cardiol* 1987; 60:1189–1190.

52. Labovitz AJ, Nelson JG, Windhorst DM, Kennedy HL, Williams GA. Frequency of mitral valve dysfunction from mitral anular calcium as detected by Doppler echocardiography. *Am J Cardiol* 1985; 55:133–137.
53. Dajani AS, Bisno AL, Chung KJ, Durack DT, Freed M, Gerber MA, Karchmer AW, Millard HD, Rahimtoola S, Shulman ST, Watanakunakorn C, Taubert KA. Prevention of bacterial endocarditis. Recommendations by the American Heart Association. *JAMA* 1990; 264:2919–2922.
54. Nair CK, Biddle P, Kaneshige A, Cook C, Ryschon K, Andersen A, Sketch MH Sr. Mitral valve replacement in patients with mitral anular calcium (abstract). *Chest* 1991; 100(Suppl):109S.
55. Sherman DG, Dyken ML, Fisher M, Harrison MJG, Hart RG. Cerebral embolism. *Chest* 1986; 89:82S–98S.
56. Aronow WS, Gutstein H, Hsieh FY. Risk factors for thromboembolic stroke in elderly patients with chronic atrial fibrillation. *Am J Cardiol* 1989; 63:366–367.
57. Benjamin EJ, Plehn JF, D'Agostino RB, Belanger AJ, Fuller DL, Comai K, Wolf PA, Levy D. Mitral annular calcification and the risk of stroke in an elderly cohort. *N Engl J Med* 1992; 327:374–379.
58. Boston Area Anticoagulation Trial for Atrial Fibrillation Investigators. The effect of low-dose warfarin on the risk of stroke in patients with nonrheumatic atrial fibrillation. *N Engl J Med* 1990; 323:1505–1511.
59. Aronow WS, Schoenfeld MR, Gutstein H. Frequency of thromboembolic stroke in persons $\geqslant$60 years of age with extracranial carotid arterial disease and/or mitral anular calcium. *Am J Cardiol* 1992; 70:123–124.
60. Aronow WS. The effect of low-dose warfarin on the risk of stroke in patients with nonrheumatic atrial fibrillation. Letter to the Editor. *N Engl J Med* 1991; 325:130.
61. Singer DE, Hughes RA, Gress DR, Sheehan MA, Oertel LB, Maraventano SW, Blewett DR, Rosner B, Kistler JP. The effect of low-dose warfarin on the risk of stroke in patients with nonrheumatic atrial fibrillation (reply to letter to the editor). *N Engl J Med* 1991; 325:131.
62. Stroke Prevention in Atrial Fibrillation Study Group Investigators. Preliminary report of the stroke prevention in atrial fibrillation study. *N Engl J Med* 1990; 322:863–868.

# 17

# Endocarditis in the Elderly

**Thomas C. Cesario**
*University of California, Irvine Medical Center, Orange, California*

**David A. Cesario**
*University of California, Irvine, California*

Endocarditis is a disease with variable manifestations. In the preantibiotic era, endocarditis predominantly occurred in the third and fourth decades (1), but numerous publications have now provided an increasing awareness of the growing proportion of older individuals afflicted with this disease.

The first comprehensive account of endocarditis in the English literature was provided by William Osler (2). Generally thought to be a result of the infection of platelet fibrin deposition on the endocardial surface (3,4) of previously damaged heart valves, the manifestations of endocarditis are many and the consequences great; however, it is acknowledged that certain organisms may infect normal heart valves. A number of recent reviews have crystallized the nature of this disease for the clinician. King and Harkness (5) have provided one such survey of the general nature of this disease process.

The overall incidence of endocarditis worldwide has been estimated to be 60 per million per year (6), with the majority of cases typically seen in males (5). The changing age incidence of this process is reviewed here.

Classically the most common predisposing factor for infection of the endocardium has been rheumatic heart disease. Of all cases, 25–60% occur on valves damaged by the consequences of rheumatic fever (5). Less common predisposing factors include congenital heart disease (10–20% of cases), mitral valve prolapse, prosthetic valves, and degenerative processes occurring on the valves. Traditionally the viridans streptococci, other strains of streptococci, and the staphylococci have accounted for the majority of cases of bacterial endocarditis (7) occurring over all age groups (8).

According to King and Harkness, endocarditis can lead to clinical manifestations in four ways: (1) constant bacteremia, (2) local invasion, (3) peripheral embolization, and (4) circulating immune complexes. These lead to the classic signs and symptoms associated with endocarditis, including changing murmurs, skin manifestations, embolic episodes, and splenomegaly. Treatment depends on identification of the appropriate organism, generally by culture of the blood, and selection of an antibiotic to which the organism is susceptible. In some cases surgery is indicated.

In past years, a number of overviews of endocarditis have appeared that have defined the character of endocarditis in the postantibiotic era. Rabinovich et al. (9) reviewed the cases of bacterial endocarditis occurring over a 40 year period at the university hospitals in Iowa. They confirmed the male predominance of the disease and that rheumatic heart disease was the major predisposing factor over the years, accounting for 68.2% of all cases. Congenital heart disease was the second most common identifiable predisposing factor, accounting for 13.1% of the cases; however, no identifiable heart disease was found in 16.3% of the cases. $\alpha$-Hemolytic streptococci accounted for 61.4% of the cases. Fever was present in every case, skin manifestations (petechiae) in 48% of the cases, clubbing in only 15%, and splenomegaly in 43%. As regards laboratory values, hematuria was present in 28% of the patients and anemia in 78%. Complications reported included embolic episodes in 55 of the 337 individuals and congestive heart failure in 25. The immediate fatality rate since 1950 was 30% for the total group, and the authors significantly noted that "age by itself did not seem to have any effect on the fatality rate."

A year later Lerner and Weinstein (10) published one of the best known endocarditis series reported in the modern era. They described 100 patients seen at the New England Medical Center in Boston. They clearly documented the rising age of patients with endocarditis occurring after the studies of Kelson and White (1) and appreciated that 60% of these individuals were over the age of 50. They again noted 56% of the patients were infected with streptococci (27% viridans streptococci) and 23% with staphylococci (20% with *Staphylococcus aureus*). In reviewing the underlying heart disease predisposing to endocarditis, these authors noted no antecedent cardiac disorder could be ascertained in 39% of the cases. Of those in whom an underlying cardiac diagnosis seemed apparent, Lerner and Weinstein reported that rheumatic heart disease was most common (40%), followed by congenital heart disease (10%) and arteriosclerotic disease (3%). They emphasized that many elderly patients with endocarditis had no knowledge of antecedent cardiac disease. In reviewing the clinical features of the disease, these authors reported 97% of the patients were febrile, 85% had murmur, 29% had petechiae, 44% had splenomegaly, and 30% had at least one episode of major embolic phenomenon. Hematuria was found in 26% of the cases, anemia in 50%, and elevated erythrocyte sedimentation rates in 90%. These authors pointed out that mortality rate did not seem affected much by age until the eighth decade of life. Of the 8 patients who were 70 or older, 7 succumbed to illness.

In 1971, Cherubin and Neu (11) reported a 30 year experience with endocarditis at Presbysterian Hospital in New York City. They reviewed the records of 656 cases of infective endocarditis seen between 1938 and 1967. They again appreciated the increasing mean age of the patients, from 31 years in 1938 to 52 years of age in 1966, and described the impact of social change on the epidemiological characteristics of endocarditis. Thus, they reported an increase in staphylococcal and fungal valvular infections secondary to increasing narcotic usage. Similarly, they appreciated a rising incidence of enterococcal disease despite the fact that *Streptococcus viridans* remained the most common causative organism for bacterial endocarditis. Rheumatic fever was the most common predisposing factor for bacterial endocarditis (38.5% of cases) in this study, followed by congenital heart disease (5.8% of the cases). They commented that "the older the patient the less frequent is an antecedent history of valvular heart disease." These authors noted an increase in aortic valve disease, a slight decrease in mitral valve disease, and a marked decline in combined aortic-mitral disease.

In 1978, Garvey and Neu (12) reported the occurrence of endocarditis at Columbia–Presbyterian Hospital for the years 1968–1973. Those years saw 154 patients admitted to that institution, with a total of 165 episodes of endocarditis. In this series, the mean age of the patients rose a further 3 years, to 55 years. Infection on prosthetic valves accounted for 20.6% of the cases, but in the cases of natural valve endocarditis, aortic involvement exceeded mitral involvement (39–35%). Rheumatic fever was again the most common predisposing factor, followed by congenital heart disease, although 65% of the cases for whom information was available had no known underlying cardiac process. Streptococci were the most common organisms producing natural valve endocarditis; however, enterococci accounted for 6.5% of the cases and *S. aureus* for 16%. Negative blood cultures were found in 11% of the patients. In 84% of the cases of natural valve endocarditis, fever was appreciated and murmurs were found in 96%. Elevated erythrocyte sedimentation rates (ESR) were noted in 86% of the cases. Major emboli occurred in 55 of the 107 cases of natural valve bacterial endocarditis, and congestive heart failure was seen in half the patients in this series. One-quarter of the cases died, but half of these were lost because the true diagnosis was not appreciated.

In 1980, Lowes et al. (13) published the experience of St. Bartholomew's Hospital, London over the years 1966–1975. These authors followed 60 patients. As found by authors before them, the age of the patients increased over reports from the preantibiotic era; thus 45% of the cases occurred in patients over the age of 50. The male–female ratio was 1:5 to 1:0. The predominant underlying heart disease was rheumatic in nature (35%), followed by congenital lesions (22%); however, no underlying disease was found in 30%. Clinically only two-thirds of the patients reported fever, but congestive heart failure, cutaneous manifestations, and splenomegaly occurred in almost half the individuals. In this period echocardiography was introduced, and 6 patients were described in whom this procedure localized the process. Blood cultures were positive in 86% of the patients from whom samples were taken, and streptococci accounted for nearly two-thirds of the isolates. Enterococci were reported in 7 instances (13%). The overall mortality in this series was 20%, but these authors suggested mortality was much higher in patients over 40 (25% versus 10% in younger patients).

Finally, Von Reyn et al. (14) in 1981 surveyed endocarditis at the Beth Israel Hospital in Boston between the years 1970 and 1977. They reported 104 instances in 94 patients and noted the advanced age of the patients (57 years mean age), the short duration of symptoms (27 days mean), and the high incidence of underlying valvular heart disease (66%). The highest percentage of cases occurred on the mitral valve (40%). Most of the cases were due to viridans streptococci, and only 5% were culture negative. Additionally, 13% of the patients had nosocomial endocarditis, 12% had prosthetic valve infections, and 18% required surgery. A total of 86% of the cases were febrile, 86% had murmurs, and 32% had splenomegaly. The overall mortality was 15% in this series. M-mode echocardiography was done in 32 patients, 6 of whom were demonstrated to have vegetations.

Thus a summary of some of the major reviews of endocarditis occurring over the last 65 years shows several changing trends. Perhaps most striking has been the advancing age of the patients, which was an almost universal finding. In addition, most of these extensive reviews found fever and murmurs to be very frequent in endocarditis patients and anemia and elevated erythrocyte sedimentation rates to be common. Other manifestations, including cutaneous findings, splenomegaly, and neurological findings, occurred in half or less of the cases. Rheumatic heart disease remained the most common predisposing factor, and streptococci, especially viridans streptococci, was the most frequent etiological agent identified.

Since the early descriptions of Osler, various authors have focused on age-related differences in the disease process. Kerr (15), in his classic monograph, noted that Gibson in 1896 remarked on the modified character of the disease in old age. Kerr himself suggested that as the population aged, arteriosclerotic valvular heart disease would become a significant antecedent cardiac lesion for bacterial endocarditis. In the later part of this review we focus on the surveys of endocarditis reported in the English literature that have examined the specifics of endocarditis in the elderly. This provides a basis for determining differences between the disease in the general population, as described earlier, and older individuals.

In 1940, Bayles and Lewis (16) reported 28 cases of endocarditis diagnosed at autopsy in people over the age of 40. The authors noted the majority of cases occurred on valves damaged by rheumatic fever but that 25% of the cases occurred on arteriosclerotic valves. They commented on the similarity of the clinical features between younger and older patients but noted the greater subtlety of the disease in the older group.

In the same year, Willis (17) described the occurrence of endocarditis in an 82 year old.

In 1945, Zeman and Siegal (18) reported 27 cases of bacterial endocarditis in patients over the age of 60. They emphasized that the features of endocarditis in the older population were more likely classified as acute. The features of acute disease have generally implied a more aggressive course with a shorter duration of symptoms. To some authors acute disease has suggested the occurrence of infection on presumably normal valves, generally caused by *S. aureus, Streptococcus pneumoniae,* or group A $\beta$-hemolytic streptococci. In recent years the utilization of the terms "acute" and "subacute" endocarditis have not been as popular. Zeman and Siegal also stressed the diagnostic difficulties encountered in older patients with bacterial endocarditis because of the frequent occurrence of other underlying disease processes.

In 1949, Traut et al. (19) reported 94 cases of bacterial endocarditis in patients over 45 years of age diagnosed at Cook County Hospital over the years 1935–1946. The vast majority of these (61%) occurred on valves damaged by rheumatic fever, but 5 occurred on atherosclerotic valves. They emphasized the infrequency of the disease in older people.

In an autopsy series Wallach et al. (20) described 13 cases of bacterial endocarditis superimposed on rheumatic valves and 17 cases imposed on valves without rheumatic disease, all of which occurred in patients over the age of 50. These authors noted that the disease in the older patients was more often incidental, not directly related to the cause of death. They further noted that the older patients more frequently had underlying genitourinary infections or other diseases (diabetes mellitus) and more often had sclerotic changes in the valves.

A year later Anderson et al. (21) emphasized the occurrence of endocarditis in older patients from St. Thomas Hospital, London. They reviewed 14 cases (18.4% of the total cases) seen from 1946 to 1954 occurring in people older than 60 years. In this group mortality was higher (50%) versus the entire group of patients with endocarditis seen at their hospital (31%). The patients included 10 with *S. viridans* infection and 4 with either negative cultures or no cultures. Virtually all patients had evening temperatures of 100°F or higher, and all had murmurs; 43% of the patients had splenomegaly, and the same number had cutaneous manifestations. They commented that endocarditis was often missed in the elderly because it was not generally realized that the disease could occur in this age group, that the disease in the aged was less severe, and that several criteria usually associated with endocarditis were not necessarily found in the aged.

Somewhat later, Gleck (22) described 10 cases of endocarditis occurring in patients over age 55. He noted that in addition to dental extractions and skin infections, genitourinary tract manipulations were precipitating events in the elderly. The subjects of this report were 6 men and 4 women. Although 3 patients had typical features of endocarditis, another 3 patients presented with changes in mental status or depression; 1 patient presented with liver disease, 1 with uremia, 1 with anorexia and weight loss, and 1 with stroke. At least 2 patients had maximum daily temperatures below 100°F. Of the 7 atypical patients, 4 died.

In the same year, Hartman and Myers (23) noted 7 of 20 patients with endocarditis to be over the age of 60. Of the 7, 4 were female, 5 were infected by *S. viridans,* one by staphylococcus, and one by enterococcus. Of these patients, 4 had rheumatic heart disease and 3 had arteriosclerotic disease; 2 patients died. These authors suggested enterococcal endocarditis was common in the older patient.

Cummings et al. (24) in 1960 noted that 18 of 55 patients with endocarditis were over age 50. Of these patients 13 died (72%), as opposed to 10 of 37 below this age (27%). Of the patients 10 were females and in all but 3 murmurs were described. Of all patients 27% had splenomegaly, but only half were reported to have fever. Streptococcal infections were seen in 6 patients, and in 1 *Proteus vulgaris* was isolated from the blood. The rest had negative cultures or no cultures were drawn.

Uwaydah and Weinberg (25), in 1965, noted the changing pattern of endocarditis. They reviewed 100 total patients seen at the Massachusetts General Hospital in Boston. In their series 38% of the cases were over the age of 60, and half of these had infection superimposed on arteriosclerotic or calcified valves. They commented on the declining incidence of rheumatic fever as a predisposition for endocarditis in the older patient. In this series 37% of the young patients died, but 68% of the older group expired.

In 1973, Habte-Gabr et al. (26) reported 57 patients over the age of 60 with endocarditis seen at the University of Iowa Hospital between 1940 and 1971. They noted endocarditis in the elderly had gradually increased. The male–female incidence was 4:1. They commented that although all the patients were febrile, half complained of weight loss, confusion, or other symptoms. These authors noted that the signs and symptoms were similar between younger and older patients. Of all patients 27% had negative cultures; however, the most common organisms isolated from in the older age group included $\alpha$-hemolytic streptococcus (40%), other streptococci (23%), and staphylococci (23%). Of the patients who were treated 56% survived. These authors stressed the varied presentation of endocarditis in the elderly, especially the prevalence of central nervous system complaints and uremia as presenting symptoms in the elderly. They emphasized the difficulty of making the true diagnosis in the elderly.

Watanakunakorn and Tan (27) reported 19 of 33 cases of staphylococcal endocarditis occurring in people over the age of 60. Presenting complaints were often nonspecific, such as anorexia and mental deterioration. Highlighting a modern risk factor for endocarditis, 2 patients were infected from indwelling intravenous catheters. In 10 patients the diagnosis was established antemortem from blood cultures, but in the others it was established at autopsy or by direct culture of surgically removed valves. All but 4 patients were febrile. Only 2 of the 10 in whom the diagnosis was made antemortem survived. At autopsy, the mitral valve was the source of the infection in 13 of the 16 cases and atherosclerosis was the predisposing cardiac condition in 8 of 16 cases.

This same group of authors also reported 20 patients with *S. viridans* endocarditis seen at the University of Cincinnati Medical Center (28) who were older than age 60. The presenting complaints of these patients were generally weakness, fatigue, and weight loss. All patients had fever, all had cardiac murmurs, 40% had splenomegaly, and 60% had cutaneous lesions. In 55% of the patients the disease involved the mitral valve, in 30% the aortic valve, and in 15% both valves. Of these patients 85% were alive 2 years after treatment, and it appeared survival was similar to that in a younger group of patients with the same disease.

Later, Applefield and Hornick (29) conducted a retrospective analysis of patients admitted to the University of Maryland Hospital between the years 1950 and 1970 with a diagnosis of endocarditis. Of 29 patients, 21% fulfilled the criteria for endocarditis and were 60 years of age or older. Among these older individuals, pyrexia of unknown origin was the presenting complaint in 48% of the cases; however, 45% presented with neurological findings, including delirium. In 10 patients no murmur was detected. In 18 individuals aortic valve disease predisposed to infection, and in 10 mitral valve disease was preexistent. Staphylococci accounted for 24% of the cases and streptococci for 41% (including 3 cases of enterococcal disease), but in 29% of the cases (8 cases in all) no organism was isolated. Of this group 72% died, but 48% had received antimicrobial therapy judged to be inappropriate.

Thell et al. (30) presented data on 42 cases of endocarditis occurring in subjects over 60 years and confirmed by autopsy or surgery. In this series, 5 cases of right-sided endocarditis were reported. The most common organisms isolated were staphylococci (33% of the cases), followed by streptococci (24% of the cases). In 37% of the cases no underlying heart disease was found, but aortic valve disease was most common in those in whom an underlying process could be identified. This included calcific aortic disease. These authors stressed that the diagnosis of endocarditis was suspected in only 38% of the cases despite that fever was present in 94% of the cases in whom it was recorded and murmurs in 68% of the patients.

Robbins et al. (31) also contributed to our understanding of endocarditis in the elderly. They reviewed 56 cases of infective endocarditis in patients 65 years of age and older. In this group, 93% were febrile, 86% had murmurs, and 36% had peripheral stigmata. They appropriately divided the cases into community-acquired and nosocomially acquired cases. Of a total of 41 community-acquired cases of endocarditis, 71% were found due to streptococci, including 6 cases of *Streptococcus faecalis;* 8 cases (20%) were due to staphylococci. Among 15 nosocomially acquired cases, 3 were due to *S. faecalis,* 7 to staphylococci (6 attributed to *S. aureus*) and 3 to fungi. Of the total cases 5 were caused by undetermined bacteria. Underlying diseases found to predispose to natural valve endocarditis in this series included 6 cases of rheumatic heart disease, 3 cases of calcific aortic valve disease, and 16 cases of atherosclerotic disease. Complications occurred in 34 individuals (64% of the patients) who developed congestive heart failure and in 20 patients (35%) who had neurological abnormalities. All patients tested had an elevated erythrocyte sedimentation rate, and two-thirds were anemic. The overall mortality in this series was 45%.

Finally, Terpenning et al. (32) compared infective endocarditis in patients over the age of 60 (53 episodes) to the disease in patients 40–60 years of age and to patients under 40 years of age (55 episodes). The percentages of cases caused by streptococci and staphylococci were approximately equal, but infection due to enterococci, *Streptococcus bovis,* and coagulase-negative staphylococci were more common in the older age group. Strikingly, 23% of the cases in the older patients were nosocomially acquired. The proportion of cases associated with various types of underlying heart disease was similar in all three groups, but the highest percentage of cases in all age groups was associated with no known underlying disease. A slightly greater percentage of the elderly group had prosthetic valves. Clinical manifestations were also similar in the various age groups, with fever present in over 80% of all individuals included regardless of age. Confusion was slightly more common in the older age group, and new or changing murmurs were present more often in the younger groups. Errors in diagnosis were significantly more common in the older age group. Echocardiograms were read as showing vegetations in 56.8% of the group under 40, 47.8% of the group 40–60 years of age, and 43.7% of the group over 65 years of age. The aortic valve was the most common valve infected overall, but the mitral was more often the site of infection in the elderly (54.7%). In the youngest age group, the tricuspid was most often infected because of the higher incidence of intravenous drug use as a predisposing factor in the process. Major neurological events were slightly more common in the elderly, and pulmonary embolic events were more frequent in the younger group. Overall mortality was significantly more common with increasing age, reaching 45% in the oldest group.

In summary, endocarditis is an evolving process that is becoming increasingly a disease of older patients. This is in part related to a declining incidence of rheumatic fever as a predisposing factor in younger patients, leaving degenerative disease as a relatively more common underlying factor. Thus older individuals constitute a greater percentage of cases. Similarly, older patients, because of more frequent underlying disease processes and a greater number of hospitalizations, are more likely to develop nosocomial infections of the sclerotic valves. Furthermore, the greater frequency of genitourinary procedures in the older patient means the older patient may more often be infected with enterococci. The major clinical manifestations in the older patient are likely to be similar. Thus the older patients still commonly have fever and some form of murmur. Peripheral manifestations (petechiae, splinter hemorrhages, Osler nodes, Janeway lesions, and so on) should be found in frequency about equal to that generally observed in other age groups and observed in the past. Common laboratory features of the disease, that is, anemia, elevated erythrocyte sedimentation rate, and hematuria, appear to be observed in the elderly with equal frequency. Confusion should be more likely in the older patient, since this is often a nonspecific response in the elderly to any physiological stress and should always force a search for infections, including endocarditis. With regard to mortality, it appears that the older patient with more frequent underlying disease and less ability to adapt to new stresses experiences a higher overall mortality from endocarditis (33). This must be extrapolated to the individual situation, however. An otherwise healthy older person with viridans streptococci on a prolapsed mitral valve may be at no greater risk of death than a younger person. In contrast, a more mature individual with underlying disease and a more difficult organism to eradicate (enterococci and methicillin-resistant coagulase-negative staphylococci) may indeed experience a higher risk of dying from the endocarditis. Finally, in the older patient it is clear the diagnosis is more difficult because clinicians are less apt to consider it until greater damage is done.

The diagnosis of endocarditis in the older adult is probably no less difficult to establish if it is considered. Blood cultures taken before empirical antibiotics, especially if endocarditis is a consideration, are certainly helpful. Echocardiography (33) in the older patient is clearly a useful diagnostic maneuver. The treatment of endocarditis in the older patient is similar to that in the younger individual (9). Care must be exerted in the older individual when using potentially toxic agents (aminoglycosides), and greater attention must be paid to renal function, toxicity monitoring, drug levels, and so on. In treating any case of endocarditis, serum cidal levels should be monitored and attempts made to keep serum levels, especially peak levels, at 1:8 or greater.

Suggested regimens for the treatment of endocarditis are listed in Table 1. Prophylaxis for bacterial endocarditis in the older patients is identical to that recommended for the younger patient (34).

**Table 1** Regimens for the Treatment of Endocarditis

| Etiology | Treatment | Duration (weeks) |
|---|---|---|
| Natural valve endocarditis | | |
| *S. viridans* | Penicillin G, 12 million U/day (divided dose) | 4 |
| Enterococci | Ampicillin, 12 g/day, and tobramicin or gentamicin, 3 mg/kg/day (divided dose) | 6 |
| Staphylococci | | |
| Coagulase positive (methicillin sensitive) | Nafcillin, 12 g/day (divided dose) | 6 |
| Coagulase negative (methicillin resistant) | Vancomycin, 500–1000 mg twice per day | 6 |
| Fastidious Gram-negative rods (e.g., *Hemophilus*) | Ampicillin, 12 g/day, and gentamicin, 5 mg/kg/day (divided dose) | 6 |
| Prosthetic valve endocarditis | | |
| Coagulase negative or positive, methicillin resistant | Vancomycin, 500–1000 mg twice per day, + gentamicin, 3 mg/kg/day, + rifampin, 300 mg every day (orally) | 6 (first 5 days only) |

All doses are intravenous unless otherwise indicated.

## REFERENCES

1. Kelson SR, White PD. Notes on 250 cases of subacute bacterial (streptococci) endocarditis studied and treated between 1927 and 1939. *Ann Intern Med* 1945; 22:40–60.
2. Osler W. Gulstonian lectures on malignant endocarditis. *Lancet* 1885; 1:415–418, 459–464, 505–508.
3. Durack TT, Beeson PB. Experimental bacterial endocarditis. Colonization of sterile vegetations. *Br J Exp Pathol* 1972; 53:44–50.
4. Freedman LR, Valone J. Experimental infective endocarditis. *Prog Cardiovasc Dis* 1979; 22:169–180.
5. King K, Harkness J. Infective endocarditis in the 1980s. *Med J Aust* 1986; 144:536–540, 588–594.
6. Freedman LR. Infective Endocarditis and Other Intravascular Infections. New York: Plenum, 1982.
7. Finland M, Barnes W. Changing etiology of bacterial endocarditis in the antibacterial area. *Ann Intern Med* 1970; 72:341–348.

8. Cantrell M, Yoshikawa T. Infective endocarditis in the aging patient. *Gerontology* 1984; 30:316–326.
9. Rabinovich S, Evans J, Smith I, January L. A long term view of bacterial endocarditis: 337 cases 1924 to 1963. *Ann Intern Med* 1965; 63:185–198.
10. Lerner P, Weinstein L. Infective endocarditis in the antibiotic era. *N Engl J Med* 1966; 274:199–206, 259–266, 323–330, 388–393.
11. Cherubin C, Neu H. Infective endocarditis at the Presbyterian Hospital in New York City from 1938–1967. *Am J Med* 1971; 51:83–96.
12. Garvey G, Neu H. Infective endocarditis an evolving disease: A review of endocarditis at Columbia Presbyterian Medical Center 1968–1973. *Medicine* (*Baltimore*) 1978; 57:105–127.
13. Lowe J, Williams G, Tabaqchali S, Hill I, Hamer J, Houang E, Shaw E, Rees G. Ten years of infective endocarditis at St. Bartholomews Hospital: Analysis of clinical features and treatment in relation to prognosis and mortality. *Lancet* 1980; 1:133–136.
14. Von Reyn CF, Levy B, Arbeit R, Friedland G, Crumpacker C. Infective endocarditis: An analysis based on strict case definitions. *Ann Intern Med* 1981; 94:505–518.
15. Kerr A. In: Puller RL, ed. Subacute Bacterial Endocarditis. Springfield, IL: Thomas, 1955 (No. 274 American Lecture Series, Monographs on Bannerstone Division of American Lectures in Internal Medicine).
16. Bayles T, Lewis W. Subacute bacterial endocarditis in older people. *Ann Intern Med* 1940; 13:2154–2163.
17. Willis F. Cardiac clinic. LXX. Clinic on subacute bacterial endocarditis afflicting an aged patient. *Proc Staf Mtg Mayo Clin* 1940; 15:270–272.
18. Zeman F, Siegal S. Acute bacterial endocarditis in the aged. *Am Heart J* 1945; 29:597–610.
19. Traut E, Carter J, Gumbiner S, Hench R. Bacterial endocarditis in the elderly, a report of 94 autopsied cases. *Geriatrics* 1949; 4:205–210.
20. Wallach J, Gless M, Lukasler L, Angust A. Bacterial endocarditis in the aged. *Ann Intern Med* 1954; 42:1206–1213.
21. Anderson J, Staffurth J. Subacute bacterial endocarditis in the elderly. *Lancet* 1955; 2:1055–1058.
22. Gleck WJ. Diagnostic aspects of subacute bacterial endocarditis in the elderly. *Arch Intern Med* 1959; 102:761–765.
23. Hartman T, Meyers W. Occurrence of bacterial endocarditis in older individuals. *Geriatrics* 1959; 14:374–379.
24. Cummings V, Furman S, Dunst M, Rubin I. Subacute bacterial endocarditis in the older age group. *JAMA* 1960; 172:137–141.
25. Uwaydah M, Weinberg A. Bacterial endocarditis—a changing pattern. *N Engl J Med* 1965; 273:1231–1234.
26. Habte-Gabr E, January L, Smith I. Bacterial endocarditis: the need for early diagnosis. *Geriatrics* 1973; 28:166–170.
27. Watanakunakorn C, Tan J. Diagnostic difficulties of staphylococcal endocarditis in geriatric patients. *Geriatrics* 1973; 28:168–173.

28. Tan J, Watanakunakorn C, Terhune C. *Streptococcus viridans* endocarditis: favorable prognosis in geriatric patients. *Geriatrics* 1973; 28:68–73.
29. Applefield M, Hornick R. Infective endocarditis in patients over age 60. *Am Heart J* 1974; 88:90–94.
30. Thell R, Martin F, Edwards J. Bacterial endocarditis in subjects 60 years of age and older. *Circulation* 1975; 51:174–182.
31. Robbins N, DeMaria A, Miller M. Infective endocarditis in the elderly. *South Med J* 1980; 73:1335–1338.
32. Terpenning M, Buggy B, Kauffman C. Infective endocarditis: Clinical features in young and elderly patients. *Am J Med* 1987; 83:626–634.
33. Melvin ET, Berger M, Lutzker L. Non-invasive methods for detection of valve vegetations in infective endocarditis. *Am J Cardiol* 1981; 47:271–278.
34. Daijani S, Bisno A, Chung K, Durack D, Freed M, Gerber M, Karchman H, Millard D, Rahimtoola S, Shulman S, Watanakunakorn C, Taubert K. Prevention of bacterial endocarditis. Recommendations of the American Heart Association. *JAMA* 1990; 264:2919–2922.

# 18

## Cardiomyopathies in the Elderly

**Michele Nanna**
*Albert Einstein College of Medicine, Bronx, New York*

**Wilbert S. Aronow**
*Mount Sinai School of Medicine, New York, New York and Hebrew Hospital Home, Bronx, New York*

### HYPERTROPHIC CARDIOMYOPATHY

Hypertrophic cardiomyopathy is a primary myocardial disorder with a hypertrophied and nondilated left ventricle (LV) not caused by other cardiovascular disease (1). Whiting et al. (2) showed that 32% of patients with hypertrophic cardiomyopathy were older than 60 years of age. Petrin and Tavel (3) reported that 83% of patients with hypertrophic cardiomyopathy were older than 50 years of age. Lever et al. (4) found that hypertrophic cardiomyopathy was more commonly diagnosed in patients 65 years or older than in patients younger than 40. Aronow and Kronzon (5) demonstrated that hypertrophic cardiomyopathy was present in 17 of 379 unselected elderly patients (4%), mean age 82 ± 8 years, in a long-term health care facility. Hypertrophic cardiomyopathy was present in 3% of elderly men and in 5% of elderly women. Of 17 elderly patients with hypertrophic cardiomyopathy, 10 (59%) had asymmetric septal hypertrophy and 7 (41%) had idiopathic hypertrophic subaortic stenosis (obstructive hypertrophic cardiomyopathy), with LV outflow tract obstruction at rest and gradients across the LV outflow tract ranging from 20 to 110 mm Hg (5). In this study, asymmetric septal hypertrophy was diagnosed when the ratio of the interventricular septum to posterior wall thickness was greater than 1.3 and the septal thickness exceeded 15 mm in the absence of other acquired or congenital heart disease likely to cause asymmetric septal hypertrophy (5).

Idiopathic hypertrophic subaortic stenosis was diagnosed when asymmetric septal hypertrophy coexisted with systolic anterior motion of the anterior mitral leaflet (5). Only systolic anterior motion that appeared independent of the motion of the posterior wall of the LV was considered significant and was included. The Doppler spectral characteristics of dynamic LV outflow tract obstruction included increased LV outflow tract velocity ($\geqslant$2.0 mm/s) and late systolic peaking of flow velocity with "ski slope" appearance (5).

Lever et al. (4) compared 28 patients 65 years or older with hypertrophic cardiomyopathy with 28 patients younger than 40 years of age with hypertrophic cardiomyopathy. Clinical findings were similar between the two groups, except for a higher prevalence of female sex, systemic hypertension, and atrial fibrillation in the elderly group. Echocardiographic findings concerning asymmetry, systolic anterior motion of the mitral valve, and a LV outflow tract gradient $\geqslant$ 20 mm Hg were similar in both groups. However, the elderly group had a predominantly ovoid cavity contour with normal septal curvature. The younger group had a predominantly crescent-shaped LV cavity and a reversed curvature of the interventricular septum. The right ventricular free wall was also more prominent in the younger group.

LV hypertrophy is more severe in younger patients with hypertrophic cardiomyopathy than in older patients with hypertrophic cardiomyopathy (6). Lewis and Maron (7) reported a group of 52 elderly patients (45 women) with obstructive hypertrophic cardiomyopathy. Echocardiographic examination showed a relatively small heart with modest LV septal hypertrophy and marked distortion of LV outflow tract morphology. LV outflow tract size at end-diastole was greatly reduced, and anterior displacement of the mitral valve within the LV cavity was marked. In most patients, anterior excursion of the mitral valve leaflets was restricted, and systolic apposition between the mitral valve and the LV septum resulted from a combination of anterior mitral valve excursion toward the LV septum and posterior excursion of the LV septum toward the mitral valve.

Topol et al. (8) reported 21 elderly patients (16 female) with a syndrome they called hypertensive hypertrophic cardiomyopathy of the elderly. Their patients had severe concentric LV hypertrophy, a small LV cavity, and supernormal indexes of LV systolic function without concurrent medical illness or coronary artery disease. Pearson et al. (9) reported 17 patients (16 female) with hypertensive hypertrophic cardiomyopathy of the elderly. All their patients had symmetrical hypertrophy with involvement of both the LV septum and the LV free wall. The increased LV outflow tract velocities were late peaking, similar to those described in hypertrophic cardiomyopathy, and localized to the LV outflow tract. LV filling was characterized by increased peak atrial velocity and decreased ratio of peak early to peak atrial velocity compared to a control group. LV end-diastolic dimension was smaller and left atrial size not different compared to a control group.

Karam et al. (10) compared 39 patients with hypertrophic cardiomyopathy and hypertension with an age-matched and gender-matched group of 39 patients with hypertrophic cardiomyopathy without hypertension. There were no significant differences in symptoms, functional class, electrocardiographic abnormalities, LV outflow tract obstruction, or most echocardiographic abnormalities, including asymmetric hypertrophy, between the two groups. However, the patients with hypertension were more likely to have a thicker posterior LV wall. These investigators suggested that hypertension makes hypertrophic cardiomyopathy worse but is not the primary cause of the disorder. They suggested that the term "hypertrophic cardiomyopathy with hypertension" was preferable to the term "hypertensive hypertrophic cardiomyopathy."

Continuous-wave Doppler echocardiography can accurately estimate the LV outflow tract gradient in patients with hypertrophic cardiomyopathy (11). Impaired LV diastolic function is the most important feature of hypertrophic cardiomyopathy. This is due to a combination of abnormalities in LV relaxation and compliance and affects both obstructive and nonobstructive forms. Abnormal LV diastolic function with abnormal Doppler diastolic indexes occurs with similar frequency in patients with hypertrophic cardiomyopathy with or without LV outflow tract obstruction and with or without cardiac symptoms (12). LV diastolic function is reduced in elderly patients with hypertrophic cardiomyopathy compared to younger patients with hypertrophic cardiomyopathy (13).

Decreased compliance in hypertrophic cardiomyopathy may be due to abnormal material properties secondary to a combination of fibrosis and cell disorganization (14–19). The fibrosis and cell disorganization, combined with an increase in LV mass, cause a shift to the left of the pressure-volume curve. Mechanisms that affect LV relaxation interfere with an active process by which calcium ions are recaptured in the sarcoplasmic reticulum, depriving the myofibrillar contractile proteins of an essential element for the actin-myosin bond.

LV diastolic filling abnormalities in hypertrophic cardiomyopathy are independent of the magnitude of LV hypertrophy and are common in patients with both marked and diffused LV hypertrophy and more mild and localized LV hypertrophy (20). These findings suggest that the primary myopathic process causing impaired LV diastolic filling in hypertrophic cardiomyopathy is not confined to the thickened portions of the LV wall. Wigle (21) concluded that impaired LV relaxation is often a more important cause of abnormal LV diastolic filling than increased passive chamber stiffness (decreased compliance) in patients with hypertrophic cardiomyopathy. However, both abnormalities may coexist.

Figures 1 through 6 illustrate M-mode echocardiographic findings (Fig. 1), two-dimensional echocardiographic findings (Figs. 2 and 3), pulsed Doppler echocardiographic findings (Fig. 4), color Doppler echocardiographic findings (Fig. 5), and continuous-wave Doppler echocardiographic findings (Fig. 6) in elderly patients with hypertrophic cardiomyopathy. Mitral annular calcification (MAC) associated with hypertrophic cardiomyopathy in the elderly is also illustrated in Figures 1 through 3.

## MITRAL ANNULAR CALCIUM

By increasing LV systolic pressure, hypertrophic cardiomyopathy may accelerate MAC. Patients with hypertrophic cardiomyopathy and MAC are older than patients with hypertrophic cardiomyopathy without MAC (22–24).

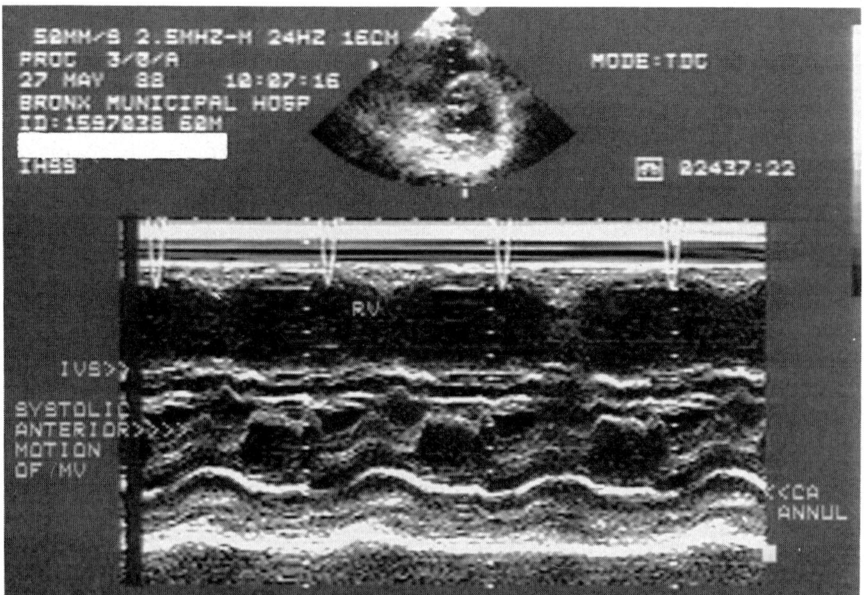


**Figure 1** M-mode echocardiogram at the mitral valve level in an elderly patient with obstructive hypertrophic cardiomyopathy. During midsystole, a smooth anterior motion of the mitral valve is noted. The mitral valve assumes a flattened curve appearance as it approaches the septum, and the contact with the septum is facilitated by the posterior motion of the septum. Mitral annular calcification is present behind the posterior leaflet. IVS = interventricular septum; RV = right ventricular cavity; MV = mitral valve; CA ANNUL = mitral annular calcification.

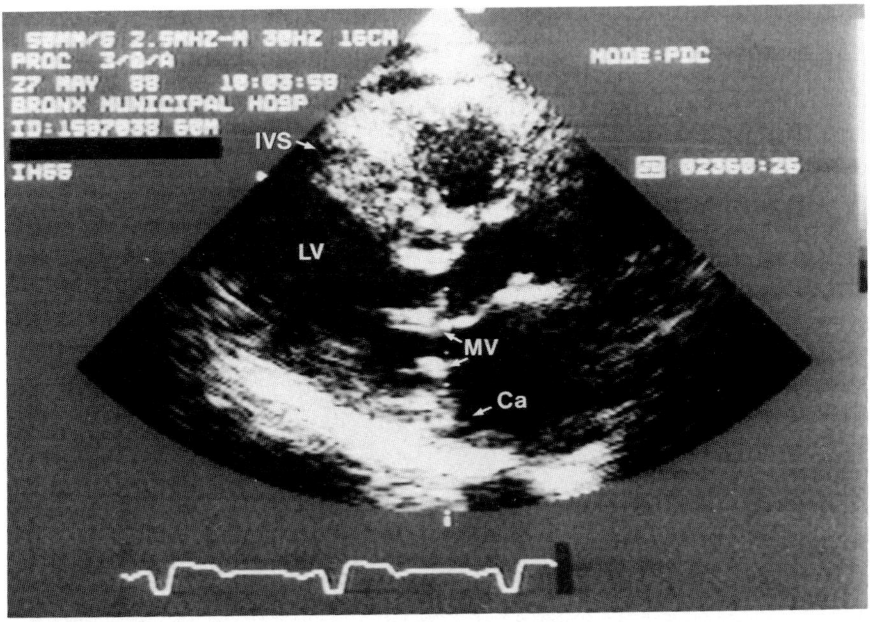


**Figure 2** Diastolic frame of a two-dimensional echocardiogram from a parasternal long-axis view in an elderly patient with hypertrophic cardiomyopathy shows a small LV chamber, a hypertrophic interventricular septum (IVS), a fibrotic mitral valve (MV), and a calcified mitral annulus (Ca).

Kronzon and Glassman (22) observed that MAC occurred in 12 of 18 patients (67%) older than 55 years with hypertrophic cardiomyopathy and in 4 of 28 patients (14%) younger than 55 years with hypertrophic cardiomyopathy ($p < 0.01$). Motamed and Roberts (23) demonstrated MAC in 30 of 100 autopsy patients (30%) older than 40 years with hypertrophic cardiomyopathy and in none of 100 patients (0%) younger than 40 years with hypertrophic cardiomyopathy. Nair et al. (24) showed that MAC was present in 12 of 42 patients (29%) with hypertrophic cardiomyopathy. Their patients with hypertrophic cardiomyopathy and MAC were older than their patients with hypertrophic cardiomyopathy without MAC. Fulkerson et al. (25) found that hypertrophic cardiomyopathy occurred in 5 of 80 patients (6%) with MAC, mean age 73 years. Aronow and Kronzon (5) showed that MAC was present in 13 of 17 elderly patients (76%) with hypertrophic cardiomyopathy and in 176 of 362 elderly patients (49%) without hypertrophic cardiomyopathy ($p < 0.025$). Lewis and Maron (7) demonstrated MAC in 52 of 52 elderly patients (100%) with hypertrophic cardiomyopathy. Calcification was severe in 39 of 52 patients (75%) and

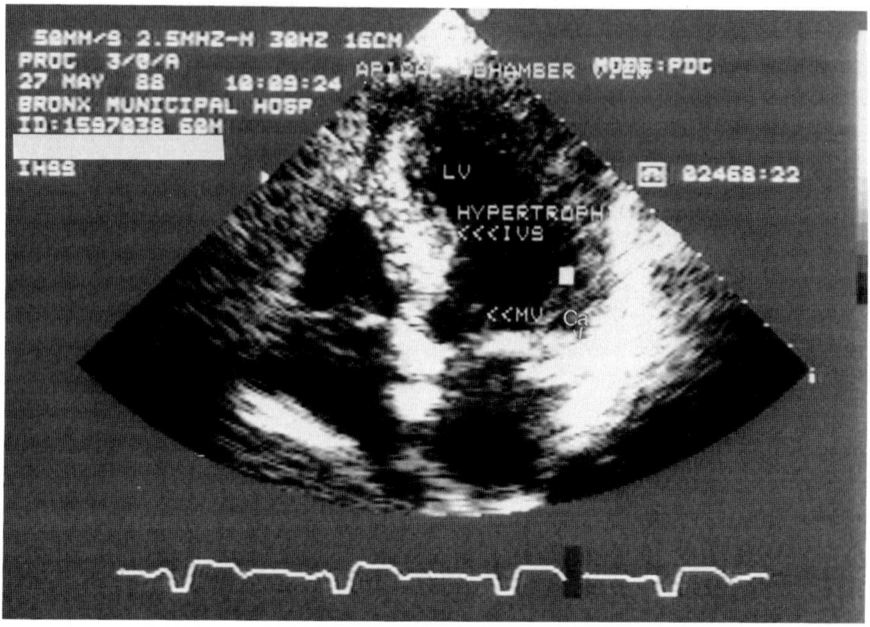


**Figure 3** Two-dimensional apical four-chamber systolic still frame from an elderly patient with obstructive hypertrophic cardiomyopathy shows hypertrophy of the interventricular septum (IVS), a small LV cavity, fibrotic mitral valve (MV) leaflets, and a calcified mitral annulus (Ca).

mild to moderate in 13 patients (25%). The sizeable deposits of calcium in the mitral annulus posterior to the mitral valve appeared to contribute to the narrowing of the LV outflow tract.

Klues et al. (26) also demonstrated that the disease process in hypertrophic cardiomyopathy is not confined to cardiac muscle. Of 94 mitral valves in patients with hypertrophic cardiomyopathy, 62 (66%) had structural abnormalities of the mitral valve unlikely to be acquired or secondary to mechanical factors. The structural abnormalities included increased mitral leaflet area and elongation of the leaflets or anomalous papillary muscle insertion directly into the anterior mitral leaflet.

## SYMPTOMS

Lever et al. (4) demonstrated in 28 elderly patients with hypertrophic cardiomyopathy that 24 (86%) had dyspnea, 17 (61%) had palpitations, 13 (46%) had angina pectoris, and 6 (21%) had syncope. Lewis and Maron (7) observed

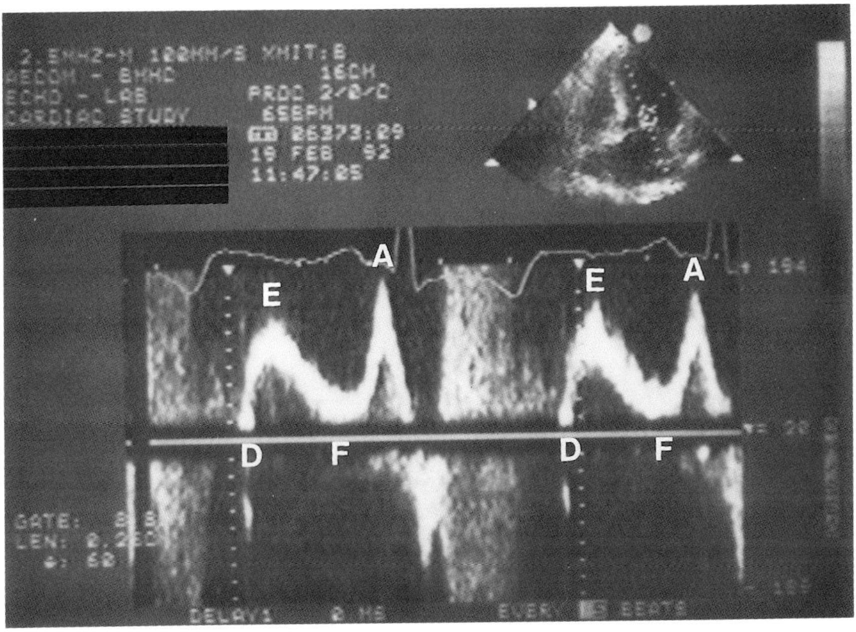


**Figure 4** LV diastolic waveforms obtained with pulsed Doppler echocardiography in an elderly patient with hypertrophic cardiomyopathy show reduced maximal flow velocity of early peak (E), slow deceleration of early diastolic flow velocity (from E to F), prolongation of early filling component (from D to F) at the expense of diastasis, and increased maximal velocity of the late peak as a result of atrial systole (A).

in 52 elderly patients with hypertrophic cardiomyopathy that 48 (92%) had exertional dyspnea and fatigue, 33 (63%) had chest pain, 22 (42%) had orthopnea or paroxysmal nocturnal dyspnea, and 12 (23%) had syncope or near-syncope. Agaston et al. (13) observed in 44 elderly patients with hypertrophic cardiomyopathy that 12 (27%) had congestive heart failure, 13 (30%) had syncope, 7 (16%) had near-syncope, and 13 (30%) had angina pectoris. Fay et al. (27) demonstrated in 95 elderly patients with hypertrophic cardiomyopathy that 47 (49%) had chest pain, 16 (17%) had syncope, 32 (34%) had New York Heart Association functional class II dyspnea, 12 (13%) had New York Heart Association functional class III dysnpea, and 24 (25%) had no symptoms.

Impaired LV filling due to LV diastolic dysfunction in patients with hypertrophic cardiomyopathy results in an elevated LV diastolic, left atrial, and pulmonary venous pressure, causing dyspnea. Syncope or-near syncope may result from an inadequate cardiac output with exertion or from cardiac arrhythmias. Angina pectoris unassociated with coronary artery disease may result from an

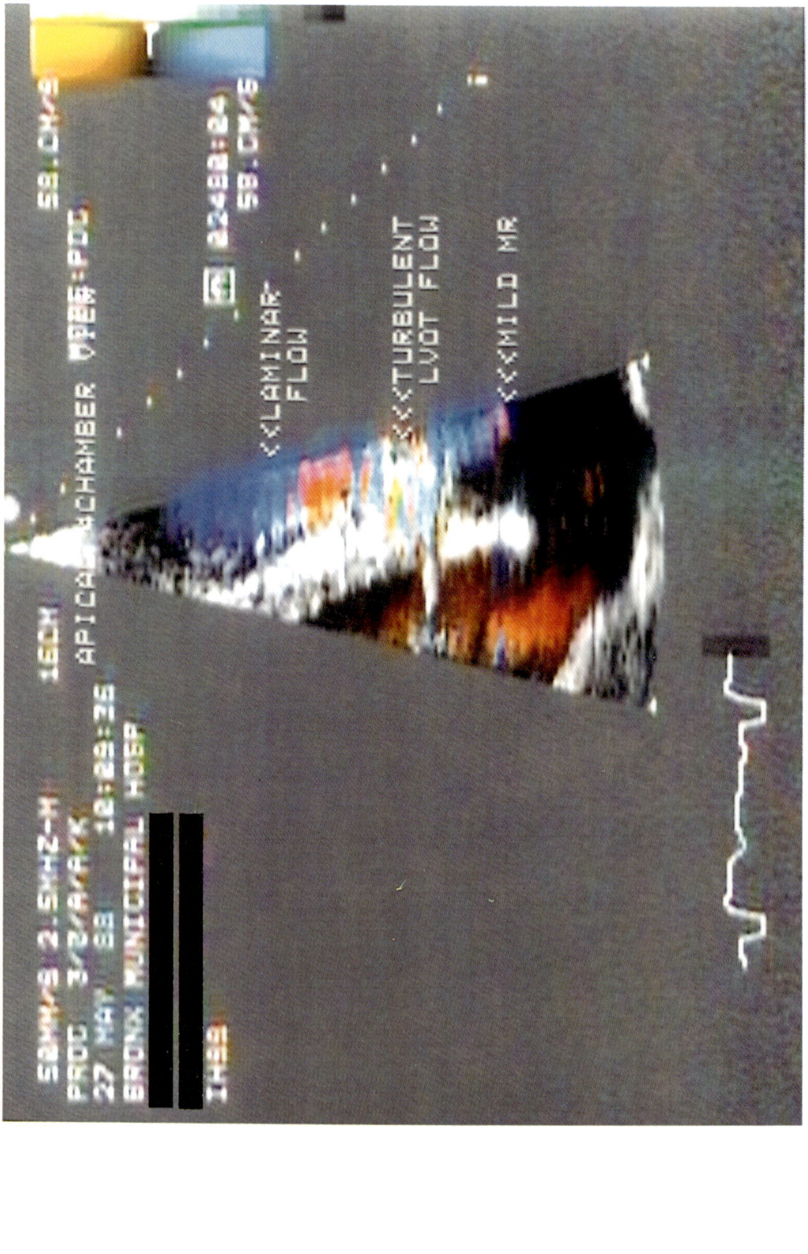


**Figure 5** Color Doppler flow display from a patient with obstructive hypertrophic cardiomyopathy shows turbulent flow in the LV outflow tract (LVOT) and mild mitral regurgitation (MR).

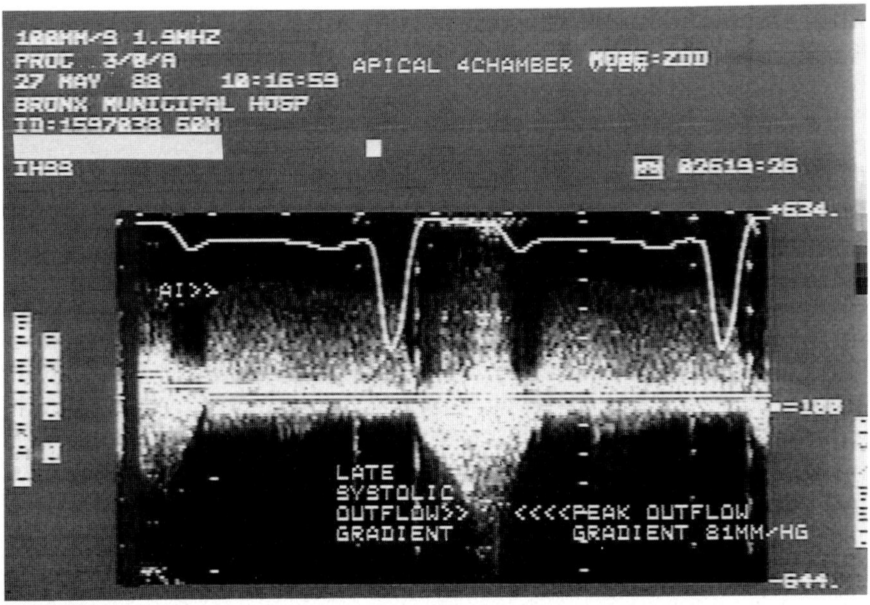


**Figure 6** Continuous-wave Doppler recording obtained in the LV outflow tract of an elderly patient with obstructive hypertrophic cardiomyopathy. Note the increased late systolic LV outflow tract velocity, which translates to a peak LV outflow tract gradient of 81 mm Hg. In diastole, a characteristic aortic insufficiency velocity pattern is noted.

increased myocardial oxygen demand and a reduced myocardial oxygen supply due to an increase in coronary vascular resistance and a decrease in coronary vascular reserve associated with LV hypertrophy (28–32). The greater the degree of LV hypertrophy, the greater is the reduction in coronary vascular reserve. The ratio of subendocardial to epicardial blood flow in the LV becomes abnormal. Intraventricular compressive forces may cause a reduction in coronary blood supply to the myocardium while myocardial oxygen demand is increased. This may result, especially during tachycardia, in subendocardial hypoperfusion and ischemia. Autopsy studies have demonstrated LV necrosis, widespread fibrosis, or transmural scarring in patients with hypertrophic cardiomyopathy (14,18,29,30). Coexistent coronary artery disease in elderly patients may also contribute to myocardial ischemia, causing chest pain.

## PHYSICAL EXAMINATION

Patients with obstructive hypertrophic cardiomyopathy may have a double apical impulse due to a prominent apical precordial impulse and a prominent presystolic apical impulse or a triple apical impulse, the third impulse being a late systolic bulge. A fourth heart sound is characteristically heard. A late systolic murmur may be due to dynamic obstruction of the LV outflow tract. Lever et al. (4) reported that a systolic murmur was heard in 26 of 28 elderly patients (93%) with hypertrophic cardiomyopathy. Fay et al. (27) stated that a systolic murmur was heard in 92 of 95 elderly patients (97%) with hypertrophic cardiomyopathy. Chandraratna and Aronow (33) concluded that the murmur of obstructive hypertrophic cardiomyopathy in patients with marked systolic anterior motion of the mitral valve is due to a composite of turbulence in the LV outflow tract and mitral regurgitation, whereas when only mild systolic anterior motion of the mitral valve is present, the systolic murmur originates in the LV outflow tract. Cassidy et al. (34) demonstrated that during handgrip exercise, the systolic murmur associated with obstructive hypertrophic cardiomyopathy becomes inaudible or decreased in intensity by auscultation. In the squatting position, the systolic murmur due to hypertrophic cardiomyopathy also decreases in intensity. The systolic murmur increases in intensity during the Valsalva maneuver or in the standing position.

The carotid arterial pulse of obstructive hypertrophic cardiomyopathy characteristically reveals a rapid initial upstroke and commonly a bifid pulse contour (34,35). Cassidy et al. (34) demonstrated a bifid carotid arterial pulse in seven of nine patients (78%) with obstructive hypertrophic cardiomyopathy. During handgrip exercise, the bifid carotid arterial pulse disappeared in five patients and greatly decreased in the other two patients.

## ELECTROCARDIOGRAM

Electrocardiographic evidence of LV hypertrophy was observed in 18 of 28 elderly patients (64%) with hypertrophic cardiomyopathy (4) and in 56 of 95 elderly patients (60%) with hypertrophic cardiomyopathy (27). Lever et al. (4) reported Q waves—anteroseptal, lateral, or both—on the electrocardiogram in 8 of 28 elderly patients (29%) with hypertrophic cardiomyopathy. Lemery et al. (36) demonstrated abnormal Q waves on the electrocardiogram in 19 of 67 patients (28%) with hypertrophic cardiomyopathy and attributed them primarily to a function of the ratio of upper anterior septal thickness to right ventricular wall thickness. Lever et al. (4) also reported in 28 elderly patients with hypertrophic cardiomyopathy that the electrocardiogram showed right bundle branch block in 4 patients (14%), left bundle branch block in 2 patients (7%), and no abnormality in 1 patient (4%).

Development of atrial fibrillation in patients with hypertrophic cardiomyopathy may cause symptomatic deterioration and increased risk of systemic embolization (7,37–40). Symptomatic deterioration is due to a rapid ventricular rate and to the loss of increased left atrial systolic filling in a LV, with impaired LV relaxation (40). Lewis and Maron (7) reported that atrial fibrillation (paroxysmal in 16 patients and chronic in 6 patients) occurred in 24 of 52 elderly patients (42%) with hypertrophic cardiomyopathy. The development of atrial fibrillation was associated with the onset of severe symptoms in 8 of 22 patients (36%) and in the progression of pre-existing symptoms in another 5 patients (23%). Lever et al. (4) showed that atrial fibrillation occurred in 7 of 28 elderly patients (25%) with hypertrophic cardiomyopathy. Spirito et al. (41) demonstrated that most patients with hypertrophic cardiomyopathy and chronic atrial fibrillation have nonobstructive hypertrophic cardiomyopathy and relatively mild LV hypertrophy.

## VENTRICULAR ARRHYTHMIAS

Spirito et al. (42) showed a strong association between magnitude of echocardiographic LV hypertrophy and ventricular tachycardia detected by 24 h ambulatory electrocardiography in patients with hypertrophic cardiomyopathy. Aronow et al. (43) found an increased prevalence of ventricular tachycardia and complex ventricular arrhythmias detected by 24 h ambulatory electrocardiography in elderly patients with echocardiographic LV hypertrophy associated with hypertrophic cardiomyopathy. Maron et al. (44) demonstrated by 24 h ambulatory electrocardiography in patients with hypertrophic cardiomyopathy that brief runs of asymptomatic ventricular tachycardia were associated with an increased risk of sudden cardiac death. At 3 years follow-up, sudden cardiac death occurred in 4 of 17 patients (24%) with asymptomatic ventricular tachycardia associated with hypertrophic cardiomyopathy and in 2 of 66 patients (3%) with hypertrophic cardiomyopathy and no ventricular tachycardia ($p < 0.02$). Aronow et al. (45) observed that ventricular tachycardia and complex ventricular arrhythmias detected by 24 h ambulatory electrocardiography in elderly patients with hypertrophic cardiomyopathy were at 2 years follow-up a risk factor for new cardiac events. Aronow et al. (46) also found at 27 months follow-up that elderly patients with hypertrophic cardiomyopathy, echocardiographic LV hypertrophy, and ventricular tachycardia or complex ventricular arrhythmias detected by 24 h ambulatory electrocardiography had an increased incidence of primary ventricular fibrillation or sudden cardiac death.

Hemodynamic and electrophysiological studies were performed by Fananapazir and Epstein (47) in 30 patients with hypertrophic cardiomyopathy who survived sudden cardiac death. Potential causes of sudden cardiac arrest were found in 30 of 30 patients (100%). Inducible sustained ventricular arrhythmias were found in 21 patients (70%): polymorphic ventricular tachycardia in 18 patients, monomorphic ventricular tachycardia in 2 patients, and ventricular fibrillation in 1 patient. Severe LV outflow tract obstruction was observed in 8 patients (27%), bradycardia in 5 patients (17%), myocardial ischemia associated with hypotension in 5 patients (17%), and atrial tachycardia causing hypotension in 4 patients (13%).

## NATURAL HISTORY

Elderly patients with hypertrophic cardiomyopathy are predisposed to develop sudden cardiac death, congestive heart failure, and syncope. Lewis and Maron (7) observed in 52 elderly patients with hypertrophic cardiomyopathy that severe symptoms were not present early in life but developed in 50 patients after age 55. Spirito and Maron (48) observed that most asymptomatic or mildly symptomatic patients with hypertrophic cardiomyopathy who die suddenly have marked and diffuse LV hypertrophy. They concluded that a relation exists between the extent of LV hypertrophy and the occurrence of sudden and unexpected cardiac death in patients with hypertrophic cardiomyopathy. Kogure et al. (49) reported that 6 of 66 patients (9%) with hypertrophic cardiomyopathy developed systemic thromboembolism during 3.7 years follow-up. All thromboembolic events occurred in patients with atrial fibrillation. Hypertrophic cardiomyopathy also predisposes to infective endocarditis (50).

A total of 95 elderly patients (mean age 71.8 years) with hypertrophic cardiomyopathy were followed for a mean duration of 4.2 years (27). The survival rates at 1 and 5 years were 95 and 76%, respectively, compared with 97 and 82%, respectively, for control subjects. Patients with class III dyspnea had a 1 year mortality rate of 36%. Advanced functional class dyspnea ($p < 0.002$), increased indexed left atrial size ($p < 0.004$), and increased indexed ventricular septal thickness ($p < 0.003$) were associated with an increased incidence of cardiac death.

## THERAPY

$\beta$-adrenergic blockers can relieve the symptoms of exertional angina pectoris, dyspnea, and light-headedness or syncope in patients with hypertrophic cardiomyopathy. In one-half to one-third of all symptomatic patients improvement of cardiac symptoms is seen after treatment with propranolol, 160–320 mg daily (37). Transient $\beta$-adrenergic hypersensitivity occurs after $\beta$-blocker withdrawal in patients with hypertrophic cardiomyopathy and is associated with clinical deterioration (51). Therefore, abrupt withdrawal of $\beta$-blockers should be avoided in patients with hypertrophic cardiomyopathy.

Calcium channel blockers, especially verapamil, have also been shown to be effective in reducing cardiac symptoms in patients with hypertrophic cardiomyopathy (40,52,53). Almost 60% of 227 patients with hypertrophic cardiomyopathy receiving verapamil (median dose 360 mg daily) because of severe cardiac symptoms despite $\beta$-blocker therapy had clinical improvement after 3–

53 months (mean 25 months) (53). β-Blockers and verapamil are contraindicated in patients with important conduction system abnormalities unless a pacemaker has been implanted. Of 47 elderly patients with severe cardiac symptoms initially treated with drugs, only 12 (26%) showed clinical improvement (7). The drug treatment included verapamil in 8 patients, propranolol in 1 patient, calcium channel blockers plus β-blockers in 2 patients, and disopyramide plus verapamil in 1 patient.

Digitalis should be avoided in patients with hypertrophic cardiomyopathy unless LV systolic dysfunction develops. Nitrates should also be avoided. Diuretics should be avoided in patients with hypertrophic cardiomyopathy and pulmonary venous congestion associated with normal LV systolic function unless administered concomitantly with a β-blocker or verapamil (37). β-Blockers or verapamil may be used to slow the ventricular rate in patients with atrial fibrillation associated with hypertrophic cardiomyopathy. Restoration of sinus rhythm in patients with atrial fibrillation should be attempted by electrical cardioversion. Once atrial fibrillation has developed, anticoagulant therapy should be started immediately and continued indefinitely (37). Patients with hypertrophic cardiomyopathy should also receive prophylactic antibiotics during procedures predisposing to infective endocarditis (50).

Of 30 patients with hypertrophic cardiomyopathy surviving cardiac arrest who underwent hemodynamic and electrophysiological evaluation, Fananapazir and Epstein (47) treated 17 of 21 patients with inducible sustained ventricular arrhythmias with an implantable defibrillator and 4 with antiarrhythmic drugs. A total of 7 patients underwent LV septal myectomy; 3 patients received antiarrhythmic drugs for atrial tachycardia; 1 patient had catheter ablation of a concealed posteroseptal accessory pathway; and 3 patients with myocardial ischemia were treated with propranolol plus verapamil (2 also had a defibrillator implanted). During 18 months follow-up (range 1–75 months), 4 patients (13%) died suddenly, and 4 (13%) received a total of 13 defibrillator shocks. The 1 year survival rate was 93%. The 1 year sudden death or shock event-free rate was 80%.

Patients with obstructive hypertrophic cardiomyopathy with severe cardiac symptoms not responding well to medical therapy should have surgical treatment. The preferred operation for most patients with obstructive hypertrophic cardiomyopathy is ventricular septal myotomy–myectomy (37,54). However, mitral valve replacement has a role in selected patients (37,55). A group of 18 severely symptomatic elderly patients with obstructive hypertrophic cardiomyopathy (LV outflow tract obstruction ⩾ 50 mm Hg) underwent surgery: 12 had ventricular septal myotomy–myectomy, and 6 had mitral valve replacement. Of 18 patients 2 (11%) died as a result of surgery. Of the 16 surgical survivors, 14 (88%) had improvement in clinical symptoms. Of the 14 patients 2 (14%) died during follow-up: 1 patient died suddenly 8 months after surgery, and 1 patient died of congestive heart failure 16 months after surgery.

## DILATED CARDIOMYOPATHY

Idiopathic dilated cardiomyopathy is a primary disease of ventricular muscle, with increased LV or biventricular volumes, without an appropriate increase in ventricular septal or free wall thicknesses, and with depression of LV systolic function (56). Other etiologic factors that can cause diffuse LV systolic dysfunction must be excluded (57). Approximately 10% of patients with dilated cardiomyopathy are older than 65 (57–61). The diagnosis of dilated cardiomyopathy can be confirmed by echocardiography. Figures 7 through 10 illustrate dilated cardiomyopathy by M-mode echocardiography (Fig. 7), by two-dimensional echocardiography (Figs. 8 and 9), and by pulsed Doppler echocardiography (Fig. 10) in elderly patients. Figure 9 also shows a large apical thrombus. Coronary angiography should be considered in patients with chest

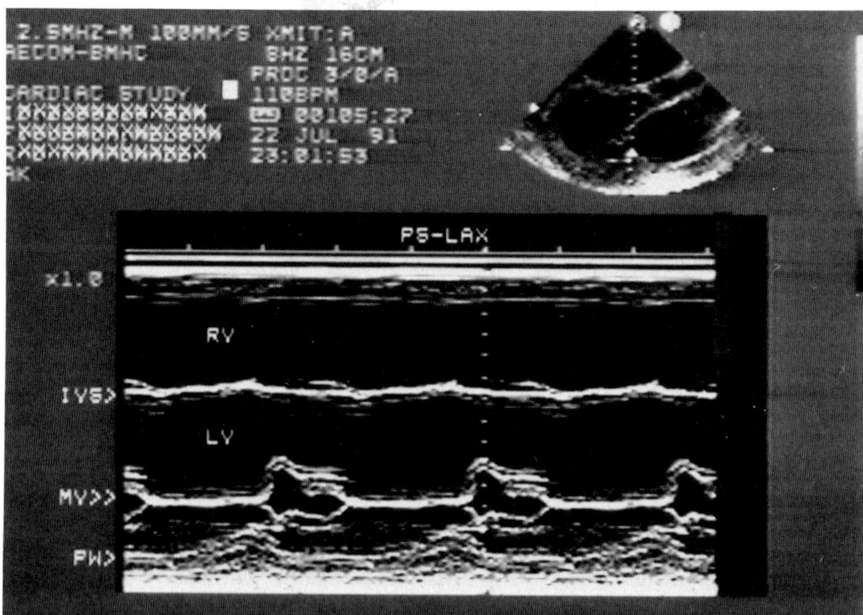


**Figure 7** M-mode echocardiogram at the mitral valve level in an elderly patient with dilated cardiomyopathy shows thinning of the interventricular septum (IVS), a markedly dilated LV cavity (LV), and increased E point septal separation. RV = right ventricle; MV = mitral valve; PW = posterior wall.

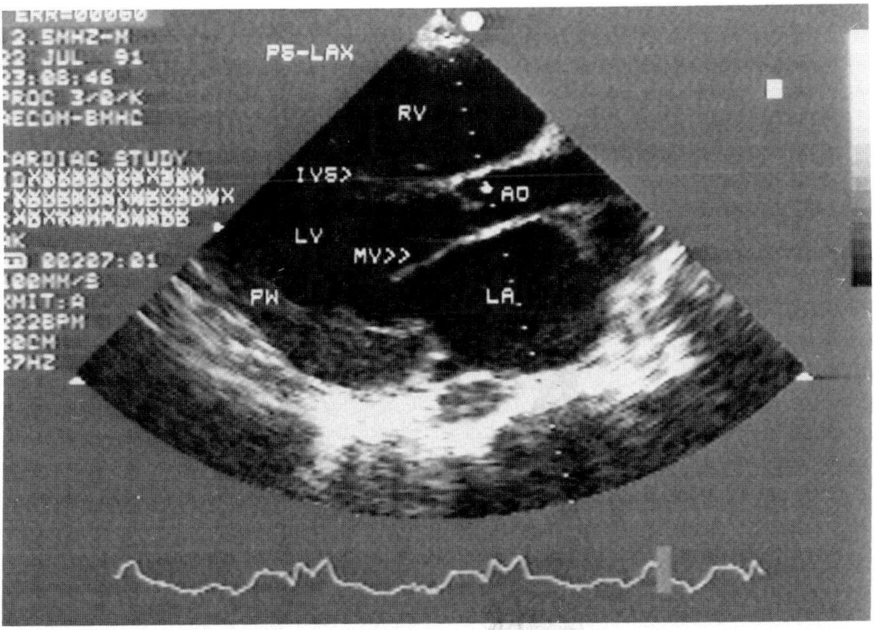


**Figure 8** Diastolic frame of a two-dimensional echocardiogram from a parasternal long-axis view in an elderly patient with dilated hypertrophic cardiomyopathy shows thinning of the interventricular septum (IVS) and a large LV cavity (LV). RV = right ventricle; AO = aorta; MV = mitral valve; PW = posterior wall; LA = left atrium.

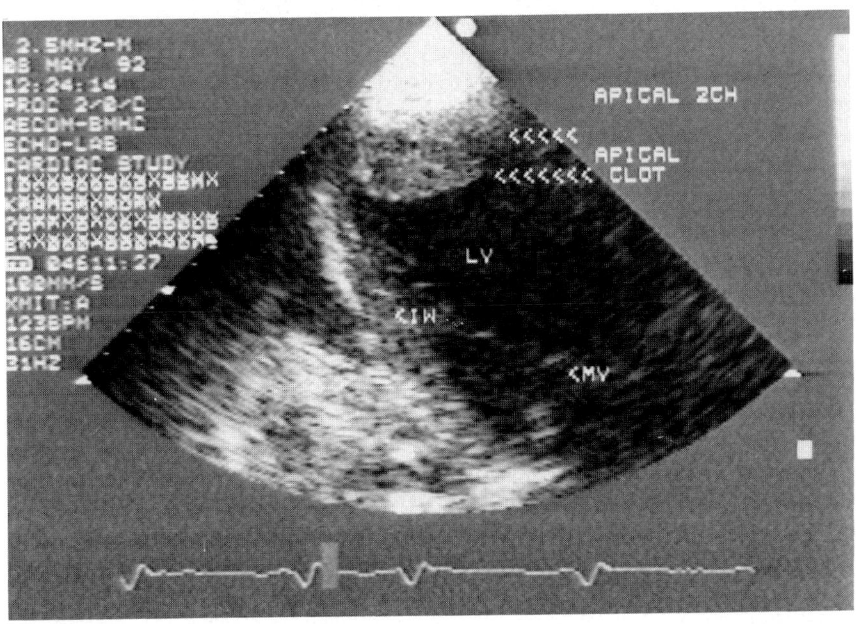


**Figure 9** Two-dimensional apical two-chamber view in an elderly patient with dilated hypertrophic cardiomyopathy shows a large apical thrombus. LV = left ventricle; IW = inferior wall; MV = mitral valve.

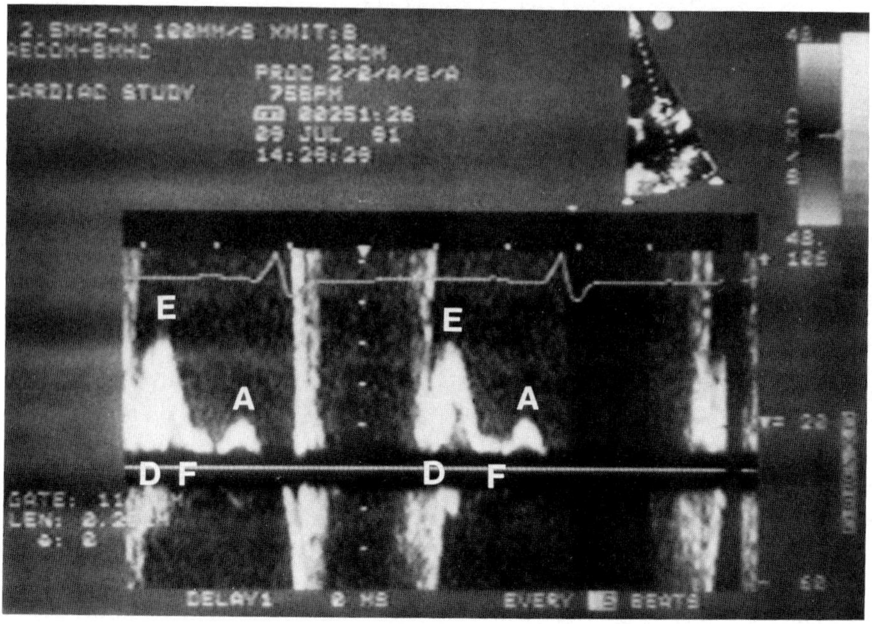


**Figure 10** LV diastolic waveforms obtained with pulsed Doppler echocardiography in an elderly patient with dilated cardiomyopathy show increased flow velocity of early peak (E), fast deceleration of early diastolic flow velocity (from E to F), shortening of early diastolic filling component (from D to F) with visible diastasis, and decreased maximal velocity of the late peak as a result of atrial systole (A).

pain considered to have dilated cardiomyopathy. Recently, transthoracic coronary echocardiography has been proposed as a useful method for distinguishing between ischemic and nonischemic dilated cardiomyopathy (62).

Symptoms due to dilated cardiomyopathy include fatigue and weakness resulting from decreased cardiac output, exercise intolerance, dyspnea due to congestive heart failure, chest pain, and syncope. Symptoms due to systemic or pulmonary emboli may also occur. Physical examination reveals moderate to severe cardiomegaly and audible third and fourth heart sounds. Signs of LV or biventricular failure may be present.

Fuster et al. (60) reported 104 patients at the Mayo Clinic with idiopathic dilated cardiomyopathy followed for 6–20 years. Of these 104 patients, 73% had congestive heart failure at the time of diagnosis, and 96% had congestive heart failure at follow-up. Systemic emboli were present in 4% of the patients at the time of diagnosis and in 18% of the patients at follow-up. Systemic thromboembolism developed in 8 of 24 patients (33%) with atrial fibrillation and in 11 of 80 patients (14%) with sinus rhythm ($p$ not significant). Systemic thromboembolism developed in 18% of patients who did not receive anticoagulant therapy and in none of those who did ($p < 0.05$). Of 104 patients 80 (77%) died at follow-up, two-thirds of the deaths occurring within 2 years.

Roberts et al. (61) reported that 148 of 152 necropsy patients (97%) with idiopathic dilated cardiomyopathy had clinical evidence of chronic congestive heart failure. Sudden death was the initial clinical manifestation in 4 patients (3%). Congestive heart failure was the initial manifestation in 114 of 152 patients (75%), and in most patients it became intractable and caused death. The mean duration from the onset of chronic congestive heart failure to known death in 120 patients was 54 months. The cause of death was chronic congestive heart failure in 58% of patients, sudden death in 27% of patients, pulmonary emboli in 9% of patients, and other in 6% of patients. Clinical evidence of pulmonary emboli was present in 39% of patients. Clinical evidence of systemic emboli was present in 20% of patients. Of 131 patients, 79 (60%) had either clinical or necropsy evidence, or both, of pulmonary or systemic emboli.

Falk et al. (63) demonstrated in 25 patients with nonischemic dilated cardiomyopathy who were not receiving anticoagulant therapy that a LV thrombus was present on initial echocardiogram in 11 patients (44%), developed during 21.5 months follow-up in 4 additional patients (16%), and disappeared in 2 patients (8%) during follow-up. Systemic thromboembolism developed in 5 of 25 patients (20%) during follow-up. Of the five thromboembolic events four occurred in patients with a LV thrombus. These 5 patients with thromboembolic events were treated with warfarin. No further embolic events occurred in these patients at 15 months follow-up.

Congestive heart failure in patients with dilated cardiomyopathy should be treated with salt restriction, diuretics, digitalis, and angiotensin-converting enzyme inhibitor therapy. $\beta$-Blocker therapy may improve symptoms in patients with dilated cardiomyopathy (64). Anticoagulants should be administered even if there is no echocardiographic evidence of LV thrombus. There is no evidence that antiarrhythmic drugs prolong life or prevent sudden cardiac death in patients with dilated cardiomyopathy. The role of endomyocardial biopsy in the diagnosis of dilated cardiomyopathy and as a guide to therapy in the elderly is unknown (57). Immunosuppressive therapy may be poorly tolerated in elderly patients with dilated cardiomyopathy (65).

## RESTRICTIVE CARDIOMYOPATHY

Restrictive cardiomyopathy may be caused by myocardial infiltrative, noninfiltrative, and storage diseases and by endomyocardial disease and is uncommon in the elderly. Primary amyloidosis is a frequent cause of restrictive cardiomyopathy but is uncommon in the elderly (57). Characteristically in cardiac amyloidosis, the ventricles are small and the atria large, with increased filling pressures and thickened walls (57). The echocardiogram shows a characteristic "sparkling" of the ventricular myocardium (Fig. 11). Stiffness of the LV in cardiac amyloidosis may cause an impaired rate of early diastolic filling of the LV. Pulsed Doppler echocardiography in restrictive cardiomyopathy due to cardiac amyloidosis shows a tall E wave and a small A wave (Fig. 12). Low QRS voltage, atrial fibrillation, and conduction defects may be present on the electrocardiogram (57). Small or absent R waves in the right precordial leads or Q waves in the inferior leads may mimic myocardial infarction. Complex ventricular arrhythmias are frequently present.

Symptoms due to cardiac amyloidosis include exertional dyspnea, fatigue, and chest pain. Peripheral edema is prominent. Congestive heart failure and postural hypotension may develop. A low systolic blood pressure, a narrow pulse pressure, jugular venous distention with prominent X and Y descents, mild to moderate cardiomegaly, a third heart sound gallop, a systolic murmur of

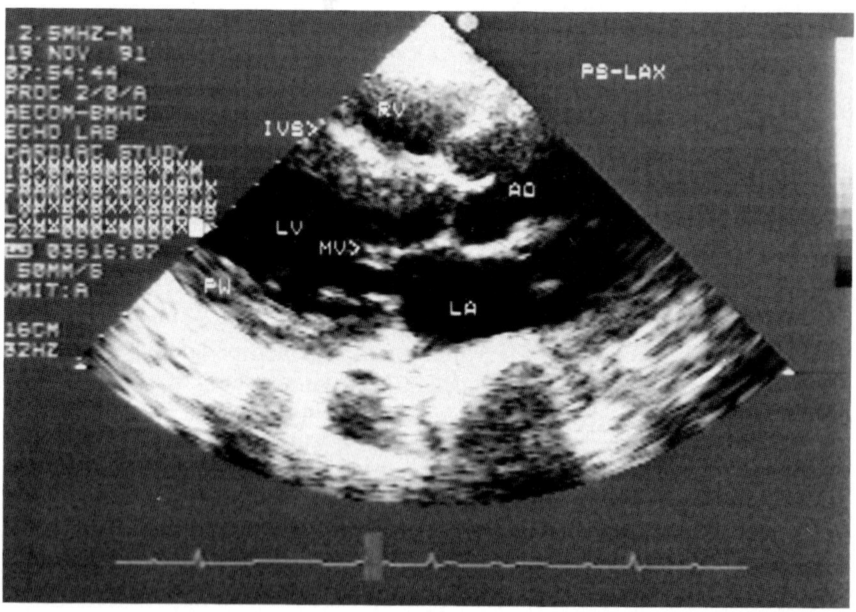


**Figure 11** Two-dimensional echocardiogram from a parasternal long-axis view in an elderly patient with cardiac amyloidosis shows a hypertrophic interventricular septum with the characteristic "sparkling" appearance of the septal myocardium. RV = right ventricle; IVS = interventricular septum; AO = aorta; LA = left atrium; MV = mitral valve; LV = left ventricle; PW = posterior wall.

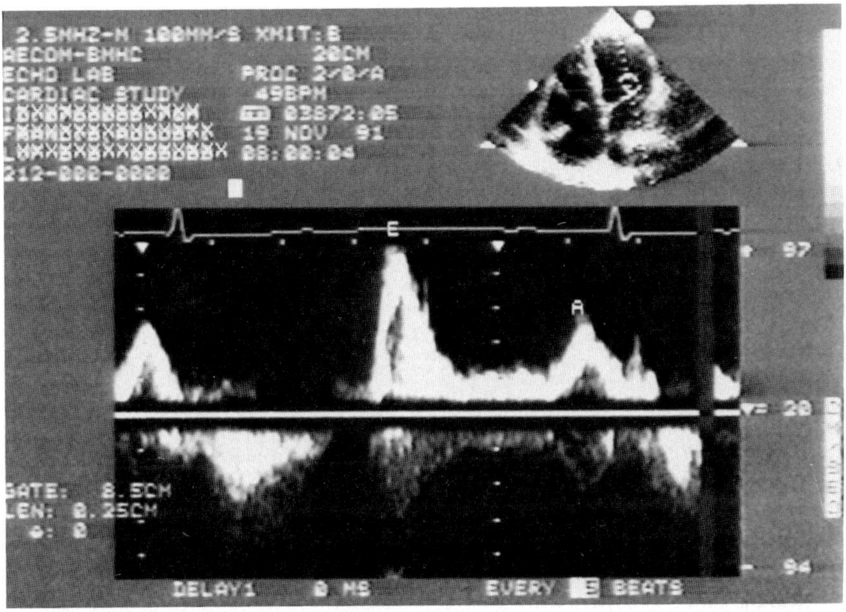


**Figure 12** LV diastolic waveforms obtained with pulsed Doppler echocardiography in an elderly patient with cardiac amyloidosis show increased flow velocity of early peak (E) and decreased maximal velocity of the late peak as a result of atrial systole (A).

tricuspid or mitral regurgitation, hepatomegaly, and peripheral edema may occur. An increase in neck vein distention with inspiration (Kussmaul's sign) may be present.

The diagnosis of cardiac amyloidosis can be confirmed by biopsy of rectal, gingival, or endomyocardial tissue (57). There is no specific treatment for cardiac amyloidosis (57). Diuretics and vasodilators should be used very cautiously in patients with congestive heart failure due to cardiac amyloidosis. Patients with cardiac amyloidosis are especially sensitive to digitalis. Patients with symptomatic conduction system abnormalities may benefit from permanent pacemaker implantation.

## REFERENCES

1. Maron BJ, Bonow RO, Cannon RO III, Leon MB, Epstein SE. Hypertrophic cardiomyopathy. Interrelations of clinical manifestations, pathophysiology, and therapy (first of two parts). *N Engl J Med* 1987; 316:780–789.

2. Whiting RB, Powell WJ, Dinsmore RE, Sanders CA. Idiopathic hypertrophic subaortic stenosis in the elderly. *N Engl J Med* 1971; 285:196–200.
3. Petrin TJ, Tavel ME. Idiopathic hypertrophic subaortic stenosis as observed in a large community hospital: Relation to age and history of hypertension. *J Am Geriatr Soc* 1979; 27:43–46.
4. Lever HM, Karam RF, Currie PJ, Healy BP. Hypertrophic cardiomyopathy in the elderly. Distinctions from the young based on cardiac shape. *Circulation* 1989; 79:580–589.
5. Aronow WS, Kronzon I. Prevalence of hypertrophic cardiomyopathy and its association with mitral annular calcium in elderly patients. *Chest* 1988; 94:1295–1296.
6. Spirito P, Maron BJ. Relation between extent of left ventricular hypertrophy and age in hypertrophic cardiomyopathy. *J Am Coll Cardiol* 1989; 13:820–823.
7. Lewis JF, Maron BJ. Elderly patients with hypertrophic cardiomyopathy: A subset with distinctive left ventricular morphology and progressive clinical course late in life. *J Am Coll Cardiol* 1989; 13:36–45.
8. Topol EJ, Traill TA, Fortuin NJ. Hypertensive hypertrophic cardiomyopathy of the elderly. *N Engl J Med* 1985; 312:277–283.
9. Pearson AC, Gudipati CV, Labovitz AJ. Systolic and diastolic flow abnormalities in elderly patients with hypertensive hypertrophic cardiomyopathy. *J Am Coll Cardiol* 1988; 12:989–995.
10. Karam R, Lever HM, Healy BP. Hypertensive hypertrophic cardiomyopathy or hypertrophic cardiomyopathy with hypertension? A study of 78 patients. *J Am Coll Cardiol* 1989; 13:580–584.
11. Sasson Z, Yock PG, Hatle LK, Alderman EL, Popp RL. Doppler echocardiographic determination of the pressure gradient in hypertrophic cardiomyopathy. *J Am Coll Cardiol* 1988; 11:752–756.
12. Maron BJ, Spirito P, Green KJ, Wesley YE, Bonow RO, Arce J. Noninvasive assessment of left ventricular diastolic function by pulsed Doppler echocardiography in patients with hypertrophic cardiomyopathy. *J Am Coll Cardiol* 1987; 10:733–742.
13. Agatston AS, Polakoff R, Hippogoankar R, Schnur S, Samet P. The significance of increased left ventricular outflow tract velocities in the elderly measured by continuous wave Doppler. *Am Heart J* 1989; 117:1320–1326.
14. Roberts WC, Ferrans VJ. Pathologic anatomy of the cardiomyopathies: Idiopathic dilated and hypertrophic types, infiltrative types, and endomyocardial disease with and without eosinophilia. *Hum Pathol* 1975; 6:287–342.
15. Ferrans VJ, Morrow AG, Roberts WC. Myocardial ultrastructure in idiopathic hypertrophic subaortic stenosis: A study of operatively excised left ventricular outflow tract muscle in 14 patients. *Circulation* 1972; 45:769–792.
16. Maron BJ, Roberts WC. Quantitative analysis of cardiac muscle cell disorganization in the ventricular septum of patients with hypertrophic cardiomyopathy. *Circulation* 1979; 59:689–706.
17. Maron BJ, Anan TJ, Roberts WC. Quantitative analysis of the distribution of cardiac muscle cell disorganization in the left ventricular wall of patients with hypertrophic cardiomyopathy. *Circulation* 1981; 63:882–894.

18. St. John Sutton MG, Lie JT, Anderson KR, O'Brien PC, Frye RL. Histopathological specificity of hypertrophic obstructive cardiomyopathy: Myocardial fibre disarray and myocardial fibrosis. *Br Heart J* 1980; 44:433–443.
19. Bulkley BH, Weisfeldt ML, Hutchins GM. Isometric cardiac contraction: A possible cause of the disorganized myocardial pattern of idiopathic hypertrophic subaortic stenosis. *N Engl J Med* 1977; 296:135–139.
20. Spirito P, Maron BJ. Relation between extent of left ventricular hypertrophy and diastolic filling abnormalities in hypertrophic cardiomyopathy. *J Am Coll Cardiol* 1990; 15:808–813.
21. Wigle ED. Impaired left ventricular relaxation in hypertrophic cardiomyopathy: Relation to extent of hypertrophy. *J Am Coll Cardiol* 1990; 15:814–815.
22. Kronzon I, Glassman E. Mitral ring calcification in idiopathic hypertrophic subaortic stenosis. *Am J Cardiol* 1978; 4:60–66.
23. Motamed HE, Roberts WC. Frequency and significance of mitral annular calcium in hypertrophic cardiomyopathy: Analysis of 200 necropsy patients. *Am J Cardiol* 1987; 60:877–884.
24. Nair CK, Kudesia V, Hansen D, Thomson V, Pagano T, Ryschon K, Sketch MH. Echocardiographic and electrocardiographic characteristics of patients with hypertrophic cardiomyopathy with and without mitral annular calcium. *Am J Cardiol* 1987; 59:1428–1430.
25. Fulkerson PK, Beaver BM, Auseon JC, Graber HL. Calcification of the mitral annulus: Etiology, clinical associations, complications and therapy. *Am J Med* 1979; 66:967–977.
26. Klues HG, Maron BJ, Dollar AL, Roberts WC. Diversity of structural mitral valve alterations in hypertrophic cardiomyopathy. *Circulation* 1992; 85:1651–1660.
27. Fay WP, Taliercio CP, Ilstrup DM, Tajik AJ, Gersh BJ. Natural history of hypertrophic cardiomyopathy in the elderly. *J Am Coll Cardiol* 1990; 16:821–826.
28. Aronow WS. Left ventricular hypertrophy. *J Am Geriatr Soc* 1992; 40:71–80.
29. Maron BJ, Wolfson JK, Epstein SE, Roberts WC. Intramural ("small vessel") coronary artery disease in hypertrophic cardiomyopathy. *J Am Coll Cardiol* 1986; 8:545–557.
30. Maron BJ, Epstein SE, Roberts WC. Hypertrophic cardiomyopathy and transmural myocardial infarction without significant atherosclerosis of the extramural coronary arteries. *Am J Cardiol* 1979; 43:1086–1102.
31. Pitcher D, Wainwright R, Maisey M, Curry P, Sowton E. Assessment of chest pain in hypertrophic cardiomyopathy using exercise thallium-201 myocardial scintigraphy. *Br Heart J* 1980; 44:650–656.
32. Cannon RO III, Rosing DR, Maron BJ, Leon MB, Bonow RO, Watson RM, Epstein SE. Myocardial ischemia in patients with hypertrophic cardiomyopathy: Contribution of inadequate vasodilator reserve and elevated left ventricular filling pressures. *Circulation* 1985; 71:234–243.
33. Chandraratna PAN, Aronow WS. Genesis of the systolic murmur of idiopathic hypertrophic subaortic stenosis. Phonocardiographic, echocardiographic, and pulsed Doppler ultrasound correlations. *Chest* 1983; 83:638–642.
34. Cassidy J, Aronow WS, Prakash R. The effect of isometric exercise on the systolic

murmur of patients with idiopathic hypertrophic subaortic stenosis. *Chest* 1975; 67:395–397.
35. Frank S, Braunwald E. Idiopathic hypertrophic subaortic stenosis. Clinical analysis of 126 patients with emphasis on the natural history. *Circulation* 1968; 37:759–788.
36. Lemery R, Kleinebenne A, Nihoyannopoulos P, Aber V, Alfonso F, McKenna WJ. Q waves in hypertrophic cardiomyopathy in relation to the distribution and severity of right and left ventricular hypertrophy. *J Am Coll Cardiol* 1990; 16:368–374.
37. Maron BJ, Bonow RO, Cannon RO III, Leon MB, Epstein SE. Hypertrophic cardiomyopathy. Interrelations of clinical manifestations, pathophysiology, and therapy (second of two parts). *N Engl J Med* 1987; 316:844–852.
38. Robinson K, Frenneaux MP, Stockins B, Karatasakis G, Poloniecki JD, McKenna WJ. *J Am Coll Cardiol* 1990; 15:1279–1285.
39. Wigle ED. Hypertrophic cardiomyopathy 1988. *Mod Concepts Cardiovasc Dis* 1988; 57:1–6.
40. Bonow RO, Frederick TM, Bacharach SL, Green MV, Goose PW, Maron BJ, Rosing DR, Epstein SE. Atrial systole and left ventricular filling in hypertrophic cardiomyopathy: Effect of verapamil. *Am J Cardiol* 1983; 51:1386–1391.
41. Spirito P, Lakatos E, Maron BJ. Degree of left ventricular hypertrophy in patients with hypertrophic cardiomyopathy and chronic atrial fibrillation. *Am J Cardiol* 1992; 69:1217–1222.
42. Spirito P, Watson RN, Maron BJ. Relation between extent of left ventricular hypertrophy and occurrence of ventricular tachycardia in hypertrophic cardiomyopathy. *Am J Cardiol* 1987; 60:1137–1142.
43. Aronow WS, Epstein S, Schwartz KS, Koenigsberg M. Correlation of complex ventricular arrhythmias detected by ambulatory electrocardiographic monitoring with echocardiographic left ventricular hypertrophy in persons older than 62 years in a long-term health care facility. *Am J Cardiol* 1987; 60:730–732.
44. Maron BJ, Savage DD, Wolfson JK, Epstein SE. Prognostic significance of 24 hour ambulatory electrocardiographic monitoring in patients with hypertrophic cardiomyopathy: A prospective study. *Am J Cardiol* 1981; 48:252–257.
45. Aronow WS, Epstein S, Koenigsberg M, Schwartz KS. Usefulness of echocardiographic abnormal left ventricular ejection fraction, paroxysmal ventricular tachycardia, and complex ventricular arrhythmias in predicting new coronary events in patients over 62 years of age. *Am J Cardiol* 1988; 61:1349–1351.
46. Aronow WS, Epstein S, Koenigsberg M, Schwartz KS. Usefulness of echocardiographic left ventricular hypertrophy, ventricular tachycardia and complex ventricular arrhythmias in predicting ventricular fibrillation or sudden cardiac death in elderly patients. *Am J Cardiol* 1988; 62:1124–1125.
47. Fananapazir L, Epstein SE. Hemodynamic and electrophysiologic evaluation of patients with hypertrophic cardiomyopathy surviving cardiac arrest. *Am J Cardiol* 1991; 67:280–287.
48. Spirito P, Maron BJ. Relation between extent of left ventricular hypertrophy and occurrence of sudden cardiac death in hypertrophic cardiomyopathy. *J Am Coll Cardiol* 1990; 15:1521–1526.
49. Kogure S, Yamamoto Y, Tomono S, Hasegawa A, Suzuki T, Murata K. High risk

of systemic embolism in hypertrophic cardiomyopathy. *Jpn Heart J* 1986; 27:475–480.
50. Roberts WC, Kishel JC, McIntosh CI, Cannon RO III, Maron BJ. Severe mitral or aortic valve regurgitation, or both, requiring valve replacement for infective endocarditis complicating hypertrophic cardiomyopathy. *J Am Coll Cardiol* 1992; 19:365–371.
51. Gilligan DM, Chan WL, Stewart R, Oakley CM. Adrenergic hypersensitivity after beta-blocker withdrawal in hypertrophic cardiomyopathy. *Am J Cardiol* 1991; 68:766–772.
52. Kaltenbach M, Hopf R, Kober G, Bussmann W-D, Keller M, Petersen Y. Treatment of hypertrophic obstructive cardiomyopathy with verapamil. *Br Heart J* 1979; 42:35–42.
53. Rosing DR, Idanpaan-Heikkila U, Maron BJ, Bonow RO, Epstein SE. Use of calcium-channel blocking drugs in hypertrophic cardiomyopathy. *Am J Cardiol* 1985; 55:185B–195B.
54. Maron BJ, Epstein SE, Morrow AG. Symptomatic status and prognosis of patients after operation for hypertrophic obstructive cardiomyopathy: Efficacy of ventricular septal myotomy and myectomy. *Eur Heart J* 1983; 4(Suppl. F):175–185.
55. Fighali S, Krajcer Z, Leachman RD. Septal myomectomy and mitral valve replacement for idiopathic hypertrophic subaortic stenosis: Short- and long-term follow-up. *J Am Coll Cardiol* 1984; 3:1127–1134.
56. Stevenson LW, Perloff JK. The dilated cardiomyopathies: Clinical aspects. *Cardiol Clin* 1988; 6:197–218.
57. Shah PM, Abelmann WH, Gersh BJ. Cardiomyopathies in the elderly. *J Am Coll Cardiol* 1987; 10:77A–79A.
58. Torp A. Incidence of congestive cardiomyopathy. *Postgrad Med J* 1978; 54:435–439.
59. Segal JP, Stapleton JF, McClellan JR, Waller BF, Harvey WP. Idiopathic cardiomyopathy: Clinical features, prognosis and therapy. *Curr Probl Cardiol* 1978; 3:1–48.
60. Fuster V, Gersh BJ, Giuliani ER, Tajik AJ, Brandenburg RO, Frye RL. The natural history of idiopathic dilated cardiomyopathy. *Am J Cardiol* 1981; 47:525–531.
61. Roberts WC, Siegel RJ, McManus BM. Idiopathic dilated cardiomyopathy: Analysis of 152 necropsy patients. *Am J Cardiol* 1987; 60:1340–1355.
62. Sawada SG, Ryan T, Segar D, Atherton L, Fineberg N, Davis C, Feigenbaum H. Distinguishing ischemic cardiomyopathy from nonischemic dilated cardiomyopathy with coronary echocardiography. *J Am Coll Cardiol* 1992; 19:1223–1228.
63. Falk RH, Foster E, Coats MH. Ventricular thrombi and thromboembolism in dilated cardiomyopathy: A prospective follow-up study. *Am Heart J* 1992; 123:136–142.
64. Waagstein F, Caidahl K, Wallentin I, Bergh C-H, Hjalmarson A. Long-term beta-blockade in dilated cardiomyopathy. Effects of short- and long-term metoprolol treatment followed by withdrawal and readministration of metoprolol. *Circulation* 1989; 80:551–563.
65. Griepp RB. A decade of human heart transplantation. *Transplant Proc* 1979; 11:285–292.

# 19

# Thyroid Heart Disease in the Elderly

**Steven R. Gambert**
*New York Medical College, Valhalla, New York*

## INTRODUCTION

The cardiovascular manifestations of both hyperthyroidism and hypothyroidism are well known and continue to serve as the focus of considerable research efforts. Cardiovascular manifestations are usually among the earliest and most consistent findings of an abnormality of the thyroid axis and are often responsible for the diagnostic testing that eventually leads to the diagnosis. This is particularly true when considering the elderly hyperthyroid population in that most of the classic signs and symptoms of hyperthyroidism are lacking at this time of life. Although there are receptors for thyroid hormone in heart tissue, thyroid hormone also affects cardiovascular function through an indirect effect on the adrenergic system, particularly in the setting of thyroid hormone excess. Age may modify some of the sequelae as well as the treatment of both hyper- and hypothyroidism, but it is important to understand the effect of these disorders on the cardiovascular system in general and consider each case individually.

## HYPERTHYROIDISM

Classic symptoms of hyperthyroidism include tachycardia, palpitations, and an increased pulse pressure. In the elderly person with hyperthyroidism, however, associated findings often include atrial fibrillation, congestive heart failure, and angina. This latter problem results from the increase in oxygen demand placed on the aged heart by excessive amounts of thyroid hormone and thus increased metabolic demands by both the heart and other body organs. A definite adrenergic contribution to the clinical manifestations of hyperthyroidism was suggested in an animal model that showed that a total or nearly total sympathetic block produced by a subarachnoid injection of procaine could successfully relieve or prevent thyroid storm (1). It was also observed that alterations in cardiovascular function in hyperthyroid dogs were ameliorated after spinal epidural procaine blockade (2). This resulted in the use of sympatholytic agents, including reserpine, guanethidine, and propranolol, to treat cardiovascular manifestations of hyperthyroidism (3–6). Since these agents are effective in reducing many of the cardiac manifestations, it appears that a significant component of these symptoms results from catecholamine–thyroid interactions. This latter phenomenon has received a great deal of attention in recent years and has been used as a model to support a membrane action for thyroid hormone because of the almost immediate effect noted on a number of systems when thyroid hormone and catecholamines interact in a synergistic manner. Interactions between thyroid hormone and the catecholamines may result from several mechanisms, including (1) an enhanced sensitivity of target cells to the activating effects of catecholamines; (2) an increase in the number of adrenergic receptor sites available to interact with catecholamines; (3) an increase in tissue levels of free catecholamines; (4) similar but separate and additive effects of thyroid hormone and catecholamines; and (5) thyroid stimulation of adrenergic nerve terminals. It has been noted for several decades that thyroid hormone is capable of potentiating both the chronotropic and pressor effects of the catecholamines (7,8). Using a model of euthyroid and hyperthyroid dogs, it was observed that thiopental anesthesia and spinal epidural block with procaine prevented the otherwise observed increase in heart rate, cardiac index, left ventricular stroke volume, and oxygen consumption noted in hyperthyroid dogs. There was also a greater increase in heart rate, cardiac index, and oxygen consumption following an infusion of either epinephrine or norepinephrine in the setting of hyperthyroidism (3). This study and several subsequent studies (7,8) were criticized for their lack of proper design and statistical analysis. More recent studies failed to demonstrate an increased sensitivity of the cardiovascular system to the action of sympathoadrenergic agents in the setting of hyperthyroidism (9–13). The parameters that were studied included blood pressure, heart rate, and contractile effects on isolated papillary muscles. In addition, studies on humans demonstrated a similar alteration in heart rate and mean atrial and arterial pressures before and after triiodothyronine ($T_3$)-induced hyperthyroidism (9,13). This is in contrast to studies that demonstrated an enhanced sensitivity to the chronotropic and arrhythmogenic effects of norepinephrine when combined with $T_3$ (14). One study reported an enhanced effect with $T_3$, but only with β-adrenergic agents (15).

Although thyroid hormone is thought to exert most of its calorigenic effects through a nuclear receptor and the process of transcription, both mitochondrial and membrane-bound receptors have been demonstrated. The membrane-bound receptor is most likely responsible for the thyroid hormone-catecholamine interaction because of the almost instantaneous synergistic response noted when catecholamines and thyroid hormone are introduced into certain systems. It has been demonstrated that chronic administration of thyroid hormone to rats increases the number but not the affinity of plasma membrane β-adrenergic receptors in heart tissue (16,17). There has been a reported decline in the α-adrenergic receptors in response to chronic thyroid hormone administration as well (16,18). Although both mechanisms may help explain some of the reported findings showing an enhanced response of cardiac tissue in the setting of hyperthyroidism, additional studies are needed before arriving at a definite conclusion. It appears that this would only partially explain the observed findings in any case, because the time it takes for new receptor formation would exceed that of the observed synergistic effect noted in certain models. Although studies have reported no change in receptors for thyroid hormone with age, none have examined cardiac tissue, and therefore no conclusions regarding an age effect can be made at this time.

Some have proposed an alteration in the synthesis and/or release of sympathetic neuronal or adrenal medullary catecholamines in the setting of hyperthyroidism to help explain, at least in part, the data demonstrating an enhanced cardiovascular response, but this has not received universal acceptance. Hearts from hyperthyroid animals have been shown to have normal or low norepinephrine concentrations and turnover (10,19). Patients who are thyrotoxic reportedly have normal plasma concentrations of epinephrine, normal or low concentrations norepinephrine, and normal rates of epinephrine and norepinephrine secretion by the adrenal (20–22). Urinary excretion of norephrine is normal or low, and the excretion of epinephrine, metanephrine, and 4-hydroxy-3-methoxylmandelic aid, the latter two representing catecholamine metabolites, are within normal range (23). A decrease in neuronal catecholamine synthesis has also been suggested based on a decrease in the plasma concentration of the enzyme dopamine β-hydroxylase (24). This makes it highly unlikely that hyperthyroidism mediates its effects by increasing endogenous catecholamine levels. It has been reported that aging is associated with higher basal levels of circulating norepinephrine. Whether the effects of hyperthyroidism are due to the same mechanism throughout life is not known at this time.

Another popular theory about why hyperthyroidism may result in an enhanced cardiovascular response relates to the way in which the catecholamines are metabolized by myocardial tissue. Although the two enzymes that metabolize catecholamines, catechol-*o*-methyltransferase and monoamine oxidase, were found not to be altered by thyroid hormone, at least in a rat model, hyperthyroidism was associated with a greater quantity of radiolabeled epinephrine and norepinephrine reaching the heart (25). There was a decrease in catecholamine binding to cardiac tissue, however, and a greater percentage of free catecholamine within the myocardium itself.

Studies have reported a decrease in the production of catecholamines in the setting of thyroid hormone excess. Nevertheless, because both thyroxine ($T_4$) and $T_3$ are concentrated and metabolized within adrenergic nerve endings, thyroid hormone may serve as a neurotransmitter, much like one of its precursors, tyrosine (26). The role of the central nervous system in regulation of cardiac function also remains a possible mechanism for the enhanced effect of thyroid hormone on the cardiovascular system. There is ample evidence showing an effect of thyroid hormone on neurotransmitters, such as $\beta$-endorphin and ACTH. Whether this may indirectly affect cardiac function remains a topic of future consideration.

Although much attention has been given to the effect that thyroid hormone may exert on cardiac tissue through a catecholamine interaction, thyroid hormone was first shown to exert a direct effect on myocardial tissue in the early part of the twentieth century (27). These studies were done before our current knowledge of receptors and cell mediators. Nevertheless, when $T_4$ was incubated with fragments of cardiac tissue from chicken embryos in the absence of adrenergic tissue, it was noted that the heart rate increased after a 12 h period. Thyroid hormone continued to exert a chronotropic effect even after pharmacological adrenergic blockade, also implying a direct effect (4,6). It is now currently agreed that the tachycardia that results from hyperthyroidism results from a combination of direct effects of thyroid hormone, as well as from an increase in adrenergic stimulation and parasympathetic inhibition.

Thyroid hormone also exerts a positive effect on cardiac contractility and inotropy. Most studies demonstrating this effect have used cat papillary muscles. Thyroid hormone increased the rate of isometric tension, decreased the time it took to achieve peak tension, and increased the velocity of muscle shortening. Since these findings were not effected by prior depletion of catecholamines, this also supports a direct effect of thyroid hormone (10). These data are consonant with those of studies using isolated atria from guinea pigs (64). There is a consensus that the majority of cardiac effects noted during the hyperthyroid state result from the direct action of thyroid hormone, with a smaller contribution from adrenergic mechanisms. With this in mind, investigators examined the dynamics of cardiac function in the setting of hyperthyroidism. It has been reported, for example in a model of hyperthyroid rabbits, that the tachycardia characteristic of hyperthyroidism is associated with an increased rate of diastolic depolarization and a decrease in the duration of the action potential in sinoatrial node cells (28). A shortening of the refractory period and a reduction in the electrical threshold of atrial cells have been implicated in the pathogenesis of cardiac arrhythmias in the setting of excess thyroid hormone (3). Although a rise in adenylate cyclase activity by thyroid hormone is the suggested mechanism for the enhanced myocardial contractility (29), not all studies have come to the same conclusion (30). This enzyme system has also been implicated in the thyroid-catecholamine interaction on cardiac function. Thyroid hormone has been reported to exert an effect on the heart through its effect on cardiac sarcoplasmic reticulum. This intracellular organelle has the capacity to accumulate and release calcium during the contractile process of the heart using calcium as a cell mediator (31,32). The ATPase system, notably Na,K-ATPase, has also been implicated in the increased effects of thyroid hormone on cardiac function, especially in ventricular tissue (33,34).

## Clinical Manifestations

Clinically, it has been noted that hyperthyroidism is commonly associated with tachycardia and atrial fibrillation. In the elderly, congestive heart failure, angina, and ventricular arrhythmias may also be seen in greater frequency. Many argue that this is due to the greater likelihood of underlying cardiovascular disease; others argue that age may alter the end-organ effect of thyroid hormone. The literature is replete with studies that demonstrate that an excess amount of thyroid hormone can lead to cardiac hypertrophy, somewhere in the range of 20–90%, depending on the species studied and the duration of exposure to excess thyroid hormone. This effect is thought to be completely reversible upon cessation of thyroid hormone stimulation (35–39). Thyroid hormone excess results in cardiac hypertrophy, but there appears to continue to be an increase in contractile function (40). Treating the hyperthyroid state with antithyroid medications has been shown capable of reversing the cardiac hypertrophy (41). Although there is no definite explanation of the pathogenesis of the cardiac hypertrophy, foci of lymphocytic and eosinophilic cells, fibrosis, and fatty infiltration have been described, along with myofibril hypertrophy. Mitochondria have been reported to be increased in number and hypertrophied, with localized areas of vacuolization and an aberrant configuration of intracellular structures (42,43).

There was no exercise-induced increase in ejection fraction in hyperthyroid subjects, in contrast to the increase usually noted (44,45). This observation was reversed upon return to the euthyroid state. Once again, no elderly subjects were studied. Although it has been demonstrated that congestive heart failure can result from hyperthyroidism even in the absence of underlying cardiovascular abnormalities and regardless of one's age, the older person is more prone to develop compromised cardiac functioning and more attention should be given to reverse the thyroid abnormality promptly before the development of a life-compromising situation. Coexisting problems, such as tachycardia and increased demand for oxygen by metabolically stimulated myocardial cells, may also lead to serious cardiac compromise, angina, cardiac ischemia, or arrythmias.

As stated previously, hyperthyroidism is classically associated with increased cardiac output, stroke volume, heart rate, and ejection time. There is a decrease in peripheral vascular resistance, a widening of the pulse pressure, and a general increase in circulating blood volume. The electrocardiogram may be normal but more commonly demonstrates a tachycardia. ST and T wave abnormalities may be noted and tend to be nonspecific. There may be evidence of cardiac ischemia, voltage changes reflecting left ventricular hypertrophy, notching and slurring of the P wave, P-R interval shortening or prolongation, Q-T interval shortening, and/or transient atrioventricular conduction abnormalities, including complete heart block (46–48). Atrial fibrillation is found in approximately 15–20% of cases, with a slower rate more commonly reported in older persons. It occurs more commonly in persons with underlying cardiovascular disease, and it appears to be more common in the setting of hyperthyroidism even in an otherwise normal heart. Of note, elderly persons who develop atrial fibrillation in the setting of hyperthyroidism have a greater chance of remaining in this rhythm despite a return to the euthyroid state compared to younger persons in whom reversibility is usually the rule. Paroxysmal supraventricular tachycardia, atrial flutter, and ventricular tachycardia are less commonly noted. Although there has been a report of a greater risk of developing the Wolff-Parkinson-White syndrome in association with hyperthyroidism (49), this finding remains uncommon.

In measuring systolic time intervals, the preejection and left ventricular ejection time are reportedly shortened during the hyperthyroid state. The ratio of preejection to ejection time, however, remains unchanged (50,51).

## Management

Many cardiac findings in the setting of hyperthyroidism appear to be well tolerated and without an apparent risk of producing an immediate crisis, but it is essential that any symptom or sign of cardiac compromise be evaluated promptly and treated as needed. In general, the goal is to treat the hyperthyroid state as quickly as possible while managing the patient in totality. Radioactive iodine therapy is the treatment of choice for most older persons with hyperthyroidism, but the time from beginning treatment with radioactive iodine until such time that euthyroidism is reached is of the order of weeks to months. Therefore, most agree that antithyroid medication should be used early in an attempt to decrease thyroid hormone production and metabolism. When an immediate effect is needed because of significantly compromised cardiac function, administration of iodine in the form of Lugol's solution can more quickly reduce circulating levels of thyroid hormone by blocking the uptake and organification process necessary for thyroid hormone production. If Lugol's solution is to be an asset, however, one must always ensure that antithyroid medication is administered before and during the iodine treatment to prevent the iodine from being converted into thyroid hormone by an already highly efficient thyroid nodule or diffusely toxic goiter, the end result being actual worsening of the hyperthyroid state. β-Blockers primarily compete with β-adrenergic receptors in the heart and other tissues, as well as reduce the conversion of thyroxine to 3,5,3′-triiodothyronine by approximately 15%. Although β-blockers have been used successfully to reduce end-organ responsiveness, caution is advised because they may precipitate cardiac failure. Reserpine and guanethidine have also been used with a great deal of success to ameliorate symptoms of tachycardia and palpitation, but once again both these agents have significant side effects for which the patient should be monitored. Both are capable of depleting tissues of catecholamines and may further depress cardiovascular reflexes, as well as induce other side effects, including altered mental function and orthostatic hypotension. In the setting of congestive heart failure, the use of diuretic therapy and digitoxin may be required until the heart becomes less of a target for the action of thyroid hormone excess. Clearly, the physician must provide close observation in all cases of hyperthyroidism in whom a compromised cardiovascular state exists, regardless of the age of the person, and seek the advice of an experienced cardiologist when uncertain concerning management. In most cases, the antithyroid medication begins working within 2 weeks, and attention can then be given to a more definitive therapy with radioactive iodine. Since it takes weeks to months for the radioactive therapy to become effective, however, it is important to continue antithyroid medications while the radioactivity has a chance to work. As the hyperthyroid condition improves, oral medication should be tapered to keep the person in a euthyroid state. Overtreatment at this time may precipitate hypothyroidism, with its own cardiac problems. Since many persons treated with radioactive iodine become hypothyroid, careful follow-up is advised, and if necessary, thyroid hormone replacement may be initiated.

## HYPOTHYROIDISM

Cardiovascular manifestations of hypothyroidism have long been recognized and classically include bradycardia, cardiomegaly, and low voltage on electrocardiographic monitoring (52,53). Congestive heart failure and evidence of cardiomyopathy are frequent diagnoses in persons with insufficient amounts of thyroid hormone. What makes the diagnosis of hypothyroidism so difficult, however, is that hypothyroidism is an age-prevalent disorder and many of the signs and symptoms resemble those of other diseases that occur with increasing frequency with advancing age. Physicians frequently treat target symptoms without regard to the etiology of the problem; for example, congestive heart failure may be treated with diuretics and digoxin for presumed atherosclerotic heart disease. The American Thyroid Association now recommends that all persons over 50 have annual screening for thyroid hormone abnormalities after studies showed the cost-benefit from such practice.

"Myxedema heart" was a term used to connote a cardiomyopathy that resulted from insufficient quantities of thyroid hormone and that was reversible with thyroid hormone replacement. It is now recognized that hypothyroidism exerts its effects on the cardiovascular system through a direct effect of thyroid hormone deficiency as well as through an indirect effect from reduced metabolism.

## Myocardial Tissue and Hypothyroidism

Studies have reported that the heart in persons with hypothyroidism may be dilated, pale, and flabby, but there is no evidence of hypertrophy (54). Histologically, swelling of the myofibrillar elements, interstitial fibrosis, basophilic degeneration, and tissue edema have been described (55). There appears to be deposition of mucopolysaccharide, likely reflecting the decline in certain enzymes necessary for the breakdown of these substances. Electron microscopic studies reveal thickening of the capillary basement membrane similar to that observed in diabetes mellitus and in persons of advanced age (56,57). Numerous other ultrastructural changes have been described, including loss of mitochondrial cristae.

## Thyroid Hormone Deficiency and Cardiovascular Function

Perhaps the most widely accepted change that has been noted in the setting of hypothyroidism is a reduction in myocardial contractility. Using isolated right ventricular papillary muscles from hypothyroid cats and dogs, a decrease was noted in isometric tension and the rate of tension development. The time it took to reach peak tension increased at all muscle lengths, and isotonic force-velocity relations were shifted downward and to the left, supporting a depressed contractile state (58,59). In all animal studies reported, congestive heart failure was not noted despite significant reductions in circulating levels of thyroid hormone. It has been postulated that decreased myocardial contractility in hypothyroidism may result from a reduction in the thyroid-adrenergic relationship, with either a diminished response to a given amount of catecholamine or a reduced amount of free catecholamine available to interact at the cardiac receptor site. Studies have reported an increase, decrease, and no change in cardiovascular sensitivity to catecholamine stimulation in the setting of hypothyroidism (60–63). Levels of norepinephrine in myocardial tissue of hypothyroid cats were not reported to be affected by thyroid status (58), and thus it appears unlikely that a lower level of catecholamine exposure to the cardiac receptor is the cause of significant cardiac effects. Studies have shown a reduction in $\beta$-adrenergic receptor activity in atria from hypothyroid rats and an increase in $\alpha$-receptor activity (64) in the same tissue. This reduction in the number and/or affinity of $\beta$-receptors in cardiac tissue could result in a depressed myocardial response. Because contractile function is depressed in isolated papillary muscles from hypothyroid rats (58), thyroid hormone deficiency seems to have a direct effect and is responsible for at least a component of the cardiovascular change induced by the hypothyroid state. It has been noted that the rate of calcium uptake and calcium-dependent ATP hydrolysis by isolated myocardial sarcoplasmic reticulum is reduced in the setting of hypothyroidism (65). A reduction in cardiac myosin ATPase activity has been described in both rat and mouse models of hypothyroidism (66–68), although not in a rabbit model (68).

Bradycardia is a well recognized accompaniment of hypothyroidism and is thought to result from the lack of thyroid stimulation of sinoatrial node cells (69), further impacted by a reduction in sympathoadrenal stimulation. A decreased rate of diastolic repolarization and a prolonged action potential duration have also been described.

## Clinical Manifestations of Hypothyroidism

Cardiac manifestations of hypothyroidism occur only in association with a significant reduction in the levels of circulating thyroid hormone. Studies using oxygen consumption as a corollary of thyroid hormone status have reported few cardiac symptoms in otherwise healthy persons until oxygen requirements decline by 75%. This is highly variable, however. Many persons with hypothyroidism have coexisting medical conditions that compromise the cardiovascular system and may lower the threshold for cardiac problems. For the most part, the reduced requirement for oxygen by the hypothyroid myocardium is protective against angina. In fact, many persons develop angina only after therapy with thyroid hormone has been initiated. Dyspnea on exertion and easy fatigability are common complaints of persons who are hypothyroid. Less frequent are complaints of orthopnea, paroxysmal noctural dyspnea, and angina. Bradycardia is common, and weak pulse, mild hypertension, distant heart sounds, and evidence of cardiomegaly are classic findings. In general, there is no change in the jugular venous pressure. In severely diminished thyroid function, however, evidence of peripheral edema, nonpitting edema of the lower extremities, pleural effusion, and even ascites may be noted and may lead one to assume that the patient has congestive heart failure (CHF). The presence of nonpitting edema should be a tip that some other process is present. The electrocardiogram may be normal despite the presence of hypothyroidism. More commonly, there is a bradycardia, flattening or inversion of the T wave, particularly in lead 11, and a low-amplitude P, QRS complex, and T wave (70). These findings may result from a direct effect of thyroid hormone deficiency, but the presence of a pericardial effusion is also known to affect the electrocardiographic picture that may accompany hypothyroidism. Although not common, incomplete and complete right bundle branch block occur with greater frequency (71). With replacement therapy, these changes return to normal and may even precede the return to normal of other clinical features of the disease.

Studies suggest that in the absence of other coexisting diseases, congestive heart failure is an extremely uncommon finding in hypothyroidism (72). In the setting of shortness of breath, pleural effusions, cardiomegaly, and other symptoms, it is often difficult to distinguish CHF from what has been termed myxedema heart. The absence of pulmonary congestion, diminished plasma volume, high protein content of the effusion, and normal resting venous, atrial, pulmonary artery, and right ventricular end-diastolic pressures is highly suggestive of myxedema itself. It has also been reported that exercise results in an increase in cardiac output and ejection fraction in persons with myxedema, in contrast to the impaired response in those with congestive failure (73,74). The hemodynamic changes associated with hypothyroidism appear to respond to thyroid hormone, but they are not very responsive to diuretic and digoxin therapy. Since in many persons both conditions occur together, there is a great deal of variability in clinical response.

## Management of Hypothyroidism

Because so many elderly persons with hypothyroidism may have underlying cardiovascular abnormalities, it is wise to begin thyroid hormone replacement therapy with a small dose of L-thyroxine (0.0125 mg daily). The use of diuretic therapy and digoxin should be reserved for persons in whom there is clear evidence of coexisting congestive heart failure. Younger persons or those with no evidence of cardiovascular compromise may be started on higher doses of L-thyroxine, although extreme caution is advised. The starting dose should be increased slowly over the next several weeks, realizing that the half-life of L-thyroxine is prolonged by both age and hypothyroidism. Because it takes approximately 5 half-lives to reach a steady state, caution is advised against too rapid a rise in dosing. In general, it is appropriate to increase the dose of thyroxine to 0.025 mg daily within 2 weeks if the dosage is well tolerated and to 0.050 mg daily within several weeks thereafter. If there are no clinical problems, the dose should be increased by 0.0125 mg increments every 4–6 weeks thereafter, depending on the age and cardiovascular status of the patient, until the level of serum thyroid stimulating hormone has declined to within the normal range or the patient develops signs of toxicity. In general, elderly persons who are hypothyroid require a replacement dose of between 0.100 and 0.125 mg L-thyroxine daily compared to an approximate dose of 0.150 mg for younger persons. L-thyroxine is the preferred thyroid hormone for replacement because $T_3$ exerts a "burst" effect on the myocardium and is less well tolerated. It also has a shorter half-life, thereby having a less equilibrated metabolic profile. USP thyroid or other combination therapies also share the disadvantage of $T_3$, a component in all these medications. In certain cases in whom severe cardiac disease exists, it may not be possible to return the patient to the euthyroid state. In all cases, close clinical observation is necessary.

## REFERENCES


1. Knight RA. The use of spinal anesthesia to control sympathetic overactivity in hyperthyroidism. *Anesthesiology* 1945; 6:225.
2. Brewster WR, Isaacs JR, Osgood PF, et al. The hemodynamic and metabolic interrelationships in the activity of epinephrine, norepinephrine, and the thyroid hormone. *Circulation* 1956; 13:1.
3. Canary JJ, Schaff M, Duffy BJ, et al. Effects of oral and intramuscular administration of reserpine in thyrotoxicosis. *N Engl J Med* 1957; 257:435.
4. Howitt G, Rowlands DJ. Beta-sympathetic blockade in hyperthyroidism. *Lancet* 1966; 1:628.
5. Shanks RG, Hadden DR, Lowe DC, et al. Controlled trial of propranolol in thyrotoxicosis. *Clin Pediatr* 1975; 14:1155.
6. Waldstein SS, West GH, Lee WY, et al. Guanethidine in hyperthyroidism. *JAMA* 1964; 189:609.
7. Harrison TS. Adrenal medullary and thyroid relationships. *Physiol Rev* 1964; 44:161.
8. Waldstein SS. Thyroid-catecholamine interrelations. *Annu Rev Med* 1966; 17:123.
9. Aoki VS, Wilson WR, Theilen EO, et al. The effects of triiodothyronine on hemodynamic responses to epinephrine and norepinephrnine in man. *J Pharmacol Exp Ther* 1967; 157:62.
10. Buccino RA, Spann JF, Pool PE, et al. Influence of thyroid state on the intrinsic contractile properties and energy stores of the myocardium. *J Clin Invest* 1967; 46:1669.
11. Cairoli VJ, Crout JR. Role of the autonomic nervous system in the resting tachycardia of experimental hyperthyroidism. *J Pharmacol Exp Ther* 1967; 158:55.
12. Levey GS, Skelton CL, Epstein SE. Influence of hyperthyroidism on the effects of norepinephrine on myocardial adenyl cyclase activity and contractile state. *Endocrinology* 1969; 85:1004.
13. Wilson WR, Theilen EO, Hege JH, et al. Effects of beta adrenergic receptor

blockade in normal subjects before, during, and after triiodothyronine-induced hypermetabolism. *J Clin Invest* 1966; 45:1159.
14. Wildenthal K. Studies of isolated fetal mouse hearts in organ culture: evidence for a direct effect of triiodothyronine in enhancing cardiac responsiveness to norepinephrine. *J Clin Invest* 1972; 51:2702.
15. Wildenthal K. Studies of fetal mouse hearts in organ culture: influence of prolonged exposure to triiodothyronine on cardiac responsiveness to isoproterenol, glucagon, theophylline, acetylcholine, and dibutyryl cyclic 3′5′-adenosine monophosphate. *J Pharmacol Exp Ther* 1974; 109:272.
16. Kunos G, Vermes-Kunos I, Nickerson M. Effects of thyroid state of adrenoreceptor properties. *Nature (Lond)* 1974; 250:779.
17. Williams LT, Lefkowitz RJ, Watanabe AM, et al. Thyroid hormone regulation of beta-adrenergic number. *J Biol Chem* 1977; 252:2787.
18. Banerjee SP, Kung LS. Beta-adrenergic receptors in rat heart: effects of thyroidectomy. *Eur J Pharmacol* 1977; 13:207.
19. Prange AJ, Meek JL, Lipton MA. Catecholamines: diminished rate of synthesis in rat brain and heart after thyroxine pretreatment. *Life Sci* 1970; 9:901.
20. Coulombe P, Dussault JH, Walker P. Plasma catecholamine concentrations in hyperthyroidism and hypothyroidism. *Metabolism* 1976; 25:973.
21. Coulombe P, Dussault JH, Letarte J, et al. Catecholamine metabolism in thyroid diseases. 1. Epinephrine secretion rate in hyperthyroidism and hypothyroidism. *J Clin Endocrinol Metab* 1976; 42:125.
22. Stoffer SS, Tian NS, Gorman CA, et al. Plasma catecholamines in hypothyroidism and hyperthyroidism. *J Clin Endocrinol Metab* 1973; 36:587.
23. Wiswell JG, Hurwitz GE, Corohno V, et al. Urinary catecholamines and their metabolites in hyperthyroidism. *J Clin Endocrinol Metab* 1963; 23:1102.
24. Nishizaway Y, Hamada N, Fujii S, et al. Serum dopamine beta hydroxylase activity in thyroid disorders. *J Clin Endocrinol Metab* 1974; 39:599.
25. Wurtman RJ, Kopin KJ, Axelrod J. Thyroid function and the cardiac disposition of catecholamines. *Endocrinology* 1963; 73:63.
26. Dratman MB. On the mechanism of action of thyroxine, an amino acid analog of tyrosine. *J Theor Biol* 1974; 46:255.
27. Markowitz C, Yater WM. Response of explanted cardiac muscle to thyroxine. *Am J Physiol* 1932; 100:162.
28. Murayama M, Goodkind MJ. Effect of thyroid hormone on the frequency-force relationship of atrial myocardium from the guinea pig. *Circ Res* 1968; 23:743.
29. Levey GS, Epstein SE. Myocardial adenyl cyclase: activation by thyroid hormones and evidence for two adenyl cyclase systems. *J Clin Invest* 1969; 48:1163.
30. Levey GS. Catecholamine sensitivity, thyroid hormone and the heart. *Am J Med* 1971; 50:413.
31. Nayler WG, Merrillees NCR, Chipperfield D, et al. Influence of hyperthyroidism on the uptake and binding of calcium by cardiac microsomal fractions and on mitochondrial structure. *Cardiovasc Res* 1971; 5:469.
32. Suko J. The calcium pump of cardiac sarcoplasmic reticulum: functional alterations at different levels of thyroid state in rabbits. *J Physiol (Lond)* 1973; 228:563.

33. Curfman GD, Crowley TJ, Smith TW. Thyroid-induced alterations in myocardial sodium and potassium-activated adenosine triphosphates, monovalent cation active transport, and cardiac glycoside binding. *J Clin Invest* 1977; 59:586.
34. Ismail-Beigi F, Edelman IS. The mechanism of the calorigenic action of thyroid hormone: Stimulation of Na+ and K+-activated adenosine-triphosphatase activity. *J Gen Physiol* 1971; 57:710.
35. Bartolome J, Huguenard J, Slotkin TA. Role of ornithine decarboxylase in cardiac growth and hypertrophy. *Science* 1980; 210:793.
36. Beznak M. Cardiovascular effects of thyroxine treatment in normal rats. *Can J Biochem* 1962; 40:1647.
37. Cohen J, Aroesty JM, Rosenfeld MG. Determinants of thyroxine-induced cardiac hypertrophy in mice. *Circ Res* 1966; 18:388.
38. Piatnek-Leunissen D, Olson RE. Cardiac failure in the dog as a consequence of exogenous hyperthyroidism. *Circ Res* 1967; 20:242.
39. Sandler G, Wilson GM. Production of cardiac hypertrophy by thyroxine in the rat. *Q J Exp Physiol* 1959; 41:282.
40. Skelton CL, Sonnenblick EH. Heterogeneity of contractile function in cardiac hypertrophy. *Circ Res* 34/35 (Suppl. II):83.
41. Nixon JV, Anderson RJ, Cohen ML. Alteration in left ventricular mass and performance in patients treated effectively for thyrotoxicosis. *Am J Med* 1979; 67:268.
42. Callas G, Hayes JR. Alterations in the fine structure of cardiac muscle mitochondria induced by hyperthyroidism. *Anat Rec* 1974; 178:539.
43. Saphir O. Myocarditis: a general review with an analysis of two hundred forty cases. *Arch Pathol* 1942; 33:88.
44. Forfar JC, Muir AL, Sawers SL, et al. Abnormal left ventricular function in hyperthyroidism. Evidence for a reversible cardiomyopathy. *N Engl J Med* 1982; 307:1165.
45. Shafer RB, Bianco JA. Assessment of cardiac reserve in patients with hyperthyroidism. *Chest* 1980; 78:269.
46. Campus S, Rappelli A, Malavasi A, et al. Heart block and hyperthyroidism. *Arch Intern Med* 1975; 135:1091.
47. Hoffman I, Lowrey RD. The electrocardiogram in thyrotoxicosis. *Am J Cardiol* 1960; 6:893.
48. Teoh PC, Chea JS, Chia BL. Effect of adrenergic blockade and specific antithyroid therapy on electrocardiographic changes in hyperthyroidism. *Am J Med Sci* 1974; 268:157.
49. Sanghvilm, Banerjee K. Wolff-Parkinson-White syndrome associated with thyrotoxicosis. *Am J Cardiol* 1961; 8:431.
50. Cohen MV, Schulman IC, Spenillo A, et al. Effects of thyroid hormone on left ventricular function in patients treated for thyrotoxicosis. *Am J Cardiol* 1981; 48:33.
51. Grossman W, Robin NI, Johnson LW, et al. The enhanced myocardial contractility of thyrotoxicosis: role of the beta adrenergic receptor. *Ann Intern Med* 1971; 74:869.
52. Fahr G. Myxedema heart. *JAMA* 1925; 84:345.
53. Zondek H. Das myxodemharz. *Munch Med Wochenschr* 1918; 65:1180.

54. Hamolsky MW, Kurland GS, Freedberg AS. The heart in hypothyroidism. *J Chron Dis* 1961; 14:558.
55. Douglas RC, Jacobson SD. Pathologic changes in adult myxedema: survey of 10 necropsies. *J Clin Endocrinol Metab* 1957; 17:1354.
56. McFadden PM, Berenson GS. Basement membrane changes in myocardial and skeletal muscle capillaries in myxedema. *Circ Res* 1972; 30:808.
57. Siperstein MD, Unger RH, Madison LL. Studies of muscle capillary basement membranes in normal subjects, diabetic, and prediabetic patients. *J Clin Invest* 1968; 47:1973.
58. Buccino RA, Spann JF, Pool PE, et al. Influence of the thyroid state on the intrinsic contractile properties and the energy stores of the myocardium. *J Clin Invest* 1967; 46:1669.
59. Taylor RR, Covell JW, Ross JR. Influence of the thyroid state on left ventricular tension-velocity relations in the intact, sedated dog. *J Clin Invest* 1969; 48:775.
60. Harrison TS. Adrenal medullary and thyroid relationships. *Physiol Rev* 1964; 44:161.
61. Waldstein SS. Thyroid-catecholamine interrelations. *Annu Rev Med* 1966; 17:123.
62. Leak D, Lew M. Effect of treatment of hypothyroidism on circulatory response to adrenaline. *Br Heart J* 1963; 25:30.
63. Margolius HS, Gaffney TE. Effects of injected norepinephrine and sympathetic nerve stimulation in hypothyroid and hyperthyroid dogs. *J Pharmacol Exp Ther* 1965; 149:329.
64. Ciaraldi T, Marinetti GV. Thyroxine and propylthiouracil effects in vivo on alpha and beta-adrenergic receptors in rat heart. *Biochem Biophys Res Commun* 1977; 74:984.
65. Suko J. The calcium pump of cardiac sarcoplasmic reticulum. Functional alterations at different levels of thyroid state in rabbits. *J Physiol (Lond)* 1973; 228:563.
66. Lifschitz MD, Kayne HL. Cardiac myofibrillar ATPase in hypophysectomized or thyroidectomized rats. *Biochem Pharmacol* 1966; 15:405.
67. Rovetto MJ, Hjalmarson AC, Morgan HE, et al. Hormonal control of cardiac myosin adenosine triphosphatase in the rat. *Circ Res* 1972; 31:397.
68. Yazaki Y, Raben MS. Effect of the thyroid state on the enzymatic characteristics of cardiac myosin. A difference in behavior of rat and rabbit cardiac myosin. *Circ Res* 1975; 36:208.
69. Freedberg AS, Papp JG, Williams EMV. The effect of altered thyroid state on atrial intracellular potentials. *J Physiol (Lond)* 1970; 207:357.
70. Douglas AH, Samuel P. Analysis of electrocardiographic patterns in hypothyroid heart disease. *N Y J Med* 1960; 60:2227.
71. Korth C, Schmidt J. Neue beobachtungen zum "myxodemherzen." *Dtsch Arch Klin Med* 1955; 202:437.
72. Aber CP, Thompson GS. The heat in hypothyroidism. *Am Heart J* 1964; 68:429.
73. Epstein SE, Beiser GD, Stampfer M, et al. Characterization of the circulatory response to maximal upright exercise in normal subjects and patients with heart disease. *Circulation* 1967; 35:1049.
74. Ertugrul A. A new electrocardiographic sign in infants and children with hypothyroidism. *Pediatrics* 1966; 37:669.

# 20

# Heart Failure in the Elderly

**Thierry H. LeJemtel and Edmund H. Sonnenblick**
*Albert Einstein College of Medicine, Bronx, New York*

## INTRODUCTION

A most troublesome issue when dealing with the syndrome of heart failure is the lack of a comprehensive definition that comprises the multifaceted aspects of the clinical syndrome. This issue becomes even more critical with heart failure in patients over 65 years of age. For example, in young and middle-aged patients, a cardinal feature of the clinical syndrome of congestive heart failure is the progressive development of exertional symptoms, such as shortness of breath and fatigue. However, shortness of breath on exertion is an extremely common complaint volunteered by over two-thirds of elderly subjects without evidence of cardiopulmonary disorder. At the opposite end, elderly patients who become symptomatic during exertion tend to curtail their daily activities, thereby matching their life-style to their ability. Therefore, they may volunteer relatively fewer exertional symptoms than their more healthy and physically active contemporaries. In such instances, elderly patients tend to consult a physician only when they become symptomatic for minimal exertion or even at rest. When compared to middle-aged patients, heart failure in the elderly tends to be diagnosed at a later stage of the disease process, when patients are decompensated or at the edge of decompensation. By diagnosing the syndrome of heart failure at a late stage in the elderly patient, control and stabilization of the symptom becomes more difficult than in younger patients and often require hospitalization. If one keeps in mind that middle-aged patients with heart failure become "symptomatic" when they have already lost half the normal peak aerobic capacity for their age and sex, one appreciates that elderly patients with congestive heart failure, whose symptoms are only picked up when they occur during minimal activities, have nearly exhausted their cardiopulmonary reserve when they are finally diagnosed as having heart failure.

In view of the substantial benefits of prolonged angiotensin converting enzyme inhibition documented in asymptomatic patients with moderate to severe left ventricular dysfunction in the prevention arm of the Studies of Left Ventricular Dysfunction (SOLVD) (1), routine echocardiography to screen for moderate to severe left ventricular dysfunction may be, from a medical and economical point of view, safer and less expensive than waiting for the elderly patient to develop decompensated heart failure requiring hospitalization. Patients with asymptomatic left ventricular dysfunction, that is, left ventricular ejection fraction $< 35\%$, who were receiving enalapril, had an over 30% reduced likelihood of developing heart failure or being admitted for management of heart failure than patients receiving placebo (1). By definition, these patients are not seeking medical attention, because symptoms, if present, are minimal. They can only be identified by systemic, noninvasive determination of left ventricular function. Recognizing systolic left ventricular dysfunction at an earlier stage would lead to initiating therapy when further progression of left ventricular dysfunction may be prevented. Later, when the left ventricle has fully dilated, the benefits of therapy are obviously limited to controlling symptoms and are purely palliative. Indeed, the appearance of symptoms in patients with heart failure is concomitant with the development of abnormalities in the peripheral circulation and possibly in skeletal muscle metabolism. During the asymptomatic phase of congestive heart failure, left ventricular dysfunction steadily progresses to the full extent, as evidenced by the lack of correlation between the severity of left ventricular dysfunction and functional capacity (2–4).

The pathophysiological mechanisms that lead to exertional symptoms in elderly patients with heart failure are complex and result from an array of abnormalities present in the heart: left ventricular systolic and/or diastolic dysfunction, mitral regurgitation, and, to a variable extent, right ventricular dysfunction, and, in the periphery, fixed and very limited ability of the skeletal muscle vasculature to dilate in response to exercise, and impaired skeletal muscle metabolism (5–8). The most surprising characteristic of the syndrome of heart failure in middle-aged men is the amount of left ventricular dysfunction that can be tolerated without resulting in symptoms of heart failure. Left ventricular ejection fractions $\leqslant 20\%$ are frequently documented in asymptomatic patients (9).

However, the issue of asymptomatic versus symptomatic heart failure in patients has become somewhat blurred. As previously mentioned, the so-called asymptomatic patients who were enrolled in the prevention arm of SOLVD had peak aerobic capacities of approximately 20 ml/kg/min, which corresponds to two-thirds of peak aerobic capacity of age- and sex-matched normal subjects (10). If one considers that a peak aerobic capacity of a patient with heart failure in functional class IV of the New York Heart Association is around 10 ml/kg/min, one realizes that the so-called aymptomatic patients have already lost half their peak aerobic reserve. Consequently, labeling patients asymptomatic or symptomatic becomes arbitrary and does not in any way reflect the extent of the pathological events that have taken place. The apparent paradox of severely depressed left ventricular dysfunction and lack of overt symptoms of heart failure can be explained in part by the status of the peripheral circulation and the skeletal muscles. Young and middle-aged patients with severely depressed left ventricular dysfunction experience only slight decreases in exercise capacity when they are physically conditioned and have a nearly normal peak reactive hyperemic response of the skeletal muscle vasculature and adequate skeletal muscle mass (11). However, elderly subjects are less likely to be conditioned in view of their sedentary life-style.

The capacity to exercise maximally appears to decline with age independently of left ventricular performance. Whereas older subjects cannot increase maximal heart rate to the same extent as younger subjects during exercise, older subjects tend to compensate by increasing left ventricular diastolic volume, thereby maintaining an adequate cardiac output response to exercise by the Starling mechanism (12,13). However, older subjects are less active and relatively deconditioned compared to younger subjects. This deconditioning probably manifests as a steady decline in the capacity of the skeletal muscle vasculature to dilate in response to maximal exercise with age (14). To what extent impairment of the peripheral circulation, which has been documented with aging, prevents complete extraction of the delivered oxygen by the active skeletal muscle is only partially understood (15). Physical abnormalities, such as reduced oxidative capacity and decreased mitochondrial volume, can also contribute to limit the ability of older subjects to widen the (atrioventricular) $O_2$ difference during maximal exercise (16). Thus, in contrast to middle-aged patients with heart failure in whom a trained peripheral skeletal muscle vasculature and metabolism may compensate for depressed left ventricular performance, elderly patients are unable to rely on such compensatory mechanisms when confronted with a decline in left ventricular function. To the contrary, the depressed left ventricular function is compounded, as far as symptoms are involved, by substantial abnormalities in the peripheral circulation and skeletal muscles. In addition, the resting systemic resistance, which tends to be higher in older patients, further depresses left ventricular performance.

Up to one-half of elderly patients diagnosed as having heart failure have normal left ventricular systolic function at rest (17–20). The clinical manifestations of the syndrome of heart failure and intact systolic function are recurrent bouts of acute pulmonary edema or left ventricular failure that commonly are attributed predominantly to left ventricular diastolic dysfunction and, to a lesser extent, a markedly reduced capacity to adequately excrete sodium. Left ventricular compliance clearly decreases in elderly patients (21,22). However, whether this is the predominant factor involved in the pathophysiology of the syndrome of congestive heart failure and normal systolic function and how much it contributes to the pathophysiology of heart failure in patients with left ventricular systolic dysfunction have not been satisfactorily resolved (17). The reduction in left ventricular compliance observed in elderly patients is related to increasing left ventricular wall thickness, which itself results from the progressive rise in systolic and diastolic blood pressure as patients age (22). In the elderly patient with congestive heart failure, increased left ventricular wall thickness clearly results from hypertrophy of individual cardiac myocytes, because the number of myocytes across the wall tends to decrease with age. Olivetti et al. (23) clearly demonstrated that the aging process was associated with a substantial loss of myocytes in the left and right ventricular myocardium of subjects who died from causes other than cardiovascular disease. This loss of myocytes was accompanied by a progressive enlargement of the remaining myocytes, which resulted in preservation of left ventricular wall thickness in both the right and left ventricles. Olivetti et al. concluded that loss of cells and enlargement of the remaining myocytes represent the structural basis for the reduced compensatory capacity of the aging heart (23). Together, loss of myocytes and hypertrophy of the remaining myocytes may contribute to the development of myocardial dysfunction and failure in the elderly.

The factors responsible for the loss of nearly 35% of the cells in the ventricle during the aging process are essentially unknown. A detrimental effect of aging on the capillary microvasculature has been described in rats (24). Moreover, a decrease in coronary vascular reserve and an increase in minimal coronary vascular resistance have been seen in the same animal (25). The loss of myocytes has been clearly documented during the aging process in humans, but it is unclear if myocyte cellular hyperplasia tends to generate the lost ventricular mass with age. Myocyte cellular hyperplasia has been documented in the hypertrophied aging rat heart in response to cell loss (26).

Changes in renal blood flow and glomerular filtration rate appear to be important determinants of the syndrome of congestive heart failure in elderly patients. The hemodynamic intrarenal compensatory mechanisms that have been documented in younger patients with congestive heart failure and include an increase in filtration fraction, resulting from an efferent vasoconstriction, have not been found to occur in elderly patients who predominantly experience afferent vasoconstriction, resulting in a marked increase in renal vascular resistance and a modest increase in filtration fraction (27). Whether this discrepancy in intrarenal hemodynamic alterations noted between elderly and younger patients with congestive heart failure results from a different pattern of neuroendocrine activation is unclear. Elderly patients with congestive heart failure tend to have a higher norepinephrine concentration and a lower activation of the renin angiotensin system than have been documented in middle-aged patients with congestive heart failure (27).

## MANAGEMENT OF HEART FAILURE IN ELDERLY PATIENTS

Therapeutic approaches may differ in elderly patients with congestive heart failure according to the onset of symptoms. Patients who have developed congestive heart failure in their late fifties or early sixties are likely to be treated with loop diuretics, nitrates, angiotensin converting enzyme inhibitors, and digoxin by the time they reach 65 years old. Therapy should not be modified in these patients, except for titrating the dose of the various medications to the changes in renal function. Indeed, over the age of 65, renal function substantially decreases and the likelihood of accumulation of the drugs, which are primarily excreted by the kidneys, steadily increases (27). It may be preferable to avoid medications with long half-lives in these patients, who because they lead less active life-styles can easily adapt to a twice-a-day medical regimen while being likely candidates for drug overdosages because of worsening cardiac and renal hemodynamic status. The goals of therapy may be different in patients who develop congestive heart failure after the age of 65 from those sought in younger patients. The primary goal in the older patient population is to control symptoms at rest and during daily activities without attempting to improve maximal functional capacity, which is of no use in the vast majority of patients who lead sedentary life-styles.

To achieve the primary goal, one cannot underestimate the importance of an adequate knowledge and understanding of a low-sodium diet by the patients. This is the cornerstone of heart failure therapy in elderly patients, especially in patients with left ventricular diastolic dysfunction. When exacerbation or new onset of myocardial ischemia or arrhythmias is ruled out as a precipitating factor, excessive sodium intake is likely to be the precipitating factor of decompensation in patients with acute left ventricular failure and normal systolic function. Strict adherence to a low-sodium diet is essential to control symptoms because pharmacological intervention aimed at improving left ventricular compliance, such as calcium antagonists, appears to have limited benefits in the absence of left ventricular outflow tract obstruction. Tailoring the dose of diuretics to sodium intake, that is, during holidays and for social events, is an effective way to prevent episodes of decompensation in these patients. The daily dose of diuretics should be rapidly downtitrated in patients with left ventricular diastolic dysfunction who need high left ventricular filling pressures to maintain an adequate stroke volume and thus do not tolerate intravascular depletion. In contrast, patients with congestive heart failure due to left ventricular systolic dysfunction tolerate higher doses of loop diuretics, which can be potentiated by concomitant administration of metolazone on an outpatient basis or intravenous dopamine at renal doses, that is, 1–2 $\mu$g/kg/min, on an inpatient basis. The goal of diuresis in patients with left ventricular systolic dysfunction whose decompensation is characterized by severe sodium and fluid retention is to generate a body weight loss of 1–2 pounds daily.

## Digitalis Glycosides

The usefulness of digitalis glycosides for the treatment of patients with congestive heart failure who are in sinus rhythm has been repeatedly questioned (28–30). Overall, long-term administration of digoxin to patients with severe congestive heart failure in sinus rhythm appears to exert beneficial effects on symptoms and functional capacity (31–34). Whereas most North American cardiologists agree with the usefulness of digoxin in the treatment of severe congestive heart failure, two issues pertinent to therapy with digoxin remain controversial. The first issue is the nature of the exact mechanisms that mediate the benefits of digoxin on symptoms and functional capacity (35). Does the efficacy of digoxin primarily result from enhanced myocardial contractility secondary to inhibition of the sodium–potassium ATPase pump, which in turn increases the availability of activator $Ca^{2+}$ for the contractile proteins, or does the efficacy of digoxin in patients with congestive heart failure relate to a normalization of impaired baroreflex mechanisms, which in turn beneficially modulate the excessive neuroendocrine activation characteristically present with the syndrome? The second issue is the safety of prolonged administration of digoxin in patients with congestive heart failure, especially the impact of long-term digitalization on survival in these patients. The effect of prolonged administration of digoxin is currently being evaluated in a large, multicenter, international trial involving several thousand patients. Independently of the results of this large trial, one should question the validity and true therapeutic interest of such an approach to determine the safety of a positive inotropic agent in the treatment of congestive heart failure.

In contrast to the adverse effects observed during vasodilator therapy, which include hypotension, worsening myocardial ischemia, and deterioration of renal function, which are readily detected, the potential adverse effects associated with positive inotropic therapy, which include cardiac afterpotentials, calcium overloading of the cardiac myocytes, and possibly exacerbation of ventricular arrhythmias, are clinically difficult to quantify in patients with congestive heart failure. The clinical response to positive inotropic therapy also appears to be highly dependent on the stage of the disease process. For example, patients who experienced the most benefit from long-term therapy with digoxin appeared to be those with massively dilated left ventricles and third heart sounds (31). For all these reasons, initiation of therapy with a positive inotropic agent requires more expertise and closer follow-up than that needed with specific or nonspecific vasodilator therapy. Whether patients with heart failure enrolled in large multicenter trials primarily aimed at determining survival are well characterized, that is, by stage of the process, etiology of heart failure, and nature of associated morbid conditions, and are followed closely to adjust medications to renal function and concomitant therapies is open to question. Consequently, although from an epidemiologic point of view large multicenter trials can undoubtedly provide an answer to the question of the safety of chronic administration of digoxin, from a therapeutic viewpoint the usefulness of this mode of treatment can go unrecognized in a subset of patients and therefore the quality of individual care may be ill served.

Long-term administration of digoxin is likely to be associated with an increased risk of side effects in elderly patients with congestive heart failure. Compared to middle-aged subjects, elderly patients with congestive heart failure are at higher risk of experiencing adverse effects during chronic administration of digoxin. The decrease in skeletal muscle mass in the elderly reduces the volume of distribution of digoxin and thereby accounts for blood levels of digoxin twice higher in elderly patients than in younger patients, for a similar dose (36,37). Decreased renal function, which is age related, may also contribute to increased serum concentration of digoxin, which predominantly is excreted by the kidney. For these reasons, elderly patients with congestive heart failure appear to be particularly prone to developing adverse effects to digoxin because of the risk of overdosage. Of note, headache, irritability, fatigue, and confusion are not uncommon symptoms of digoxin overdose in elderly patients with congestive heart failure. When serum digoxin concentrations are maintained below 1 ng/ml, the risk of overdosage is low, improvement in left ventricular performance increases, as evidenced by a rise in ejection fraction, and clinical benefits are consistently observed (38,39). Whereas elderly patients with atrial fibrillation and congestive heart failure are the most likely to benefit from prolonged administration of digoxin, patients with dilated left ventricles, third heart sounds, and severe symptoms are also candidates for long-term digoxin therapy.

## Angiotensin Converting Enzyme Inhibition

In view of the results of the SAVE trial and the substantial impact of enalapril on morbidity in the prevention arm of the SOLVD, angiotensin converting enzyme inhibitors appear to be a pharmacological intervention that impedes the spontaneous deterioration of the syndrome of congestive heart failure (1,40). In this regard, angiotensin converting enzyme inhibitors appear to be of greater therapeutic interest as a first-line drug than diuretics, which do not alter the progression of the syndrome but, to the contrary, may stimulate the activity of the renin-angiotensin-aldosterone system. The impact of prolonged angiotensin converting enzyme inhibition on survival at an early stage of the syndrome of heart failure, when the heart is only mildly dilated, has not been clearly established (41). When patients with recent myocardial infarction are not selected on the basis of depressed left ventricular function, administration of enalapril for 6 months does not favorably alter the survival curve compared to placebo (42). However, the earlier angiotensin converting enzyme inhibition is initiated during the dynamic process of left ventricular dysfunction, the longer the follow-up period is needed to demonstrate an effect because of the low incidence of fatal events. In addition, during the conduct of randomized trials of angiotensin converting enzyme inhibitors versus placebo, it is now unethical to withhold open-label therapy with angiotensin converting enzyme inhibitors in patients who developed symptoms of congestive heart failure not controlled by loop diuretics. Thus, by intention-to-treat analysis, the likelihood of detecting a potential effect of angiotensin converting enzyme inhibition is reduced by the patients who are crossed over.

Angiotensin converting enzyme inhibitors should be prescribed to symptomatic patients with left ventricular dysfunction. However, whether angiotensin converting enzyme inhibitors should be routinely prescribed in asymptomatic patients with minimal left ventricular dysfunction has not been established. The results of SAVE indicate that when the left ventricular ejection fraction is lower than 40%, angiotensin converting enzyme inhibitors are beneficial (40). Interestingly, the benefits of angiotensin converting enzyme inhibition were not readily apparent in patients with ejection fractions above 30% in the SOLVD (1). From these results one can extrapolate that angiotensin converting enzyme inhibitors, although of little use in patients with normal or nearly normal left ventricular dimension, should be given to patients when their left ventricles start to dilate. Direct measurement of left ventricular end-diastolic dimension by two-dimensional echocardiography may be a more sensitive index to establish the need for angiotensin converting enzyme inhibition therapy than left ventricular ejection fraction, which may be normal if the stroke volume is somewhat increased, even though the left ventricle is dilated. Besides their beneficial effects in preventing further left ventricular dilatation, angiotensin converting enzyme inhibitors have been shown in both the SAVE and SOLVD to reduce the incidence of coronary events, that is, myocardial infarction and hospitalization for unstable angina, by 20–30% (1,40). Although the mechanisms that mediate these protective effects of angiotensin converting enzyme inhibitors are not understood, this further argues for initiating angiotensin converting enzyme inhibition therapy as soon as left ventricular dilatation is detected.

The clinical benefits of angiotensin converting enzyme inhibitors have been well documented in patients with left ventricular systolic dysfunction at daily doses that are, overall, greater than those routinely prescribed to patients with heart failure. Whether lower doses of angiotensin converting enzyme inhibitors produce the same benefits is currently unclear, but clinical experience favors initiation of therapy with a low dose and gradually increasing the dose over the next few weeks. The role of angiotensin converting enzyme inhibitors in the therapy of patients with left ventricular diastolic dysfunction is still not completely understood. These drugs may prevent further left ventricular hypertrophy and thereby increase left ventricular compliance as well as enhance urinary sodium excretion, but the efficacy of angiotensin converting enzyme inhibitors in the clinical setting has not been demonstrated in double-blind, randomized trials.

## PHYSICAL CONDITIONING

As mentioned earlier, the peripheral circulation and skeletal muscles of elderly patients with heart failure are poorly conditioned. The benefits of physical training have been demonstrated in middle-aged and older patients with heart failure (43,44). However, it is doubtful that elderly patients can undergo rigorous physical training on the treadmill or bicycle ergometer. In these patients, segmental training, limb by limb, may offer the local benefits of conventional physical training on the peripheral circulation and skeletal muscles, without stressing the heart, and may be better tolerated by patients who frequently are limited by joint disorders.

## SUMMARY

From a pathophysiological standpoint, the syndrome of congestive heart failure appears in the elderly to be characterized by a substantial impairment of left ventricular filling and urinary sodium excretion, as well as markedly deconditioned peripheral circulation and skeletal muscle. Impairment in left ventricular filling, that is, diastolic dysfunction, is the cause of heart failure in approximately 50% of elderly patients. Decreased capacity to excrete sodium may also play an important role in the pathophysiology of heart failure as a result of diastolic dysfunction. In elderly patients with left ventricular systolic dysfunction, the periphery is grossly deconditioned and thus, as far as symptoms are concerned, magnifies the limitations already imposed by the depressed left ventricular performance. Angiotensin converting enzyme inhibitors initiated at low dose should be considered first-line therapy in patients with left ventricular systolic dysfunction because they are the only agents that have been demonstrated to impede the progression of the syndrome. In patients with left ventricular diastolic dysfunction, careful monitoring of sodium intake and adjustments of diuretic dosages are essential to controlling the episodes of sudden decompensation.

## REFERENCES

1. SOLVD Investigators. Effect of enalapril on mortality and the development of heart failure in asymptomatic patients with reduced left ventricular ejection fractions. *N Engl J Med* 1992; 327:685–691.
2. Franciosa JA, Ziesche S, Wilen M. Functional capacity of patients with chronic left ventricular failure: Relationship of bicycle exercise performance to clinical and hemodynamic characterization. *Am J Med* 1979; 67:460–466.
3. Franciosa JA, Park M, Levine BT. Lack of correlation between exercise capacity and indexes of resting left ventricular performance in heart failure. *Am J Cardiol* 1981; 47:33–39.
4. Benge W, Litchfield RL, Marcus ML. Exercise capacity in patients with severe left ventricular dysfunction. *Circulation* 1980; 61:955–959.
5. LeJemtel TH, Maskin CS, Lucido D, Chadwick BJ. Failure to augment maximal limb blood flow in response to one-leg versus two-leg exercise in patients with severe heart failure. *Circulation* 1986; 74:245–251.
6. Wilson JR, Fink L, Maris J, Ferraro N, Power-Vanwart J, Eleff S, Chance B. Evaluation of energy metabolism in skeletal muscle of patients with heart failure with gated phosphorus-31 nuclear magnetic resonance. *Circulation* 1985; 71:57–62.
7. Massie B, Conway M, Yonge R, Frostick S, Ledingham J, Sleight P, Radda G, Rajagopolan B. Skeletal muscle metabolism in patients with congestive heart failure: Relation to clinical severity and blood flow. *Circulation* 1987; 76:1009–1019.
8. Zelis R, Sinoway LI, Musch TI. Why do patients with congestive heart failure stop exercising? *J Am Coll Cardiol* 1988; 12:359–361.
9. Litchfield RL, Kerber RE, Benge WJ, Mark AL, Sopko J, Bhatnagar RK, Marcus ML. Normal exercise capacity in patients with severe left ventricular dysfunction: Compensatory mechanisms. *Circulation* 1982; 66:129–134.
10. Liang C-S, Stewart DK, LeJemtel TH, Kirlin PC, McIntyre KM, Cahill WL, Galvao M, Boichot H, Woods P, Held P, for the SOLVD Investigators. Depressed peak aerobic capacity in asymptomatic patients with reduced left ventricular ejection fraction (abstract). *Circulation* 1990; 82(4):III–325.
11. Jondeau G, Katz SD, Zohman L, Goldberger M, McCarthy M, Bourdarias J-P, LeJemtel TH. Active skeletal muscle mass and cardiopulmonary reserve: Failure to attain peak aerobic capacity during maximal bicycle exercise in patients with severe congestive heart failure. *Circulation* 1992; 86.
12. Rodeheffer RJ, Gerstenblith G, Becker LC, Fleg JL, Weisfeldt ML, Lakatta EG. Exercise cardiac output is maintained with advancing age in healthy human subjects: Cardiac dilatation and increased stroke volume compensate for a diminished heart rate. *Circulation* 1984; 69(2):203–213.

13. Higginbotham MB, Morris KG, Williams RS, Coleman RE, Cobb FR. Physiologic basis for the age-related decline in aerobic work capacity. *Am J Cardiol* 1986; 57:1374–1379.
14. Jordfeldt L, Wahren J. Leg blood flow during exercise in man. *Clin Sci* 1971; 41:459–473.
15. Blomqvist CG. Cardiovascular adaptations to physical training. *Annu Rev Physiol* 1983; 45:169–189.
16. Scheuer J, Tipton CM. Cardiovascular adaptations to physical training. *Annu Rev Physiol* 1977; 39:221–251.
17. Sonnenblick EH, Yellin E, LeJemtel TH. Congestive heart failure and intact systolic ventricular performance. *Heart Failure* 1988; 4(4/5):164–173.
18. Aronow WS, Ahn C, Kronzon I. Prognosis of congestive heart failure in elderly patients with normal versus abnormal left ventricular systolic function associated with coronary artery disease. *Am J Cardiol* 1990; 66:1257–1259.
19. Wong WF, Gold S, Fukuyama O, Blanchette PL. Diastolic dysfunction in elderly patients with congestive heart failure. *Am J Cardiol* 1989; 63:1526–1528.
20. Aronow WS, Kronzon I. Effect of enalapril on congestive heart failure treated with diuretics in elderly patients with prior myocardial infarction and normal left ventricular ejection fraction. *Am J Cardiol* 1993; 71:602–604.
21. Bryg RJ, Williams GA, Labovitz AJ. Effect of aging on left ventricular diastolic filling in normal subjects. *Am J Cardiol* 1987; 59:971–974.
22. Lakatta EG. Changes in cardiovascular function with aging. *Eur Heart J* 1990; 11(Suppl. C):22–29.
23. Olivetti G, Melissari M, Capasso JM, Anversa P. Cardiomyopathy of the aging human heart. Myocyte loss and reactive cellular hypertrophy. *Circ Res* 1991; 68:1560–1568.
24. Anversa P, Hiler B, Ricci R, Guideri G, Olivetti G. Myocyte cell loss and myocyte hypertrophy in the age rat heart. *J Am Coll Cardiol* 1986; 8(6):1441–1448.
25. Hachamovitch R, Wicker P, Capasso JM, Anversa P. Alterations of coronary blood flow and reserve with aging in Fischer 344 rats. *Am J Physiol* 1989; 256:H66–H73.
26. Anversa P, Palackal T, Sonnenblick EH, Olivetti G, Meggs LG, Capasso JM. Myocyte cell loss and myocyte cellular hyperplasia in the hypertrophied aging rat heart. *Circ Res* 1990; 67:871–885.
27. Cody RJ. Characteristics of the elderly patient with congestive heart failure. *Am J Geriatr Cardiol* 1992; 1:30–41.
28. Fleg JL, Gottlieb SH, Lakatta EG. Is digoxin really important in treatment of compensated heart failure? A placebo-controlled crossover study in patients with sinus rhythm. *Am J Med* 1982; 73:244–250.
29. Aronow WS, Starling L, Etienne F. Lack of efficacy of digoxin in treatment of compensated congestive heart failure with third heart sound and sinus rhythm in elderly patients receiving diuretic therapy. *Am J Cardiol* 1986; 58:168–169.
30. Aronow WS. Clinical use of digitalis. *Comp Ther* 1992; 18(2):38–41.
31. Lee DC-S, Johnson RA, Bingham JB, et al. Heart failure in outpatients. A randomized trial of digoxin versus placebo. *N Engl J Med* 1982; 306:699–705.
32. Guyatt GH, Sullivan MJJ, Fallen EJ, et al. A controlled trial of digoxin in congestive heart failure. *Am J Cardiol* 1988; 61:371–375.

33. Arnold SB, Byrd RC, Meister W, et al. Long-term digitalis therapy improved left ventricular function in heart failure. *N Engl J Med* 1980; 303:1443–1448.
34. Mooradian AD, Grieff VL, Bressler R, Reed RL, Marcus FI. Digitalis in the elderly. University of Arizona Grand Rounds. *J Am Geriatr Soc* 1989; 37:873–882.
35. Gheorghiade M, Ferguson D. Digoxin. A neurohormonal modulator in heart failure? *Circulation* 1991; 84:2181–2186.
36. Passmore AP, Johnston GD. Digoxin toxicity in the aged. Characterising and avoiding the problem. *Drugs Aging* 1991; 1(5):364–379.
37. Aronow WS. Digoxin or angiotensin converting enzyme inhibitors for congestive heart failure in geriatric patients. Which is the preferred treatment? *Drugs Aging* 1991 1(2):98–103.
38. Luchi RJ, Taffet GE, Teasdale TA. Congestive heart failure in the elderly. *J Am Geriatr Soc* 1991; 39:810–825.
39. Ware HA, Snow E, Luchi JM, et al. Effect of digoxin on ejection fraction in elderly patients with congestive heart failure. *J Am Geriatr Soc* 1984; 32:631–000.
40. Pfeffer MA, Braunwald E, Moye LA, Basta L, Brown EJ Jr, Cuddy TE, Davis BR, Geltman EM, Goldman S, Flaker GC, Klein M, Lamas GA, Packer M, Rouleau J, Rouleau JL, Rutherford J, Wertheimer JH, Hawkins CM, on behalf of the SAVE Investigators. Effect of captopril on mortality and morbidity in patients with left ventricular dysfunction after myocardial infarction. *N Engl J Med* 1992; 327:669–677.
41. Mitchell GF, Pfeffer MA. Left ventricular remodeling after myocardial infarction: Progression toward heart failure. *Heart Failure* 1992; 8(2):55–69.
42. Swedberg K, Held P, Kjekshus J, Rasmussen K, Ryden L, Wedel H, on behalf of the CONSENSUS II Study Group. Effects of the early administration of enalapril on mortality in patients with acute myocardial infarction. *N Engl J Med* 1992; 327:678–684.
43. Sullivan MJ, Higginbotham MB, Cobb FR. Exercise training in patients with severe left ventricular dysfunction. Hemodynamic and metabolic effects. *Circulation* 1988; 78:506–515.
44. Coats AJS, Adamopoulos S, Radaelli A, McCance A, Meyer TE, Bernardi L, Solda PL, Davey P, Ormerod O, Forfar C, Conway J, Sleight P. Controlled trial of physical training in chronic heart failure. Exercise performance, hemodynamics, ventilation and autonomic function. *Circulation* 1992; 85:2119–2131.

# 21

# Management of Supraventricular Tachycardia in the Elderly

**Kevin J. Ferrick and John D. Fisher**
*Albert Einstein College of Medicine and Montefiore Medical Center, Bronx, New York*

## INTRODUCTION

Over the last 15 years, significant advances have been made in the ability to detect, diagnose, and treat a broad spectrum of complex arrhythmias. Although much of the emphasis during this time has focused on the management of sustained ventricular tachycardia and patients with aborted sudden cardiac death, equally dramatic advances have been made in the management of supraventricular arrhythmias including, atrial fibrillation, atrial flutter, atrioventricular (AV) node reentry, and AV reciprocating tachycardia. The following reviews the most common supraventricular arrhythmias, with emphasis on their current management. The putative mechanisms responsible for these arrhythmias are discussed, along with current tenets of acute and chronic management. Currently available diagnostic modalities and their potential role in patients with paroxysmal or infrequent arrhythmias are also reviewed. Finally, some of the recently appreciated risks associated with pharmacological therapy are discussed.

## REENTRY AS THE BASIS OF SUPRAVENTRICULAR ARRHYTHMIAS

The term "supraventricular arrhythmias" constitutes a wide variety of arrhythmias that arise primarily from a level superior to the division of the common bundle of His into left and right bundle branches and/or activate the ventricles utilizing the native conduction pathways (i.e., His-Purkinje network) as an integral part of the circuit. The vast majority of supraventricular arrhythmias are thought to be based on reentry, as apart from abnormal or enhanced automaticity, which account for a minority (less than 5%) of clinically significant arrhythmias (1). For a reentrant circuit to result in a sustained arrhythmia, three basic requirements must be fulfilled. These include (1) physical contiguity of two electrophysiologically (but not necessarily anatomically) distinct tissues, (2) unidirectional block of conduction in one of the electrophysiological "pathways," and (3) slow conduction in part of the pathway, to allow repolarization and subsequent conduction along the initial depolarized path (2–4). If a critical balance is maintained, with the leading wave front timed to engage tissue capable of sustaining conduction, a sustained arrhythmia perpetuates. Often the latent substrate for supraventricular arrhythmias based upon reentry is "activated" by properly timed atrial or ventricular premature depolarizations, which allow the dissociation of the conduction properties of the two component pathways, resulting in initiation of a sustained circuit. The hallmark of these arrhythmias is their paroxysmal nature, insofar as they are based upon a latent substrate that can be provoked by a variety of factors, including atrial and ventricular premature depolarizations, ischemia, changes in sympathetic tone, scarring, and even pharmacological agents (5–9). Abnormalities of automaticity, either enhanced or triggered, are believed to be responsible for the minority of these arrhythmias (10).

## SPECTRUM OF SUPRAVENTRICULAR ARRHYTHMIAS

The most common supraventricular arrhythmia is atrial fibrillation, with an estimated prevalence of over 1 million (11). It is characterized by a continuous depolarization of the atrium, with often rapid and irregularly irregular conduction to the ventricle. Although the mechanism of this arrhythmia has in the past been controversial, work by Allessie, Moe, and others has suggested that it is reentrant in nature (11–14). In the absence of pharmacological therapy and in the setting of normal AV nodal conduction, the mean ventricular response to atrial fibrillation in a patient free of medication is often in the 150–170 bpm range.

The second most common supraventricular arrhythmia is atrial flutter, and this may represent one end of a continuous spectrum with atrial fibrillation. Once again, studies have suggested that the mechanism of this rhythm is reentry (15,16). This rhythm is characterized by a rapid regular rate of atrial depolarization, often 300 bpm, although this can vary from between 220 and 350 bpm, depending upon the patient. The usual form of atrial flutter is characterized electrophysiologically by organized atrial activity (so-called F waves), which resemble a "sawtooth" or "picket fence" pattern as seen in standard leads II, III, and AVF. Atrial flutter most commonly conducts to the ventricle with a 2:1 pattern, such that the ventricular rate during flutter is often 150 bpm and is usually characterized by a normal QRS morphology. There appears to be a continuous spectrum between atrial flutter and atrial fibrillation, and it has been demonstrated that atrial flutter can degenerate into atrial fibrillation and then reorganize into atrial flutter (17). Atrial mapping studies have suggested that the common form of atrial flutter involves a counterclockwise depolarization of the atrium, moving from an inferior to posterior to superior direction (16). The uncommon form of atrial flutter is usually more rapid (atrial rates in the 400 bpm range) and is usually characterized by a positive F wave in the inferior leads (superior to inferior direction).

AV nodal reentrant tachycardia accounts for approximately 60% of the supraventricular arrhythmias termed paroxysmal supraventricular tachycardia (PSVT) (18). It is often characterized as a narrow complex tachycardia that is regular in nature, exhibiting rates in the 150–180 bpm range, although in younger individuals rates of the 200–240 bpm range may be seen (19,20). A hallmark of this arrhythmia is its regularity. A 12-lead electrocardiogram during PSVT in two-thirds of patients does not show evidence of discreet P wave activity, because the atrium and ventricle are simultaneously depolarized, with the larger amplitude QRS masking the presence of P wave (atrial) activity. In approximately 30% of patients with AV node reentry, there is evidence of discreet atrial activity in the ST segment following the QRS. This occurs when the retrograde conduction time to the atrium is slow in comparison with antegrade conduction to the ventricle. In approximately 6% of patients with AV node reentry, the retrograde conduction time to the atrium is slow enough so that the "R-P" interval (as measured from the onset of the QRS to the onset of retrograde P wave activity) is >50% of the succeeding R-R interval. In this circumstance, differentiating an AV node reentrant tachycardia from either an intraatrial tachycardia or sinus node reentry can be difficult.

Paroxysmal supraventricular tachycardia secondary to accessory pathway conduction occurs in approximately 30% of patients with sustained PSVT (18). Accessory pathway conduction can either be overt, as in the Wolff-Parkinson-White syndrome, or concealed, because accessory pathways can be capable of either unidirectional or bidirectional conduction. Unidirectional retrograde conduction is electrocardiographically silent (i.e., one does not see evidence of delta waves); however, such accessory pathways are capable of sustaining a macroreentrant tachycardia, so-called AV reciprocating tachycardia, which involves antegrade conduction from atrium to ventricle utilizing the His-Purkinje system, with retrograde conduction mediated by the accessory pathway. This mechanism is identical to that utilized in so-called orthodromic tachycardia related to Wolff-Parkinson-White syndrome. In patients with Wolff-Parkinson-White syndrome, during sinus rhythm the ventricle is depolarized as a fusion between antegrade conduction across the AV node and antegrade conduction across the accessory pathway. Although the majority of PSVT related to Wolff-Parkinson-White syndrome (estimated prevalence of 0.3% in the general population, with equal prevalence in the young and the elderly) involves orthodromic tachycardia, in a minority of patients the sustained arrhythmia involves antegrade conduction across the bypass tract, with retrograde conduction along the His-Purkinje and AV node (so-called antidromic tachycardia) (21–23). This presents as a maximally preexcited QRS and is often mistaken for ventricular tachycardia. It generally responds to the same maneuvers as orthodromic tachycardia.

## MAKING THE DIAGNOSIS

Appropriate management of supraventricular tachycardia requires making the correct arrhythmic diagnosis. Among the points essential to interpretation of arrhythmia is defining whether the observed QRS are wide or narrow, as well as assessing the regularity of each successive QRS. The relationship (if any) of atrial depolarization to that of the QRS complexes can yield important information about the mechanism of arrhythmia. The majority of supraventricular arrhythmias conduct to the ventricle with a narrow QRS, assuming normal baseline conduction. A wide QRS supraventricular tachycardia can of course occur in the setting of preexisting conduction disturbances (right bundle branch block and left bundle branch block), as well as rate-related conduction disturbances. As the relative refractory period of His-Purkinje and ventricular tissue is directly proportional to the preceding R-R interval, atrial fibrillation often manifests the so-called Ashman's phenomenon (24). This presents as wide QRS complexes that are supraventricular in nature, occurring when close coupled QRS complexes follow a preceding pause. Because the relative refractory period of the right bundle branch is somewhat longer than that of the left bundle branch, the majority of "Ashman's beats," and indeed rate-related aberration in general, are of right bundle branch morphology. More specifically, approximately 85% of bundle branch aberrancy is right bundle in nature, with the remaining 15% presenting as left bundle branch block aberration. Therefore, wide complex tachycardias that are left bundle branch block in morphology are more likely, from a statistical perspective, to be of ventricular origin. Supraventricular tachycardias with bundle branch block aberration generally have QRS durations $< 140$ ms and most often exhibit a normal frontal plane axis. Moreover, a 12-lead electrocardiogram of aberrated PSVT will demonstrate a "classic" right bundle or left bundle branch block, not a nonspecific intraventricular conduction deficit (i.e., QRS that looks like right bundle branch block in lead I but manifests a left bundle branch block pattern in $V_1$). Such characteristics as extremely wide QRS, exhibiting an abnormal frontal plane axis and so-called concordance across the precordium (where lead $V_1$ has a morphology similar to that seen in lead $V_2$, $V_3$, and so on), strongly favor a ventricular origin of the tachycardia.

As mentioned, establishing the relationship between atrial activity and QRS depolarization is important in determining the type of supraventricular arrhythmia. The hallmark of atrial fibrillation is the absence of discreet atrial activity in the setting of a chaotic and irregularly irregular baseline, and the ventricular response to atrial fibrillation is classically irregular, although this may be difficult to appreciate at rapid ventricular rates. Approximately 60% of PSVT secondary to AV node reentry is free of evidence of atrial activity insofar as the atrium and ventricle are depolarized simultaneously. When one observes retrograde atrial activity following the QRS, as evidenced by a high-frequency depolarization in the ST segment or proximal T wave, 50% of these tachycardias represent AV node reentry; the remaining 50% represent so-called AV reciprocating tachycardia, with retrograde conduction mediated by an accessory pathway. If the R-P interval is >50% of the R-R interval, intraatrial tachycardia or sinus node reentry should be suspected (18). Invasive electrophysiological study, by determining the atrial activation sequence during tachycardia and its relationship to ventricular depolarization, can help to determine the mechanism of a patient's tachycardia more definitively (Figs. 1 and 2).

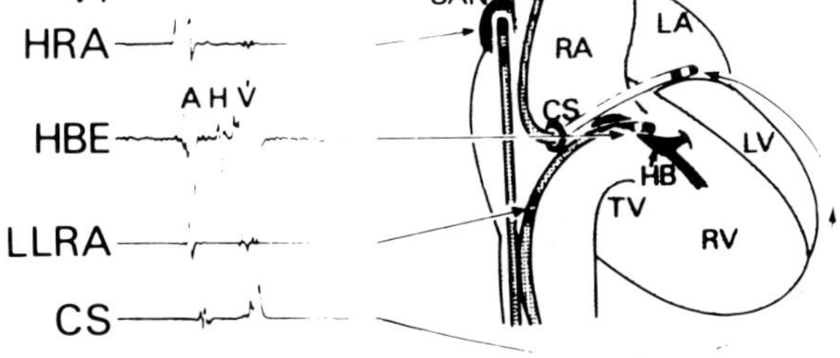


**Figure 1** Catheter placement for routine electrophysiological study. Intracavitary electrograms are displayed. Normal ranges for intracardiac conduction intervals are shown.

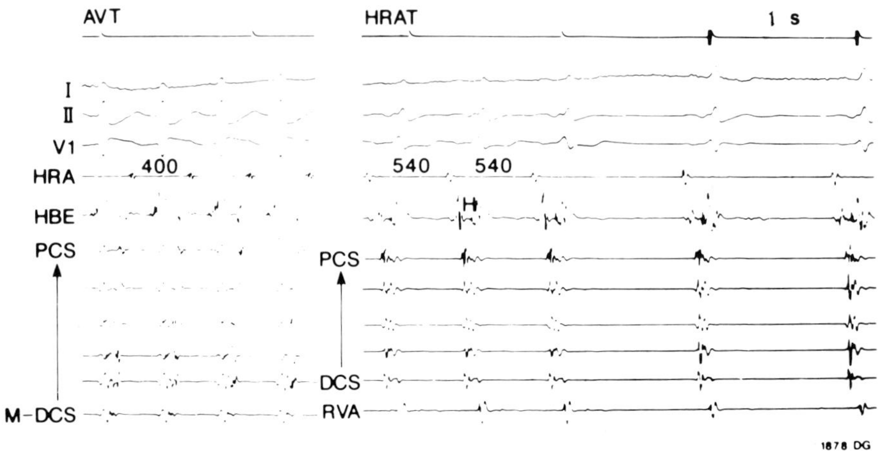


**Figure 2** Electrograms taken from a patient with two forms of paroxysmal supraventricular tachycardia. Surface electrocardiograms are displayed, along with intracavitary electrograms from the high right atrium (HRA), His bundle region (HBE), and numerous sites in the mid- and distal coronary sinus (M-DCS). On the left, AV reciprocating tachycardia demonstrating the presence of a left-sided accessory pathway is seen, with evidence of early atrial activation in the distal coronary sinus. On the right, a high right atrial tachycardia is shown, demonstrating high to low atrial activation sequencing.

## ACUTE MANAGEMENT OF SUPRAVENTRICULAR TACHYCARDIA

The acute management of any arrhythmia must involve assessment of the patient's hemodynamic status. This is of extreme importance in the elderly patient with underlying cardiovascular disease. In a setting in which the patient is compromised, that is, hypotensive, in severe congestive heart failure, or with persistent anginal type of chest pain, the treatment of choice is DC cardioversion. This should be done under brief anesthesia using a short-acting barbiturate or benzodiazepam, such as diazepam or midazolam. AV reciprocating tachycardia and AV node reentrant tachycardia are often vulnerable to 25 or 50 J synchronized shocks, but atrial fibrillation usually requires higher energies of 100 J or more. DC cardioversion is usually effective in terminating an acute episode of sustained supraventricular tachycardia, although it does not preclude arrhythmia recurrence. DC cardioversion is not of use in frequently recurring arrhythmias or rhythms thought to be secondary to enhanced automaticity, such as multifocal atrial tachycardia.

If the patient is tolerating the arrhythmia well, one should attempt to ascertain the specific nature of the arrhythmia to help guide specific treatment. The

**Table 1** Maneuvers Used to Accentuate Atrial Activity

| |
|---|
| Recording leads II, III, AVF, $V_1$ |
| Carotid massage |
| Valsalva maneuver |
| Lewis leads |
| Double speed, standard |
| Esophageal lead |
| Intraatrial recording |

importance of establishing the relationship, if any, between atrial and ventricular activity in this assessment was discussed previously. Vagal maneuvers (i.e., Valsalva maneuver and carotid massage), by transiently increasing the level of AV block, can be used to differentiate the type of arrhythmia. Atrial fibrillation and atrial flutter, for example, often exhibit a slowed ventricular response to carotid massage, allowing clear fibrillatory or flutter waves to be seen, whereas abrupt termination of the arrhythmia is often the response of AV reciprocating or AV node reentrant tachycardia. Other maneuvers that can assist in accentuating atrial activity are listed in Table 1. The following agents are often utilized in acute management of paroxysmal supraventricular tachycardia (Table 2).

## Adenosine

A purine nucleoside with a half-life of approximately 1.5 s, this agent exhbits a relatively selective electrophysiological effect on the AV node. Administered initially as a 6 mg bolus to be followed by 12 mg if the initial dose is ineffective, adenosine is extremely effective in slowing AV nodal conduction and terminating PSVT secondary to AV node reentry or AV reciprocating tachycardia in

**Table 2** Options in the Acute Management of Paroxysmal Supraventricular Tachycardia

| |
|---|
| Pharmacological therapy |
|   Adenosine |
|   Verapamil |
|   β-blockers |
|   Digoxin |
|   Procainamide |
| Pacing |
| Cardioversion |

more than 85% of patients (25–27). Transient atrial fibrillation, presumably due to the shortening of the atrial refractory period by adenosine, has been described. Its effect on atrial fibrillation and atrial flutter is modest; however, transient slowing of the ventricular response is often seen. In view of its relative specificity for the AV node, adenosine has been advocated as a "pharmacological probe" to help better elucidate the mechanism of specific arrhythmias. Side effects include transient flushing and chest pain; however, because of its extremely short half-life, these side effects are self-limited (28–30). It is therefore particularly useful in elderly patients with underlying left ventricular dysfunction who might otherwise not tolerate other agents.

## Verapamil

Introduced in the early 1980s, verapamil is successful in terminating AV node reentrant tachycardia and AV reciprocating tachycardia in 60–90% of patients (31,32). It is administered as an initial dose of 10 mg over 2 min, although in elderly patients, who may be more prone to its hypotensive effect, an initial dose of 5 mg is recommended. The half-life of the intravenous agent is 20–30 min, and it is in general well tolerated, although transient hypotension is not uncommon. Verapamil has an effect on both the sinus and AV node, and it can be useful in slowing the ventricular response to atrial fibrillation and atrial flutter. Continuous infusion of intravenous verapamil can be used to mitigate the ventricular response to atrial fibrillation in patients who do not absorb or cannot take oral medications. Verapamil should be avoided in patients with atrial fibrillation and evidence of preexcitation (Fig. 3). Intravenous diltiazem was recently approved by the U.S. Food and Drug Administration (FDA) for the temporary control of rapid ventricular response to both atrial fibrillation and atrial flutter, as well as for the conversion of PSVT to sinus rhythm.

## β-Blocking Agents

These agents exhibit a negative chronotropic as well as a negative dromotropic (slowing AV node conduction) effect, such that the response to supraventricular arrhythmias is similar to that seen with verapamil, although the response rate appears less with these agents. Intravenous β-blockers should not be used in combination with intravenous verapamil because of the negative inotropic effects of these agents. β-Blocking agents can also be effective in preventing atrial fibrillation in patients undergoing open-heart surgery (33–35).

## Digoxin

With a time to peak onset of 90 min, intravenous digoxin is not very effective in rapidly controlling supraventricular arrhythmias. This agent acts primarily by

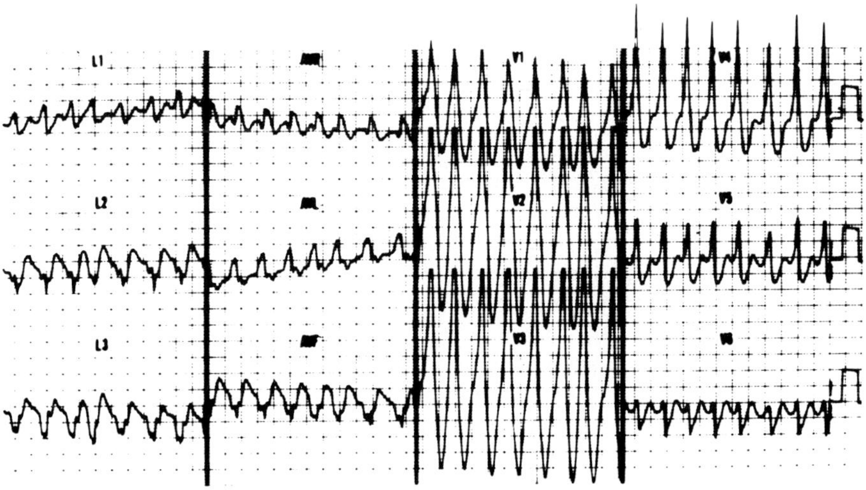

**Figure 3** A 12-lead electrocardiogram demonstrating atrial fibrillation in a patient with Wolff-Parkinson-White syndrome. Of note, the irregularly irregular QRS complexes demonstrate varying degrees of preexcitation (so-called concertina effect).

slowing conduction through the AV node. Although there have been reports of conversion with atrial fibrillation to sinus rhythm after digoxin administration, recent reports suggest that the conversion rate to sinus rhythm after digoxin is similar to that seen with placebo (36–38).

## Procainamide

A sodium channel blocking agent that moderately prolongs the refractory period of atrial and ventricular tissue (a so-called Ia agent of the Vaughn/Williams classification), procainamide can be effective in converting atrial fibrillation and atrial flutter to sinus rhythm. It can be administered intravenously at a rate of 20 mg/min to a target dose of 10–15 mg/kg. This agent can also be effective in terminating AV node reentrant tachycardia, as well as AV reciprocating tachycardia, although the effect of procainamide on the AV node is modest (39,40). Hypotension and QRS widening can be seen with IV administration, so that careful attention must be paid to the infusion rate of the drug.

## Pacing Maneuvers

In suitable candidates, programmed stimulation of the atrium or ventricle using overdrive, underdrive, or premature extrastimuli can be used to terminate reentrant arrhythmias. Conversion rates in the 60–80% range have been reported (41,42). Pacing maneuvers are ineffective in terminating atrial fibrillation, although atrial flutter can be entrained and terminated by rapid atrial pacing (43).

## CHRONIC THERAPY

Historically, the mainstay of chronic therapy for sustained supraventricular arrhythmias has been pharmacological (Table 3). Broadly speaking, the available agents can be subdivided into those agents whose predominant electrophysiological effect is upon the AV node and those that affect working myocardial cells ("atrial stabilizing effect"). This classification is not absolute, however, insofar as many agents exhibit both types of effects, although perhaps not of equal magnitude. Historically, digoxin and quinidine have constituted the mainstay of therapy for a variety of supraventricular arrhythmias, the former agent confining its primary electrophysiological effect to the AV node and the latter acting as an "atrial stabilizing" agent (44–46). Indeed quinidine, with its vagolytic effect, can actually enhance AV nodal conduction, and therefore its use as monotherapy for atrial fibrillation has not been advocated. However, the last 15 years has seen a variety of newer agents with either AV nodal blocking and/or atrial stabilizing characteristics (Table 3).

### Agents with Predominant Effects on the AV Node

Both verapamil and diltiazem, as calcium channel antagonists, have been shown to affect AV nodal conduction (47–52). These agents have demonstrated success rates in the 55–70% range in chronically controlling recrudescence of PSVT. Their use in atrial fibrillation is largely limited to moderation of ventricular

**Table 3** Options for Chronic Management of Supraventricular Tachycardia

| |
|---|
| Pharmacological |
| "AV nodal" agents |
| Atrial stabilizing agents |
| Anticoagulation |
| Nonpharmacological |
| Pacing |
| Ablation |
| Surgery |

response, and although effective at rest, they often fail to control ventricular rates during modest activity (50,51). Although generally well tolerated, these agents can cause annoying side effects, including peripheral edema, constipation, and nausea. Hypotension and exacerbation of congestive heart failure have been reported with verapamil administration secondary to its negatively inotrophic effect (53–55). When administered acutely to patients with wide complex tachycardias mistakenly believed to represent PSVT with aberration, verapamil has resulted in cardiovascular collapse and cardiac arrest. $\beta$-Blocking agents are effective in reducing the frequency of PSVT and have been shown to exhibit a significant effect in controlling the ventricular response to atrial fibrillation. In postoperative patients, $\beta$-blocking agents appear to be effective in preventing atrial fibrillation (52,54).

## Agents with Atrial Stabilizing Effects

### *Class Ia Agents*

Quinidine, procainamide, and disopyramide are agents that exhibit moderately potent sodium channel antagonist activity and also moderately prolong the effective refractory period of atrial and ventricular tissue. These drugs have been used to treat both paroxysmal supraventricular tachycardia and paroxysmal atrial fibrillation (PAF). Of these drugs, however, only quinidine is approved by the Food and Drug Administration for this indication. Although agents of this type have efficacy rates of approximately 50–60% for the maintenance of sinus rhythm in patients with paroxysmal atrial fibrillation, as well as control of recurrence of paroxysmal supraventricular tachycardia, side effects limit their long-term use (55–58). Positive antinuclear antibody titers develop in the majority of individuals treated with long-term procainamide, and a lupuslike syndrome can occur in these patients. Hematological abnormalities have been reported in patients treated with either procainamide or quinidine (thrombocytopenia and neutropenia), but this appears to be less common with disopyramide. Nausea, abdominal discomfort, and diarrhea occur in 5–15% of patients treated with quinidine. In view of the negative inotropic effects of disopyramide, its use should be avoided in individuals with a history of congestive heart failure (59). Frequently, anticholinergic side effects (dry mouth, urinary hesitancy, and blurred vision) can be ameliorated through the use of a cholinergic agent, such as pyridostigmine. Mestinon-SR in doses of 90 mg administered on either an every 8 h or every 6 h regimen has been shown to effectively ameliorate these symptoms (60). Recently, concerns over the safety of quinidine in the treatment of atrial fibrillation have been raised by a retrospective metaanalysis by Coplen et al., which demonstrated a threefold excess mortality in patients treated with quinidine for paroxysmal atrial fibrillation compared with controls (58).

### *Class Ic Agents*

Flecainide, a class Ic antiarrhythmic agent, was first introduced in 1985 for the treatment of ventricular arrhythmias. This agent was recently approved by the Food and Drug Administration for use in the treatment of a variety of supraventricular arrhythmias. As an agent of the Ic class, with potent sodium channel blocking effect, flecainide markedly slows cardiac conduction by blunting the upstroke during phase 0 of cardiac depolarization (61–64). At normal heart rates, flecainide exerts a minimal effect on the refractory period; at more rapid rates, however, flecainide markedly prolongs action potential duration and refractoriness. The drug in normal individuals has a half-life of elimination of approximately 20 h. It is metabolized in the liver and excreted by the kidney both as inactive metabolites and as unchanged drug. Flecainide has been demonstrated to reduce the frequency of episodes of PSVT and to prolong the interval between episodes in susceptible patients when compared with placebo. Flecainide has also been demonstrated to be effective in approximately 31% of treated patients in preventing recurrent paroxysmal atrial fibrillation. It has been demonstrated to increase by greater than fourfold the interval between episodes of paroxysmal atrial fibrillation compared with control.

Flecainide has also been demonstrated to be effective in preventing both the clinical recurrence and induction by programmed stimulation of paroxysmal supraventricular tachycardia in patients with Wolff-Parkinson-White syndrome (64). Success rates of up to 75% have been reported during short-term treatment with this agent. In general, flecainide is well tolerated in the vast majority of treated patients. Adverse cardiac effects have been reported to occur in 7% of patients treated for supraventricular arrhythmias (4% of those with PSVT and 10% of those with PAF). These cardiac effects have included increasingly frequent supraventricular tachycardia (proarrhythmia), conduction disturbances, and congestive heart failure. Sudden death has rarely been reported in patients treated with flecainide for supraventricular arrhythmias. The majority of these cardiac effects have occurred within 4 weeks of initiating therapy, and most have occurred in the setting of known structural heart disease. Noncardiac side effects include dizziness, blurred vision, light-headedness, and nausea.

When used to treat patients with asymptomatic ventricular arrhythmias following myocardial infarction (during the Cardiac Arrhythmia Suppression Trial), flecainide was associated with a 2.2-fold increase in 10 month mortality (from 2.3 to 5.1%) (65). However, the data for patients treated with flecainide for supraventricular arrhythmias suggest that the risk of proarrhythmia is much less (66). A recent study that compared patients treated with either flecainide or encainide with patients treated at a tertiary medical center with a variety of agents for supraventricular tachycardia failed to demonstrate evidence of excess mortality in patients treated with agents of the Ic class (63). Nevertheless, in view of concerns over potential proarrhythmia, flecainide is not recommended for the treatment of patients with significant structural heart disease, and if chronic therapy with flecainide is considered, exercise testing should be performed in an attempt to exclude exertional proarrhythmia. Because flecainide has negative inotropic effects, it should not be used in patients with congestive heart failure or significantly reduced ejection fractions. The recommended starting dose for the treatment of PSVT and paroxysmal atrial fibrillation is 50 mg every 12 h. The dosage can be titrated upward in increments of 50 mg twice per day every 4 days. The maximum recommended daily dose is 300 mg (i.e., 150 mg twice per day).

## Agents with Class III Effects

The primary electrophysiological effect of these agents is to prolong action potential duration markedly. Electrocardiographically, this results in QRS prolongation, mild QT prolongation in parallel with the degrees of QRS prolongation, and no effect on the "J-T interval." Agents of this class include amiodarone and sotalol, the latter agent also exhibiting a mild to moderate $\beta$-blocking effect. Amiodarone, an agent with an extremely long half-time of accumulation (67), has been demonstrated in a number of European studies to be extremely effective in treating both paroxysmal atrial fibrillation and PSVT (68–70). However, the use of this agent in the United States for these indications has been extremely limited. At the present time, the Food and Drug Administration approves the use of amiodarone only for life-threatening ventricular arrhythmias in view of its broad profile of side effects, some of which are potentially life threatening (i.e., hepatic failure and pulmonary fibrosis). Amiodarone also possesses mild class I effect and is effective in mitigating the ventricular response to atrial fibrillation. Sotalol, an agent that has been available in Europe for over 20 years and which was approved by the FDA in 1993 for the treatment of life-threatening ventricular arrhythmias, combines a nonselective $\beta$-blocking effect with a class III effect. It has been demonstrated to be effective in maintaining sinus rhythm after DC cardioversion, as well as in controlling the ventricular response in patients with chronic atrial fibrillation (71–73). It exhibits a modest negative inotropic effect and has a low incidence of central nervous system effects secondary to its hydrophilic properties (74). Although it is believed to have a limited potential for proarrhythmia, torsades de pointes has been reported during its use, especially at higher doses (75). Its use is contraindicated in patients with severe congestive heart failure.

## Anticoagulation in Atrial Fibrillation

It is well established that patients with rheumatic valvular disease and chronic atrial fibrillation are at significantly increased risk for stroke (approximately

17-fold) (76). It has been more recently appreciated that individuals with chronic atrial fibrillation and nonrheumatic heart disease are at approximately 5-fold increased risk for stroke compared with the general population (77,78). Anticoagulation therapy has been demonstrated to significantly reduce the incidence of stroke in patients over the age of 60 by approximately 60% (79,80). The role of aspirin in reducing stroke risk is controversial (81), and in the recently reported Stroke Prevention in Atrial Fibrillation Study, the beneficial effect of aspirin was not seen in patients over the age of 75 (82). Individuals in the absence of structural heart disease or with paroxysmal atrial fibrillation may not require chronic anticoagulation (see Chap. 9 for further discussion).

## NONPHARMACOLOGICAL MANAGEMENT OF SUPRAVENTRICULAR ARRHYTHMIAS

In view of the limited efficacy, the potential for proarrhythmia, and the cumulative toxicity of long-term pharmacological therapy for arrhythmias, it is not surprising that over the last 20 years much attention has focused on the nonpharmacological management of sustained, symptomatic arrhythmias. In the early 1970s, great enthusiasm was mustered for the use of implantable pacemakers in the management of recurrent supraventricular arrhythmias. This was followed by the development of surgical procedures for the treatment of PSVT. More recently, surgical techniques for the treatment of automatic atrial tachycardias, as well as atrial fibrillation, have been reported. Additionally, with the advent of the use of radiofrequency energy, catheter ablation techniques have now assumed center stage for the chronic management of a variety of supraventricular arrhthymias. Although still considered investigational at most centers, if initial success rates persist, ablative techniques may become the gold standard for long-term treatment. The following attempts to highlight the major advances and limitations of these differing approaches.

### Antitachycardia Pacing

With the development of sophisticated electrophysiological testing techniques that provided greater understanding of the mechanisms responsible for sustained arrhythmias, coupled with the availability of multiprogrammable pacemakers, it appeared in the early and mid-1970s that antitachycardia pacing would become a major therapeutic modality for supraventricular arrhythmias. Pacemakers can be utilized in an attempt to prevent tachycardia occurrence by pacing at rates more rapid than that of baseline sinus rhythm (i.e., overdrive suppression), thereby reducing the number of premature complexes that often serve to trigger an arrhythmia (83–85). They can also improve hemodynamics during incessant tachycardia, for example by pacing the atrium to produce 2:1 atrioventricular conduction and thereby effectively slow the ventricular rate during tachycardia (86–88). Devices can also be utilized to assess the continuing efficacy of a pharmacological regimen. Specially designed pacemakers capable of performing noninvasive programmed stimulation allow such studies to be performed without the need for repeat catheterization. These devices can therefore be useful to identify the need for alterations in ongoing therapy, if such therapy is proven to be ineffective. However, the preeminent role of pacemakers for the treatment of supraventricular arrhythmias is the use of automated detection and termination algorithms to terminate recurrent episodes effectively. Currently available devices can define the presence of tachycardia by using characteristics of rate, mode of onset, and rate stability, such that a programmed sequence of pacing can be utilized in an attempt to terminate an arrhythmic event (89–92). A variety of complex pacing algorithms using pacing stimuli in a variety of patterns (single, multiple, bursts, incremental-decremental sequencing, and so on) have been used for this purpose (Fig. 4). Unfortunately, the long-term efficacy of antitachycardia pacing for PSVT is only fair. A series from Montefiore Medical Center (92) suggests 93% efficacy at 1 year; however, this declines to 86% at 2–4 years and ultimately to 68% at 8 years (Fig. 5). This progressive inefficacy is often due to the development of chronic atrial fibrillation or the precipitation of atrial fibrillation during attempts at rhythm termination. Other series have suggested that even in the absence of atrial fibrillation, implanted devices often need to be adjusted during follow-up to maximize algorithm efficacy (89). These factors suggest that antitachycardia pacing for PSVT may be most appropriate for patients with a limited life expectancy or whose car-

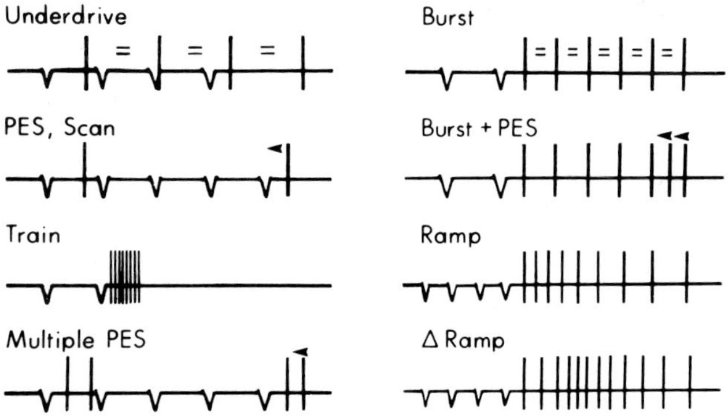


**Figure 4** Different antitachycardia pacing algorithms that can be used to terminate PSVT. PES = premature extrastimuli. Arrows connote an automated change in timing interval, with stimuli brought closer to the last detected QRS or pacing stimulus.

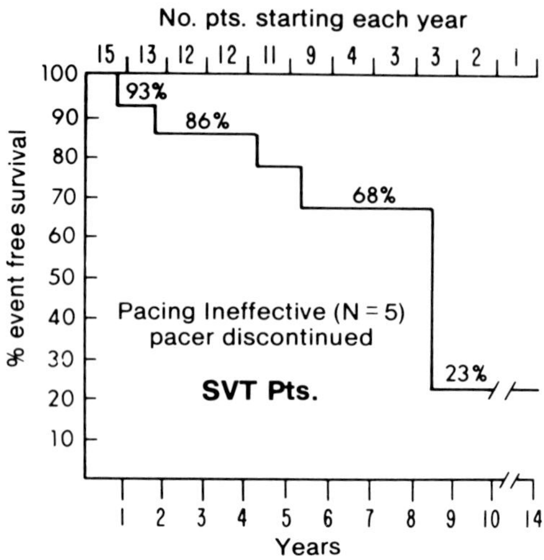


**Figure 5** Actuarial survival of effective antitachycardia pacing in patients treated for PSVT. (Reproduced with permission from Fisher et al., Ref. 92.)

diovascular status precludes more definitive therapy (i.e., surgery and catheter ablation).

## Surgical Techniques

Surgical techniques have been developed over the last 15 years to treat a variety of supraventricular arrhythmias. Indeed, surgical therapy has been considered by some have become the gold standard in the management of supraventricular tachycardia secondary to accessory pathways (Wolff-Parkinson-White syndrome and concealed bypass tracts). Success rates in excess of 95% with a surgical mortality of less than 1% have been consistently reported from centers that have performed this form of surgery since the mid-1970s (21–26,93–97). The surgical technique involves intraoperative confirmation of accessory pathway location, often using a computer-assisted mapping system with a multipole band electrode (Fig. 6). Although the original technique as described by Sealy and colleagues involved a combination of blunt and sharp dissection using an endocardial approach (i.e., incising from within the atrium out to the epicardial fat pad (93)), more recent techniques have involved epicardial dissection in concert with the application of cryolesions using nitrous oxide. Using the technique described by Guiraudon and others, the need for cardiopulmonary bypass can be avoided in many instances (94). Either right or left free-wall accessory pathway locations are particularly suited to this epicardial approach, whereas difficulties

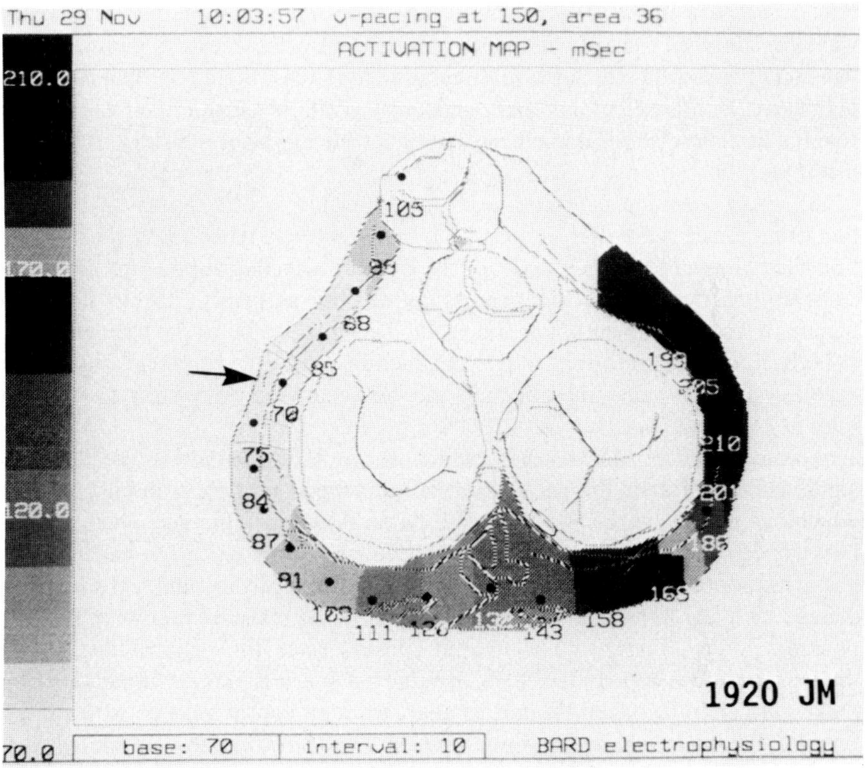


**Figure 6** Computer-generated intraoperative atrial activation sequence map in a patient with Wolff-Parkinson-White syndrome. Arrow identifies the earliest site of atrial activation during ventricular pacing, confirming the presence of a left lateral bypass tract. Light-colored areas demonstrate areas of early activation, with darker areas coming progressively later. Numbers located along the AV groove represent local V-A conduction times in milliseconds.

can arise in effectively ablating pathways in the posterior-septal region using solely an epicardial approach. This is secondary to the variable location of pathways in this region, which limit effective delivery of cryotherapy. High success rates coupled with major morbidity rates approaching the limits of general anesthesia alone make the surgical approach to Wolff-Parkinson-White syndrome extremely attractive. Successfully treated patients are "cured" of the arrhythmia in the broadest sense of the word and can be free of the need for chronic antiarrhythmic therapy and its attendant toxicities. Accurate pre- and intraoperative mapping is essential to the successful application of these techniques, because up to 10% of individuals may have multiple accessory pathways; in addition, a significant number of patients with accessory pathways may have other substrates for supraventricular arrhythmias, including dual AV nodal pathways. Definition of coronary anatomy to allow concomitant myocardial revascularization is useful in elderly patients with angina or a history of myocardial infarction.

AV node reentrant tachycardia is also amenable to direct surgical intervention using either sharp dissection, which can effectively interrupt the atrial insertion sites of input to the AV node, or through the selective application of cryolesions around the triangle of Koch, as defined by the central fibrous body, the tendon of Todaro, the coronary sinus, and the septal leaflet of the tricuspid valve (98–102). With monitoring of AV conduction during the application of serial cryolesions, AV nodal modification can be accomplished with a low risk of high-degree AV block.

Automatic atrial tachycardias, which account for a minority of clinically significant atrial arrhythmias, can often be mapped to a focal point of origin, which can then be surgically removed. Often these arrhythmias, which encompass a spectrum of different sites of enhanced automaticity (i.e., so-called paroxysmal atrial tachycardia, inappropriate sinus tachycardia, and chronic atrial ectopic tachycardia), have historically proven to be resistant to a wide range of pharmacological therapy. The overall success rates for surgical therapy for these arrhythmias approaches 90%, as reported in a small series of patients from Duke University Medical Center, as apart from an approximately 34% success rate for medical therapy in similar patients (103,104). Because uncontrolled automatic atrial tachycardia can be associated with the development of a dilated cardiomyopathy, early surgical intervention of these arrhythmias has been advocated. Long-term efficacy of surgical treatment, however, may be limited by the development of enhanced automaticity in other areas of the atrium, resulting in recrudescence of atrial tachycardia. There are limited data on the long-term efficacy of these procedures.

Cox recently developed a procedure for the surgical treatment of atrial fibrillation (105). This so-called "maze" procedure involves a series of anatomically defined incisions that attempt to "channel" the wave front of atrial depolarization in a path from the sinus to the AV node such that localized reentry cannot occur (Fig. 7). Conceptually, this provides organized atrial contraction synchronized to the sinus node, as well as an intact chronotropic response to activity. As electromechanical coupling exists in the atrium following this procedure, the risk of embolic phenomena should be reduced. This is in contradistinction to the so-called corridor operation proposed by Guiraudon et al., in which the majority of atrial tissue is electrically separated from a direct "corridor" connecting sinus and AV node (106). This latter procedure allows chronotropic competence by electrically "connecting" the sinus and AV node; the bulk of the atria remain fibrillating following this procedure such that the risk of

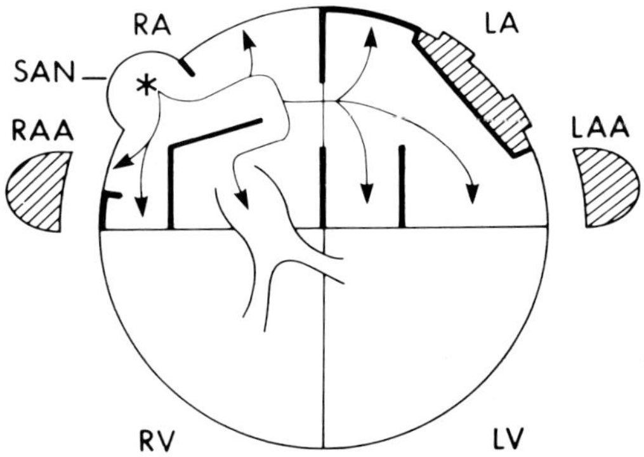


**Figure 7** Suggested rationale behind the surgical incisions used for the Maze procedure. Incisions (heavy lines) are placed to "channel" the wave front of depolarization from the sinus node to the AV node region. Incisions are placed such that the wave front cannot "double back" on itself to form a localized area of reentry and recrudescence of atrial fibrillation.

emboli persists and anticoagulation following the operation is required. Sinus node dysfunction has developed in a subset of patients following both operations, and it is unclear whether this is a result of intraoperative damage to the sinus node or sinus node artery or reflects the natural history of sick sinus syndrome in atrial fibrillation. Postoperatively, patients undergoing the maze procedure often develop significant volume overload secondary to a depletion of atrial natriuretic factor such that vigorous diuresis during the postoperative period is mandatory.

## Catheter Ablation Techniques

Catheter ablation was first reported in 1982 for the treatment of refractory supraventricular arrhythmias (107), although the first report of an ablative procedure was in 1979 by Vedel et al., when high-degree AV block was inadvertently produced during an electrophysiological study after cardioverting a sustained hemodynamically unstable tachycardia (108). The authors hypothesized that part of the defibrillating current passed through the intracavitary catheter, resulting in His bundle ablation. The first energy source used for ablative techniques was direct current, which utilized a conventional defibrillator to deliver energy to the patient. With this technique, the output from a defibrillator is channeled through the distal electrode of an intracavitary catheter (as cathode), using a backplate positioned on the posterior chest as the anodal sink. The energy delivered has a damped sinusoidal morphology, with resultant tissue injury from the procedure secondary to thermal and barotrauma, as well as direct electrical injury (109). Although in a given patient the direct contribution of each factor may be variable, it is believed by many that current flux created by the discharge is likely to be the major determinant of damage (110,111). Cellular studies in dogs undergoing DC shock ablation demonstrate local hemorrhage and contraction band necrosis. Chronically, volume loss, fibrosis, and fatty infiltration are common.

During ablation using a conventional electrophysiology catheter, currents up to 40 A occur, along with voltages in the range of 1000–2000 V. Defibrillator outputs of 300–400 J are used. This causes arcing, with the formation of a plasma arc. Significant localized barotrauma occurs, with transient increases in localized pressure to the $\leqslant$150 atm range (110).

DC shock ablation was first used in the management of atrial fibrillation to control ventricular response. Applying energy to the region of the AV node (with the catheter positioned to record an atrial electrogram that is larger than the ventricular electrogram and with a diminutive His bundle spike), applications of up to 360 J can create high-degree AV block in approximately two-thirds of patients. An additional 15–20% of patients following the procedure demonstrate effective slowing of ventricular response either in the absence of pharmacological therapy or during pharmacological therapy that was previously ineffective. Thus, DC shock ablation is effective in approximately 85% of patients in whom previous attempts at pharmacological therapy were ineffective in controlling the ventricular response to atrial fibrillation (107,109,111). The major "down side" of DC shock ablation for the management of atrial fibrillation is the need for permanent pacemaker implantation, insofar as the majority of patients treated become pacemaker dependent. With the advent of rate-responsive pacemakers, after DC shock ablation of the AV node a patient can be left with virtually physiological rate responsivity to exercise. Nevertheless, insofar as DC shock ablation of the AV node does not restore sinus rhythm, such patients should be anticoagulated indefinitely to reduce the embolic risk associated with atrial fibrillation.

DC shock ablation is performed under brief general anesthesia, optimally with chemically induced muscular paralysis using an agent like succinylcholine to prevent muscular contraction during the procedure. Complications reported with AV node ablation using DC energy are infrequent but include transient ventricular arrhythmias, including ventricular tachycardia and ventricular fibrillation immediately following the procedure, which can require DC cardioversion for termination. Tamponade secondary to atrial perforation has been reported, albeit rarely (112), such that whenever DC shock ablation is performed, a cardiac surgeon should be on standby in the event of cardiac perforation.

DC shock ablation can also be used to ablate appropriately located accessory pathways (109,111–116). Early attempts at ablating left lateral accessory pathways were associated with a significant risk of coronary sinus rupture and tamponade (112). This presumably occurs secondary to barotrauma in the relative confines of the coronary sinus. The risk of such trauma is significantly less with right-sided tracts: by positioning the endocavitary catheter in the right atrium at the level of the AV junction, transient increases in pressure during ablation can be dissipated in the distensible right atrium. However, spasm of the right coronary artery has been reported (115). DC shock ablation can be used to ablate accessory pathways in the posterior septal location. Using this technique, the ablating catheter is positioned at the os of the coronary sinus, with the current flux directed from the catheter tip to an indifferent anterior or posterior electrode (Fig. 8). Morady et al. reported success in approximately two-thirds of patients treated with DC shock ablation for posterior septal accessory pathways. The risk of cardiac tamponade in this setting is approximately 1% (113).

Over the last 3 years, however, enthusiasm for DC shock ablation has waned with the advent of radiofrequency energy. Using this technique, localized lesions are created as a result of resistive heating of tissue at the site of the catheter tip. Using this more controllable energy source, arcing and subsequent barotrauma do not occur. With average impedances of approximately 100 Ω, 50 V at 0.5 A are applied to the target area for between 30 and 60 s. The lesions created using this form of energy are more focal, and selective AV nodal modification has been described that can result in control of AV node reentrant tachycardia without causing complete AV block. Jackman and others have described the selective modification of the AV nodal "slow pathway" with success rates of 85–90% in controlling PSVT (117–120). Morady and others have described using a somewhat different catheter location to ablate the AV nodal "fast

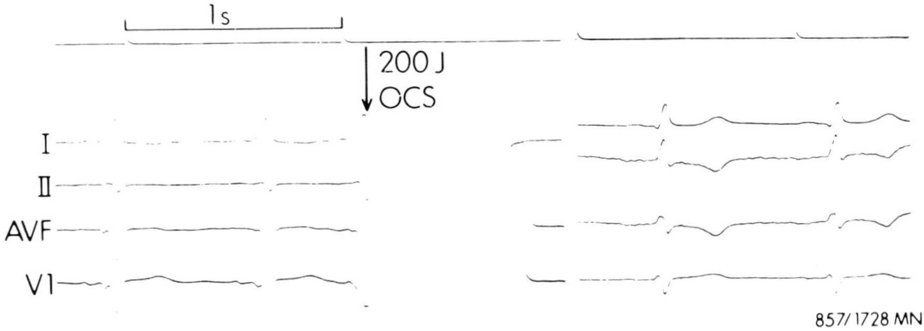


**Figure 8** Surface electrocardiograms immediately before (left) and after (right) DC shock ablation in a patient with Wolff-Parkinson-White syndrome. Delta waves with a pseudoinferior wall myocardial infarction pattern are seen in leads 2 and AVF preablation. Following the application of a 200 J shock via a catheter positioned at the os of the coronary sinus (OCS), delta waves are not seen and the initial vector of depolarization of the QRS in leads 2 and AVF is now positive.

pathway," with similar success rates (118). The risk of high-degree AV block with fast pathway ablation is of the order of 1–2% and may be higher than that associated with slow pathway ablation.

Radiofrequency energy can also be used to ablate accessory pathways and thereby "cure" AV reciprocating tachycardia. A major advantage in this regard is that by avoiding arcing and the resultant barotrauma, ablation can be attempted for virtually all accessory pathway locations with minimal risk of cardiac perforation (121–123). Ablation of left-sided accessory pathways involves placing a specially designed ablating catheter with a large 4 mm distal electrode tip into the femoral artery and advancing it retrogradely across the aortic valve to position the tip either over or under the mitral valve apparatus at the level of the AV junction. The earliest site of atrial activation during reciprocating tachycardia can then be assessed using the ablating catheter either alone or in concert with a catheter positioned in the coronary sinus. Jackman and others have described recording accessory pathway depolarizations (Fig. 9) using a special orthogonal electrode array on the catheter positioned on the coronary sinus. By targeting this accessory pathway depolarization (so-called "Kent potential"), success rates in excess of 90% in ablating accessory pathway conduction have been reported (Fig. 10) (121). As in AV nodal modification, radiofrequency energy is directed between the distal ablating catheter tip and in an indifferent electrode usually placed on the patient's back (a commercially available patch used during routine electrophysiological studies or one of similar design used by

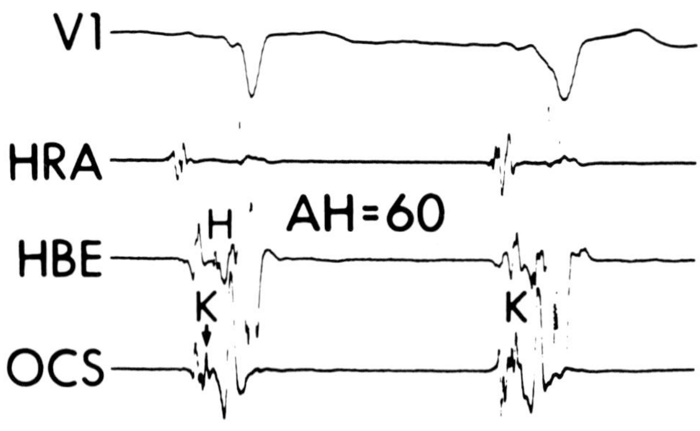


**Figure 9** Intracavitary electrograms from a patient with Wolff-Parkinson-White syndrome. Notice the high-frequency deflection from a recorded catheter positioned at the os of the coronary sinus representing a Kent potential (K). A His bundle electrogram (H) is recorded from a catheter positioned in the His bundle region. The AH interval during sinus rhythm is normal at 60 ms. HRA = high right atrium, HBE = His bundle electrogram, OCS = os of coronary sinus.

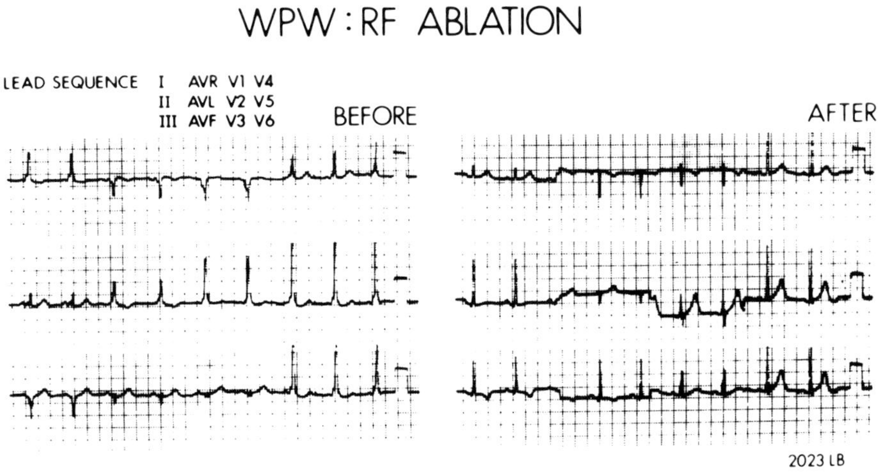


**Figure 10** Example of 12-lead electrograms, before and after radiofrequency ablation of an accessory pathway. Notice the absence of delta wave activity following the procedure.

surgical electrocautery devices). The impedance across the system is monitored during radiofrequency energy application, with ablation halted at the first sign of an impedance rise. Impendance rises are often associated with localized eschar formation along the catheter tip, resulting in diminution of current flow. The use of a large-tip electrode has been shown to minimize impedance rises; when they occur, however, the catheter must be removed and the tip cleaned of debris.

In view of the discrete nature of the lesions formed by radiofrequency energy application, mapping must be precise. It is not uncommon for repeat applications of RF energy to be used before successful pathway ablation or AV node modification. Although there have been reports of successful ablation in studies lasting less than 4 h (118), it is not uncommon for diagnostic electrophysiological studies involving ablation attempts to run in excess of 12 h. Total x-ray exposure time for both the patient and the operator can be significant, and the long-term sequelae of this have not been adequately characterized (123).

Catheter ablation techniques can also be applied to the management of automatic atrial tachycardia, as well as atrial flutter. The common form of atrial flutter appears to involve a macroreentrant circuit with a zone of slow conduction in the posterior right atrium near the os of the coronary sinus. Successful ablation of atrial flutter has been reported with both DC shock ablation and radiofrequency ablation; however, success rates may be less than those for PSVT secondary to AV node reentry or accessory pathway conduction (124,125).

Intracavitary DC shocks have been described as effective in cardioverting atrial fibrillation to sinus rhythm, and there have been reports suggesting that this may result in long-term maintenance of sinus rhythm in a minority of patients. The mechanism behind the successful conversion to sinus rhythm is unknown; however, it may be related to barotrauma and the transient "stretching" of the right atrium.

The management of supraventricular tachyarrhythmias has undergone a marked evolution in the last decade. Although options for pharmacological therapy have significantly broadened during this time, the most striking advancements have been in the nonpharmacological realm, with impressive developments in surgical and ablative modalities of therapy. In view of the potential toxicity and limited efficacy of pharmacological therapy, if the initial successes of nonpharmacological therapy are confirmed, these techniques may become the modalities of choice for the treatment of sustained arrhythmias in the elderly.

## ACKNOWLEDGMENT

We express our appreciation to Ms. Sandra Lenofsky for her excellent secretarial support in manuscript preparation.

## REFERENCES

1. Cranefield PF, Wit AL, Hoffman BF. Genesis of cardiac arrhythmias. *Circulation* 1973; 47:190–204.
2. Hoffman BF, Cranefield PF. The physiologic basis of cardiac arrhythmias. *Am J Med* 1964; 37:670–684.
3. Vaughan Williams EM. Subdivision of class I drugs. In: Reiser H, Horowitz L, eds. Mechanisms and treatment of cardiac arrhythmias: Relevance for basic studies to clinical management. Baltimore: Urban & Schwarzenbert, 1985:165–172.
4. Rosen MR, Wit AL. Arrhythmogenic actions of antiarrhythmic drugs. *Am J Cardiol* 1987; 59:10E–18E.
5. Fisch C. Relation to electrolyte disturbances to cardiac arrhythmias. *Circulation* 1973; 47:409–419.
6. Chen CM, Gettes LS. Combined effects of rate, membrane potential and drugs on maximum rate of rise ($V_{max}$) of action potential upstroke of guinea pig papillary muscle. *Circ Res* 1976; 38:464–469.
7. Rosen M, Merker C, Pippenger C. The effects of lidocaine on the canine ECG and electrophysiologic properties of Purkinje fibers. *Am Heart J* 1976; 91:191–202.
8. Selzer A, Wray HW. Quinidine syncope. Paroxysmal ventricular fibrillation occurring during treatment of chronic atrial arrhythmias. *Circulation* 1964; 30:17–26.
9. Olshansky B, Martins J, Hunt S. *N*-acetylprocainamide causing torsades de pointes. *Am J Cardiol* 1982; 50:1439–1445.

10. Cranefield PF. Action potentials, afterpotentials and arrhythmias. *Circ Res* 1977; 41:415–423.
11. Albert JS, Peterson P, Godtfredsen J. Atrial fibrillation: Natural history, complications and management. *Annu Rev Med* 1988; 39:41–52.
12. Moe GK, Abidson JA. Atrial fibrillation as a self-sustaining arrhythmia independent of focal discharge. *Am Heart J* 1959; 58:59–70.
13. Moe GK. On the multiple wavelet hypothesis of atrial fibrillation. *Arch Int Pharmacodyn Ther* 1962; 140:183–188.
14. Allessie MA, Lammers WJEP, Bonke FIM. Experimental evaluation of Moe's multiple wavelet hypothesis of atrial fibrillation. In: Zipes DP, Jalife J, eds. Cardiac Arrhythmias. New York: Grune & Stratton, 1985:265–276.
15. Allessie MA, Lammers WJEP, Bonke FIM. Intra-atrial reentry as a mechanism for atrial flutter by acetylcholine and rapid pacing in the dog. *Circulation* 1984; 70:123–135.
16. Boineau JP, Schussler RB, Mooney CR. Natural and evoked atrial flutter due to circus movement in dogs. *Am J Cardiol* 1980; 45:1167–1181.
17. Ange DT, Rubenfire M, Drake EH. Conversion of atrial flutter to atrial fibrillation with carotid sinus pressure. *J Electrocardiol* 1962; 377–380.
18. Josephson ME. Paroxysmal supraventricular tachycardia. An electrophysiologic approach. *Am J Cardiol* 1978; 41:1123–1126.
19. Wu D. Chronic electrophysiologic study in patients with recurrent paroxysmal tachycardia: A new method for developing successful oral antiarrhythmic therapy. In: Kulbertus HE, ed. Reentrant Arrhythmias. Baltimore: University Park Press, 1976.
20. Wu D, Denes P, Amay-Y-Leon F, Dhingra R, Wyndham C, Bauernfeind R, Latif P, Rosen K. Clinical electrocardiographic and electrophysiologic observations in patients with paroxysmal supraventricular tachycardia. *Am J Cardiol* 1978; 41:1045–1051.
21. Gallagher JJ, Sealy WC, Cox JL. Results of surgery for pre-excitation caused by accessory atrioventricular pathways in 267 consecutive cases. In: Josephson ME, Wellens HJJ, eds. Tachycardias: Mechanisms, diagnosis and treatment. Philadelphia: Lea & Febiger, 1984:259–269.
22. Cox JL, Gallagher JJ, Cain ME. Experience with 118 consecutive patients undergoing surgery for the Wolff-Parkinson-White syndrome. *J Thorac Cardiovasc Surg* 1985; 90:490.
23. Kramer JB, Corr PB, Cox JL, Witkowski F, Cain M. Simultaneous computer mapping to facilitate intraoperative localization of accessory pathways in patients with Wolff-Parkinson-White syndrome. *Am J Cardiol* 1985; 56:571–576.
24. Godaux JL, Ashman R. Auricular fibrillation with aberration simulating ventricular paroxysmal tachycardia. *Am Heart J* 1947; 34:366–367.
25. DiMarco JP, Sellers TD, Berne RM, West GA, Berlardinelli L. Adenosine: Electrophysiologic effects and therapeutic use for terminating paroxysmal supraventricular tachycardia. *Circulation* 1983; 68:1254–1263.
26. DiMarco JP, Miles W, Akhtar M, Milstein S, Sharma A, Platia E, McGovern B, Scheinman M, Grovier W. Adenosine for paroxysmal supraventricular tachycardia: Dose ranging and comparison with verapamil. *Ann Intern Med* 1990; 113:104–110.

27. Garratt CJ, Linker NJ, Griffith MJ, Ward DE, Camm AJ. Comparison of adenosine and verapamil for termination of paroxysmal junctional tachycardia. *Am J Cardiol* 1989; 64:1310–1316.
28. Camm AH, Garratt CJ. Drug therapy: Adenosine and supraventricular arrhythmias. *N Engl J Med* 1991; 325:1621–1629.
29. Sylven C, Jonzon B, Brandt R, Beermann B. Adenosine-provoked angina pectoris-like pain—time characteristics, influence of autonomic blockade and naloxone. *Eur Heart J* 1987; 8:738–743.
30. Sylven C, Jonzon B, Edlund A. Angina pectoris-like pain provoked by i.v. bolus of adenosine: Relationship to coronary sinus blood flow, heart rate and blood pressure in healthy volunteers. *Eur Heart J* 1989; 10:48–54.
31. Rinkenberger RL, Prystowsky EN, Heger JJ, Troup PJ, Jackman WM, Zipes DP. Effects of intraveous and chronic oral verapamil administration in patients with supraventricular tachyarrhythmias. *Circulation* 1980; 62:996–1010.
32. Rankin AC, Rae AP, Oldroyd KG, Cobbe SM. Verapamil or adenosine for the immediate treatment of supraventricular tachycardia. *Q J Med* 1990; 74:203–208.
33. Kowey PR, Friehling TD, Marinchak RA. Electrophysiology of beta blockers in supraventricular arrhythmias. *Am J Cardiol* 1987; 60:32–38.
34. Jewitt DE, Singh BN. The role of beta-adrenergic blockage during and after myocardial infarction. *Prog Cardiovasc Dis* 1974; 16:421–440.
35. Duff H, Roden DM, Brorson L, et al. Electrophysiologic actions of high plasma concentrations of propranolol in human subjects. *J Am Coll Cardiol* 1983; 2:1134–1140.
36. Falk RH, Jeffrey IL. Digoxin for atrial fibrillation. A drug whose time has gone. *Ann Intern Med* 1991; 114:573–575.
37. Wofford JL, Ettinger WH. Risk factors and manifestations of digoxin toxicity in the elderly. *Am J Emerg Med* 1991; 9:11–15.
38. Batker HE, Toft P, Klitgaard NA, Simonsen EE. Influence of physical exercise on serum digoxin concentration and heart rate in patients with atrial fibrillation. *Br Heart J* 1991; 65:337–341.
39. Boahene KA, Lein GJ, Yee R, Sharma AD, Fujimura O. Termination of acute atrial fibrillation in the Wolff-Parkinson-White syndrome by procainamide and propafenone: Importance of atrial fibrillatory cycle length. *J Am Coll Cardiol* 1990; 16:1408–1414.
40. Kus T, Derakhchan K, Bouchard C, Page P. Effects of procainamide on refractoriness, conduction and excitable gap in canine atrial reentrant tachycardia. *PACE* 1991; 14:1707–1713.
41. Furman S. Therapeutic uses of atrial pacing. *Am Heart J* 1973; 86:835–840.
42. Fisher JD, Kim SG, Furman S, Matos J. Role of implantable pacemakers in control of recurrent ventricular tachycardia. *Am J Cardiol* 1982; 49:194–206.
43. Waldo AL, MacLean WAH, Karp RB. Continuous rapid atrial pacing to control recurrent or sustained supraventricular tachycardias following open heart surgery. *Circulation* 1976; 54:245–250.
44. Singh BN, Hauswirth O. Comparative mechanisms of action of antiarrhythmic drugs. *Am Heart J* 1974; 87:367–378.
45. Campbell TJ. Subclassification of class I antiarrhythmic drugs. In: Vaughan Wil-

liams EM, Campbell TJ, eds. Anti-arrhythmic Drugs. Berlin: Springer-Verlag, 1988:135–155.

46. Colatsky TJ. Mechanism of action of lidocaine and quinidine on action potential duration in rabbit cardiac Purkinje fibers: an effect on steady-state sodium currents? *Circ Res* 1982; 50:17–27.
47. DiMarco JP, Miles W, Akhtar M, Milstein S, Slarma A, Platia E, McGovern B, Scheinman M, Grovier W. Adenosine for paroxysmal supraventricular tachycardia: Dose ranging and comparison with verapamil. *Ann Intern Med* 1990; 113:104–110.
48. Garratt CJ, Linker NJ, Griffith MJ, Ward DE, Camm AJ. Comparison of adenosine and verapamil for termination of paroxysmal junctional tachycardia. *Am J Cardiol* 1989; 64:1310–1316.
49. Talajic M, Nayebpour M, Jing W, Nattel S. Frequency-dependent effects of diltiazem on the atrioventricular node during experimental atrial fibrillation. *Circulation* 1989; 80:380–389.
50. Ellenbogen KA, Dias VC, Plumb VJ, Heywood JT, Mirvis DM. A placebo-controlled trial of continuous intravenous diltiazem infusion for 24-hour heart rate control during atrial fibrillation and atrial flutter: a multicenter study. *J Am Coll Cardiol* 1991; 18:891–897.
51. Lundstrton T, Rydden L. Ventricular rate control and exercise performance in chronic atrial fibrillation: effects of diltiazem and verapamil. *J Am Coll Cardiol* 1990; 16:86–90.
52. Kowey PR, Taylor JE, Rials SJ, Marinchak RA. Meta-analysis of the effectiveness of prophylactic drug therapy in preventing supraventricular arrhythmia early after coronary artery bypass grafting. *Am J Cardiol* 1992; 69:963–965.
53. Kirk CR, Gibbs JL, Thomas R, Radley-Smith R, Qureshi SA. Cardiovascular collapse after verapamil in supraventricular tachycardia. *Arch Dis Child* 1987; 62:1265–1266.
54. Fuller JA, Adams GG, Buxton B. Richmond. Atrial fibrillation after coronary artery bypass grafting: is it a disorder of the elderly? *J Thorac Cardiovasc Surg* 1989; 97:821–825.
55. Boisel JP, Wolf E, Gillet J. Controlled trial of long-acting quinidine for maintenance of sinus rhythm after conversion of sustained atrial fibrillation. *Eur Heart J* 1981; 2:49–55.
56. Ewy GA, Ulfers L, Hager WD, Rosenfeld A, Roesoe W, Goldman S. Response of atrial fibrillation to therapy: Role of etiology and left atrial diameter. *J Electrocardiol* 1980; 13:119–124.
57. Karlson BW, Torstensson I, Abjorn C, Jawsson S, Peterson L. Disopyramide in the maintenance of sinus rhythm after electroconversion of atrial fibrillation. *Eur Heart J* 1988; 9:284–290.
58. Coplen SE, Antman EM, Berlin JA, Hewitt P, Chalmers T. Efficacy and safety of quinidine therapy for maintenance of sinus rhythm after cardioversion: A meta-analysis of randomized control trials. *Circulation* 1990; 82:1106–1116.
59. Podrid PI, Schoeneberger A, Lown B. Congestive heart failure caused by oral disopyramide. *N Engl J Med* 1980; 302:614–617.
60. Teichman SL, Fisher JD, Matos JA, Kim SG. Disopyramide-pyridostigmine:

Report of a beneficial drug interaction. *J Cardiovasc Pharmacol* 1985; 7:108–113.
61. Morganroth J, Horowitz LN. Flecainide: Its proarrhythmic effect and expected changes on the surface electrocardiogram. *Am J Cardiol* 1984; 53:89B–94B.
62. Wiseman MN, Elstob JE, Camm AJ, Nathan AW. A study of the use of flecainide acetate in the long-term management of cardiac arrhythmias. *PACE* 1990; 13:767–775.
63. Pritchett EL, Wilkinson WE. Mortality in patients treated with flecainide and encainide for supraventricular arrhythmias. *Am J Cardiol* 1991; 67:976–980.
64. Pritchett EL, DaTorre SD, Platt ML, McCarville SE, Hougham AJ. Flecainide acetate treatment of paroxysmal supraventricular tachycardia and paroxysmal atrial fibrillation: dose-response studies: The flecainide supraventricular tachycardia study group. *J Am Coll Cardiol* 1991; 17:297–303.
65. Echt DS, Liebson PR, Brent M, Peters RW, Obias-Manno D, Barket AH, Arensberg D, Baker A, Friedman L, Greene L, Huther ML, Richardson DW, and the CAST Investigators. Mortality and morbidity in patients receiving encainide, flecainide or placebo: The cardiac arrhythmia suppression trial. *N Engl J Med* 1991; 324:781–788.
66. Henthorn RW, Waldo AL, Anderson JL. Flecainide acetate prevents recurrence of symptomatic paroxysmal supraventricular tachycardia. *Circulation* 1991; 83:119–125.
67. Mitchell LB, Syse DG, Gillis AM, Duff JH. Electropharmacology of amiodarone therapy initiation. Time courses of onset of electrophysiologic and antiarrhythmic effects. *Circulation* 1989; 80:34–42.
68. Gold RL, Haffajee K, Charos G, Baker S, Alpert J. Amiodarone for refractory atrial fibrillation. *Am J Cardiol* 1986; 57:124–127.
69. Mason JW. Amiodarone. *N Engl J Med* 1987; 316:455–466.
70. Singh BN, Zipes DP, eds. Proceedings of the symposium: Amiodarone. Basic concepts and clinical applications. *Am Heart J* 1983; 106:787–964.
71. Juul-Moller S, Edvardsson N, Rehnqvist-Ahiberg N. Sotalol versus quinidine for the maintenance of sinus rhythm after direct current conversion of atrial fibrillation. *Circulation* 1990; 82:1932–1939.
72. Camm AJ, Paul V. Sotalol for paroxysmal supraventricular tachycardias. *Am J Cardiol* 1990; 65:67A–73A.
73. Suttorp MJ, Kingma JH, Tjon JG, van Hemel NM, Koomen EM, Defauw JA, Adan AJ, Ernst SM. Efficacy and safety of low- and high-dose sotalol versus propranolol in the prevention of supraventricular tachyarrhythmias early after coronary artery bypass operations. *J Thorac Cardiovasc Surg* 1990; 100:921–926.
74. Antonaccio MJ, Gomoll A. Pharmacology, pharmacodynamics and pharmacokinetics in sotalol. *Am J Cardiol* 1990; 65:12A–21A.
75. Soyka LF, Wirtz C, Spangenberg RB. Clinical safety profile of sotalol in patients with arrhythmias. *Am J Cardiol* 1990; 65:74A–81A.
76. Chesebro JH, Fuster V, Halperin JL. Atrial fibrillation—risk marker for stroke. *N Engl J Med* 1990; 323:1556–1558.

77. Aronow WS, Gutstein H, Hsieh FY. Risk factors for thromboembolic stroke in elderly patients with chronic atrial fibrillation. *Am J Cardiol* 1989; 63:366–367.
78. Petersen P. Thromboembolic complications of atrial fibrillation and their prevention: A review. *Am J Cardiol* 1990; 75:24C–28C.
79. The Boston area anticoagulant trial for atrial fibrillation investigators. The effect of low-dose warfarin on the risk of stroke in patients with nonrheumatic atrial fibrillation. *N Engl J Med* 1990; 323:1505–1511.
80. Connolly SJ. Canadian atrial fibrillation anticoagulation (CAFA) study, abstracted. *Circulation* 1990; 82(Suppl.III):111–108.
81. Petersen P, Boysen G, Godtfredsen J, Andersen E, Andersen B. Placebo-controlled, randomised trial of warfarin and aspirin for prevention of thromboembolic complications in chronic atrial fibrillation: The Copenhagen AFASAK study. *Lancet* 1989; 1:175–179.
82. SPAF Study Group Investigators. Preliminary report of the stroke prevention in atrial fibrillation study. *N Engl J Med* 1990; 322:863–868.
83. Preston TA, Haynes RE, Gavin WA, Hessel EA. Permanent rapid atrial pacing to control supraventricular tachycardia. *PACE* 1979; 2:331–334.
84. Begemann MJS, Bennekers JH, Kingma JH. Prevention of tachycardia initiation by programmed stimulation. *J Electrophysiol* 1987; 4:350–356.
85. Davies DW, Butrous GS, Spurrel RAJ, Camm AJ. Pacing techniques in the prophylaxis of junctional reentry tachycardia. *PACE* 1987; 10:519–532.
86. Arbel ER, Cohen HC, Langendorf R, Glick G. Successful treatment of drug-resistant atrial tachycardia and intractable congestive heart failure with permanent coupled atrial pacing. *Am J Cardiol* 1978; 41:336–340.
87. Waldo AL, Krongrad E, Kupersmith J, Levine OR, Bowman FO, Hoffman B. Ventricular paired pacing to control rapid ventricular heart rate following open heart surgery. *Circulation* 1986; 53:176–181.
88. Fisher JD, Kim SG, Mercando AD. Electrical devices for the treatment of arrhythmias. *Am J Cardiol* 1988; 61:45A–57A.
89. Holt P, Crick JCP, Sowton E. Antitachycardia pacing: A comparison of burst overdrive, self-searching and adaptive table scanning programs. *PACE* 1986; 9:490–497.
90. Spurrell RAJ, Sowton E. An implanted atrial synchronous pacemaker with a short atrioventricular delay for the prevention of paroxysmal supraventricular tachycardias. *J Electrocardiol* 1976; 9:89–96.
91. Schluter M, Kunze KP, Kuck KH. Train stimulation at the atria for prevention of atrioventricular tachycardia: Dependence on accessory pathway location. *J Am Coll Cardiol* 1987; 9:1288–1293.
92. Fisher JD, Johnston DR, Furman S, Mercando A, Kim SG. Long-term efficacy of antitachycardia devices. *Am J Cardiol* 1987; 60:1311–1316.
93. Cobb FR, Blumenschein SD, Sealy WB. Successful surgical interruption of the bundle of Kent in a patient with Wolff-Parkinson-White syndrome. *Circulation* 1968; 38:1018–1025.
94. Guiraudon GM, Klein GJ, Sharma AD, Yee R, McLellan DG. Surgical treatment of supraventricular tachycardia: A five-year experience. *PACE* 1986; 9:1376–1380.

95. Lowe JE. Surgical treatment of the Wolff-Parkinson-White syndrome and other supraventricular tachyarrhythmias. *J Cardiac Surg* 1986; 1:117.
96. Mahomed Y, King RD, Zipes D, Niles W, Prystowsky E, Heger J, Brown W. Surgical division of Wolff-Parkinson-White pathways utilizing the closed-heart technique: A 2 year experience in 47 patients. *Ann Thorac Surg* 1988; 45:495–504.
97. Cox JL, Boineau JP, Schussler RB, Ferguson TB, Cain ME, Lindsay BD, Corr PB, Kater KM, Lappas DG. Successful surgical treatment of atrial fibrillation: Review and clinical update. *JAMA* 1991; 266:1976–1980.
98. Pritchett ELC, Anderson RW, Benditt DG, Kasell J, Harrison L, Wallace A, Sealy W, Gallagher J. Reentry within the atrioventricular node: Surgical cure with preservation of atrioventricular conduction. *Circulation* 1979; 60:440–446.
99. Holman WL, Ikeshita M, Lease JG, et al. Cryosurgical modification of retrograde atrioventricular conduction: Implications for the surgical treatment of atrioventricular node reentry tachycardia. *J Thorac Cardiovasc Surg* 1986; 91:826.
100. Fujimara O, Guiraudon GM, Yee R, Sharma A, Klein G. Operative therapy of atrioventricular node reentry and results of an anatomically guided procedure. *Am J Cardiol* 1989; 64:1327–1334.
101. Cox JL, Holman WL, Cain ME. Cryosurgical treatment of atrioventricular node reentrant tachycardia. *Circulation* 1987; 76:1329–1336.
102. Cox JL, Ferguson TB Jr. Surgery for atrioventricular node reentry tachycardia: The discrete cryosurgical technique. *Semin Thorac Cardiovasc Surg* 1989; 1:47.
103. Hendry PJ, Packer DL, Anstadt MP, Plunkett MD, Lowe JE. Surgical treatment of automatic atrial tachycardias. *Ann Thorac Surg* 1990; 49:253–260.
104. Yee R, Guiraudon GM, Gardner MJ, Gulamhusein SS, Klein GJ. Refractory paroxysmal sinus tachycardia: Management by subtotal right atrial exclusion. *J Am Coll Cardiol* 1984; 3:400–404.
105. Cox JL. The surgical treatment of atrial fibrillation. IV. Surgical technique. *J Thorac Cardiovasc Surg* 1991; 101:584–592.
106. Guiraudon GM, Capbell CS, Jones DL. Combined sinoatrial node atrioventricular isolation: A surgical alternative to His bundle ablation in patients with atrial fibrillation. *Circulation* 1985; 72:111–220.
107. Gallagher JJ, Svenson RH, Kasell JH, German LD, Bardy GH, Broughton A, Critelli G. Catheter technique for closed-chest ablation of the atrioventricular conduction system: A therapeutic alternative for the treatment of refractory supraventricular tachycardia. *N Engl J Med* 1982; 194–200.
108. Vedel J, Frank R, Fontaine G, Fournial JF, Grosgogeat Y. Bloc auriculo-ventricular intra-hisien definitif induit au cours d'une exploration endoventriculaire droite. *Arch Mal Coeur* 1979; 72:107–112.
109. Scheinman MM, Laks MM, DiMarco J, Plumb V. Current role of catheter ablative procedures in patients with cardiac arrhythmias: A report for health professionals from the subcommittee on electrocardiography & electrophysiology. *Circulation* 1991; 83:2146–2156.
110. Bardy GH, Coltorti F, Ivey TD, Alverness C, Rackson M, Hansen K, Steward R, Greene HL. Some factors affecting bubble formation with catheter-mediated defibrillator pulses. *Circulation* 1986; 73:525–538.

111. Fisher JD, Brodman R, Waspe LE, Kim SG. Nonsurgical electrical ablation (fulguration) of tachycardias. *Circulation* 1987; 75(III):194–199.
112. Fisher JD, Brodman R, Kim SG, Matos JA, Brodman E, Wallerson D, Waspe LE, Johnston DR, Scavin GM. Attempted nonsurgical electrical ablation of accessory pathway via the coronary sinus in the Wolff-Parkinson-White syndrome. *J Am Coll Cardiol* 1984; 4:685–694.
113. Morady F, Scheinman MM, Winston SA, DiCarlo LA, Davis JC, Griffin JC, Ruder M, Abbott JA, Eldar M. Efficacy and safety of transcatheter ablation of posteroseptal accessory pathways. *Circulation* 1985; 72:170–177.
114. Bardy GH, Ivey TD, Coltorti F, Steward RB, Johnson G, Greene HL. Developments, complications and limitations of catheter-mediated electrical ablation of posterior accessory atrioventricular pathways. *Am J Cardiol* 1988; 61:309–316.
115. Hartzler GO, Giorgi LV, Diehl AM, Hamaker WR. Right coronary spasm complicating electrode catheter ablation of a right lateral accessory pathway. *J Am Coll Cardiol* 1985; 6:250–253.
116. Evans GT Jr, Schienman MM, Zipes DP, Benditt D, Breithardt G, Levy S, Prystowsky E, Josephson M, Morady F, Ruskin J. The percutaneous cardiac mapping and ablation registry: Final summary of results. *PACE* 1988; 11:1621–1626.
117. Jackman WM, Wang X, Friday KJ, Fizgerald DM, Roman C, Moulton K, Margolis PD, Bowman AJ, Kuck KH, Naccarelli GV, Pitha JV, Dyer J, Lazzara R. Catheter ablation of atrioventricular junction using radiofrequency current in 17 patients: Comparison of standard and large-tip catheter electrodes. *Circulation* 1991; 83:1562–1576.
118. Calkins H, Sousa J, El-Atassi R, Rosenheck S, de Buitleir M, Kou WH, Kadish AH, Langberg JJ, Morady F. Diagnosis and cure of the Wolff-Parkinson-White syndrome or paroxysmal supraventricular tachycardias during a single electrophysiologic test. *N Engl J Med* 1992; 324:1612–1618.
119. Lee MA, Morady F, Kadish A, Schamp DJ, Chin MC, Scheinman MM, Griffin JC, Lesh MD, Pederson D, Goldberger J, Calkins H, deBuitleir M, Kou MH, Rosenheck S, Sousa J, Langberg JJ. Catheter modification of the atrioventricular junction with radiofrequency energy for control of atrioventricular nodal reentry tachycardia. *Circulation* 1991; 83:827–835.
120. Yeung-La-Wah JA, Alison JF, Lonergan L, Leather R, Kerr CR. High success rate of atrioventricular node ablation with radiofrequency energy. *J Am Coll Cardiol* 1992; 18:1753–1758.
121. Jackman WM, Wang X, Friday KJ, Roman CA, Moulton KP, Beckman KJ, McClelland JH, Twidale N, Hazlitt A, Prior MI, Margolis PD, Calame JD, Overholt ED, Lazzara R. Catheter ablation of accessory atrioventricular pathways (Wolff-Parkinson-White syndrome) by radiofrequency current. *N Engl J Med* 1992; 324:23.
122. Schluter M, Geiger M, Siebels J, Duckeck W, Kuck KH. Catheter ablation using radiofrequency current to cure symptomatic patients with tachyarrhythmias related to an accessory atrioventricular pathway. *Circulation* 1991; 84:1644–1661.
123. Calkins H, Niklason L, Sousa J, El-Atassi R, Langberg J, Morady F. Radiation exposure during radiofrequency catheter ablation of accessory atrioventricular connections. *Circulation* 1991; 84:2376–2382.

124. Chauvin M, Brechenmacher C. Endocardial catheter fulguration for treatment of atrial flutter. *Am J Cardiol* 1988; 61:471–472.
125. Chauvin M, Brechenmacher C. A clinical study of the application of endocardial fulguration in the treatment of recurrent atrial flutter. *PACE* 1989; 12:219–223.

# 22

# Ventricular Arrhythmias and Cardiopulmonary Resuscitation in the Elderly

**Donald D. Tresch**
*Medical College of Wisconsin and University of Wisconsin, Milwaukee, Wisconsin*

**Ranjan K. Thakur**
*University of Western Ontario, London, Ontario, Canada*

## SIGNIFICANCE OF VENTRICULAR ARRHYTHMIAS

The management of ventricular arrhythmias, regardless of the age of the patient, is one of the most complex and frustrating cardiac problems facing the physician in the 1990s. The problem can be even more challenging when encountering the elderly patient with such arrhythmias. Ventricular arrhythmias are known to increase with age. Various studies (1–6) have reported a prevalence of 70–80% in healthy patients over the age of 60 years. The frequency of ventricular premature contractions (VPC) is often high, and complex forms are common in this age group, even though the patient is usually asymptomatic. The frequency and complexity of VPC are even higher in the elderly patient with underlying heart disease.

Aronow and associates (5) reported the prevalence of ventricular arrhythmias on 24 h Holter monitoring to be 81% in 453 nonselected nursing home patients over the age of 62 years (mean age 82). Of patients with left ventricular ejection fraction (LVEF) < 50%, 67% demonstrated complex arrhythmias, compared to 52% of patients with LVEF > 50%. Ventricular tachycardia (VT) was found in 14% of patients with LVEF < 50% and in 8% of patients with a LVEF > 50%.

In a study of 24 h Holter monitoring of healthy subjects from the Baltimore Longitudinal Study of Aging, Fleg and Kennedy (6) reported ventricular arrhythmias occurred in 80% of 98 subjects aged 60–85 years, with 17% of the group demonstrating at least 100 VPC in 24 h. Half the group demonstrated complex ventricular arrhythmias. Ventricular tachycardia was seen more frequently in subjects age 70 and older. No significant differences were found in the prevalence of ventricular arrhythmias between men and women or between hypertensive and normotensive subjects.

Because of the increased prevalence of ventricular arrhythmias in the elderly population, with most elderly persons asymptomatic and unaware of underlying cardiac disease, it has been questioned whether these arrhythmias have any prognostic significance. It has been well documented that ventricular arrhythmias in patients without significant underlying cardiac disease are not predictive of increased mortality (7–12). Kennedy and associates (7) reported 73 asymptomatic, apparently healthy persons who demonstrated ventricular arrhythmias on 24 h Holter monitoring. The patients' ages ranged from 18 to 72 years, with a mean age of 46 ± 13 years. A frequency of VPC per hour ranged from a mean of 78 to 1994 beats per hour; complex ventricular ectopy was found in 63% of the subjects, and VT was present in 26%. At 6 years mean follow-up, only 5 subjects experienced cardiovascular events: 2 subjects had myocardial infarctions (MI); 1 had heart failure; 1 had cardiac arrest; and 1 had syncope. The authors concluded that the long-term prognosis of asymptomatic healthy persons with frequent and complex ventricular ectopy is similar to that of the healthy U.S. population and suggests no increased risk of death.

Other studies (8–12) support the Kennedy group's findings in both young and elderly persons with ventricular arrhythmias; even when more complex ventricular arrhythmias are documented, the prognosis appears to be favorable in the absence of underlying heart disease. In a study of nursing home patients (12), Aronow and associates reported no significant correlation of complex ventricular arrhythmias, including VT, and new cardiac events in elderly patients who had no evidence of heart disease. Fleg and Lakatta (13), in a study of exercise stress testing in elderly persons, also found that elderly persons without heart disease had an excellent prognosis, even if they demonstrated exercise-induced VT.

The favorable outcome of asymptomatic elderly persons with ventricular arrhythmias who do not demonstrate significant underlying cardiac disease may not apply to elderly patients with structural heart disease. Studies (14–22) have demonstrated ventricular arrhythmias to be predictive of total mortality and sudden death in patients with cardiac disease. In one of the first studies assessing the predictive value of ventricular ectopy, Ruberman and associates (14) found that the presence of complex ventricular ectopy (runs, early beats, or bigeminal or multiform beats) on 1 h monitoring in post-MI men under the age of 75 years was associated with a risk of sudden cardiac death three times that in patients without complex ventricular ectopy. In this study the prevalence of ventricular ectopy increased with age, with the increased prevalence due to the increase in complex beats. The frequency of complex beats in 1 h increased from 18% in men under 55 to 35% in men 65–74 years of age. The probability of total death also increased sharply with increasing age, as did sudden cardiac death; however, the presence of complex ventricular ectopy was determined to be an independent risk for all forms of death, including sudden cardiac death.

More recently, Bigger and associates (22) reported a multicenter study in which the predictive value of ventricular ectopy as determined by 24 h electrocardiographic recording was assessed in 766 post-MI patients. As in the Ruberman group's study, a strong association was found between the frequency and the repetitiveness of VPC and total death. Paired VPC were associated with a greater than threefold increase in the odds of dying compared with no VPC; runs of VT were associated with a five- to sixfold increase in dying. The patients in this study were all under 70 years of age.

Even though numerous studies have demonstrated a positive correlation between mortality, including sudden death, and frequency and complexity of ventricular ectopy, the sensitivity and predictive value of these findings are poor. Shen and Hammill (23), in reviewing the literature, calculate the sensitivity of VPC, defined as 10 or more per hour, as a predictor of sudden cardiac death in post-MI patients to range from 25 to 54%, and the positive predictive value ranged from 9 to 15%. The presence of nonsustained VT appeared to be a better predictor; in most studies the total mortality following an MI ranged from 7 to 15% for patients without nonsustained VT, compared to 14–38% for patients with nonsustained VT, at a follow-up varying from 12 to 36 months (23). The risk of sudden death was two to three times higher in patients with than in patients without nonsustained VT (23).

Specific studies concerning the prognostic value of ventricular arrhythmias in elderly patients are sparse, although it appears that the predictive value is similar to that reported in studies of younger patients. As previously noted, Aronow and associates (5) found ventricular arrhythmias to be very prevalent in elderly nursing home patients, and in a prospective study (12), ventricular arrhythmias were predictive of mortality. At 2 years mean follow-up, only 8% of 176 nursing home patients without complex ventricular ectopy and a normal LVEF had new cardiac events. The percentage of patients having new cardiac events increased to 81% in patients with paroxysmal VT and an abnormal LVEF.

In a study of 101 elderly subjects over 75 years of age (range 75–95) living independently in the community, Martin and associates (24) found the presence of VPC to be highly predictive of mortality. Of the 27 subjects who demonstrated VPC at the rate of greater than 10 per hour at the initial examination, 17 (63%) had died at 5 years follow-up. In comparison, 27 (36%) of the 74 subjects without VPC or with fewer than 10 per hour died. The subjects were considered "healthy," although many of the subjects had symptoms that could have been referrable to cardiovascular disease. Thus, it is possible that the high correlation of VPC and mortality in these elderly subjects reflected the presence of underlying heart disease.

In addition to ventricular arrhythmias, left ventricular dysfunction has been shown to be a predictor of total mortality and sudden cardiac death. The relationship of ventricular ectopy and left ventricular dysfunction as a predictor of total mortality and sudden cardiac death has been controversial. Some investigators have concluded that ventricular arrhythmias are so strongly associated with left ventricular dysfunction that this association accounts for the relationship between ventricular arrhythmias and sudden death (2,25,26). Recent studies (14–16,18,22) have now documented that both ventricular arrhythmias and left ventricular dysfunction are independent predictors of mortality, including sudden cardiac death, in patients with coronary artery disease. Results from the Multicenter Post-Infarction Research Group (22) demonstrated a 2 year mortality rate in patients with both LVEF less than 30% and more than 3 VPC per hour to be 38%, whereas the 2 year mortality rate of the remaining patients was 10%. The odds of dying within 2 years were almost six times as great for patients with a LVEF under 30% and more than 3 VPC per hour, compared with all other patients. In the Multicenter Investigation of the Limitation of Infarct Size Study (16), the incidence of sudden death was 18% in patients with both left ventricular dysfunction (ejection fraction $< 0.40$) and frequent VPC (10 or more per hour), approximately 11 times that of patients with neither of these findings.

As in the studies of patients with coronary artery disease, ventricular arrhythmias and left ventricular systolic dysfunction in patients with nonischemic heart disease have also been demonstrated to be predictors of total mortality and sudden death (27–29). Most studies have shown that the more severe the left ventricular dysfunction and the more malignant the ventricular arrhythmias, the worse is the prognosis. Holmes and associates (27), in assessing the predictive value of ventricular arrhythmias in patients with ischemic or nonischemic cardiomyopathy, found mortality to be directly related to the severity of ventricular arrhythmias. All patients had severe congestive heart failure. At 25 months follow-up a 59% mortality was noted in patients with complex ventricular arrhythmias, compared to a mortality of only 11% in patients with simple ventricular arrhythmias. The age range of the patients was 34–78 years (mean 56 years).

In a study of generally young patients with hypertrophic cardiomyopathy, Maron et al. (29) reported an approximately 25% occurrence of sudden death or cardiac arrest (an increased mortality rate of 8.6%) in 17 patients with hypertrophic cardiomyopathy who demonstrated VT on 24 h Holter monitoring, compared to a 3% rate of sudden death or cardiac arrest (annual rate of 1.0%) in 66 patients without VT. The patients' ages ranged from 9 to 65 years, mean 38. Similar results have been reported by other investigators (30) who studied older patients with hypertrophic cardiomyopathy.

Besides left ventricular ejection fraction, left ventricular hypertrophy (LVH) must be considered when assessing elderly patients with ventricular arrhythmias. Left ventricular hypertrophy, which is so common in elderly patients, has been found to be associated with ventricular arrhythmias and is a predictor of mortality (31–33). Messerli and associates (31) reported that patients aged 56–72 years, mean 68 years, with LVH had a 24 h VPC rate 40–50 times higher than that of patients without LVH, and this higher prevalence was closely related to the degree of LVH. The number of complex VPC was also related to the presence of LVH. In reference to mortality, the Framingham Heart Study (32) reported the risk of sudden death in patients with LVH to be five to six times higher than that in patients without LVH. Aronow and associates (33), in an attempt to correlate LVH and ventricular arrhythmias to sudden death, found that the incidence of sudden death and ventricular fibrillation at 24 months mean follow-up increased from 4% in elderly nursing home patients without LVH or complex ventricular ectopy to 29% in patients with LVH and complex ventricular ectopy. The incidence of sudden death and ventricular fibrillation increased to 57% in those nursing home patients with VT and LVH.

## ROLE OF ELECTROPHYSIOLOGICAL STUDIES AND SIGNAL-AVERAGED ELECTROCARDIOGRAPHY

Recently, electrophysiological studies (EPS) and signal-averaged electrocardiography have been used to stratify patients with ventricular arrhythmias into high- and low-risk groups for sudden cardiac death. Most studies (34–39) of EPS have demonstrated the inducibility of VT to range from 11 to 44% in post-MI patients. In some studies mortality has also been found to be significantly higher among patients with inducible VT compared to patients in whom VT could not be induced (37,39). Other studies have not substantiated these findings (36,38). Although the sensitivity and specificity in these studies have been acceptable, the positive predictive values varied substantially (23,40). On the basis of the data, it appears that the role of EPS in post-MI patients remains unclear, and no conclusions can be made about the value of EPS as a predictor for sudden cardiac death in elderly patients who have had a MI (23,40).

Signal-averaged electrocardiography is a new, noninvasive method, using a computer, of detecting high-frequency, low-amplitude potentials at the end of the QRS complex (41). It is thought that these abnormal ventricular late potentials originate from damaged myocardial tissue and may be a marker for spontaneous and inducible VT, plus sudden death, in patients who have had an acute

MI. The prevalence of these late potentials after MI in most studies (42–49) varied from 26 to 52% and appeared to be dependent on many factors, including recording techniques (45), time relationship to MI (47), and location of MI (45). Nevertheless, some studies have demonstrated the risk of sudden cardiac death or sustained VT in patients post-MI with late potentials to be 4–10 times greater than that in patients without late potentials (42,44–49). The frequency of inducible VT was also significantly increased in patients with late potentials compared to patients without late potentials (42). Unfortunately, the findings of studies of signal-averaged electrocardiography suggest that the use of signal-averaged electrocardiography for identification of patients at risk for sudden cardiac death is associated with a high proportion of false positive results (23). Thus, as with EPS, the routine use of signal-averaged electrocardiography at the present time cannot be recommended in elderly patients with ventricular arrhythmias.

Some investigators consider the combination of ventricular arrhythmias on Holter monitoring, assessment of left ventricular dysfunction, and late potentials on signal-averaged electrocardiography to provide the best predictor of sudden cardiac death or sustained VT (either spontaneous or inducible) in post-MI patients (44,46,47). Gomes and associates (44) found that the presence of any two of the three abnormal assessments (presence of late potentials, LVEF $<$ 40%, and 10 VPC per hour, couplets, and triplets), or all three, was associated with an arrhythmia event rate of 36–50% during a 12.6 month follow-up period. The combination of two abnormalities that were the best predictors of arrhythmia events was the presence of late potentials and abnormal LVEF. When these two tests were normal, no arrhythmic events were noted. Other studies (46,47,49) have reported similar findings. El-Sherif and associates (47) found a 37% event rate in patients who demonstrate late potentials and an abnormal LVEF, whereas the incidence of an arrhythmic event was only 1% when these two tests were normal. When late potentials were present in association with both an abnormal LVEF and high grades of ventricular ectopy on 24 h Holter monitoring recording, the arrhythmic event rate was 50% for a 1 year period.

## TREATMENT OF VENTRICULAR ARRHYTHMIAS

The objective of antiarrhythmic therapy in elderly patients should be, as in younger patients, to relieve arrhythmic symptoms and to prevent death while minimizing drug-related side effects. When confronting the symptomatic elderly patient, it is important to confirm that the patient's symptoms are related to the arrhythmia. Not uncommonly, elderly patients have concomitant diseases that may be the etiology of the patient's symptoms, with the ventricular arrhythmias a coincidental finding. Also, symptoms related to the ventricular arrhythmia should be severe and incapacitating, or the arrhythmias life threatening, before specific antiarrhythmic therapy is initiated.

## Antiarrhythmic Drug Therapy

Empirical antiarrhythmic drug therapy has been shown by many studies (50–57) to be ineffective in reducing sudden cardiac death and total mortality of patients with ventriclar arrhythmias, and in some studies, the drug therapy has been not only ineffective, but detrimental (Table 1). Specific drug trials in elderly patients are sparse. In a prospective study of 406 elderly nursing home patients, mean age 82 years (range 62–100), with ventricular arrhythmias, Aronow and associates (56) demonstrated that the use of quinidine and procainamide was ineffective in preventing sudden cardiac death, total cardiac death, or total death. At 24 months mean follow-up, 21% of 222 patients started on antiarrhythmic drugs and 23% of 186 patients on no antiarrhythmic drugs sustained sudden cardiac death. Of patients taking either quinidine or procainamide 65% died, compared to 63% of patients on no antiarrhythmic drugs. In addition to the lack of efficacy of the drug therapy, patients on the antiarrhythmic drugs developed a significant number of side effects.

In addition to the dismal results of these earlier studies, the results of the recent Cardiac Arrhythmic Suppression Trial (CAST) (57) have raised further questions about the benefit of the suppression of spontaneous ventricular arrhythmias following MI using antiarrhythmic drugs. A greater than threefold increase in arrhythmic deaths and nonfatal cardiac arrests was found in post-MI patients treated with the class IC antiarrhythmic drugs flecainide and encainide compared to patients who received placebo. Approximately 35% of the patients in the study were older than 65 years of age.

On the basis of the results of the many studies that have failed to document any objective efficacy of drug therapy in improving mortality in patients with ventricular arrhythmias, plus the results of the recent CAST, it is difficult to justify the empirical use of antiarrhythmic drugs in most elderly patients with ventricular arrhythmias. The $\beta$-adrenergic blocking agents, however, are one group of drugs that needs to be considered when evaluating the elderly patient with ventricular arrhythmias. Studies (58–62) assessing the use of $\beta$-blockers (with exception of $\beta$-blockers with significant intrinsic agonist activity, such as pindolal and oxprenolol) in post-MI patients have found the drugs to be beneficial in reducing total mortality, sudden death, and recurrent MI. Data pooled from the major studies reveal a reduction of 28% in total mortality and a 33% reduction in sudden death, and these studies have demonstrated $\beta$-blockers to be as beneficial in elderly patients as in younger patients. Gunderson et al. (62) reported a reduction of 25% in mortality and a 39% reduction in reinfarction rate in post-MI patients aged 65–75 years. There was no significant difference in the reduction in mortality or reinfarction between patients 65–75 years of age compared to patients under 65 years of age.

Even though the specific mechanism by which $\beta$-blockers reduce sudden cardiac death is not known, the benefit of $\beta$-blocker therapy in post-MI elderly

**Table 1** Efficacy of Antiarrhythmic Therapy in Survivors of Myocardial Infarction

| Drug | Total number of patients | Age range, years (mean) | Follow-up (months) | Mortality (%) | | *P* value |
|---|---|---|---|---|---|---|
| | | | | Placebo | Drug | |
| Procainamide (50) | 70 | (59) | 6 | 17 | 17 | NS |
| Phenytoin (52) | 568 | <40–70[a] | 12 | 9 | 8 | NS |
| Tocainide (53) | 112 | (—)[b] | 6 | 9 | 9 | NS |
| Mexilitine (51) | 630 | 30–74 (60) | 9 | 5 | 8 | NS |
| Aprindine (54) | 143 | 31–87 (61) | 12 | 22 | 17 | NS |
| Encainide (57) Flecainide (57) | 1455 | (61)[c] | 10 | 3 | 8 | 0.0003 |

[a] 46% of patients between 56 and 70 years of age.
[b] Data not reported.
[c] Approximately 35% of patients older than 65 years of age.

patients is so overwhelming that it behooves the physician to consider myocardial ischemia as a possible etiology of the arrhythmia when confronting elderly patients with ventricular arrhythmias. In many elderly patients myocardial ischemia may be "silent" and stress testing (exercise or pharmacological) is necessary to elicit and document the ischemia (see Chapter 11). In post-MI elderly patients who demonstrate ventricular arrhythmias but fail to demonstrate symptomatic or silent ischemia, β-blockers are still indicated and should be the first line of therapy, unless contraindicated.

Despite the overwhelming benefits of β-blockers in post-MI patients, it has been shown that β-blockers are used disproportionately in elderly patients. Forman and associates (63), in a study assessing the use of β-blockers in post-MI elderly patients, found that a β-blocker was prescribed in 31% of post-MI patients 70 years or older compared to 49% of patients younger than 70 years; in only 14% of patients 80 years or older was a β-blocker prescribed. As expected, contraindications to using a β-blocker were more common in the elderly patients; 61% of patients 80 years or older had contraindications compared to only 30% of patients 50–59 years of age. After adjusting for patients with contraindications, however, it was still found that age of the patient was a significant factor in prescribing a β-blocker drug; a β-blocker was prescribed in 64% of patients under the age of 70 years, whereas a β-blocker was prescribed for only 36% of patients 70 or older. The authors concluded that the age-associated decrease in the use of β-blockers is disproportionate to the prevalence of comorbidity.

Other etiologies that play a role in causing ventricular arrhythmias and that should be considered in elderly patients are heart failure and electrolyte abnormalities. Heart failure should always be considered as playing a role in causing arrhythmias and, when present, treated vigorously.

When considering the use of a specific antiarrhythmic drug in elderly patients with ventricular arrhythmias, whether empirical or guided by EPS, the risk-benefit ratio must be considered. As previously discussed, symptoms related to ventricular arrhythmias should be severe and incapacitating or the arrhythmias life threatening before antiarrhythmic drugs are administered. Besides the cardiac side effects, including proarrhythmia, conduction defects, and negative inotropy, the noncardiac side effects of the antiarrhythmic drugs must also be considered. Table 2 lists the comparable efficacy of antiarrhythmic drugs in controlling life-threatening ventricular arrhythmias and the side effects of the drugs.

In reference to the use of antiarrhythmic drugs specifically in the elderly, it is well known that there are normal aging changes that affect how drugs are absorbed (66), metabolized (67), and excreted (68). Also, elderly patients are more likely to have multiple diseases and are more likely to be taking multiple medications that increase the risk of drug side effects. Even though elderly patients are more prone to develop side effects than younger patients, studies have demonstrated that patient age alone is not a risk factor for developing side

**Table 2** Comparison of Efficacy and Side Effects of Antiarrhythmic Drugs in Treating Ventricular Arrhythmias

| Drug by class | Efficacy LTVA | Risk of organ toxicity | Risk of proarrhythmia | Risk of CHF |
|---|---|---|---|---|
| I: Moricizine | $2^+$ | Low/none | Low | $1^+$ |
| IA | | | | |
| Quinidine | $2^+$ | Moderate | High | 0 |
| Procainimide | $2^+$ | High | — | $1^+$ |
| Disopyramide | $1^+$ | Low | — | $4^+$ |
| IB | | | | |
| Tocainide | $1^+$ | High | — | 0 |
| Mexiletine | $1^+$ | Low | Possible | 1 |
| IC | | | | |
| Encainide | $2^+$ | Low | Highest | $1^+$ |
| Flecainide | $2^+$ | Low | Highest | $4^+$ |
| Propafenone | $2^+$ | Low | — | $3^+$ |
| II: $\beta$-blocker | 0 | Low | None | $2^+$ |
| III: Amiodarone | $3^+$ | Highest | — | $1^+$ |
| IA + IB | $2^+$ | Moderate | High | 1 |

CHF = congestive heart failure; LTVA = life-threatening ventricular arrhythmias.
*Source*: Adapted from Morganroth and Horowitz (64) and Morganroth (65).

effects from antiarrhythmic drugs, and age alone does not predict the immediate efficacy or the long-term outcome of therapy (69). Therefore, elderly patients with ventricular arrhythmias must be assessed and treated individually.

## Aggressive Approach to Management in Elderly Patients

The use of invasive interventions for both evaluation and treatment has been shown to be beneficial in the management of patients with life-threatening ventricular arrhythmias. Programmed ventricular stimulation has been assessed as beneficial in guiding antiarrhythmic drug therapy in patients who have had spontaneous and induced VT (70,71) and in patients who have been resuscitated from cardiac arrest (72–74). Cardiac surgery, including coronary artery bypass surgery (CABG), ventricular resection, and ablation, is considered beneficial in patients with life-threatening ventricular arrhythmias (75,76). More recently, repeated studies (77–80) have demonstrated the use of the automatic internal cardioverter-defibrillator (AICD) to be the most effective therapy in preventing sudden death in patients with symptomatic life-threatening ventricular arrhythmias.

Even though an aggressive approach appears beneficial in patients with life-threatening arrhythmias, most physicians are hesitant to subject elderly patients to such interventions. Compared to younger patients, elderly patients are known to have increased complications associated with interventional diagnostic testing (81) and are more likely to have higher operative morbidity and mortality (81,82). Tresch and associates (83,84), however, have shown that an aggressive approach in managing patients with life-threatening ventricular arrhythmias is as beneficial in elderly patients as in younger patients (Table 3). A group of 49 elderly patients, age range 68–84 years, and 44 younger patients, age range 44–53 years, who were referred to the Johns Hopkins Arrhythmia Service for treatment of recurrent life-threatening ventricular tachyarrhythmias were studied (83). More than 80% of the elderly patients had at least one MI before the onset of the life-threatening arrhythmia, in comparison to 57% of the younger patients, and twice as many elderly patients had a history of heart failure. Patients underwent coronary angiographic studies and EPS testing before initiation of definitive treatment. Anatomically, elderly patients demonstrated more severe coronary artery disease, with 80% of the elderly patients having three-vessel disease compared to 30% of the younger patients. Therapy consisted of programmed ventricular stimulation-directed antiarrhythmic drug therapy, cardiac surgery (CABG and/or left ventricular resection), and implantation of AICD. Despite the difference in cardiac history and anatomical disease, there was no significant difference in complications from the aggressive evaluation or treatment between the two age groups, and long-term survival was comparable. Surgical mortality, however, was higher in the elderly patients.

More recently, Tresch and associates (84) studied a group of 54 elderly patients, age range 66–80 years (mean 70), in whom AICD were implanted for life-threatening ventricular arrhythmias. The outcome of the elderly patients was compared to that of a group of 79 younger patients, age range 18–65 years (mean 53), treated in a similar manner. All patients in each age group underwent extensive evaluation, including coronary angiography and repeated EPS testing. The majority of patients in each age group had coronary artery disease, and left ventricular function was significantly impaired; mean left ventricular ejection was 35% in the younger patients and 31% in the elderly patients. An AICD device was implanted in all patients, and 37% of elderly patients and 29% younger patients had concomitant heart surgery. Concomitant heart surgery consisted of CABG, left ventricular resection, and left ventricular cryoablation. No significant difference was noted in complications from the evaluation or therapy (medical or surgical) between the age groups, and at a mean follow-up of 25 months only 1 younger patient and 3 elderly patients died suddenly. It was concluded that AICD is very effective in the treatment of life-threatening ventricular arrhythmias, and this benefit applies to elderly patients as well as younger patients.

**Table 3** Interventional Therapy for Life-Threatening Ventricular Arrhythmias in Elderly Patients

| Study | Number of patients | F/U (months)[a] | Age (years)[a] | LVEF (%) | Procedures | | | Mortality | | |
|---|---|---|---|---|---|---|---|---|---|---|
| | | | | | CABG | LV resection | AICD | Early | Late | Total SD |
| Tresch et al. (83) | | | | | | | | | | |
| Younger | 44 | 25 | 50 | 37 | 10 | 10 | 16 | 2 | 12 | 11[b] |
| Elderly | 49 | 25 | 70 | 32 | 16 | 7 | 22 | 8 | 11 | 8[b] |
| Tresch et al. (84) | | | | | | | | | | |
| Younger | 79 | 26 | 53 | 36 | 20 | 12 | 79 | 2 | 14 | 1[b] |
| Elderly | 54 | 26 | 70 | 31 | 20 | 2 | 54 | 2 | 9 | 3[b] |
| Scott et al. (85) | | | | | | | | | | |
| Younger | 30 | 12–36 | $<60$ | —[c] | —[c] | —[c] | 30 | —[c,d] | —[c,d] | 2[e] |
| Elderly | 20 | 12–36 | $\geq 70$ | 35 | —[c] | —[c] | 20 | —[c,d] | —[c,d] | 1[e] |

[a]Mean values
[b]Includes early and late deaths
[c]No information given
[d]No difference between age groups
[e]Late sudden death
AICD = automatic internal converter defibrillator; CABG = coronary artery bypass grafting; SD = sudden death.

Similar results were found by Scott and associates (85) in a study comparing the use of AICD in elderly patients 70 years or older and patients under 60 years with life-threatening ventricular arrhythmias (Table 3). No difference was found between the age groups in operative mortality or complications. Four elderly patients required concomitant cardiac pacemakers. At 1–3 years of follow-up there was no significant difference between the age groups in patient hospital readmissions, and only one elderly patient died suddenly, compared to two younger patients.

## SUDDEN CARDIAC DEATH AND CARDIOPULMONARY RESUSCITATION

The prevalence of sudden cardiac death increases with age (86,87). In many elderly persons sudden cardiac death may be the terminal event following years of cardiac symptoms; however, in other elderly persons sudden cardiac death may be the first manifestation of cardiac disease in a supposedly healthy person.

In the last few years, the issues of whether cardiopulmonary resuscitation (CPR) is beneficial in the elderly and whether CPR should be performed in this age group have attracted considerable attention from both the medical profession and the general public. Results of studies have been variable and conflicting. However, the studies have demonstrated that many factors influence the success of CPR in elderly persons, and patient age may not be the major determinant.

Determinants besides patient's age that appear to influence the success of CPR in elderly persons are (1) patient setting (in-hospital, out-of-hospital, or long-term care facility) at the time of cardiac arrest, (2) type of arrhythmia at the time of the arrest, (3) prearrest characteristics of the patient, including functional and mental status, medical illnesses, and medications, and (4) patient symptoms at the time of the arrest.

### In-Hospital Cardiac Arrest

The percentage of hospitalized patients sustaining cardiac arrest and surviving to discharge following CPR varies from approximately 7 to 20%, depending on the study (Table 4) (88–92). Patient age has not been found to be a determinant of survival in many studies, although some recent studies have reported very low survival rates in older persons sustaining cardiac arrest and receiving CPR.

In an early study, Fusgen and Summa (88) prospectively studied 335 patients hospitalized in three hospitals in Nuremberg, Germany in 1974 who sustained cardiac arrest and received CPR. Of 96 patients younger than 60 years 11% survived, compared to 5% of 239 patients over age 60. Of men under 60 years 17% survived compared to 5% of men over 60 years. In contrast, none of the women under 60 years survived compared to 6% of the women over 60 years. The

**Table 4** Success Rate for CPR in Hospitalized Patients

| Study (location, year) | % Patients surviving to discharge | | |
|---|---|---|---|
| | All | Younger | Older |
| Fusgen and Summa (Nuremberg, 1974) (88) | | | |
| All rhythms | 7 | 11 | 5 |
| VF | — | — | — |
| Gulati et al. (Lancashire, 1982) (89) | | | |
| All rhythms | 17 | 18 | 17 |
| VF | 23 | — | — |
| Bedell et al. (Boston, 1981–1982) (90) | | | |
| All rhythms | 14[a] | — | — |
| VF | 27[a] | — | — |
| Taffet et al. (Houston, 1984–1985) (91) | | | |
| All rhythms | — | 16 | 0 |
| VF | — | — | 0 |
| Murphy et al. (Boston, 1977–1987) (92) | | | |
| All rhythms | — | — | 6.5 |
| VF | — | — | 21 |

VF = ventricular fibrillation.
[a] Patient's age not a significant determinant of survival.
*Source*: Reprinted from Tresch et al. (105), with permission.

authors did not classify specific cardiac rhythms at the time of the arrest, although they stated that none of the patients over 70 years who demonstrated asystole survived. The chance of surviving for all patients regardless of age was greatest when the arrest was associated with an acute MI and worse in patients with multiple diseases. The authors concluded that multiple pathology rather than age seemed to be the decisive factor influencing success of resuscitation.

Gulati and associates (89), in another European prospective study, assessed the success of CPR in a geriatric hospital in Lancashire, England during a 10 month period in 1982. Of 52 elderly patients, mean age 76 years, range 64–91, who sustained cardiac arrest, 27% were initially resuscitated and 17% survived to be discharged. Patient age was not a determinant of survival in this study, although cardiac rhythm was strongly predictive of survival. Of patients who demonstrated ventricular fibrillation (VF), 23% survived, compared to only 5% of patients with asystole. Evaluation of the survivors following hospital discharge did not reveal any significant neurological or functional change from the prearrest state.

In one of the larger prospective studies of CPR in hospitalized patients, Bedell and associates (90) analyzed the success of CPR in 294 consecutive patients in Beth Israel Hospital, Boston during an 18 month period from 1981 through 1982. Of the 294 patients, 41 patients (14%) survived to be discharged and 33 (11%) were alive at 6 months of follow-up. In this study, patient age ranged from 18 to 101 years, with a mean age of 70 years. Patient age was not a significant predictor of outcome. As in Gulati's study, patients demonstrating VF at the time of the arrest had the best chance of surviving compared to patients with other rhythms: 27% of patients with VF survived, compared to only 8% of the patients with other rhythms. Other predictors of survival included severity of the patient's prearrest illnesses, level of the patient's prearrest activity, and the duration of CPR, plus whether intubation was necessary during CPR.

In contrast to these earlier studies (88–90), two recent retrospective studies reported patient age to be a major determinant of survival (91,92). In a retrospective study of CPR in a Veterans Administration Medical Center in Houston, Texas between 1984 and 1985, Taffet et al. (91) found that patients 70 years or older could be initially resuscitated as successfully as patients under 70 years. However, 16% of 261 patients under 70 years survived to be discharged, whereas none of 68 patients 70 years or older survived. The reason for the poor survival in the elderly was unclear; however, using multivariate analysis, the presence of sepsis, cancer, increased age, increased number of medications administered, and absence of a witness were all predictive of poor outcome. Specific cardiac rhythms at the time of the arrest were not reported.

In another retrospective study, Murphy and associates (92) analyzed CPR in 503 patients over the age of 69 years sustaining cardiac arrest between 1977 and 1987 in the city of Boston. Patients were subdivided by location of the arrest—in-hospital and out-of-hospital. Of the five health institutions included in the study, three were long-term care facilities. In 92 (36%) of the 259 hospitalized patients CPR was initially successful, although only 17 (6.5%) of the patients survived to be discharged. Approximately 50% of survivors at the time of the hospital discharge were found to be more functionally impaired, compared to their prearrest functional status, and less than 50% of the survivors were discharged to their homes. The patients not discharged to their homes were transferred to a rehabilitation hospital or long-term care facility. Prearrest patient clinical characteristics that significantly favored survival were a hematocrit greater than 35% and fewer than three acute illnesses. There was a trend, although the difference was not significant, that patients with moderate to severe functional impairment or any mental impairment had worse outcomes than those without such impairments. Characteristics at the time of the arrest that influenced survival were the specific cardiac rhythm, whether the arrest was witnessed or unwitnessed, and the duration of CPR. Of patients who demonstrated VT or VF 21% survived, compared to only 2.6% of the patients with other rhythms. In this study it was found that only 53 (26%) of these elderly hospitalized patients demonstrated VT or VF; the remainder of the patients had electromechanical dissociation (EMD), asystole, or junctional rhythms at the time of the arrest. Only 1 patient whose arrest was not witnessed survived, and only 3% of the patients survived if CPR lasted more than 5 min. Murphy and associates concluded that CPR is rarely effective in hospitalized elderly patients whose cardiac arrest is not witnessed and whose arrest is not related to ventricular arrhythmias.

## Out-of-Hospital Cardiac Arrest

In the Murphy and associates' study (92) of CPR in elderly patients in the city of Boston, the success of CPR in patients who sustained out-of-hospital cardiac arrest was even more dismal than that found in hospitalized patients. Less than 1% of 244 elderly patients who received CPR following out-of-hospital cardiac arrest survived. As reported in their study of hospitalized elderly patients, VF was not a common rhythm in the out-of-hospital elderly patients sustaining cardiac arrest; only 28% of the patients demonstrated VF.

In contrast to the Boston study, the results of other studies (93–100) of elderly patients who sustained out-of-hospital cardiac arrest and received CPR have been more encouraging (Table 5). Tresch and associates (93), in a study of 1345 consecutive patients residing in the Milwaukee area who sustained cardiac arrest and received CPR by paramedics, found that patients over 70 years could be initially resuscitated and hospitalized as successfully as patients under 70 years. However, 16% of 932 patients less than 70 years of age survived compared to 9% of 613 patients over 70 years. As in the other studies, initial documented cardiac arrhythmia at the time of the arrest was a significant determinant of survival. Of the younger patients, 23%, and 16% of the elderly patients in the Milwaukee study survived if the initial documented rhythm was VF, whereas less than 4% of both age groups survived if the rhythm was asystole or EMD. Even in the patients 80 years or older, 14% survived if the rhythm was VF; as in the Boston study, however, VF was not a common rhythm in the elderly patients.

Tresch and associates (94) analyzed a subset of 381 persons whose out-of-hospital cardiac arrest was witnessed by Milwaukee paramedics (the arrest occurred after arrival of the paramedics). Compared to their other study, survival was significantly improved in this subset of patients whose arrest was witnessed by paramedics: 47% of the younger patients and 24% of the elderly patients survived if the rhythm was VF. Besides rhythm, patient symptoms before the arrest were found to be a significant determinant of survival. Approximately 60% of the younger and elderly patients survived if they complained of chest pain before the arrest and demonstrated VF at the time of the arrest. Patients who complained of dyspnea were less likely to survive, as were patients who did not demonstrate VF at the time of the arrest. When comparing the age

**Table 5** Success Rate for CPR in Out-of-Hospital Patients

| Study (location, year) | % Patients surviving to discharge | | |
|---|---|---|---|
| | All | Younger | Older |
| Tresch et al. (Milwaukee, 1983–1985) (93) | | | |
| All rhythms | 13 | 16 | 9 |
| VF | 20 | 23 | 16 |
| Tresch et al. (Milwaukee, 1980–1985) (94)[a] | | | |
| All rhythms | 17 | 24 | 10 |
| VF | 44 | 47 | 24 |
| Murphy et al. (Boston, 1977–1987) (92) | | | |
| All rhythms | — | — | 0.8 |
| VF | — | — | 2 |
| Bonnin et al. (Houston, 1987) (96) | | | |
| All rhythms | — | — | 6 |
| VF | 14 | 14 | 15 |
| Denes et al. (St. Paul, 1987–1988) (97) | | | |
| All rhythms | — | — | — |
| VF | 17 | 16 | 18 |
| Eisenberg et al. (King County, WA, 1975–1989) (98,99) | | | |
| All rhythms | 19 | 22 | 9 |
| VF | 29 | 32 | 20 |
| Longstreth et al. (Seattle, 1970–1980) (100) | | | |
| All rhythms | 12 | 14 | 10 |
| VF | 24 | 27 | 21 |
| Applebaum et al. (Baltimore, 1987) (102) | | | |
| All rhythms | — | — | 11 |
| VF | — | — | — |

VF = ventricular fibrillation.
[a] Patients' arrests witnessed by paramedics.
*Source*: Reprinted from Tresch et al. (105), with permission.

groups, it was found that elderly patients more commonly complained of dyspnea, whereas younger patients more commonly complained of chest pain before the arrest, and as in the other studies, VF was more common in the younger patients and bradyasystole was more common in elderly patients. Regardless of the patient's age, patients with chest pain before the arrest were more likely to have VF at the time of the arrest, whereas patients with dyspnea were more likely to demonstrate bradyasystole at the time of the arrest.

The explanation for the difference in the prevalence of the specific cardiac rhythm at the time of the arrest and the difference in symptoms before the arrest between the age groups is unclear. Tresch and associates (94,95) have reported that compared to younger patients, elderly patients who sustain out-of-hospital cardiac arrest more commonly have a history of heart failure and more commonly are taking digitalis and diuretics. The authors have hypothesized that the cardiac arrest in elderly patients may commonly be related to abnormal left ventricular function with underlying heart failure, which would explain the dyspnea in the elderly patients before the arrest and might also explain the bradyasystole noted at the time of the arrest. In comparison to the elderly patients, the cardiac arrest in younger patients may more commonly be related to acute myocardial ischemia or infarction manifested as acute chest pain with the development of VF and cardiac arrest.

In reference to residual functional and neurological impairment in patients who survive cardiac arrest, Tresch and associates (95) did not find any significant difference in impairment between elderly and younger survivors. Furthermore, there was no significant difference in long-term survival between elderly and younger patients; approximately 65% of both age groups were alive at 2 years following hospital discharge. Of the total survivors at the time of hospital discharge 14% required placement in a long-term care facility. All but one of the patients discharged home were functioning at the prearrest state at the time of follow-up evaluation.

Other recent studies have corroborated Tresch's findings, and in certain studies, the results have even been more encouraging. Bonnin et al. (96), in a prospective study of the Houston paramedic experience, found a survival of 6% in 177 consecutive patients over 70 years of age who received CPR following out-of-hospital cardiac arrest during a 6 month period, the survival increasing to 15% in 59 patients who demonstrated VF or VT. The prevalence of VF or VT in the elderly patients at the time of the arrest was 33%, similar to that reported by Tresch and associates (93). Denes et al. (97) reported similar results in a study of paramedics in St. Paul, Minnesota. Of 82 patients over 70 years 18% survived out-of-hospital cardiac arrest if the cardiac rhythm was VF or VT, compared to a 16% survival of 116 patients under 70 years of age who demonstrated VF or VT. Eisenberg and associates (98,99), reporting on the largest patient series in the United States, found that 111 (20%) of 569 patients 75 years or older who sustained out-of-hospital cardiac arrest in King County, Washington from 1975 through 1989 survived if the cardiac rhythm was VF. A more recent study by Longstreth and associates (100) reported a 24% survival rate in 493 patients 70 years or older who received CPR following out-of-hospital cardiac arrest in Seattle if the cardiac rhythm at the time of the arrest was VF. There was no significant difference in survival between patients older and younger than 70 years, and age was not a significant determinant of survival until the ninth decade. No significant difference was found between the age groups in the survivors' prearrest to postarrest functional status; approximately

3% of patients in each group were discharged to nursing homes. As found in other studies, both young and old patients who demonstrated asystole and EMD at the time of the arrest had very little chance of surviving. In the Seattle study a significant difference in the prevalence of VF between the age groups was not found.

## Nursing Home Cardiac Arrest

Data concerning the success of CPR following cardiac arrest in nursing homes is sparse (Table 6). Approximately 16% of the out-of-hospital arrests in the Murphy study (92) occurred in nursing homes, and none of the patients survived. Kaiser et al. (101), in a retrospective analysis of cardiac arrests in a Rochester long-term care institution between 1977 and 1985, found that 9 (28%) of 32 patients who received CPR following cardiac arrest survived for 24 h; 5 patients (16%) survived longer than 30 days, and at 6 months 3 (9%) were still alive. More recently, Applebaum and associates (102) analyzed the success of CPR in 696 persons 65 years or older who sustained cardiac arrest in Baltimore city or county during 1987. Of the persons 117 were residing in nursing homes; the other 580 were nonnursing home residents living in the community. Only 2 of the nursing home patients (2%) survived, compared to 61 of the nonnursing home residents (11%). Awoke et al. (103) reported similar dismal results in a

**Table 6** Success Rates for CPR in Nursing Home Patients

| | Patients surviving to discharge | |
|---|---|---|
| Study (location, year) | Number | Number surviving (%) of total) |
| Kaiser et al. (Rochester, 1977–1985) (101): | | |
| total rhythms | 32 | 5 (16)[a] |
| Murphy et al. (Boston, 1977–1987) (92): | | |
| total rhythms | 41 | 0 |
| Applebaum et al. (Baltimore, 1987) (102): | | |
| total rhythms | 177 | 2 (2) |
| Awoke et al. (Washington, D.C., 1987–1990) (103): | | |
| total rhythms | 45 | 0 |
| Neahring et al. (Milwaukee, 1986–1989) (104): | | |
| Total rhythms | 196 | 10 (5) |
| VF | 39 | 6 (15) |
| VF + witnessed arrest | 22 | 6 (27) |

VF = ventricular fibrillation; VT = ventricular tachycardia.
[a] Alive at 30 days.
*Source*: Reprinted from Tresch et al. (105), with permission.

study of CPR in a long-term care facility in Washington, D.C. during 1987–1990. None of the 45 patients who sustained cardiac arrest and received CPR survived. Neither the Applebaum nor the Awoke study analyzed all the patients' prearrest characteristics or cardiac rhythms at the time of the arrest. Both investigators concluded that because of the poor outcome, CPR should be eliminated in nursing homes.

In a study of CPR in Milwaukee nursing homes (196 consecutive patients), Neahring and associates (104) found two significant determinants of survival. As in their previous studies of out-of-hospital cardiac arrest, the initial documented cardiac rhythm at the time of the arrest influenced survival, and the other determinant of survival was whether the arrest was witnessed or not witnessed. Of the nursing home patients who demonstrated VF 15% survived, compared to only 2.5% of patients with other rhythms, and 8% of patients whose arrest was witnessed survived, compared to 2% of patients whose arrest was not witnessed. Further investigation of these two determinants of survival demonstrated that the determinants were interactive. When both determinants were present (arrest witnessed and VF documented) the survival rate was 27%, whereas for other combinations the survival rate was only 2.3%. The presence of only one favorable predictor was not associated with a higher survival rate than the absence of both predictors. Patient age, mental or function status, hematocrit, creatinine, presence of pulmonary disease, cancer, or cardiovascular disorders were not significant predictors associated with survival. Analyzing the functional status of survivors, there was no significant difference in prearrest and postarrest status, although many of the survivors had severe functional and neurological impairments before the arrest. Of the survivors 50% had been diagnosed as demented before the arrest. Follow-up of the survivors demonstrated that 40% of survivors survived for longer than 12 months.

On the basis of the results of their study, which demonstrated that only nursing home patients whose arrest is witnessed and who demonstrate VF benefit from CPR, Neahring and associates (104) concluded that guidelines could now be suggested concerning the use of CPR in nursing homes. In nursing home patients who desire CPR, CPR should only be initiated in those patients whose arrest is witnessed and should only be continued in patients who demonstrate VF.

Finally, from the available studies of CPR it appears that, in general, elderly persons do not fare as well as younger persons who receive CPR following cardiac arrest. There is a subset group of elderly patients in whom CPR can be gratifying, however. The main determinant of survival appears to be the initial documented cardiac rhythm at the time of the arrest. Numerous studies have reported a survival rate of approximately 15–20% in patients over the age of 70 who demonstrate VF or VT at the time of cardiac arrest, whether the patients are hospitalized or reside in the community. Most studies have failed to demonstrate a significant difference in neurological or functional impairment between elderly survivors and younger survivors, and the majority of elderly survivors are capable of returning to normal living. At the present time more data concerning CPR in nursing homes are needed before a definitive conclusion can be reached. Most studies have demonstrated very poor survival rates; however, some studies have reported survival in a subset of nursing home patients to be no different from that of elderly persons residing in the community who sustain cardiac arrest and receive CPR. Even so, since many nursing home patients are severely impaired, both mentally and functionally, the issue of CPR in this setting is more complex than a simple survival analysis would indicate.

## REFERENCES

1. Camm AJ, Evans KE, Ward DE, Martin A. The rhythm of the heart in active elderly subjects. *Am Heart J* 1980; 99:598–603.
2. Kantelip JP, Sage E, Duchene-Marullaz P. Findings on ambulatory electrocardiographic monitoring in subjects older than 80 years. *Am J Cardiol* 1986; 57:398–401.
3. Glasser SP, Clark PI, Applebaum JH. Occurrence of frequent complex arrhythmias defected by mandatory monitoring. Findings in an apparently healthy asymptomatic elderly population. *Chest* 1979; 75:565–568.
4. Clarke JM, Shelton JR, Hamer J, Taylor S, Venning GR. The rhythm of the normal human heart. *Lancet* 1976; 2:508–512.
5. Aronow WS, Epstein S, Schwartz KS, Koenigsberg M. Prevalence of arrhythmias detected by ambulatory electrocardiographic monitoring and of abnormal left ventricular ejection fraction in persons older than 62 years in a long-term health care facility. *Am J Cardiol* 1987; 59:368–369.
6. Fleg JL, Kennedy HL. Cardiac arrhythmia in a healthy elderly population. Detection by 24-hour ambulatory electrocardiography. *Chest* 1982; 81:302–307.
7. Kennedy HL, Whitlock JA, Sprague MK, Kennedy LJ, Buckingham TA, Goldberg RJ. Long-term follow-up of asymptomatic healthy subjects with frequent and complex ventricular ectopy. *N Engl J Med* 1985; 312:193–197.
8. Kirkland JL, Lye M, Faragher EB, dos Santos AGR. A longitudinal study of the prognostic significance of ventricular ectopic beats in the elderly. *Gerontology* 1983; 29:199–201.
9. Montague TJ, McPherson DD, MacKenzie BR, Spencer CA, Nanton MA, Horacek BM. Frequent ventricular ectopic activity without underlying cardiac disease: analysis of 45 subjects. *Am J Cardiol* 1983; 52:980–984.
10. Bjerregaard P. Premature beats in healthy subjects 40–79 years of age. *Eur Heart J* 1982; 3:493–503.
11. Gordon JB, Evans LC, Beckwith GH, McCall MM, Simpson RJ, Foster JR. Followup of complex ventricular arrhythmias in healthy young adults and children (abstract). *Clin Res* 1979; 2:170A.
12. Aronow WS, Epstein S, Koenigsberg M, Schwartz K. Usefulness of echocardiographic abnormal left ventricular ejection fraction, paroxysmal ventricular tachy-

cardia and complex ventricular arrhythmias in predicting new coronary events in patients over 62 years of age. *Am J Cardiol* 1988; 61:1349–1351.

13. Fleg JL, Lakatta EG. Prevalence and prognosis of exercise-induced nonsustained ventricular tachycardia in apparently healthy volunteers. *Am J Cardiol* 1984; 54:762–764.
14. Ruberman W, Weinblatt E, Goldberg JD, Frank CW, Shapiro S. Ventricular premature beats and mortality after myocardial infarction. *N Engl J Med* 1977; 297:750–757.
15. Moss AJ, Davis HT, DeCamilla J, Bayer LW. Ventricular ectopic beats and their relation to sudden and nonsudden cardiac death after myocardial infarction. *Circulation* 1979; 60:998–1003.
16. Mukharji J, Rude RE, Poole WK, et al., MILIS Study Group. Risk factors for sudden death after acute myocardial infarction: two-year follow-up. *Am J Cardiol* 1984; 54:31–36.
17. Schulze RA Jr, Strauss HW, Pitt B. Sudden death in the year following myocardial infarction. Relation to ventricular premature contractions in the late hospital phase and left ventricular ejection fraction. *Am J Med* 1977; 62:192–199.
18. Kostis JB, Byington R, Friedman LM, Goldstein S, Furberg C, Bhat Study Group. Prognostic significance of ventricular ectopic activity in survivors of acute myocardial infarction. *J Am Coll Cardiol* 1987; 10:231–242.
19. Anderson KP, DeCamilla J, Moss AJ. Clinical significance of ventricular tachycardia (3 beats or longer) detected during ambulatory monitoring after myocardial infarction. *Circulation* 1978; 57:890–897.
20. Follansbee WP, Michalson EL, Morganroth J. Nonsustained ventricular tachycardia in ambulatory patients: Characteristics and association with sudden cardiac death. *Ann Intern Med* 1980; 92:741–747.
21. Kleiger RE, Miller JP, Thanavaro S, Province MA, Martin TF, Oliver GC. Relationship between clinical features of acute myocardial infarction and ventricular runs 2 weeks to 1 year after infarction. *Circulation* 1981; 63:64–70.
22. Bigger JT Jr, Fleiss JL, Kleiger R, Miller JP, Rolintsky LM, Multicenter Post-Infarction Research Group. The relationships among ventricular arrhythmias, left ventricular dysfunction, and mortality in the 2 years after myocardial infarction. *Circulation* 1984; 69:250–258.
23. Shen WK, Hammill SC. Survivors of acute myocardial infarction: who is at risk for sudden cardiac death? *Mayo Clin Proc* 1991; 66:950–962.
24. Martin A, Benbow LJ, Butrous GS, Leach C, Camm AJ. Five-year follow-up of 101 elderly subjects by means of long-term ambulatory cardiac monitoring. *Eur Heart J* 1984; 5:592–596.
25. Califf RM, McKinnis RA, Burks J, et al. Prognostic implications of ventricular arrhythmias during 24 hour ambulatory monitoring in patients undergoing cardiac catheterization for coronary artery disease. *Am J Cardiol* 1982; 50:23–31.
26. Califf RM, McKinnis RA, McNeer JF, et al. Prognostic value of ventricular arrhythmias associated with treadmill exercise testing in patients studied with cardiac catheterization for suspected ischemic heart disease. *J Am Coll Cardiol* 1983; 2:1060–1067.

27. Holmes J, Kubo SH, Cody RJ, Kligfield P. Arrhythmias in ischemic and nonischemic dilated cardiomyopathy: prediction of mortality by ambulatory electrocardiography. *Am J Cardiol* 1985; 55:146–151.
28. Meinertz T, Hofmann T, Kasper W, et al. Significance of ventricular arrhythmias in idiopathic dilated cardiomyopathy. *Am J Cardiol* 1984; 53:902–907.
29. Maron BJ, Savage DD, Wolfson JK, Epstein SE. Prognostic significance of 24 hour ambulatory electrocardiographic monitoring in patients with hypertrophic cardiomyopathy: a prospective study. *Am J Cardiol* 1981; 48:252–257.
30. McKenna WJ, England D, Doi YL, Deanfield JE, Oakley CM, Goodwin JF. Arrhythmias in hypertrophic cardiomyopathy. I. Influence on prognosis. *Br Heart J* 1981; 46:168–172.
31. Messerli FH, Ventura HO, Elizardi DJ, et al. Hypertension and sudden death: increased ventricular ectopic activity in left ventricular hypertrophy. *Am J Med* 1984; 77:18–22.
32. Kannel WB, Gordon T, Offutt D. Left ventricular hypertrophy by electrocardiogram: prevalence, incidence, and mortality in the Framingham Study. *Ann Intern Med* 1969; 71:89–101.
33. Aronow WS, Epstein S, Koenigsberg M, Schwartz KS. Usefulness of echocardiographic left ventricular hypertrophy, ventricular tachycardia and complex ventricular arrhythmias in predicting ventricular fibrillation or sudden cardiac death in elderly patients. *Am J Cardiol* 1988; 62:1124–1125.
34. Roy D, Marchand E, Theroux P, Waters DD, Pelletier GB, Bourassa MG. Programmed ventricular stimulation in survivors of an acute myocardial infarction. *Circulation* 1985; 72:487–494.
35. Santarelli P, Bellocci F, Loperfido F. Ventricular arrhythmias induced by programmed ventricular stimulation after acute myocardial infarction. *Am J Cardiol* 1985; 55:391–394.
36. Marchlinski FE, Buxton AE, Waxman HL, Josephson ME. Identifying patients at risk of sudden death after myocardial infarction: value of the response to programmed stimulation, degree of ventricular ectopic activity and severity of left ventricular dysfunction. *Am J Cardiol* 1983; 52:1190–1196.
37. Richards DA, Cody DV, Denniss AR, Russell PA, Young AA, Uther JB. Ventricular electrical instability: a predictor of death after myocardial infarction. *Am J Cardiol* 1983; 51:75–80.
38. Hamer A, Vohra J, Hunt D, Sloman G. Prediction of sudden death by electrophysiologic studies in high risk patients surviving acute myocardial infarction. *Am J Cardiol* 1982; 50:223–229.
39. Bhandari AK, Hong R, Kotlewski A, et al. Prognostic significance of programmed ventricular stimulation in survivors of acute myocardial infarction. *Br Heart J* 1989; 61:410–416.
40. Bhandari AK, Rahimatoda SH. Invasive electrophysiologic testing and Holter monitoring in infarction survivors. In: Gersh BJ, Rahimatoda SH, eds. Acute Myocardial Infarction. New York: Elsevier, 1991:409–422.
41. Breithardt G, Becker R, Serpal L, et al. Non-invasive detection of late potentials in man: a new marker for ventricular tachycardia. *Eur Heart J* 1981; 2:1–11.

42. Denniss AR, Richards DA, Cody DV, et al. Prognostic significance of ventricular tachycardia and fibrillation induced at programmed stimulation and delayed potentials detected on the signal-averaged electrocardiograms of survivors of acute myocardial infarction. *Circulation* 1986; 74:731–745.
43. Breithardt G, Borggrefe M, Haarten K. Role of programmed ventricular stimulation and non-invasive recording of ventricular late potentials for the identification of patients at risk of ventricular arrhythmias after acute myocardial infarction. In: Zipes DP, Jalife J, eds. Cardiac Electrophysiology and Arrhythmias. Orlando, FL: Grune & Stratton, 1984:553–561.
44. Gomes JA, Winters SL, Stewart D, Horowitz S, Milner M, Barreca P. A new noninvasive index to predict sustained ventricular tachycardia and sudden death in the first year after myocardial infarction: based on signal-averaged electrocardiogram, radionuclide ejection fraction and Holter monitoring. *J Am Coll Cardiol* 1987; 10:349–357.
45. Gomes JA, Winters SL, Martinson M, et al. The prognostic significance of quantitative signal-averaged variables relative to clinical variables, site of myocardial infarction, ejection fraction and ventricular premature beats: a prospective study. *J Am Coll Cardiol* 1989; 13:377–384.
46. Kuchar DL, Thorburn CS, Sammel NL. Prediction of serious arrhythmic events after myocardial infarction: signal-averaged electrocardiogram, Holter monitoring, and radionuclide ventriculography. *J Am Coll Cardiol* 1987; 9:531–538.
47. El-Sherif N, Ursell SN, Bekheit S, et al. Prognostic significance of the signal-averaged electrocardiogram depends on the time of recording in the post infarction period. *Am Heart J* 1989; 118:256–264.
48. Cripps T, Bennett ED, Camm AJ, Ward DE. High-gain signal-averaged electrocardiogram combined with 24-hour monitoring in patients early after myocardial infarction for bedside prediction of arrhythmia events. *Br Heart J* 1988; 60:181–187.
49. Steinberg JS, Regan A, Sciacca RR, Bigger JT, Fleiss JL. Predicting arrhythmic events after acute myocardial infarction using the signal-averaged electrocardiogram. *Am J Cardiol* 1992; 69:13–21.
50. Nielson BL, Clausen J, Nielsen JS. Can procainamide improve the prognosis of patients with ventricular arrhythmias after myocardial infarction? *Dan Med Bull* 1978; 25:121–125.
51. Impact Research Group. International Mexiletine and placebo antiarrhythmic coronary trial. I. Report on arrhythmia and other findings. *J Am Coll Cardiol* 1984; 4:1148–1163.
52. Collaborative Group. Phenytoin after recovery from myocardial infarction. *Lancet* 1971; 1055–1057.
53. Ryden L, Arnman K, Conradson TB, Hafvendahl S, Mortensen O, Smedgard P. Prophylaxis of ventricular tachyarrhythmias with intravenous and oral tocainide in patients with and recovering from acute myocardial infarction. *Am Heart J* 1980; 100:1006–1012.
54. Gottlieb SH, Achuff SC, Mellits ED, et al. Prophylactic antiarrhythmic therapy of high-risk survivors of myocardial infarction: lower mortality at one month but not at one year. *Circulation* 1987; 75:792–799.

55. Peter T, Ross D, Duffield A, et al. Effect on survival after myocardial infarction of long-term treatment with phenytoin. *Br Heart J* 1978; 40:1356–1360.
56. Aronow WS, Mercando AD, Epstein S, Kronzon I. Effect of quinidine or procainamide versus no antiarrhythmic drug on sudden cardiac death, total cardiac death, and total death in elderly patients with heart disease and complex ventricular arrhythmias. *Am J Cardiol* 1990; 66:423–428.
57. Cardiac Arrhythmia Suppression Trial. Preliminary report: effect of encainide and flecainide on mortality in a randomized trial of arrhythmia suppression after myocardial infarction. *N Engl J Med* 1989; 321:406–412.
58. Norwegian Multicenter Study Group. Timolol-induced reduction in mortality and reinfarction in patients surviving acute myocardial infarction. *N Engl J Med* 1981; 304:801–807.
59. Olsson G, Rehnqvist N, Sjogren A, Erhardt L, Lundman T. Long-term treatment with metoprolol after myocardial infarction: effect on three year mortality and morbidity. *J Am Coll Cardiol* 1985; 5:1428–1437.
60. Beta Blocker Heart Attack Trial Research Group. A randomized trial of propranolol in patients with acute myocardial infarction. *JAMA* 1983; 250:2814–2819.
61. Hjalmarson A, Elmfeldt D, Herlitz J, et al. Effect on mortality of metoprolol in acute myocardial infarction. *Lancet* 1981; 2:823–826.
62. Gundersen T, Abrahamsen AM, Kjershus J, et al. Timolol related reduction in mortality and reinfarction in patients ages 65–75 years surviving acute myocardial infarction. *Circulation* 1982; 66:1179–1184.
63. Forman DE, Wei JY. Is the use of beta blocker therapy decreased in the elderly (abstract)? *J Am Geriatr Soc* 1991; 39:A49.
64. Morganroth J, Horowitz LN. Antiarrhythmic drug therapy 1988: for whom, how, and where? *Am J Cardiol* 1988; 62:461–465.
65. Morganroth J. Comparative safety of antiarrhythmic drugs. *Choices Cardiol* 1991; 5:12–14.
66. Lany PP. Modifying drug disease in elderly patients. In: Covington TR, Walker JN, eds. Current Geriatric Therapy. Philadelphia: W. B. Saunders, 1984:42–46.
67. Myers M, Meier DE, Walsh JR. General principles. In: Cassel CK, Walsh JR, eds. Geriatric Medicine. New York: Springer-Verlag, 1984:605–617.
68. Reidenberg MM, Camacho M, Kluger J, et al. Aging and renal clearance of procainamide and acetylprocainamide. *Clin Pharmacol Ther* 1980; 28:732–735.
69. Hohnloser SH, Raeder EA, Podrid PJ, et al. Predictors of antiarrhythmic drug efficacy in patients with malignant ventricular tachyarrhythmias. *Am Heart J* 1987; 114:1–7.
70. Ruskin JN, Schoenfeld MH, Garan H. Role of electrophysiologic techniques in the selection of antiarrhythmic drug regimens for ventricular arrhythmias. *Am J Cardiol* 1983; 52:41C–46C.
71. Swerdlow CD, Winkle RA, Mason JW. Determinants of survival in patients with ventricular tachyarrhythmias. *N Engl J Med* 1983; 308:1436–1442.
72. Wilber DJ, Garan H, Finkelstein D, et al. Out-of-hospital cardiac arrest: use of electrophysiologic testing in the prediction of long-term outcome. *N Engl J Med* 1988; 318:19–24.
73. Ruskin JN, DiMarco JP, Garan H. Out-of-hospital cardiac arrest: electrophysiolo-

gic observations and selection of long-term antiarrhythmic therapy. *N Engl J Med* 1980; 303:607–613.

74. Morady F, Scheinman MM, Hess DS, Sung RJ, Shen E, Shapiro W. Electrophysiologic testing in the management of survivors of out-of-hospital cardiac arrest. *Am J Cardiol* 1983; 51:85–89.
75. Tresch DD, Wetherbee JN, Siegel R, et al. Long-term follow-up of survivors of prehospital sudden cardiac death treated with coronary bypass surgery. *Am Heart J* 1985; 110:1139–1145.
76. Manolis AS, Rastegar H, Payne D, Cleveland R, Estes NAM III. Surgical therapy for drug-refractory ventricular tachycardia: results with mapping-guided subendocardial resection. *J Am Coll Cardiol* 1989; 14:199–208.
77. Winkle RA, Mead RH, Ruder MA, et al. Long-term outcome with the automatic implantable cardioverter-defibrillator. *J Am Coll Cardiol* 1989; 13:1353–1361.
78. Tchou PJ, Kadri N, Anderson J, Caceres JA, Jazayeri M, Akhtar M. Automatic implantable cardioverter-defibrillators and survival of patients with left ventricular dysfunction and malignant ventricular arrhythmias. *Ann Intern Med* 1988; 109:529–534.
79. Kelly PA, Cannom DS, Garan H, et al. The automatic implantable cardioverter-defibrillator: efficacy, complications and survival in patients with malignant ventricular arrhythmias. *J Am Coll Cardiol* 1988; 11:1278–1286.
80. Troup PJ. Implantable cardioverters and defibrillators. *Curr Probl Cardiol* 1989; 14:673–843.
81. Gersh BJ, Kronmal RA, Frye RL, et al. Coronary arteriography and coronary artery bypass surgery: morbidity and mortality in patients ages 65 years or older. *Circulation* 1983; 67:483–490.
82. Rose DM, Gelbfish J, Jacobowitz IJ, et al. Analysis of morbidity and mortality in patients 70 years of age and over undergoing isolated coronary artery bypass surgery. *Am Heart J* 1985; 110:341–346.
83. Tresch DD, Platia EV, Guarnieri T, Reid PR, Griffith LSC. Refractory symptomatic ventricular tachycardia and ventricular fibrillation in elderly patients. *Am J Med* 1987; 83:399–404.
84. Tresch DD, Troup PJ, Thakur RK, et al. Comparison of efficacy of automatic implantable cardioverter defibrillator in patients older and younger than 65 years of age. *Am J Med* 1991; 90:717–724.
85. Scott J, Aarons D, Juanteguy J, Veltri EP. Automatic implantable cardioverter/defibrillator in the elderly (abstract). *J Am Coll Cardiol* 1991; 17:329A.
86. Kannel WB, Thomas HE Jr. Sudden coronary death: the Framingham study. *Ann N Y Acad Sci* 1982; 382:3–21.
87. Kuller L, Lilienfeld A. Epidemiological study of sudden and unexpected deaths due to arteriosclerotic heart disease. *Circulation* 1966; 34:1056–1068.
88. Fusgen I, Summa JD. How much sense is there in an attempt to resuscitate an aged person? *Gerontology* 1978; 24:37–45.
89. Gulati RS, Bhan GL, Horan MA. Cardiopulmonary resuscitation of old people. *Lancet* 1983; 267–269.
90. Bedell SE, Delbanco TL, Cook EF, Epstein FH. Survival after cardiopulmonary resuscitation in the hospital. *N Engl J Med* 1983; 309:569–576.

91. Taffet GE, Teasdale TA, Luchi RJ. In-hospital cardiopulmonary resuscitation. *JAMA* 1988; 260:2069–2072.
92. Murphy DJ, Murray AM, Robinson BE, Compion EW. Outcomes of cardiopulmonary resuscitation in the elderly. *Ann Intern Med* 1989; 111:199–205.
93. Tresch DD, Thakur RK, Hoffmann RG, Brooks HL. Comparison of outcome of resuscitation of out-of-hospital cardiac arrest in persons younger and older than 70 years of age. *Am J Cardiol* 1988; 61:1120–1122.
94. Tresch DD, Thakur RK, Hoffmann RG, Aufderheide TP, Brooks HL. Comparison of outcome of paramedic-witnessed cardiac arrest in patients younger and older than 70 years. *Am J Cardiol* 1990; 65:453–457.
95. Tresch DD, Thakur RK, Hoffmann RG, Olson D, Brooks HL. Should the elderly be resuscitated following out-of-hospital cardiac arrest? *Am J Med* 1989; 86:145–150.
96. Bonnin MJ, Pepe PE, Clark PS. Survival prognosis for the elderly after out-of-hospital cardiac arrest (abstract). *Ann Emerg Med* 1989; 18:469.
97. Denes P, Long L, Madison C, Gorham J, Carruthers N, Luxemberg M. Resuscitation from out-of-hospital ventricular tachycardia/fibrillation (VT/VF): the effect of age on outcome (abstract). *Circulation* 1990; 82:III–81.
98. Eisenberg MS, Cummins RO, Larsen MP. Cardiopulmonary resuscitation in the elderly. *Ann Intern Med* 1990; 113:408–409.
99. Eisenberg MS, Horwood BT, Cummins RO, et al. Cardiac arrest and resuscitation: a tale of 29 cities. *Ann Emerg Med* 1990; 19:179–186.
100. Longstreth WT Jr, Cobb LA, Fahrenbruch CE, Copass MK. Does age affect outcomes of out-of-hospital cardiopulmonary resuscitation? *JAMA* 1990; 264:2109–2110.
101. Kaiser TE, Kayson EP, Campbell RG. Survival after cardiopulmonary resuscitation in a long-term care institution (abstract). *J Am Geriatr Soc* 1986; 34:909.
102. Applebaum GE, King JE, Finucane TE. The outcome of CPR initiated in nursing homes. *J Am Geriatr Soc* 1990; 38:197–200.
103. Awoke S, Mouton CP, Parrott M. Outcomes of skilled CPR in long term care facility: futile therapy? *J Am Geriatr Soc* 1992; 40:6:593–595.
104. Neahring J, Tresch D, Mark D, Duthie E, Kartes S, Aufderheide T. Outcomes of cardiopulmonary resuscitation (CPR) in nursing homes: who should receive CPR (abstract)? *J Am Coll Cardiol* 1992; 19:377A.
105. Tresch DD. CPR in the elderly: when should it be performed? *Geriatrics* 1991; 46:47–56.

# 23

# Bradyarrhythmias and Cardiac Pacemakers in the Elderly

**Anthony D. Mercando**
*Columbia University, College of Physicians and Surgeons, New York, New York;*
*and Albert Einstein College of Medicine and Montefiore Medical Center, Bronx, New York*

## DIAGNOSIS

*Bradycardia* is used to describe any slow heart rhythm, but such rhythms are always caused by specific abnormalities in cardiac impulse formation or conduction. Although mean heart rates decline with age, the prevalence and significance of bradyarrhythmias in the elderly remain controversial (1–4). Degenerative disease in the sinus node can lead to pathological sinus bradycardia, sinus arrest, or sinus exit block. Sick sinus syndrome is a condition that includes one or several abnormalities in sinus node or atrioventricular (AV) node function.

AV block and block in the His-Purkinje system can occur as a result of ischemic heart disease or various degenerative processes. Baroreceptor and autonomic abnormalities can produce symptomatic sinus slowing or AV node block. Bradyarrhythmias are in the differential diagnosis of syncope and presyncope in the elderly. The identification of bradycardia as a cause of syncope is crucial because pacemaker therapy usually relieves the problem.

### History

Bradycardia should be suspected in patients who present with symptoms of syncope, presyncope, episodes of light-headedness, or palpitations. Patients should be questioned about the relationship of these symptoms to time of day, activity, and position, since the causes of bradycardias are usually intermittent or precipitated by specific events. Often there are associated symptoms, such as dyspnea or chest pain, that can give a clue to the etiology of an arrhythmia. The patient should be asked to tap out any associated palpitations to help in differentiating rapid from slow arrhythmias and regular from irregular rhythms. If symptoms are associated with activity or rapid palpitations, a bradycardia is unlikely to be an isolated cause of the patient's complaints. History of associated illness, such as thyroid disease, and use of sedative drugs or medications that can produce bradycardia (such as $\beta$-blockers, digoxin, or calcium channel blockers) should be elicited (5). Family members should be instructed to take the patient's pulse during episodes and to comment on the regularity and rate of the pulse.

## Physical Examination

During an arrhythmia, pulse rate, rhythm, and blood pressure abnormalities may be detected. In addition, AV dissociation and variability of systolic blood pressure from beat to beat may give clues to the types of arrhythmia. The changes associated with AV dissociation may be seen as abnormalities in the venous pulse, such as intermittent high-volume A waves.

## Electrocardiography

The findings obtained during history and physical examination may be nonspecific, and the diagnosis of symptomatic bradyarrhythmias rests with demonstration of the abnormality by electrocardiography (possibly with carotid sinus massage) and electrophysiological testing. Because of the intermittent nature of sinus node and conduction system abnormalities, a single 12-lead electrocardiogram (ECG) or a longer ECG rhythm strip are usually inadequate to make a diagnosis. The twenty-four hour ambulatory (Holter) recordings should be obtained early in the evaluation of the patient. Careful evaluation of the rate and relationship of P waves and QRS complexes should be made. All pauses greater than 1.5 s on Holter monitoring should be examined to identify the mechanism of the event. In all cases, symptoms should be correlated with ECG abnormalities, and the patient should be instructed to keep a detailed diary of symptoms during the time of the Holter recording. Pauses of greater than 2–3 s may occur in normal individuals. If the event does not produce symptoms and is due to sinus node dysfunction or some types of AV block, a pacemaker is not indicated. Lack of heart rate increase with exercise may be pathological and could result in presyncope.

In many individuals, 24 or 48 h of Holter monitoring may be inadequate to identify symptomatic bradycardias. In these cases, a patient-activated event recorder or continuous memory loop recorder may be useful. These recorders store several seconds or minutes of ECG data when an event button is activated.

The stored tracing can be sent to a central location via telephone after the patient has recovered from the event. The 24 h memory loop recorders are more cumbersome, since they remain on the patient for prolonged periods of time (up to 1 month or more), but the importance of correlating symptoms to ECG abnormalities is so crucial that their use may be necessitated.

## Provocative Testing

When the preceding techniques fail to provide a diagnosis, exercise testing, carotid sinus massage, or pharmacological testing can be employed. All such tests are generally insensitive and nonspecific, so they must be used in concert with other diagnostic tests. Failure of the sinus node rate to increase with exercise has been reported in sick sinus syndrome (6). An abnormally long pause during carotid sinus massage (greater than 3 s) may indicate hypersensitive carotid sinus reflex, but this may occur in asymptomatic elderly patients (7). Determination of *intrinsic heart rate* following autonomic blockade with propranolol and atropine may identify sinus node function that falls outside population-determined norms. Since all these tests fail to correlate abnormalities with symptoms, however, their usefulness is limited.

## Electrophysiological Testing

The technique of electrophysiological testing can be useful in the diagnosis and management of a wide variety of atrial and ventricular arrhythmias (8). Wires are usually inserted via a subclavian or femoral vein, with electrodes in the high right atrium and the right ventricular apex, and via the right femoral vein across the tricuspid valve, with electrodes in the region of the bundle of His (Fig. 1). Recordings are made from these sites and from others as necessary. By analyzing conduction times, sites of block can be defined; by pacing the atrium and ventricle, the integrity of the conduction system can be studied and arrhythmias can be reproduced.

Sinus node function is usually evaluated during electrophysiological testing using sinus node recovery time and sinoatrial conduction time. The sinus node recovery time examines the ability of the sinus node to recommence firing after overdrive suppression with atrial pacing. A normal value in most laboratories is less than 1500 ms or, when corrected for the baseline sinus rate, varies from laboratory to laboratory between 350 and 550 ms. Sinoatrial conduction time is an indirect measurement of the time it takes for an impulse to travel into and then exit from the sinus node. The sensitivity of these techniques, even when combined, is only about 64%, with a specificity of about 88% (9).

Atrial conduction, AV node function, and His-Purkinje system function are assessed by measuring intracardiac conduction intervals and by atrial pacing. An electrophysiological study can be useful in identifying the site of atrioven-

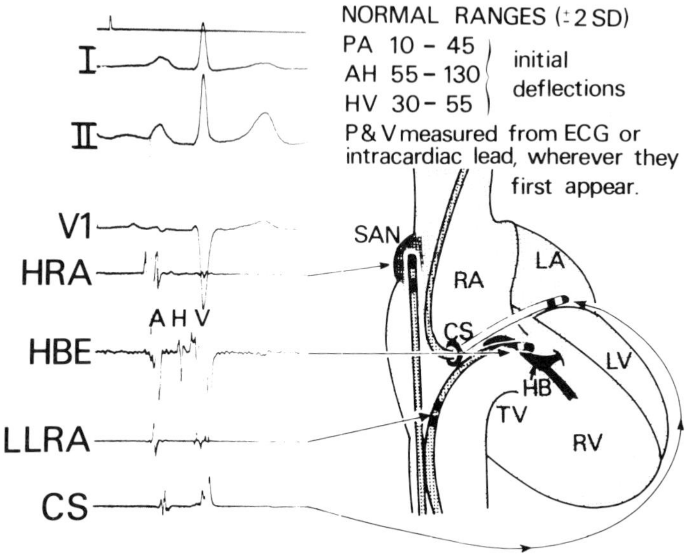


**Figure 1** Surface electrocardiograms and intracardiac electrograms recorded during an electrophysiological study. Arrows show location of electrodes in the heart. I, II, VI = standard surface ECG leads; HRA = high right atrium; HBE = His bundle electrogram; LLRA = low lateral right atrium; CS = coronary sinus; P = P wave; V = ventricular depolarization. (From Fisher JD. *Prog Cardiovasc Dis* 1981; 24:25–90. Used with permission.)

tricular block and in assessing the competence of the His-Purkinje system at rest and during pacing.

An electrophysiological study should be performed in patients with suspected sinus node disease or AV block who are symptomatic with syncope or presyncope and in whom the relationship between symptoms and a bradyarrhythmia has not been established. Patients who have symptoms documented to be due to bradyarrhythmias or patients with degrees of heart block that require permanent pacing (see indications for cardiac pacing, later) do not require an electrophysiological study. When the site of AV block cannot be determined by electrocardiography or Holter monitoring and differentiation of the site would help in the decision to implant a pacemaker, a His bundle study should be performed. This may be necessary in patients with fixed 2:1 AV block and bundle branch block or in patients with Mobitz type II block with a normal QRS in whom block in the bundle of His is suspected. The use of electrophysiological testing to diagnose patients with syncope of undetermined origin is discussed in Chapter 24.

## NORMAL CARDIAC CONDUCTION SYSTEM

The understanding of bradyarrhythmias and their management is enhanced by a knowledge of the specialized cardiac conduction system (Fig. 2). Normal cardiac activation originates in a group of cells in the high right atrium, known as the sinus node. The node is composed of nodal cells, which are the source of normal impulse formation, transitional cells, which may form the pathway for impulse conduction to the atrium, and working atrial myocardial cells, which extend into the node from surrounding atrial tissue. The sinus node receives innervation from postganglionic adrenergic and cholinergic nerve endings. Vagal stimulation slows sinus node discharge and prolongs conduction times within the node. Adrenergic stimulation increases sinus rate. From the sinus node, the normal cardiac impulse travels through atrial tissue and possibly through internodal and interatrial pathways, although this latter point is controversial (10,11). Conduction from right to left atrium appears to travel preferentially over a band of muscle fibers known as Bachmann's bundle.

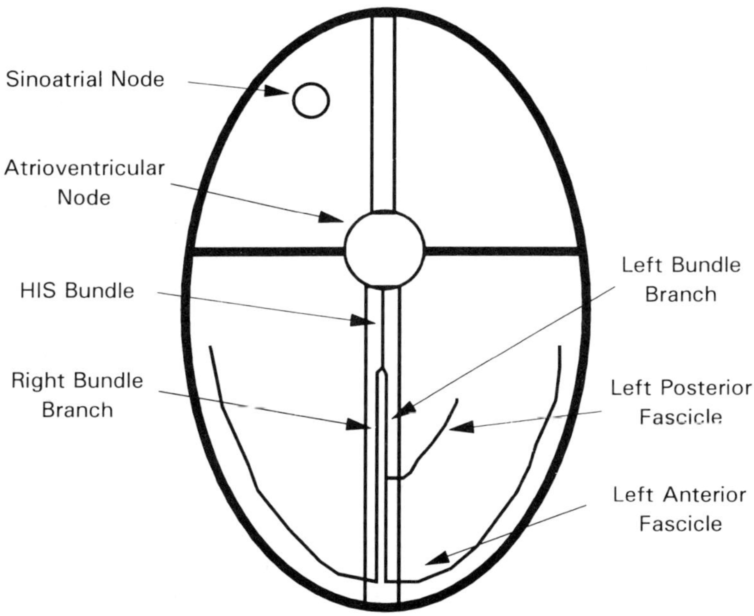


**Figure 2** Components of the cardiac conduction system (see text).

The signal eventually reaches the AV node, located in the lower part of the right atrium near the septal leaflet of the tricuspid valve, anterior to the ostium of the coronary sinus. The AV node conducts the impulse from the atrium to the bundle of His. In normal hearts, the remainder of the interface between atria and ventricles is electrically insulated. In patients with Wolff-Parkinson-White syndrome, this insulator and the AV node are short-circuited via a bypass tract known as a Kent bundle.

AV nodal tissue exhibits a characteristic known as decremental conduction: the more rapidly impulses stimulate and attempt to pass through the AV node, the more slowly the node will conduct, even to the point of intermittent block. Like the sinus node, the AV node is richly innervated by cholinergic and adrenergic nerve endings. Vagal stimulation increases AV node conduction time and can produce block. Sympathetic stimulation shortens AV node conduction time and refractory periods.

From the AV node, the cardiac impulse travels to the bundle of His, the first part of the specialized ventricular conduction system. From the bundle of His, the impulse travels through the bundle branches and eventually to terminal Purkinje fibers. These fibers form interweaving branches on the endocardial surface of both ventricles and allow rapid transmission of the impulse to the entire ventricular myocardium in a period of 60 to 100 ms. Without the specialized ventricular conduction system, muscle conduction of the cardiac impulse would require longer periods of time, typically of the order of 120 to 160 ms. The anatomy of the bundle branches is variable between individuals, although the most common configuration is that of a main right bundle branch and a left bundle branch that bifurcates into an anterior and a posterior fascicle.

Bradyarrhythmias can result from abnormalities in impulse formation in the sinus node or impulse conduction in the sinus node, atrial myocardium, AV node, bundle of His, or bundle branches. Total or subtotal destruction of the sinus node or transitional zone tissue may be found in patients with sick sinus syndrome. Inflammatory and degenerative changes can also be seen in some cases. AV nodal block may be due to infiltration of the node by fibrosis or calcification from adjacent structures (Lev's disease), like that in calcific aortic stenosis. The ventricular conduction system can be affected by degeneration caused by chronic ischemic heart disease or by a sclerotic degenerative process (Lenegre's disease) (12).

## SINUS NODE DYSFUNCTION

### Sinus Bradycardia

Sinus bradycardia is defined as a sinus node rhythm with a rate of less than 60 bpm. The arrhythmia may result from excessive vagal tone or diminished sympathetic tone, medications, such as $\beta$-blockers, digoxin, or calcium channel blockers, or because of sick sinus syndrome and its associated anatomical abnormalities. Well-trained athletes can exhibit sinus bradycardia, but this is a less common cause in the elderly population. Sinus bradycardia can also occur during sleep, with manipulation of the eye during surgery, or secondary to hypothyroidism, hypothermia, intracranial tumors, meningitis, or increased intracranial pressure. Excessive vagal tone, as is seen during intense vomiting, can also produce symptomatic sinus bradycardia. Besides $\beta$-blockers and calcium channel blockers, lithium and clonidine have been reported to cause sinus bradycardia. $\beta$-Blocker eye drops may be absorbed and produce sinus slowing or AV node block (13).

The ECG during sinus bradycardia shows normal-appearing P waves before each QRS complex and occurring at a rate less than 60 bpm. Normal-appearing P waves imply that the impulse originates in the sinus node. There can be coexisting AV block, which further lowers the ventricular rate.

Treatment of sinus bradycardia is usually not necessary, unless the patient is symptomatic during the periods of slow rhythm. In the acute setting, such as following a myocardial infarction, symptomatic patients can be treated with 0.5 mg intravenous (IV) atropine, repeated every 5 min up to 2 mg. If atropine fails, 1–10 $\mu$g/min of IV isoproterenol can be started cautiously while awaiting pacemaker therapy. Isoproterenol should be avoided in patients with myocardial ischemia, since it can increase myocardial oxygen demand and is proarrhythmic even at low doses. In the acute setting, an external transthoracic pacemaker or transvenous temporary pacemaker can be employed. If the patient exhibits chronic symptomatic sinus bradycardia not attributable to medications, permanent pacing is the treatment of choice.

## Sinus Arrest

Sinus arrest occurs because of an abnormality in impulse formation caused by medications or any of the disease processes mentioned previously. Bradycardia occurs if lower pacemakers such as the AV node, fail to produce an appropriate escape rhythm.

On the ECG, P waves are identified before each QRS and are normal in configuration, as they are in sinus bradycardia. The tracing shows a pause in the sinus rhythm, with a P-P interval that is not equal to a multiple of the patient's basic P-P interval (Fig. 3).

Treatment for asymptomatic sinus arrest is usually not required. For symptomatic patients, treatment is similar to that outlined for sinus bradycardia.

## Sinoatrial Exit Block

Sinoatrial exit block represents an abnormality in impulse conduction from the sinus node to surrounding atrial tissue. It can be caused by medications, includ-

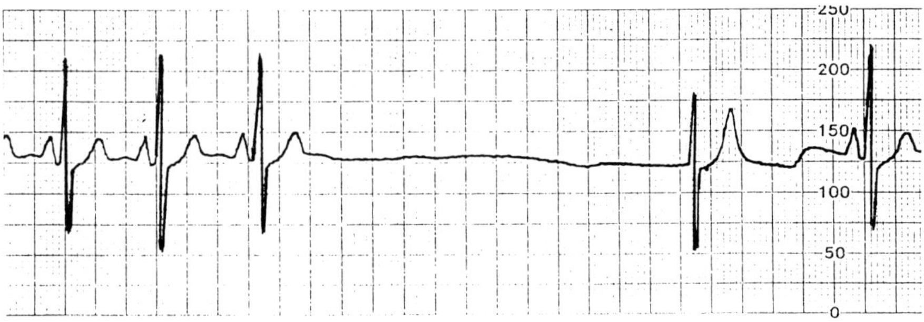


**Figure 3** Sinus arrest. The escape beat is from the AV node, and the peaked T wave following this beat implies that a P wave is buried in the T wave.

ing type IA antiarrhythmics, such as quinidine and procainamide. The arrhythmia can also be caused by the other sinus node abnormalities described earlier. On the ECG, there is a pause in the sinus rhythm, which is equal to a multiple of the underlying P-P interval.

The treatment for patients with symptomatic sinoatrial exit block is similar to that for sinus bradycardia. For asymptomatic patients no treatment is required and the block may be transient, resolving after any offending medications are discontinued.

## Sick Sinus Syndrome

Sick sinus syndrome includes a number of abnormalities of sinus node, atrial myocardial, or AV node abnormalities. It is often considered synonymous with the bradycardia–tachycardia syndrome, which consists of paroxysmal regular or irregular atrial tachycardias alternating with episodes of bradyarrhythmias, but is only one manifestation of sick sinus syndrome. Also included in the definition are persistent sinus bradycardia not caused by medications, episodes of sinus arrest or sinus exit block, abnormalities of sinus node and atrial function in conjunction with AV conduction abnormalities (such as atrial fibrillation with slow ventricular response), or any combination of these conditions (Fig. 4). The etiology of sick sinus syndrome is probably multifactorial, varying from patient to patient. There may be inflammatory or degenerative changes in the sinus node and perinodal tissues. Autonomic abnormalities are also common (14,15).

Treatment of sick sinus syndrome can be problematic, since medications used to suppress or slow chronic or paroxysmal atrial tachycardias may exacerbate the associated bradycardias. Digoxin in particular can cause profound bradyarrhythmias in these patients. Often, ventricular pacing must be used with drug therapy to treat patients with the bradycardia-tachycardia syndrome.

Although prophylactic pacing is not indicated, patients who require digoxin, $\beta$-blockers, calcium channel blockers, or antiarrhythmic medications should be monitored after these medications are started. If long ventricular pauses occur or if patients become symptomatic, they should receive permanent pacing.

## CAROTID SINUS HYPERSENSITIVITY

Hypersensitive carotid sinus syndrome is defined as ventricular asystole of greater than 3 s during carotid sinus stimulation, although the definition is arbitrary. Studies have shown conflicting results regarding the significance of the 3 s pause during carotid sinus massage (16–18). Hypersensitive carotid sinus response can be found in elderly patients complaining of syncope or presyncope, but many of these patients have multiple causes for their symptoms.

The cause of hypersensitive carotid sinus syndrome is not known but may involve an abnormal baroreceptor set point, excessive release of acetylcholine, inadequate cholinesterase to metabolize the acetylcholine, or abnormal central autonomic response.

Carotid sinus hypersensitivity may manifest clinically following carotid stimulation from head turning or from tight collars. On the ECG during carotid sinus stimulation, either sinus arrest or sinus exit block is found. Although AV node block can occur, it is infrequent because the sinus slowing masks its manifestation.

Atropine can blunt the cardioinhibitory effects of carotid sinus hypersensitivity, but long-term treatment requires ventricular pacing. Medications, such as $\beta$-blockers, calcium channel blockers, digitalis, and clonidine, should be avoided in patients who do not have an implanted ventricular pacemaker.

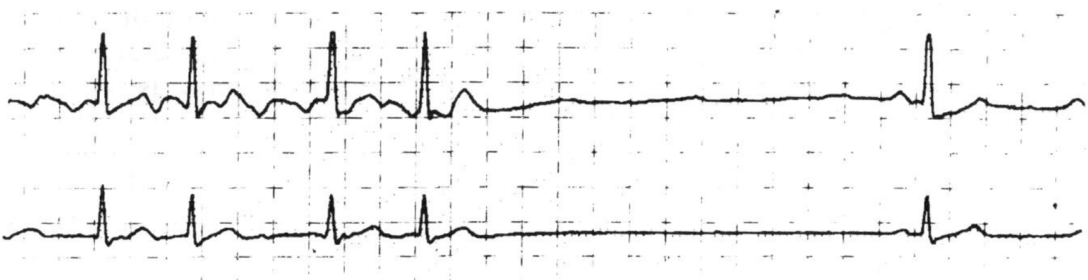

**Figure 4** Long sinus pause after spontaneous conversion of atrial fibrillation to sinus rhythm in a patient with sick sinus syndrome. Prolonged recovery of the sinus node is characteristic of this condition and can also produce long pauses following electrical cardioversion.

## ATRIOVENTRICULAR BLOCK

Atrioventricular block is a nonphysiological delay in conduction or a lack of conduction of the electrical impulse from atria to ventricles. Block can result from abnormal conduction in any part of the electrical system of the heart. Blocks that occur during a period of time in which the AV conduction system should be refractory (for example, an atrial premature contraction that occurs early after a normally conducted beat) must be excluded. The causes of block have been discussed previously and include ischemic heart disease, degenerative and infiltrative diseases, drug toxicities, and excess vagal activity. Atrioventricular block can be paroxysmal or fixed. A patient can exhibit different degrees of AV block at different times and under different pathophysiological conditions.

Electrocardiographic criteria are used to define degrees of block. *First-degree block* refers to a delay in AV conduction without nonconduction. On the ECG, normal sinus P waves are each followed by QRS complexes but with a P-R interval that is prolonged at greater than 0.20 s. Occasionally, the P-R interval can be as long as 1.0 s. P-R interval prolongation can be due to slowed conduction in the atrium (prolonged P-A interval), in the AV node (prolonged A-H interval), or in the His-Purkinje system (prolonged H-V interval). The presence of a narrow QRS usually indicates disease in the AV node, but first-degree AV block with a widened QRS morphology does not localize disease to the AV node or the His-Purkinje system (19).

*Second-degree AV block* is manifested by intermittent lack of conduction from atria to ventricles. Type I second-degree AV block (also called Wenckebach block) is usually but not always due to disease in the AV node and produces a gradual prolongation of P-R intervals in successive beats until a P wave is completely blocked for one beat (Fig. 5). Type II second-degree block, which usually involves disease below the AV node in the His-Purkinje system, produces intermittent block in AV conduction without prior prolongation of the P-R interval (Fig. 6). Type I block is usually considered benign, since AV node disease is the usual site of block and the prognosis is good. There is less tendency for the process to progress to complete heart block and frank syncope.

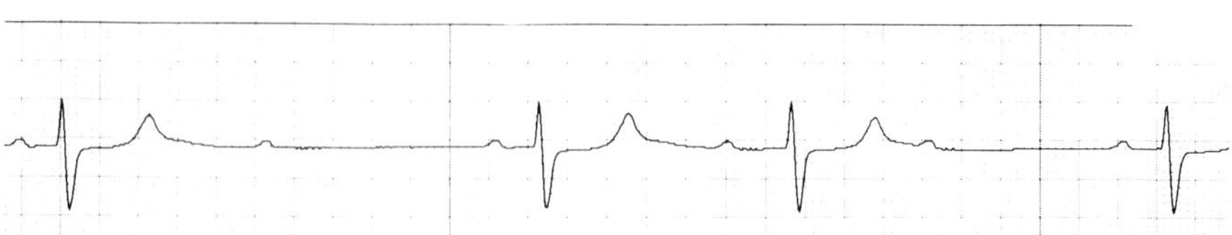

**Figure 5** Second-degree AV block, type I (Wenckebach). Note the prolongation of the P-R interval before the blocked P wave.

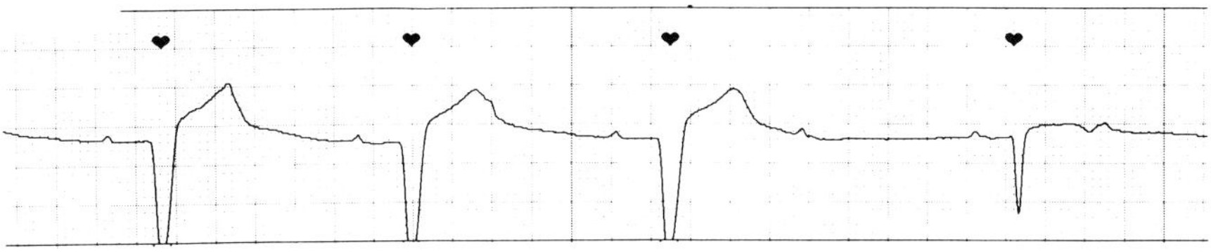

**Figure 6** Second-degree AV block, type II. Note that the P-R intervals are not prolonged before the blocked P wave.

Type I block can occur with inferior wall myocardial infarction and tends to be transient. Patients are generally asymptomatic, and temporary or permanent pacing is not required. Type II block occurs more commonly after anterior wall myocardial infarction and usually indicates a large area of myocardial damage. Type II block also leads to complete heart block more frequently than type I and consequently produces more symptoms. Temporary and permanent pacing are usually indicated for type II block because of this propensity to advance to complete heart block. Following anterior wall myocardial infarction, mortality remains high, despite permanent pacing, because of the association with extensive myocardial damage.

There is a special case of second-degree block in which every other P wave is blocked. This is known as 2:1 block. Since two successive P-R intervals cannot be examined, it is not possible to further classify the rhythm as type I (Wenckebach) or type II second-degree block. When the QRS interval is narrow, the block is usually in the AV node. When the QRS interval is wide, the block can be in either the AV node or the His-Purkinje system. In such cases, it is necessary to examine long rhythm strips or 24 h Holter recordings in an attempt to find evidence for Wenckebach or non-Wenckebach conduction.

The term "high-grade AV block" is used by many cardiologists but is not uniformly defined. Usually the term refers to a situation in which multiple consecutive P waves are blocked. Usually, the P-R interval does not change in conducted beats, so this rhythm resembles type II second-degree AV block.

In *third-degree* or *complete AV block,* there is a total lack of conduction and communication between atria and ventricles. The atrial rhythm does not affect the ventricular rhythm, which is produced by an escape focus in the AV node (junctional escape rhythm) or, more commonly, in the ventricle (idioventricular escape rhythm). The ECG during complete heart block usually exhibits three features: (1) nonconducted P waves; (2) atrioventricular dissociation (atrial and ventricular rhythms are independent); and (3) a regular ventricular response due to the escape rhythm (Fig. 7).

An algorithm can be constructed to aid in the correct identification of the degree of heart block based on the surface electrocardiogram (Fig. 8). By

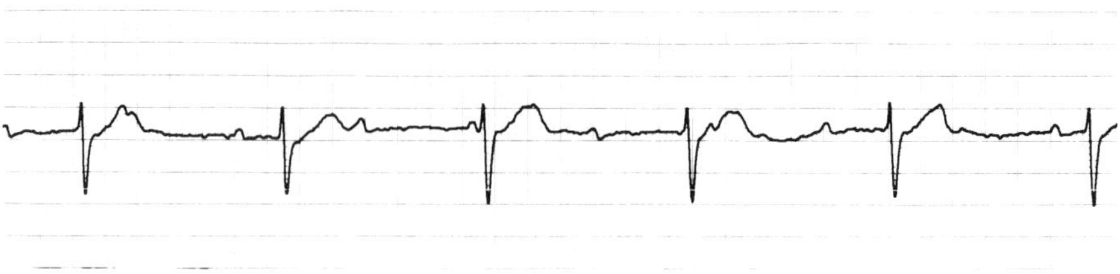

**Figure 7** Complete heart block, with narrow complex escape rhythm (AV nodal escape). Note the blocked P waves, A-V dissociation, and regular ventricular response (from the escape rhythm).

answering several simple yes-no questions, an accurate diagnosis can be established. One must first determine whether there are blocked P waves. If there are none and the P-R interval is greater than 0.20 s, the patient has first-degree AV block. If there are blocked P waves, then the P-R intervals must be examined. The algorithm does not require that an assessment be made of whether a particular P wave is causing a QRS. Simply identify a QRS, find the P wave that precedes that QRS, and define that as a P-R interval. If the intervals are not vari-

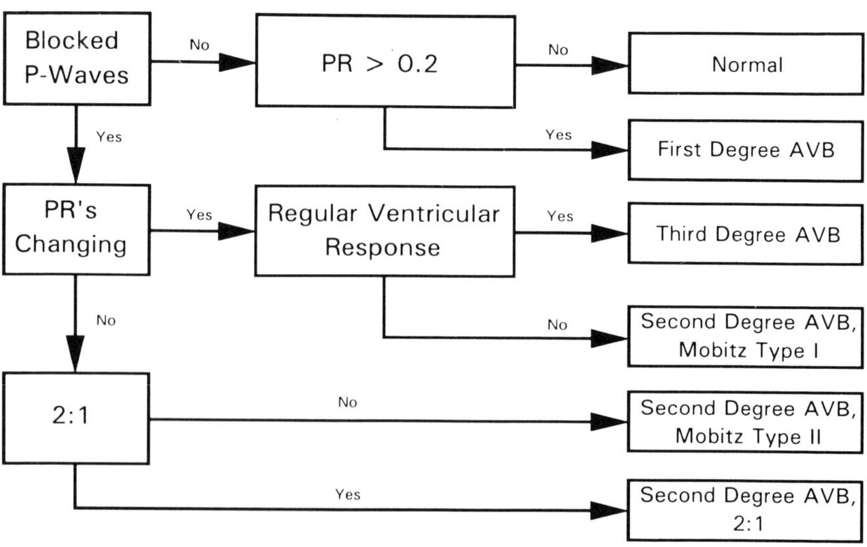


**Figure 8** Algorithm for the ECG diagnosis of heart block (see text).

able, then the special case of second-degree block with 2:1 conduction must be excluded. If 2:1 conduction is present, it is not possible to further categorize the block as Mobitz type I or Mobitz type II, and the diagnosis of second-degree AV block, 2:1 is made. If the patient has constant P-R intervals and is not in 2:1 block, then the diagnosis of second-degree AV block, Mobitz type II, is made. If the P-R intervals are changing and the ventricular rhythm is not regular, then the diagnosis of second-degree AV block, Mobitz type I, is present. If the ventricular response is regular, then the criteria for third-degree (complete) AV block have been met.

Electrophysiological testing can be used to identify the site of the atrioventricular block. In the nonmedicated state, the patient's rhythm is recorded and the P-A, A-H, and H-V intervals are determined (Fig. 1). Lack of a His bundle depolarization following a blocked P wave signifies that the AV node is the site of the block. Presence of the His bundle signal following a blocked P wave indicates that the impulse has traveled through the AV node, has stimulated the bundle of His, and has blocked below that point. Block below the bundle of His generally requires permanent pacing.

First-degree block alone does not require treatment. Second-degree block, Mobitz type I, in an asymptomatic patient does not require treatment. Symptomatic Mobitz I can be treated acutely with temporary pacing and eventually with permanent pacing. A permanent pacemaker should be used only after possible causative medications have been discontinued. Permanent pacing is indicated in patients with symptomatic and probably asymptomatic Mobitz type II block and probably in Mobitz II block acquired during an acute myocardial infarction. Even with permanent pacing, however, the mortality rate in this group of patients with anterior wall myocardial infarction remains high. Acquired third-degree block requires permanent pacing, since the patient is dependent upon an escape rhythm that may be unreliable. If the patient exhibits symptoms with complete heart block, a temporary pacemaker should be inserted while the patient waits for definitive therapy with a permanent pacemaker.

## PACEMAKER THERAPY FOR BRADYCARDIAS

### Indications

Indications for permanent pacemaker implantation have been developed by the American Heart Association and the American College of Cardiology (20), and the Health Care Financing Administration has published guidelines for reimbursement for pacemaker implantation. In general, permanent pacing is indicated to treat symptomatic bradyarrhythmias. If a causative drug can be identified and stopped, this should be done. Pacing should be undertaken only if the symptomatic arrhythmia persists. When symptoms cannot be temporally related to a bradyarrhythmia, controversies regarding indications for implantation exist.

Group I indications are those in which a permanent pacemaker is considered acceptable and necessary if the cause is not transient. These include acquired complete heart block with symptoms, such as syncope, seizures, congestive heart failure, dizziness, or limited exercise tolerance; symptomatic Mobitz type II second-degree AV block; symptomatic Mobitz type I second-degree block with hemodynamic instability related to the block; symptomatic sinus bradycardia, with heart rate less than 50 bpm, and documented hemodynamic instability related to the bradycardia; symptomatic sinus bradycardia or atrial fibrillation, with slow ventricular response resulting from required long-term drug treatment and without acceptable alternative drugs; symptomatic sinus node dysfunction (sick sinus syndrome); sinus node dysfunction without symptoms when the bradycardia leads to potentially life-threatening ventricular arrhythmias; and patients with severe carotid sinus hypersensitivity and syncope.

Group II indicators are those with some divergence of opinion but in which the pacemaker can assist in the management of the patient. These indications include asymptomatic acquired complete heart block; bifascicular or trifascicular block with syncope after other causes of syncope have been excluded; prophylactic use after acute myocardial infarction during which the patient exhibited transient Mobitz type II second-degree block or complete heart block; asymptomatic Mobitz type II second-degree AV block; mildly symptomatic sinus bradycardia secondary to required long-term drug treatment; and for overdrive pacing in some patients with recurrent ventricular tachyarrhythmias.

Group III indications are those in which pacing is not routinely indicated and scientific evidence cannot support its use. These include syncope of unidentifiable origin; asymptomatic sinus bradycardia; asymptomatic sinoatrial node block or sinus arrest; asymptomatic ventricular pauses during atrial fibrillation; bradycardia during sleep; asymptomatic right bundle branch block with left anterior hemiblock; asymptomatic Mobitz type I second-degree AV block; and first-degree AV block. Asymptomatic type I second-degree AV block in which the block is located in or below the bundle of His may be an indication for permanent pacing, but supra-Hisian block is not.

## Modes of Cardiac Pacing and Cardiac Pacemaker Codes

The earliest cardiac pacemakers were simple devices that paced the ventricle or atrium without the ability to sense the patient's underlying heart rhythm. As the technology advanced, the ability to sense the patient's native heart beat was added, as was dual-chamber pacing. In the 1980s, multiprogrammability became common, allowing adjustments in many pacemaker parameters using an external programming device. Several newer pacemakers have the capability of providing antitachycardia therapy. Most recently, some pacemakers can modulate their pacing rates using physiological sensors (such as activity, acceleration, body temperature, and minute ventilation) that are independent of sinus node activity.

A pacemaker code system was developed by committees of the Intersociety Commission for Heart Disease Resources and the North American Society of Pacing and Electrophysiology (Table 1). The code initially consisted of three positions: the first to indicate the chambers paced, the second the chambers sensed, and the third the response that the pacemaker exhibited to a sensed event. A fourth position was added to identify programmability and rate modulation, and an optional fifth position indicates antitachycardia functions. The original pacemakers with no sensing capabilities are identified as VOO or AOO. A ventricular demand pacemaker is designated VVI and, with rate modulation, VVI,R. The same pacemaker used in the atrium is designated AAI or AAI,R. The pacemaker that senses atrial activity but paces the ventricle following the atrial sensing is designated VAT. Such a pacemaker is useful in treating a patient with complete heart block in whom sinus node activity is normal and can be used to modulate the ventricular pacing rate (AV synchronous pacemaker). A pacemaker that paces both chambers but senses only the ventricle is designated DVI and is useful in a patient with symptomatic sinus bradycardia in whom AV synchrony is desired (AV sequential pacemaker). A pacemaker that combines both dual-chamber pacing with dual-chamber sensing is designated DDD and is capable of tracking atrial activity and providing AV synchrony under all conditions. This is the most common dual-chamber mode used in modern pacemakers. Rate modulation has been added to DDD pacing (DDD,R) and is useful in patients with an inadequate sinus node response to exercise. Dual-chamber pacing is not appropriate for patients with frequent atrial tachyarrhythmias, in particular atrial fibrillation, but VVI pacing with rate modulation (VVI,R) is useful for maintaining heart rate response and increasing cardiac output with exercise.

Programming rate-modulated parameters should involve the use of some form of exercise testing to achieve an optimum rate response prescription. These devices typically allow the physician to determine a threshold level for rate modulation and a slope of heart rate increase in response to the sensed physiological parameter.

## PACEMAKER FOLLOW-UP

Although modern pacemakers and leads are extremely reliable, periodic evaluation of the pacemaker-lead-patient system is required. Initial thresholds for stimulation of the heart may change with time or with partial or complete

**Table 1** Pacemaker Code

| Chamber paced | Chamber sensed | Response to sensed event | Programmability and rate modulation | Antitachycardia functions |
|---|---|---|---|---|
| O = None | O = None | O = None | O = None | O = None |
| A = Atrium | A = Atrium | T = Triggered | P = Simple | P = Pacing (antitachycardia) |
| V = Ventricle | V = Ventricle | I = Inhibited | M = Multiprogrammable | |
| D = Dual | D = Dual | D = Dual | C = Communicating | S = Shock |
| | | | R = Rate modulation | D = Dual |

dislodgment of the implanted leads. Follow-up is also required to predict impending battery depletion to allow elective replacement of the pulse generator when the time arrives. Pacemakers are usually followed via telephone and/or patient visits. Single- and dual-chamber pacemakers are checked twice in the first month after implantation. Following this, single-chamber pacemakers should be checked every other month from months 2 to 36 postimplantation and monthly thereafter. Dual-chamber pacemakers should be checked monthly from months 2 to 6, every other month from months 7 to 36, and monthly thereafter. It is our practice to perform at least yearly threshold and telemetry checks in the office in patients whose routine checks are done via telephone monitoring. The telephone monitor permits transmission of a rhythm strip in the free-running mode and with magnet application but does not give information about sensitivity or output thresholds in most cases. Some pacemakers allow threshold checking via telephone.

The follow-up also involves patient reassurance and answering questions that the patient or family members may have regarding the pacemaker.

## FUTURE OF CARDIAC PACING

The future promises devices with more sophisticated (but more "user friendly") programming capabilities, more reliable and more physiological metabolic rate sensors, and more capacity for providing useful telemetric information from the patient. Great strides are being made in the application of devices to the treatment of atrial and ventricular tachyarrhythmias using antitachycardia pacing, low-energy cardioversion, and high-energy defibrillation. Because of the high incidence of bradyarrhythmias in patients with tachyarrhythmias, implantable cardioverter-defibrillators will possess backup bradycardia pacing capabilities.

## CONCLUSIONS

Bradycardias and the sick sinus syndrome, symptomatic and asymptomatic, are common in elderly individuals. Treating patients for such arrhythmias involves careful history taking, physical examination, and diagnostic testing. Correlating symptoms with abnormalities of the rhythm can be challenging and in some cases impossible. However, such a correlation is important to allow proper therapy by medications and implanted devices. There is debate about the use of pacemakers for certain indications, but the demonstration of bradycardia-induced symptoms usually makes the decision straightforward.

## REFERENCES

1. Agruss NS, Rosen EY, Adolph RJ, Fowler NO. Significance of chronic sinus bradycardia in elderly people. *Circulation* 1972; 46:924–930.

2. Camm AJ, Evans KE, Ward DE, Martin A. The rhythm of the heart in active elderly subjects. *Am Heart J* 1980; 99:598–603.
3. Fleg JL, Kennedy HL. Cardiac arrhythmias in a healthy elderly population: Detection by 24-hour ambulatory electrocardiography. *Chest* 1982; 81:302–307.
4. Kostis JB, Moreyra AE, Amendo MT, DiPietro J, Cosgrove N, Kuo PT. The effect of age on heart rate in subjects free of heart disease. Studies by ambulatory electrocardiography and maximal exercise stress testing. *Circulation* 1982; 65:141–145.
5. Sagie A, Strasberg B, Kusnieck J, Sclarovsky S. Symptomatic bradycardia induced by the combination of oral diltiazem and beta-blockers. *Clin Cardiol* 1991; 14: 314–316.
6. Holden W, McAnulty JH, Rahimtoola SH. Characterization of heart rate response to exercise in the sick sinus syndrome. *Br Heart J* 1978; 40:923–930.
7. Peretz DI, Abdulla A. Management of cardioinhibitory hypersensitive carotid sinus syncope with permanent cardiac pacing: A seventeen year prospective study. *Can J Cardiol* 1985; 1:86–91.
8. Fisher JD. The role of electrophysiologic testing in the diagnosis and treatment of patients with known and suspected bradycardias and tachycardias. *Prog Cardiovasc Dis* 1981; 24:25–90.
9. American College of Cardiology/American Heart Association Task Force on assessment of diagnostic and therapeutic cardiovascular procedures (Subcommittee to assess clinical intracardiac electrophysiologic studies). Guidelines for clinical intracardiac electrophysiologic studies. *Circulation* 1989; 80:1925–1939.
10. James TN, Sherf L, Schlant RC, Silverman ME. Anatomy of the conduction system of the heart. In: Hurst JW, ed. The Heart, 5th ed. New York: McGraw-Hill, 1982, pp. 46–56.
11. Anderson RH, Becker AE. Gross anatomy and microscopy of the conducting system. In: Mandel WJ, ed. Cardiac Arrhythmias, Their Mechanisms, Diagnosis and Management. Philadelphia: J. B. Lippincott, 1980.
12. Lev M. Anatomic basis for atrioventricular block. *Am J Med* 1964; 37:742.
13. VanBuskirk EM. Adverse reactions from timolol administration. *Ophthalmology* 1980; 87:447–450.
14. Kang PS, Gomes JA, Kelen G, El-Sherif N. Role of autonomic regulatory mechanism in sinoatrial conduction and sinus node automaticity in sick sinus syndrome. *Circulation* 1981; 64:832–838.
15. Gomes JA, Kang PS, El-Sherif N. Effects of digitalis on the human sick sinus node after pharmacologic autonomic blockade. *Am J Cardiol* 1981; 48:783–788.
16. Hilgard J, Ezri MD, Denes P. Significance of ventricular pauses of three seconds or more detected on twenty-four hour Holter recordings. *Am J Cardiol* 1985; 55:1005–1008.
17. Ector H, Rolies L, DeGeest H. Dynamic electrocardiography and ventricular pauses of three seconds and more: Etiology and therapeutic implications. *PACE* 1983; 6:548–551.
18. Volkman H, Schnerch B, Kuhnert H. Diagnostic value of carotid sinus hypersensitivity. *PACE* 1990; 13:2065–2070.
19. Sokoloff NM. Bradyarrhythmias: AV conduction disturbances. *Geriatrics* 1985; 40:83–86.

20. Frye RL, Collins JJ, DeSanctis RW, Dodge HT, Dreifus LS, Fisch C, Geths LS, Gillette PC, Parsonnett V, Reeves J, et al. Guidelines for permanent cardiac pacemaker implantation. A report of the joint American College of Cardiology/American Heart Association Task Force on assessment of cardiovascular procedures (Subcommittee on pacemaker implantation). *Circulation* 1984; 70:331A–339A.

# 24

## Syncope in the Elderly

**Wishwa N. Kapoor**
*University of Pittsburgh, Pittsburgh, Pennsylvania*

Syncope is defined as a sudden transient loss of consciousness with associated loss of postural tone. Patients must regain consciousness spontaneously and not require electrical or chemical cardioversion. Diseases that cause syncope range from common benign problems to severe life-threatening disorders. As a result, the clinical approach to this problem frequently involves hospital admission and performance of a wide variety of diagnostic tests. Although evaluation is often focused on explaining the symptom by a single disease process, this may not apply to the elderly since multiple physiological processes and age-related changes may contribute to syncope. The purpose of this review is to describe the pathophysiology and etiologies of syncope and provide a practical goal-directed evaluation of elderly patients with this symptom.

### EPIDEMIOLOGY

The incidence and prevalence of syncope in the elderly general population is not known. In one study of 771 very elderly individuals (mean age of 87 years), there was a prevalence of 23% over 10 years (1). A two-year prospective follow-up of this population revealed a yearly incidence of 6% and recurrence rate of 30%. Only 67 patients had developed syncope during this follow-up. Analysis of survival of the patients who developed syncope showed no difference in mortality between patients with cardiac, noncardiac, or syncope of unknown etiology.

In a study of 210, mostly community-dwelling elderly patients (mean age 71 years), a cause of syncope was not established in 40% of patients (2). Patients with a cardiac cause of syncope had a higher mortality than those with noncardiac cause of syncope or unknown cause but there was no difference in mortality between young and elderly with cardiac causes. In multivariate analysis, in patients with noncardiac cause or unknown cause of syncope, a history of congestive heart failure, older age, and male sex were important prognostic factors.

## PATHOPHYSIOLOGY

The vast majority of causes of syncope result from transient decrease in cerebral blood flow to those parts of the brain subserving consciousness (brainstem reticular activating system). During hypotension, there is a reduction in cerebral blood flow and cerebral oxygen utilization. Studies on experimental cardiac arrest and acute anoxia in humans have shown that after 5–15 s there was loss of consciousness, pallor, and muscle relaxation. More prolonged cerebral ischemia (> 15 s) was associated with generalized tonic spasm and incontinence.

There are four general mechanisms of transient cerebral hypoperfusion that may result in syncope: (1) vasomotor instability associated with disorders that decrease systemic vascular resistance or venous return or both; (2) critical reduction of cardiac output due to obstruction of blood flow within the heart or pulmonary circulation; (3) cardiac arrhythmias leading to transient decline in cardiac output; and (4) cerebrovascular disease with focal or generalized decreased cerebral perfusion.

Rarely, normal or even increased cerebral blood flow can be associated with loss or alteration of consciousness when there is a lack of essential nutrients necessary for cerebral metabolism. These states include hypoglycemia, hypoxemia, and hypercarbia; however, these disorders more frequently lead to somnolence and coma than syncope. Additionally, seizures occasionally mimic syncope; in these instances, cerebral blood flow may be normal and loss of consciousness results from an abnormal electrical discharge.

Lipsitz has noted that multiple pathologic abnormalities in the elderly may be particularly important in causing a reduction in cerebral blood flow and leading to syncope (3,4). It is well known that patients 65 years of age or older have an average of 3.5 chronic diseases (5). These coexisting conditions include coronary artery disease, diabetes mellitus, congestive heart failure, chronic obstructive lung disease, renal insufficiency, and others. Furthermore, elderly patients are often taking multiple medications. Thus, multiple comorbid conditions in these settings may make elderly persons more prone to syncope, while one factor alone may not be sufficient to lead to loss of consciousness.

Several physiological impairments that are a result of aging may also be important in predisposing elderly patients to syncope (4). These processes include:

1. Decreased baroreceptor response. Baroreflex sensitivity is known to diminish with aging. In normal, young individuals, cerebral blood flow is maintained by increasing heart rate and vascular tone in the setting of hypotension. In the elderly, the baroreflex response is decreased, predisposing patients to hypotension and syncope. Examples of problems include higher sensitivity of the elderly to the effects of vasodilators and a diminished ability to respond to hypotension from volume loss, hemorrhage, upright posture, and Valsalva's maneuver.
2. Decreased heart rate response. Aging may be associated with decreased cardiac sensitivity to adrenergic stimulation. This may be due to a defect in sympathetic responsiveness that develops with aging. Blunted heart rate response may occur with upright posture, exercise, hypoxia, and hypercarbia. Because of this blunted response, adjustment to ordinary circumstances may be impaired, predisposing the elderly to syncope.
3. Decreased ability to maintain extracellular volume. In the elderly, there is a diminished ability of the kidney to conserve sodium in the face of salt restriction and decreased basal plasma levels of renin and aldosterone. These changes may make the elderly more susceptible to orthostatic hypotension and syncope. As a result, the effects of diuretics, salt restriction, and upright posture may be more pronounced in the elderly.

## ETIOLOGIES OF SYNCOPE

Because of multiple chronic diseases, medication, and age-related physiological changes, syncope is common and assigning an etiology is often difficult. Furthermore, evaluation of syncope in the elderly is complicated by atypical presentation of disease, since the symptoms of common or serious illnesses may present in a nonspecific fashion. Thus, a careful and meticulous evaluation of the elderly is necessary to arrive at the cause of the patient's symptoms. Table 1 shows a list of major etiologies of syncope. A brief discussion of these entities will be provided first, since they are important in determining an approach to the evaluation of this problem.

### Vasovagal Syncope

Vasovagal syncope is characterized by a sudden fall in blood pressure in association with autonomic and humoral activity such as pallor, nausea, sweating,

**Table 1** Etiologies of Syncope

| | |
|---|---|
| Vasodepressor | Seizure |
| Situational | Psychogenic |
| Micturition syncope | Anxiety disorder |
| Defecation syncope | Panic disorder |
| Cough syncope | Somatization |
| Swallow syncope | Depression |
| Drug-induced syncope | |
| Orthostatic hypotension | |
| Cerebrovascular disease | |
| Carotid sinus syncope | |
| Glossopharyngeal neuralgia | |
| Trigeminal neuralgia | |
| CARDIAC DISEASES | |
| Obstruction to Flow | |
| Obstruction to left ventricular outflow: aortic stenosis and hypertrophic cardiomyopathy, left atrial myxoma, mitral stenosis | |
| Obstruction to pulmonary flow: pulmonic stenosis, pulmonary hypertension, pulmonary embolism, Tetralogy of Fallot, right atrial myxomas | |
| Pump failure: myocardial infarct, unstable angina, coronary spasm | |
| Cardiac tamponade | |
| Aortic dissection | |
| Arrhythmias | |
| Bradyarrhythmias | |
| Sinus node disease | |
| Second and third degree atrioventricular block | |
| Pacemaker malfunction | |
| Drug-induced bradyarrhythmias | |
| Tachyarrhythmias | |
| Ventricular tachycardia | |
| Torsades de pointes (e.g., associated with congenital long QT syndromes or acquired QT prolongation) | |
| Supraventricular tachycardia | |

Reprinted from Kapoor WN. Diagnostic evaluation of syncope. *Am J Med* 1991; 90:91–106.

mydriasis, bradycardia, and hyperventilation. Vasodepressor syncope occurs both in the young and the elderly, often in response to fear or injury. Examples of predisposing factors include fatigue, prolonged standing, venipuncture, blood donation, and heat. Vasovagal syncope may also occur without any identifiable predisposing factors and may be provoked by standing still in an upright posture in susceptible individuals.

Vasovagal syncope is preceded by evidence of an increase in sympathetic activity and a decrease in vagal activity immediately prior to loss of consciousness. During this phase, blood pressure and heart rate increase. This is abruptly followed by hypotension and often bradycardia. The hypotension is due to vasodilatation in the skeletal muscles as well as other tissues due to the inhibition of sympathetic vasoconstrictor activity. The vasodilatation is in large part mediated by reflexes initiated by the stimulation of cardiac mechanoreceptors. The mechanism of excitation is probably an increased force of ventricular contraction in the setting of reduced ventricular filling.

Although vasovagal syncope is more common in young individuals, recent studies with upright tilt table testing show that it may also be a common cause of syncope in elderly patients who present with syncope of unknown etiology.

## Situational Syncope

### *Micturition Syncope*

Micturition syncope has been described in the young and the elderly. Loss of consciousness in healthy young men occurs after rising from bed in the early morning hours, during or immediately after urination. Predisposing factors include reduced food intake, recent upper respiratory tract infection, fatigue, and ingestion of alcohol. Older patients (mean age 60 years) with multiple acute and chronic medical problems have been reported with micturition syncope (6). No cause for micturition syncope could be implicated, but the majority of elderly patients have had orthostatic hypotension.

A combination of physiological changes during sleep and micturition may act together, leading to a decline in cerebral blood flow during urination. Physiological changes include sudden decompression of the bladder, leading to hypotension and circulatory collapse; a decline of blood pressure and heart rate mediated by decreased peripheral resistance during sleep; vagal stimuli associated with micturition; and Valsalva's maneuver associated with a decrease in venous return. In the elderly, orthostatic hypotension may be aggravated by one or more of the aforementioned physiological changes leading to micturition syncope.

### *Defecation Syncope*

Syncope in association with defecation in one study was associated with a variety of gastrointestinal tract (Meckel's, ruptured appendix) and cardiovascular diseases (ventricular arrhythmias), as well as orthostatic hypotension and transient ischemic attacks (7). No specific associated disorder could be identified in approximately half of the patients. Cases of association with pulmonary embolism have been reported (8).

The mechanism of defecation syncope may be hypotension and/or bradycardia due to the combined effects of defecation with the physiological changes secondary to sleep in the setting of acute or chronic medical disorders.

### *Cough Syncope*

Syncope after paroxysms of severe cough is described primarily in middle-aged men with acute or chronic lung disease. At least two mechanisms are suggested: (1) coughing may produce extremely high intrathoracic pressure, resulting in a decreased venous return and cardiac output; (2) it is also recognized that intrathoracic pressure during cough is transmitted to the subarachnoid space, and the resulting extremely high pressure within the cranium may reduce cerebral blood flow and cause syncope.

Rare case reports have associated cough syncope with Mobitz II or complete AV block, obstructive cardiomyopathy, hypersensitive carotid sinus syndrome, herniated-cerebellar tonsils, severe bilateral carotid artery disease, and Arnold Chiari malformation.

### *Swallow Syncope*

Generally, patients who have reported syncope during or immediately after swallowing have had structural abnormalities of the esophagus or the heart (9–11). Examples of esophageal disorders include diverticula, diffuse esophageal spasm, achalasia, and stricture. Cardiac conditions have included acute rheumatic carditis on digitalis, acute myocardial infarction, and a calcified mass over the aortic valve and septum. Bradyarrhythmias have been found to be the cause of swallow syncope and include sinus arrest, complete AV block, nodal or sinus bradycardia, and sinoatrial block. Vagolytic agents or pacemakers have reportedly abolished symptoms.

## Drug-Induced Syncope

Drug-induced syncope is due to alteration of vascular volume or tone (e.g., antihypertensive agents, nitrates), arrhythmias (e.g., digoxin toxicity, torsades de pointes associated with prolonged QT interval), or an allergic or anaphylactic reaction. Drugs are responsible for 2–9% of symptoms in patients presenting with syncope. The most common drugs causing syncope include nitrates, beta blockers, and vasodilators (Table 2).

## Orthostatic Hypotension

Several homeostatic adjustments in the brain and reflexes in the systemic circulation are responsible for maintaining blood pressure. Upon standing, approximately 500 ml of blood is pooled in the lower extremities and the splanchnic circulation. This reduction in venous return to the heart results in decreased car-

**Table 2** Common Drugs Causing Syncope

| | |
|---|---|
| Vasodilators | Psychoactive drugs |
| Nitrates | Phenothiazines |
| Calcium channel blockers | Antidepressants |
| ACE inhibitors | (e.g., tricyclic agents, MAO inhibitors) |
| Others (e.g., prazosin, hydralazine) | CNS depressants (e.g., barbiturates) |
| Drugs associated with torsades de pointes | Other mechanisms |
| Quinidine | Vincristine and other neuropathic drugs |
| Procainamide | Digitalis |
| Disopyramide | Insulin |
| Flecainide | Marijuana |
| Encainide | Alcohol |
| Amiodarone | Cocaine |
| Sotalol | |
| Diuretics | |

ACE = angiotensin converting enzyme; CNS = central nervous system; MAO = monoamine oxidase inhibitor.
Reprinted from Kapoor WN. Diagnostic evaluation of syncope. *Am J Med* 1991; 90:91–106.

diac output, which leads to stimulation of aortic, carotid, and cardiopulmonary baroreceptors. This results in an increase in sympathetic outflow and a decrease in parasympathetic activity, leading to an increase in heart rate and vascular resistance to maintain systemic blood pressure (12).

A wide variety of disorders and drugs are associated with orthostatic hypotension. Decreased intravascular volume and adverse effects of drugs are the most common causes of symptomatic orthostatic hypotension (12). Orthostatic hypotension is also an important manifestation of autonomic dysfunction, which may result from a wide variety of diseases and drugs (13) (Table 3).

Idiopathic orthostatic hypotension is a rare illness that affects men five times more than women, and is often associated with other autonomic disturbances such as sphincter disturbances, impotence, impaired erection and ejaculation, and impaired sweating. Plasma norepinephrine levels are markedly reduced at rest and remain unchanged upon standing, suggesting a peripheral dysfunction.

Shy–Drager syndrome is associated with autonomic failure and involvement of the corticospinal, extrapyramidal, and cerebellar tracts including a Parkinsonlike syndrome. Laryngeal stridor, as well as cholinergic dysfunction affecting the vagal, ocular, bladder, and sweat glands, has also been reported. A diffuse degenerative process has been well described but no specific etiology is

**Table 3** Causes of Orthostatic Hypotension

1. Primary
   (a) Pure autonomic failure (idiopathic orthostatic hypotension)
   (b) Autonomic failure with multiple system atrophy (Shy and Drager syndrome)
   (c) Autonomic failure with Parkinson's disease
2. Secondary
   (a) General medical disorders: diabetes; amyloid; alcoholism
   (b) Autoimmune disease: acute and subacute dysautonomia; Guillain-Barré syndrome; mixed connective tissue disease; rheumatoid arthritis; Eaton-Lambert syndrome; systematic lupus erythematosus
   (c) Carcinomatous autonomic neuropathy
   (d) Metabolic disease: porphyria; Fabry's disease; Tangier disease; $B_{12}$-deficiency
   (e) Hereditary sensory neuropathies, dominant or recessive
   (f) Infections of the nervous system: syphilis; Chagas' disease; HIV infection; botulism; herpes zoster
   (g) Central brain lesions: vascular lesion or tumors involving the hypothalamus and midbrain, for example, craniopharyngioma; multiple sclerosis; Wernicke's encephalopathy
   (h) Spinal cord lesions
   (i) Familial dysautonomia
   (j) Familial hyperbradykinism
   (k) Renal failure
   (l) Dopamine $\beta$-hydroxylase deficiency
   (m) Aging
3. Drugs
   (a) Selective neurotoxic drugs; alcoholism
   (b) Tranquillizers: phenothiazines; barbiturates
   (c) Antidepressants: tricyclics; monoamine oxidase inhibitors
   (d) Vasodilator hypotensive drugs: prazosin; hydralazine
   (e) Centrally acting hypotensive drugs: methyldopa; clonidine
   (f) Adrenergic neuron blocking drugs: guanethidine
   (g) $\alpha$-Adrenergic blocking drugs: phenoxybenzamine; labetalol
   (h) Ganglion-blocking drugs: hexamethonium; mecamylamine
   (i) Angiotensin-converting enzyme inhibitors: captopril; enalapril; lisinopril

Adapted from *Autonomic Failure*, Second edition, 1988 (Bannister SR, ed.), Oxford University Press, p. 8.

known. Norepinephrine levels are normal at rest but remain unchanged upon standing, suggesting an inability to stimulate normally functioning peripheral neurons.

Lesions of the spinal cord caused by neck trauma and other disorders, such as transverse myelitis, syringomyelia, and various tumors, may also result in severe orthostatic hypotension. Orthostatic hypotension may also be a manifestation of peripheral neuropathy that involves sympathetic fibers. This may be associated with diseases such as diabetes mellitus, amyloidosis, porphyria, chronic alcoholism, and pernicious anemia. Acute infectious neuropathy (e.g., Guillain-Barré syndrome) may also cause orthostatic hypotension.

Central lesions that may result in orthostasis include parasellar and posterior fossa tumors, cerebral infarcts, and Wernicke's encephalopathy.

## Cerebrovascular Disease

Syncope is an unusual manifestation of TIAs. Only about 15% of patients with vertebrobasilar TIA have drop attacks or syncope. Syncope and drop attacks are generally accompanied by other neurological symptoms of ischemia in the vertebrobasilar distribution. Syncope is generally not a manifestation of carotid artery ischemia unless accompanied by disease of the vertebral arteries. Transient ischemic attacks may result from atherosclerotic disease, inflammatory disorders (e.g., giant cell arteritis, systemic lupus erythematosus), aortic arch syndrome, dissection of extracranial arteries, cardiac diseases leading to emboli (e.g., rheumatic heart disease, myxoma), anomalies of the cervical spine, and others (14). Subclavian steal syndrome due to subclavian artery stenosis and reversal of blood in the ipsilateral vertebral artery to supply blood flow to the arm is also rarely associated with syncope. A difference in blood pressure in two arms (usually $\geqslant$ 20 mm Hg) and pulse intensity are helpful diagnostically (15).

"Faint sensation" is reported in 12–18% of patients with migraine (16). Common migraine may result in syncope and orthostatic hypotension possibly due to a defect in the noradrenergic nervous system described during migraine attack. Migraines may also lead to a vasovagal reaction due to pain.

## Carotid Sinus Syncope

Carotid sinus syncope is primarily a disorder of the elderly. The carotid sinus baroreceptors consist of sensory nerve endings located in the internal carotid artery just above the bifurcation of the common carotid artery. Afferent impulses travel via the sinus nerve of Hering and join the glossopharyngeal, cervical sympathetic, and vagus nerves to the sensory nucleus of the vagus (solitary tract) and the vasomotor center. Efferent pathways include sympathetic adrenergic nerves to the heart, resistance and capacitance vessels, and cardiac vagus nerve (17).

Three types of carotid sinus hypersensitivity are recognized (17). Cardioinhibitory response is widely defined as cardiac asystole of $\geqslant$ 3 s. The pure vasodepressor type is defined as a systolic blood pressure decline of $\geqslant$ 50 mm Hg (in the absence of significant bradycardia). A mixed type consists of a combination of cardioinhibitory and vasodepressor response. The prevalence of carotid sinus hypersensitivity in an asymptomatic population is reported to be 5–25%, occurring in the elderly, and is found 2–4 times more commonly in men. The cardioinhibitory variety accounts for 34–78% and the vasodepressor variety for 5–10% of cases of carotid sinus hypersensitivity.

From 5–20% of individuals with abnormal carotid sensitivity suffer spontaneous loss of consciousness, termed carotid sinus syncope. Attacks may be precipitated by factors that exert pressure on the carotid sinus (tight collar, shaving, sudden turning, etc.), but a history of this is obtained in only a quarter of patients with this syndrome. The majority have coronary artery disease and hypertension. Predisposing factors include neck pathology, such as enlarged lymph nodes, scar tissue, carotid body tumors, parotid, thyroid, and head and neck tumors. Possible association with digitalis, alpha methyldopa, and propranolol is reported.

Commonly, massage is done in the supine position, and occasionally repeated in the sitting and standing positions if the vasodepressor variety is suspected and the supine test is negative. Electrocardiographic and blood pressure monitoring is needed during testing. Mixed response (cardioinhibitory and vasodepressor) is diagnosed when carotid sinus massage is performed after bradycardia is abolished with atropine or atrioventricular sequential pacing. The duration of massage has varied from 5–40 s, but recent recommendations are for a limit of 5 s (17). Simultaneous bilateral massage should never be done. At least 15 s should be allowed between massage from one side to the other. Complications of carotid sinus massage include prolonged asystole, ventricular fibrillation, transient or permanent neurological deficit, and sudden death. Complication rates are not available but are considered extremely low; however, in patients with cerebrovascular disease the test should be done only if all other diagnostic modalities are exhausted and the pretest probability of carotid sinus syncope remains high.

Carotid sinus syncope is diagnosed in patients who are found to have carotid sinus hypersensitivity if they have (1) loss of consciousness related to activities that press or stretch the carotid sinus; or (2) recurrent syncope with a negative workup. Symptom reproduction during carotid sinus massage is generally not necessary (17).

## NEURALGIA

Syncope has been reported during an attack of glossopharyngeal or trigeminal neuralgia. In most instances, syncope is due to asystole or bradycardia and rarely due to a vasodepressor reaction (18,19).

## Seizure

A seizure disorder is often considered in the differential diagnosis of syncope. It is well recognized that convulsion may occur after hypotension and cerebral ischemia. For example, 12% of patients with vasovagal syncope after blood donation develop convulsions. Furthermore, experimental cerebral ischemia of more than 15 s is regularly associated with seizurelike activity. Confusion after loss of consciousness supports a diagnosis of seizure rather syncope (20).

## Psychiatric Illnesses

Psychiatric illnesses are important causes of syncope but they are more often found in younger patients. Generalized anxiety may produce hyperventilation and vasodepressor reactions resulting in loss of consciousness. Syncope is also a manifestation of panic disorder, accounting for up to 9% of the presenting somatic complaints in this illness (21). Approximately 4.5% of patients with somatization disorder have loss of consciousness consistent with syncope. Major depression has also been associated with syncope (22).

## Cardiac Diseases

Syncope is primarily due to disorders that result in severe obstruction to cardiac output or rhythm disturbances.

### *Obstruction to Flow*

Table 1 shows a list of structural diseases of the heart that may critically reduce cerebral blood flow and result in syncope. Exertional syncope is a common manifestation of heart disease in which cardiac output is fixed and does not rise (or even falls) with exercise. Syncope occurs in up to 42% of patients with severe aortic stenosis, commonly with exercise (23). The mechanisms of exertional syncope in aortic stenosis are similar to loss of consciousness associated with other states of left ventricular outflow obstruction. Systemic vascular resistance normally decreases with exercise, which is due to arteriolar dilatation. Normally, the decline in peripheral vascular resistance results in a compensatory response that leads to an increase in cardiac output, thus maintaining arterial pressure. However, when there is a severe outflow obstruction, cardiac output may not increase, leading to hypotension and syncope. Additionally, in patients with aortic stenosis, reflex vasodilatation may occur since high intraventricular pressure may stimulate ventricular mechanoreceptors, leading to hypotension and syncope. Syncope is prognostically important in the natural history of aortic stenosis; average survival is 2–3 years after onset of syncope in the absence of valve replacement.

The pathophysiological mechanism of syncope in hypertrophic cardiomyopathy is similar. Syncope is reported in as many as 30% of patients with hypertrophic cardiomyopathy. Left ventricular outflow obstruction can worsen by an increase in contractility, a decrease in size, or decrease in afterload or distending pressure. Thus, conditions such as Valsalva's maneuver, severe coughing paroxysm, or specific drugs (e.g., digitalis) may precipitate hypotension and syncope. Ventricular tachycardia is reported in approximately 25% of adult patients with hypertrophic cardiomyopathy and constitutes an important cause of syncope in this disease (24,25).

Effort syncope is reported in up to 30% of patients with primary pulmonary hypertension and also occurs with severe pulmonic stenosis. Cardiac output may not increase due to limitations to right ventricular outflow. This, in association with lowered peripheral resistance with exercise, may lead to hypotension and syncope. Patients with congenital heart disease (e.g., tetralogy of Fallot, patent ductus arteriosus, and interventricular or interatrial septal defects) may have syncope with effort or crying due to sudden reversal of a left-to-right shunt and fall in arterial oxygen saturation.

Atrial myxomas may result in obstruction of the mitral or tricuspid valve, leading to symptoms of cardiac failure and rarely syncope. Syncope, dyspnea, and cardiac murmurs that change with body position are particularly suggestive of myxoma (26). Mitral stenosis may rarely lead to syncope that may be due to severe obstruction to outflow, atrial fibrillation with rapid ventricular response, pulmonary hypertension, or a cerebral embolic event.

Of elderly patients with acute myocardial infarction, 5–12% may present with syncope rather than chest pain. Mechanisms responsible for syncope include: (1) sudden pump failure leading to hypotension; and (2) rhythm disturbance that may include ventricular tachycardia or bradyarrhythmias. Bradyarrhythmias due to excessive parasympathetic tone are reported in up to 17% of patients with acute myocardial infarction. These arrhythmias usually occur in inferior or posterior myocardial infarction due to vascular occlusion of branches that supply the sinus or AV node. Unstable angina and coronary artery spasm also have been rarely associated with syncope (27).

Syncope occurs in 5% of patients with aortic dissection. Loss of consciousness is often due to rupture into the pericardial space, resulting in sudden cardiac tamponade (28).

Syncope is reported in 10–15% of patients with pulmonary embolism and is more commonly associated with massive embolism. Pulmonary embolism may result in acute right ventricular failure, and increased right ventricular filling pressure and decreased stroke volume. Subsequent decreased cardiac output and hypotension leads to loss of consciousness. Consciousness is regained when the embolus breaks and migrates distally in the pulmonary artery. Transient sinus bradycardia and AV block, possibly due to parasympathetic reflex in patients with recurrent pulmonary embolism and chronic corpulmonale, are also reported, as well as syncope due to right atrial thromboembolism.

### *Arrhythmias*

Sinus bradycardia may be from excessive vagal tone, decreased sympathetic tone, or sinus node disease. Sinus bradycardia occurs with eye surgery, myxedema, intracranial and mediastinal tumors, and with a large number of parasympathomimetic, sympatholytic, beta blockers, and other drugs. Conjunctival instillation of beta blockers may also cause symptomatic bradycardia.

Syncope is reported in 25–70% of patients with sick sinus syndrome. Electrocardiographic manifestations include sinus bradycardia, pauses, arrest, or exit block. Additionally, supraventricular tachycardia or atrial fibrillation may occur in association with bradycardia, or atrial fibrillation may be associated with slow ventricular response (tachycardia–bradycardia syndrome).

Ventricular tachycardias are an important cause of syncope and commonly occur in the setting of known organic heart disease. Torsades de pointes and syncope occur in the setting of syndromes of congenital prolongation of Q-T interval (with or without deafness) as well as acquired long QT syndromes associated with drugs, electrolyte abnormalities, and central nervous system disorders (29). Antiarrhythmic drugs are the most common cause of torsades de pointes as reported with quinidine (quinidine syncope), procainamide, disopyramide, flecainide, encainide, amiodarone, and sotalol (30).

Syncope may also be associated with other tachyarrhythmias such as atrial fibrillation or flutter with rapid ventricular response, AV nodal reentrant tachycardia, and supraventricular tachycardia in patients with Wolff-Parkinson-White syndrome (31).

## DIAGNOSTIC EVALUATION

The most important elements in the evaluation of syncope are determining whether the patient had syncope and then planning a workup to define the etiology of loss of consciousness.

A history from the patient and the witness, if present, is needed to separate syncope from other entities such as dizziness, vertigo, drop attacks, coma, and seizure. A particularly important issue is the distinction between syncope and seizure. A study comparing the clinical symptoms of patients with syncope and seizure showed that a wide variety of symptoms were associated with seizures, including blue face (or not pale), frothing at the mouth, tongue biting, disorientation, aching muscles, sleepiness after event, and unconsciousness for a period of more than 5 min. On the other hand, symptoms associated with syncope were sweating or nausea before the event and no disorientation after the event. Disorientation after the episode is much more frequently reported by patients with seizure than syncope (20).

### History, Physical Examination, and Baseline Laboratory Tests

Once it has been determined that the patient had syncope, a history and physical examination are crucial in choosing diagnostic tests to ascertain the etiology.

A detailed account of syncope, the events leading to loss of consciousness, and symptoms following the episode are crucial to diagnosing specific entities. In diagnosing vasovagal syncope, precipitating factors, in conjunction with autonomic symptoms, lead to diagnosis (6–11). Syncope during or immediately after micturition, cough, defecation, and swallow are well described and easily diagnosed by history. Syncope associated with neurological symptoms of brain stem ischemia suggest transient ischemic attacks, basilar artery migraines, and subclavian steal syndrome (14–16). A detailed drug history is important (Table 2). A wide variety of other clinical presentations may suggest specific entities that need to be confirmed. Examples include syncope with arm exercise (suggesting subclavian steal syndrome syncope), syncope in a deaf child with effort or emotional distress (suggesting long QT syndromes), and syncope with flushing and itching (suggesting systemic mastocytosis) (32). A detailed description of these entities can be found elsewhere (32,33).

Physical examination is used to diagnose specific entities and exclude others. In the elderly, orthostatic hypotension, cardiovascular findings, and neurological examination are critical in this regard.

Orthostatic hypotension is generally defined as a decline of 20 mm Hg or more in systolic pressure and often of 10 mm Hg or more in diastolic pressure upon assuming an upright position. However, this finding is reported in up to 24% of the elderly and is frequently not associated with symptoms. Thus, the clinical diagnosis of orthostatic hypotension should incorporate the presence of symptoms in association with a decrease in systolic blood pressure, and often diastolic blood pressure as well. Symptoms due to orthostatic hypotension include dizziness or light-headedness, blurring or loss of vision, a sense of profound weakness, and syncope. These symptoms are often worse upon arising in the morning and may be especially prominent after meals or exercise. A systolic blood pressure decline of $\geqslant$ 20 mm Hg after a meal has been reported in as high as 36% of elderly nursing home residents, occurring at 45–60 min in most patients (34). This decline is often asymptomatic, but occasionally may lead to syncope and presyncope.

There are no standardized methods for detection of orthostatic hypotension. Supine blood pressure and heart rate should be measured after the patient has been lying down for at least 5 min. Standing measurements should be obtained immediately and for at least 2 min. These measurements should be carried out for 10 min if there is a high suspicion of orthostatic hypotension but a drop in blood pressure is not found earlier (35). Orthostatic hypotension may be missed if only sitting blood pressure is obtained (12).

Several cardiovascular findings are crucial diagnostically. Differences in the pulse intensity and blood pressure (generally $>$ 20 mm Hg) in the two arms are suggestive of aortic dissection or subclavian steal syndrome. Special focus on cardiovascular examination for aortic stenosis, idiopathic hypertrophic subaortic stenosis, pulmonary hypertension, myxomas, and aortic dissection may uncover clues to these entities.

In recent studies, in those patients in whom a diagnosis could be assigned, the history and physical examination identified a potential cause in 49–85% (36–41). Furthermore, organic cardiac diseases causing syncope (e.g., aortic stenosis, idiopathic hypertrophic subaortic stenosis, pulmonary embolism) and neurological diseases (e.g., subclavian steal syndrome) are strongly suspected by the history and physical examination. Testing for these diseases should be selective and based upon findings of a careful history and physical examination. In one study, suggestive findings on history and physical examination were helpful in assigning the ultimate cause of syncope by directed testing in 8% of additional patients (37).

Table 4 shows the results in the elderly as compared to the young (2). In the elderly, arrhythmias were more often diagnosed as the etiology as compared to the young. Several entities were primarily found in the elderly and included aortic stenosis, TIA's, and carotid sinus syncope.

Initial laboratory blood tests rarely yield diagnostically helpful information (36–41). In studies that included patients with seizure, 2–3% had hypoglycemia, hyponatremia, hypocalcemia, or renal failure (36–41). These tests were confirmatory of clinical suspicion of these electrolyte abnormalities and in one study only one unexpected finding was discovered (hyponatremia with seizures) (9). Bleeding as a cause of syncope was diagnosed clinically, but was confirmed by a complete blood count or hemoccult tests (36–41).

## Arrhythmia Detection

### *ECG/Rhythm Strip*

An abnormal electrocardiogram is found in 50% of patients with syncope but is rarely diagnostic of the cause of syncope (37). In 2–11% of patients with syncope, a cause is assigned by initial electrocardiogram or a rhythm strip (36–41). Furthermore, initial abnormalities on electrocardiogram such as bundle branch block, Wolfe-Parkinson-White syndrome, or unsustained ventricular tachycardia may guide further diagnostic testing for arrhythmic syncope. Finally, the finding of a normal ECG may help guide further evaluation since arrhythmias are less likely in patients with a normal ECG. In one study of the elderly, ECG led to a diagnosis in 9% of patients as compared to 4% of the young group (Table 5) (2).

Exercise treadmill testing can be used for provoking exercise-induced tachyarrhythmias when they are suspected clinically (e.g., patients with exertional syncope). However, this test is rarely useful for arrhythmia detection in most patients with syncope.

**Table 4** Causes of Syncope

| | Young (patients) | Elderly (patients) |
|---|---|---|
| | *n* | *n* |
| Cardiovascular Causes of Syncope | | |
| Ventricular tachycardia | 13[a] | 33 |
| Sick sinus syndrome | 3 | 12[a] |
| Carotid sinus syncope | 0 | 5 |
| Supraventricular tachycardia | 5 | 0 |
| Bradycardia | 1 | 2 |
| Second-degree atrioventricular block | 1 | 1 |
| Complete heart block | 1 | 5 |
| Pacemaker malfunction | 2 | 1 |
| Aortic stenosis | 0 | 8 |
| Myocardial infarction | 1 | 4 |
| Dissecting aortic aneurysm | 1 | 0 |
| Pulmonary embolus | 2 | 0 |
| Pulmonary hypertension | 2 | 0 |
| Total | 32 | 71 |
| Noncardiovascular Causes of Syncope | | |
| Vasodepressor | 29 | 3 |
| Orthostatic hypotension | 17 | 18 |
| Situational | 17 | 15 |
| Drug-induced | 2 | 7 |
| Transient ischemic attack | 1 | 7 |
| Seizure | 3[a] | 3[a] |
| Subclavian steal | 0 | 2 |
| Trigeminal neuralgia | 0 | 1 |
| Psychiatric | 3[a] | 0 |
| Total | 72 | 56 |

[a] Diagnoses made on follow-up: ventricular tachycardia (one patient), sick sinus syndrome (one patient), seizure disorder (two young patients, three elderly patients), and conversion reaction (one patient).

## *Prolonged Electrocardiographic Monitoring*

In the elderly, arrhythmias were diagnosed more frequently by monitoring as compared to the young (Table 5) (2). However, the use of electrocardiographic monitoring (Holter) in diagnosing arrhythmias is often problematic since the vast majority of detected arrhythmias are brief and produce no symptoms (42). Furthermore, a wide variety of brief arrhythmias are reported in otherwise asymptomatic elderly individuals. The sensitivity and specificity of ambulatory

**Table 5** Diagnostic Studies that Established a Cause of Syncope

| | Young (patients) | Elderly (patients) |
|---|---|---|
| | *n* | *n* |
| History and physical examination | 38 | 25 |
| Electrocardiography | 4 | 9 |
| Electrocardiographic monitoring | 8 | 17[a] |
| Electroencephalography | 0.5 | 0.5 |
| Carotid massage | 0 | 2 |
| Electrophysiologic studies | 1 | 2 |
| Cardiac catheterization | 2 | 4 |
| Cerebral angiography | 0 | 1 |
| Stress test | 1 | 0 |

[a] $p = 0.008$

From Kapoor W, Snustad D, Peterson J, Wieand HS, Cha R, Karpf M. Syncope in the elderly. *Am J Med* 1986; 80:419–428.

monitoring for diagnosis of arrhythmic syncope are not known because of the lack of criteria for abnormal results or a gold standard that is independent of arrhythmias diagnosed by monitoring. Table 5 shows a summary of the studies that have reported on monitoring for evaluation of syncope and dizziness (37,42–49). These studies were chosen if they reported at least 12 h of monitoring and noted symptoms during the monitoring period. Symptomatic correlation with an arrhythmia was found in 4% of the patients. In an additional 17%, no arrhythmias were found but patients had symptoms. In some of these patients, symptoms may be similar to the presenting syncope and thus arrhythmias can be excluded as an etiology. In approximately 13% of the patients, asymptomatic arrhythmias are found and in 69% of the patients, no arrhythmias are recorded during monitoring. Since arrhythmias may be episodic, lack of finding arrhythmias does not exclude a rhythm disturbance as a cause of syncope.

Monitoring longer than 24 h is not likely to increase the yield of symptomatic arrhythmias. In one study, although there was an increased yield of brief arrhythmias after the first 24 h (14.7% were abnormal during the first 24 h, 11% during the second 24 h, and 4.2% during the third 24 h), none of the arrhythmias during the second and third 24 h were associated with symptoms (49).

More prolonged monitoring for weeks to months is also possible using patient-activated intermittent loop recorders. This type of a recorder can capture arrhythmias during a syncopal episode if the patient activates it after regaining consciousness. The device can record 4–5 min of retrograde electrocardiographic rhythm strip. The experience with this recorder has been limited. In one study of patients with multiple recurrences of syncope (median of 10 episodes), 7 of the 57 patients had an arrhythmia found with recurrent symptoms of which 3 were due to neurally mediated syncope (50). Seven others had negative findings, therefore excluding arrhythmias as a cause of syncope. However, in 18 patients there were technical problems with use of the recorder resulting in an inability to arrive at a diagnosis. Thus, at the current time, patient-activated loop monitors appear to be useful in a small subset of patients who have high probability of recurrences.

### *Electrophysiologic Studies*

The indications for electrophysiologic studies in patients with syncope have not been systematically defined. These tests are more likely to be abnormal in patients with underlying heart disease, as follows (51–61):

1. Patients with structural heart disease including coronary artery disease, prior myocardial infarction, congestive heart failure, valvular heart disease, and hypertrophic cardiomyopathy.
2. ECG abnormalities, such as bundle branch block or Wolf-Parkinson-White.
3. Abnormalities on ambulatory monitoring such as unsustained ventricular tachycardia.

Predictors of a negative electrophysiologic study in patients with syncope include: the absence of heart disease; an ejection fraction > 40%; normal electrocardiogram and Holter monitoring; absence of injury during syncope; and multiple or prolonged (> 5 min) episodes of syncope (60).

In the reported studies of findings from electrophysiologic testing in patients with unexplained syncope (Table 6), approximately 45% have had inducible ventricular tachycardia, 22% supraventricular tachycardia, 28% conduction disturbance (abnormal sinus node, atrioventricular node, or His-Purkinje function), and 5% other abnormalities (including hypervagotonia and carotid hypersensitivity). These data do not include results of studies on special subsets as those with bundle branch block (62), carotid sinus hypersensitivity (63), excess vagal tone (64), and electrophysiologic studies with upright tilt (65). In the elderly, a study of 75 patients who were 75 years old or older showed electrophysiologic testing to be abnormal in 68% (66). The abnormalities consisted of sinus node disease in 55%, His-bundle conduction abnormalities in 39%, and inducible ventricular tachycardia in 14% (66).

A problem in using electrophysiologic testing has been the clinical significance of abnormal findings in assigning an etiology of syncope. The problems include:

The finding of prolonged sinus node recovery time has low sensitivity for diagnosis of sinus node dysfunction (18–69%), although it is reported to have

**Table 6** Results of Electrophysiologic Testing in Patients with Syncope of Unknown Etiology

| | No. Patients | Abnormal EP (%) | EP Abnormality (%)[a] | | | |
|---|---|---|---|---|---|---|
| | | | SVT | VT | Conduction[b] | Other[c] |
| DiMarco (51) | 25 | 68 | 6 | 53 | 18 | 24 |
| Gulamhusein (52) | 34 | 18 | 50 | 0 | 50 | 0 |
| Hess (53) | 32 | 56 | 61 | 6 | 33 | 0 |
| Akhtar (54) | 30 | 53 | 0 | 68 | 32 | 0 |
| Olshansky (55) | 105 | 37 | 32 | 68 | 10 | 0 |
| Doherty (56) | 119 | 66 | 29 | 40 | 11 | 20 |
| Teichman (57) | 150 | 75 | 11 | 22 | 54 | 13 |
| Denes (58) | 89 | 71 | 21 | 21 | 58 | 12 |
| Bass (59) | 70 | 53 | 7 | 80 | 13 | 0 |
| Krol (60) | 104 | 30 | 6 | 68 | 26 | 0 |
| Sra (83) | 86 | 34 | 17 | 73 | 10 | 0 |
| Total No; Mean % | 844 | 51 | 22 | 45 | 28 | 5 |

VT = Ventricular tachycardia; SVT = Supraventricular tachycardia; EP = Electrophysiologic testing.

[a] Patients have more than one abnormality.

[b] Includes abnormal sinus node, atrioventricular node, or His-Purkinje function.

[c] Includes hypervagotonia, carotid sinus hypersensitivity.

high specificity (88–100%) (67–68). The usefulness of other tests of sinus node function (e.g., sinoatrial conduction time) is controversial (69,70). Various tests for atrioventricular nodal conduction and refractoriness are also difficult to interpret and the sensitivity and specificity of these findings are not known. These tests vary considerably with autonomic tone and are thus not likely to be sensitive or specific.

A markedly prolonged H-V interval and block between H and V with atrial pacing is more likely to be a marker of significant conduction disease associated with bradyarrhythmias and syncope. There is, however, no consensus regarding the length of H-V interval that is considered significant (criteria have ranged from > 55 ms to > 100 ms).

Supraventricular tachycardias are rarely initiated in patients without a prior history of these arrhythmias. Atrial fibrillation or flutter may be occasionally initiated, especially if aggressive induction procedures are used. In these situations the false positive rate for these arrhythmias may be high (69,70).

The finding of sustained monomorphic ventricular tachycardia has a sensitivity and specificity of ≥ 90% for presence of spontaneous ventricular tachycardia and thus is considered important diagnostic information. However, induction of polymorphic ventricular tachycardia is often a nonspecific response to an aggressive ventricular stimulation protocol (67,69,70). The importance of nonsustained ventricular tachycardia is also controversial (67,69,70).

In general, the following findings in patients with syncope are considered abnormal and potentially important in the etiology of the loss of consciousness: sustained monomorphic ventricular tachycardia; sinus node recovery time $\geqslant$ 3 s; pacing-induced infranodal block; H-V interval $>$ 100 ms; and paroxysmal supraventricular tachycardia with symptomatic hypotension (and symptoms similar to spontaneous syncope).

Mortality at 3–5 years is higher in patients with positive findings. This has largely been attributed to underlying heart disease which is more prevalent in patients with abnormal findings (51–61). At 3 years mortality rates as high as 61% and sudden death rates of 48% have been reported in patients with abnormal studies as compared to 15% and 9% in the negative group (59). Sixty-three percent of patients with ventricular tachycardia by electrophysiologic study have been reported to have a 5-year mortality rate (58).

The recurrence of syncope (over 11–36 months) is lower in patients with abnormal electrophysiologic studies (0–32%) as compared to 8–80% in patients with normal findings, although some of the largest studies do not show differences in recurrence rates (51–61). Recurrence of syncope (at a mean of 26 months) in the elderly with positive electrophysiologic results was 16% as compared to 25% in the negative group (66).

The risks of electrophysiologic studies include hematoma, excessive bleeding, vascular dissection, venous thrombosis, pulmonary emboli, and pneumothorax (71). The complication rate has been estimated at 1–2%, and long-term sequelae from these complications appear to be uncommon. There is a very small risk of cardiac perforation and mortality. Electrophysiologic studies were estimated in 1984 to cost more than $2,000 per patient (43), not including hospital costs. The average duration of hospital stay depends upon the underlying abnormalities and can range from 5–10 days in most cases.

What is the current role of electrophysiologic studies in syncope? A thorough clinical and noninvasive evaluation using a history and physical examination, electrocardiogram, ambulatory monitoring, and other noninvasive or directed tests is needed prior to the consideration of electrophysiologic studies. If an etiology of syncope is determined by noninvasive evaluation, management decisions can be made. In patients without heart disease, upright tilt testing and neuropsychiatric evaluation should be utilized in the workup especially in those with recurrent syncope. In the group of patients with unexplained syncope and organic heart disease, electrophysiologic testing may be useful to define potential arrhythmias and select specific therapy. In these patients, evaluation of underlying heart disease may be needed prior to electrophysiologic testing since issues regarding treatment of underlying cardiac disease are equally important in the management of these patients.

Some centers have used signal-averaged electrocardiogram as a screening test for ventricular tachycardia in selecting patients for electrophysiologic studies. Signal-averaging, a computer-based technique, is used to reduce random noise in the ECG and to enhance detection of low-amplitude signals in the terminal portion of QRS complex. Detection of low-amplitude signals (late potentials) by this technique has been reported to have a sensitivity of 73–89% and specificity of 89–100% for prediction of inducible sustained ventricular tachycardia in patients with syncope (72,73). The overall usefulness of this technique in managing patients presenting with syncope is still not totally clear. Complete electrophysiologic studies are generally needed to evaluate syncope when the decision is made to perform this test since other abnormalities (conduction system disease and supraventricular tachycardia) as well as multiple abnormalities are often of concern.

## Upright Tilt Testing

Vasovagal syncope can be induced by keeping susceptible individuals upright on a tilt table with or without chemical stimulation using isoproterenol. The mechanism of tilt-induced syncope is not entirely understood. Inhibitory reflexes originating from the heart are widely believed to be responsible for this type of syncope (74). This reflex originates in the cardiac sensory receptors (mechanoreceptors) located primarily in the inferior and posterior wall of the left ventricle. These receptors may be stimulated by stretch, cardiac distention, forceful, rapid systolic contraction, or chemical substances. The stimulation of receptors leads to increased neural discharges through unmyelinated C fibers to the medulla (vasomotor center) leading to enhanced parasympathetic and decreased sympathetic activity. The end result is the development of sudden bradycardia and/or hypotension.

Upright posture leads to pooling of blood in the lower limbs resulting in decreased venous return. Normal compensatory responses to orthostatic stress is reflex tachycardia, more forceful contraction of the ventricles, and vasoconstriction. However, in individuals susceptible to vasovagal syncope, this forceful ventricular contraction in the setting of a relatively empty ventricle may activate the cardiac mechanoreceptors, triggering reflex hypotension and/or bradycardia (75). Catecholamine release (as may occur with anxiety, fear, and panic), by increasing ventricular contraction, may also activate the nerve endings responsible for triggering this reflex.

There are two varieties of upright tilt testing protocols: passive tilt testing (76–81) and tilt testing in conjunction with intravenous isoproterenol (82–86). Blood pressure monitoring is performed using cuff blood pressure measurements or continuous intraarterial blood pressure recording. ECG is monitored continuously. After measurements of supine baseline blood pressure and heart rate, patients are suddenly brought to an upright position. As shown in Table 7,

**Table 7** Upright Tilt Testing in Patients with Syncope of Unknown Etiology

| | Patients | | | Controls | | | |
|---|---|---|---|---|---|---|---|
| Author | Total n | Positive n | Positive % | Total n | Positive n | Positive % | Tilt angle |
| Passive tilt | | | | | | | |
| Kenny (76) | 15 | 10 | 67 | 10 | 1 | 10 | 40 |
| Fitzpatrick (77) | 71 | 53 | 75 | 27 | 2 | 7 | 60 |
| Strasberg (78) | 40 | 15 | 38 | 10 | 0 | 0 | 60 |
| Raviele (79) | 30 | 15 | 50 | 8 | 0 | 0 | 60 |
| Abi-Samra[a] (80) | 151 | 63 | 42 | 15 | 0 | 0 | 60 |
| Brignole (81) | 35 | 9 | 26 | 35 | 2 | 6 | 60 |
| Tilt testing in conjunction with isoproterenol | | | | | | | |
| Almquist (82) | 18 | 13 | 87 | 18 | 2 | 11 | 80 |
| Sra (83) | 57 | 34 | 60 | — | — | — | 70 |
| Grub (84) | 25 | 15 | 75 | 6 | 0 | 0 | 80 |
| Pongigline (85) | 20 | 16 | 80 | — | | — | 90 |
| Kapoor (86) | 20 | 15 | 75 | 20 | 9 | 45 | 80 |

[a] Duration of tilting 20 min; all of the other passive protocols up to 60 min.

angles of 40–60° are used. The rates of induction of syncope with upright tilt testing is lower with lower angles of tilt testing. The optimal duration of tilting with passive protocol is not well known; 45 min was recommended in one study since this consisted of a mean plus 2 standard deviations for abnormal responses (77). The endpoints of a positive tilt test are the development of syncope or presyncope in association with hypotension and/or bradycardia.

Tilt table testing with isoproterenol involves an initial passive phase of 10–30 min. If an endpoint of testing is not reached, the patient is brought to a supine position for 5 min. Isoproterenol infusion is started and the patient is then brought to upright position. The duration of upright tilt testing, the dose of isoproterenol, and the increments in subsequent doses have been variable. Patients are kept in an upright position generally for 5–30 min. If endpoints do not occur, the patient is rapidly lowered to a supine position. In some protocols, the infusion rate of isoproterenol is increased with repeated brief periods of tilting. The test is ended upon development of hypotension and/or bradycardia in association with syncope or presyncope, side effects, intolerance to medications, or development of marked tachycardia (heart rate > 150 bpm) (82).

Table 7 summarizes the results of upright tilt testing in syncope of unknown origin. Studies of the passive test show a rate of positive response of 26–75%. Test protocols using isoproterenol show a positive response of 60–87%. The sensitivity of upright tilt testing has not been widely studied. Sensitivity is defined as the proportion of patients with disease (i.e., vasovagal syncope) who have a positive test. There is limited information on upright tilt testing in patients who have a clinical diagnosis of vasovagal syncope. These studies show that the sensitivity of this test may be approximately 70% (87). The specificity of the test has been evaluated in a limited number of subjects in reports of upright tilt testing. Specificity has been reported to be 89–100% in most studies. In one study of young healthy normal individuals, the specificity was 55% (86). In 20–30% of patients this test is not reproducible (77).

A study of tilt testing in 10 elderly patients showed that vasovagal syncope was provoked by upright tilt testing in 5 of 10 patients. The specificity of this test in the elderly is not known (88).

What is the role of tilt table testing in evaluating syncope? In patients without heart disease in whom the history, physical examination, and initial electrocardiogram do not lead to an etiology of syncope, upright tilt testing may define a potential diagnosis. Furthermore, in patients who have underlying heart disease and do not have evidence of arrhythmias based on electrocardiographic monitoring and electrophysiologic studies, this test may provide a specific diagnosis. The only endpoint of clinical importance is the development of symptoms that are similar or identical to the patient's prior symptoms.

The severity and natural history of vasovagal syncope is variable. Patients may have a large number of events at one period of time which may diminish or resolve spontaneously. There are rare patients who continue to have episodes over many years. Thus, the frequency and severity of events are important in devising treatment plans for the patient. Because treatments may have potential side effects, they should be reserved for patients who have frequent or disabling symptoms.

Several types of therapies have been tried for patients with vasovagal syncope. No randomized trials are available, but a decrease in recurrence of syncope or resolution of symptoms has been reported. Beta blockers (e.g., metoprolol and atenolol) are the most commonly used drugs (82–84). The mechanism of action of beta blockers is not fully understood but they may diminish cardiac contractility inhibiting the activation of cardiac mechanoreceptors. Anticholinergic agents such as transdermal scopolamine may be particularly useful in patients with profound bradycardia during upright tilt testing. Disopyramide has been reported to decrease recurrence of syncope (89). This drug has anticholinergic and negative inotropic effects that may inhibit activation of cardiac mechanoreceptors. Theophylline has rarely been used (90,91). The mechanism of action of theophylline in the treatment of vasovagal syncope is not known but a blockade of effects of adenosine, which has vasodilatory effects, is postulated. Measures to expand volume have been used and include increased salt intake, custom-fitted counter pressure support garments from ankle to waist, and fludrocortisone acetate (0.1–1 mg per day). Potential side effects may include recumbent hypertension, hypokalemia, fluid retention, and congestive heart failure. Finally, atrioventricular pacing may be considered in patients with significant bradycardia in response to upright tilt testing (76,92). Even in these patients, the initial treatment of choice is pharmacologic treatment. The pacemaker should be reserved for those who fail drug therapy.

### Low Yield Tests

A wide variety of other tests are rarely helpful in assigning an etiology for syncope (Table 8). Skull films, lumbar puncture, radionuclide brain scan, and cerebral angiography have not yielded diagnostic information for a cause of syncope in the absence of clinical findings suggestive of a specific neurological process (93). In one study, glucose tolerance testing did not lead to a diagnosis of hypoglycemia in patients with syncope. Studies of EEG in syncope have shown that in 1% of patients an epileptiform was found; almost all of these were suspected clinically (36–41,93,94). Head CT scans are rarely useful to assign an etiology, but are needed if subdural bleeding due to head injury is suspected or in patients suspected of having a seizure as a cause of loss of consciousness (37).

## APPROACH TO EVALUATION

A careful history and physical examination form the cornerstone of the evaluation of patients with syncope and identify the vast majority of the causes of syncope. Furthermore, history and physical examination may reveal findings suggestive of specific entities as possible causes (e.g., findings of aortic stenosis or neurological signs and symptoms suggestive of a seizure disorder) that may require further noninvasive or invasive tests for establishing a diagnosis and initiating treatment.

**Table 8** Low Yield Diagnostic Tests

| |
|---|
| Blood Tests |
| Routine blood tests (CBC, electrolytes, BUN, creatinine) |
| Glucose tolerance test |
| Neurological Tests |
| Lumbar puncture |
| Skull x-rays |
| Carotid noninvasive studies |
| EEG |
| Head CT scan |

An electrocardiogram is generally needed for the initial evaluation of patients with syncope, the cause of which is not apparent from the history and physical examination. Although the diagnostic yield of electrocardiogram for arrhythmias or suspicion of myocardial infarction is low, abnormalities can be acted upon quickly if found.

In patients in whom a cause of syncope is not determined by the history, physical examination, and initial electrocardiogram, further diagnostic testing can be approached by stratifying patients into those with and without heart disease.

Patients with known heart disease such as coronary artery disease, congestive heart failure, valvular heart disease, obstructive cardiomyopathy, and bundle branch block have a higher likelihood of arrhythmias. In elderly patients without clinical heart disease and unexplained syncope, cardiac assessment with stress testing or echocardiogram may be needed to define the presence of occult heart disease. Prolonged electrocardiographic monitoring provides an initial step in the evaluation of these patients. If prolonged monitoring is nondiagnostic, these patients may be candidates for electrophysiologic studies. The findings of electrophysiologic studies can be used to select potential therapy. In the elderly, diseases may present in an atypical fashion or multiple abnormalities may be important in causing syncope. Thus, clinical assessment should be particularly focused at these issues. If multiple abnormalities are found that could have led to loss of consciousness, a trial of empiric treatment of those factors may be warranted prior to considering an invasive workup.

Patients with negative electrophysiologic studies have a favorable prognosis and thus empiric therapy (with a pacemaker or antiarrhythmic drugs) is not justified. A large proportion of patients with negative electrophysiologic studies may have vasovagal syncope. Upright tilt testing may define a potential etiology. Therapy of vasovagal syncope can be initiated in patients with recurrent or disabling symptoms.

In the elderly patients without heart disease and with a normal electrocardiogram, the likelihood of arrhythmias is low. A large proportion of these patients may have vasovagal syncope which can be investigated using upright tilt testing. If there is clinical suspicion of arrhythmias, ambulatory monitoring or loop monitoring (when there is recurrent syncope) may help define an etiology. The yield of electrophysiologic studies is low in this group. These studies are not needed in the vast majority of the patients.

## REFERENCES

1. Lipsitz LA, Wei JY, Rowe JW. Syncope in an elderly, institutionalized population: prevalence, incidence, and associated risk. *Q J Med* 1985; 55:45–55.
2. Kapoor W, Snustad D, Peterson J, Wieand HS, Cha R, Karpf M. Syncope in the elderly. *Am J Med* 1986; 80:419–428.

3. Lipsitz LA. Syncope in the elderly. *Ann Intern Med* 1983; 99:92–105.
4. Lipsitz LA, Pluchino FC, Wei JY, Rowe JW. Syncope in institutionalized elderly: the impact of multiple pathological conditions and situational stress. *J Chron Dis* 1986; 39:619–630.
5. Besdine RW. Geriatric medicine: an overview. *Annu Rev Gerontol* 1980; 1:135–153.
6. Kapoor WN, Peterson JR, Karpf M. Micturition syncope. *JAMA* 1985; 253:796–798.
7. Kapoor W, Peterson J, Karpf M. Defecation syncope. A symptom with multiple etiologies. *Arch Intern Med* 1986; 146:2377–2379.
8. Kollef MH, Schachter DT. Defecation syncope caused by pulmonary embolism. Letter. *Ann Intern Med* 1990; 113:86.
9. Levin B, Posner JB. Swallow syncope. Report of a case and review of the literature. *Neurology* 1972; 22:1086–193.
10. Kunis RL, Garfein OB, Pepe AJ, et al. Deglutition syncope and atrioventricular block selectivity induced by hot food and liquid. *Am J Cardiol* 1985; 55:613.
11. Kadish AH, Wesler L, Marchlinski FE. Swallowing syncope: Observations in the absence of conduction system or esophageal disease. *Am J Med* 1986; 81:1098–2000.
12. Lipsitz L. Orthostatic hypotension in the elderly. *N Engl J Med* 1989; 321:952–6.
13. Bannister SR, ed. Antonomic Failure: A Textbook of Clinical Disorders of the Autonomic Nervous System, 2nd ed. New York: Oxford Medical Publishers, 1988:1–20.
14. Ausman JI, Shrontz CE, Pearce JE, Diaz FG, Crecelius JL. Vertebrobasilar insufficiency. A review. *Arch Neurol* 1985; 42:803–808.
15. Fields WS, Lemak NA. Joint study of extracranial arterial occlusion. VII. Subclavian steal—a review of 168 cases. *JAMA* 1972; 222:1139–1143.
16. Sacquegna T, Cortelli P, Baldrati A, Carolis P, Tinuper P. Impairment of consciousness and memory in migraine: A review. *Headache* 1987; 27: 30–33.
17. Strasberg B, Sagie A, Erdman S, Kusniec J, Sclarvosky S, Agmon J. Carotid Sinus Hypersensitivity and the Carotid Sinus Syndrome. *Progr Cardiovasc Dis* 1989; 5:379–391.
18. St. John JN. Glossopharyngeal neuralgia associated with syncope and seizures. *Neurosurgery* 1982; 10:380–383.
19. Kapoor WN, Jannetta PJ. Trigeminal neuralgia associated with seizure and syncope. *J Neurosurg* 1984; 61:594–595.
20. Hoefnagels WAJ, Padberg GW, Overweg J, van der Velde EA, Roos RAC. Transient loss of consciousness: the value of the history for distinguishing seizure from syncope. *J Neurosurg* 1991; 238:39–43.
21. Katon W. Panic disorder and somatization. Review of 55 cases. *Am J Med* 1984; 77:101–106.
22. Linzer M, Felder A, Hackel A, Maria I, Melville MI, Krishnan KR. Psychiatric syncope. *Psychosomatics* 1990; 31:181–188.
23. Lombard JT, Selzer A. Valvular aortic stenosis. A clinical and hemodynamic profile of patients. *Ann Intern Med* 1987; 106:292–298.

24. Kowey PR, Eisenberg R, Engel TR. Sustained arrhythmias in hypertrophic obstructive cardiomyopathy. *N Engl J Med* 1984; 310:1566–69.
25. Fananapazir L, Tracy CM, Leon MB, et al. Electrophysiologic abnormalities in patients with hypertrophic cardiomyopathy. *Circulation* 1989; 80:1259–68.
26. Markel ML, Waller BF, Armstrong WF. Cardiac myxoma. A review. *Medicine* 1987; 66:114–25.
27. Igarashi Y, Yamazoe M, Suzuki K, et al. Possible role of coronary artery spasms in unexplained syncope. *Am J Cardiol* 1990; 65:713–717.
28. DeSanctis RW, Doroghazi RM, Austen WG, Buckley MJ. Aortic dissection. *N Engl J Med* 1987; 317:1060–1067.
29. Jackman WM, Friday KJ, Anderson JL, Aliot EM, Clarm M, Lazzara R. The long QT syndromes: a critical review, new clinical observations and a unifying hypothesis. *Prog Cardiovasc Dis* 1988; 31:115–72.
30. Laakso M, Aberg A, Savola J, Pentikainen PJ, Pyorala K. Diseases and drugs causing prolongation of the QT interval. *Am J Cardiol* 1987; 59:862–865.
31. Paul T, Guccione P, Garson A. Relation of Syncope in Young Patients with Wolff-Parkinson-White Syndrome to Rapid Ventricular Response During Atrial Fibrillation. *Am J Cardiol* 1990; 65:318–21.
32. Ross RT. Syncope. Philadelphia: W. B. Saunders, 1988:113–117.
33. Kapoor WN. Hypotension and syncope. In: Braunwald E, ed., Heart Disease. A Textbook of Cardiovascular Medicine. Philadelphia: W. B. Saunders, 1991:875–886.
34. Vaitkevicius PV, Esserwein DM, Maynard AK, O'Connor FC, Fleg JL. Frequency and importance of postprandial blood pressure reduction in elderly nursing-home patients. *Ann Intern Med* 1991; 115:865–870.
35. Atkins D, Hanusa B, Sefcik T, Kapoor W. Syncope and orthostatic hypotension. *Am J Med* 1991; 91:179–185.
36. Kapoor W, Karpf M, Wieand S, Peterson J, Levey G. A prospective evaluation and follow-up of patients with syncope. *N Engl J Med* 1983; 309:197–204.
37. Kapoor W. Evaluation and outcome of patients with syncope. *Medicine* 1990; 69:160–175.
38. Eagle KA, Black HR. The impact of diagnostic tests in evaluating patients with syncope. *Yale J Biol Med* 1983; 56:1–8.
39. Silverstein MD, Singer DE, Mulley A, Thibault GE, Barnett GO. Patients with syncope admitted to medical intensive carc units. *JAMA* 1982; 248:1185–1189.
40. Martin GJ, Adams SL, Martin HG, et al. Prospective evaluation of syncope. *Ann Emerg Med* 1984; 13:499–504.
41. Day SC, Cook EF, Funkenstein H, Goldman L. Evaluation and outcome of emergency room patients with transient loss of consciousness. *Am J Med* 1982; 73:15–23.
42. DiMarco JP, Philbrick JT. Use of ambulatory electrocardiography (Holter) monitoring. *Ann Intern Med* 1990; 113:53–68.
43. Jonas S, Klein I, Dimant J. Importance of Holter monitoring in patients with periodic cerebral symptoms. *Ann Neurol* 1977; 1:470–4.
44. Boudoulas H, Schaael SF, Lewis RP, Robinson JL. Superiority of 24-hour outpa-

tient monitoring over multi-stage exercise testing for the evaluation of syncope. *J Electrocardiol* 1979; 12:103–8.
45. Clark PI, Glasser SP, Spoto E. Arrhythmias detected by ambulatory monitoring: lack of correlation with symptoms of dizziness and syncope. *Chest* 1980; 77:722–5.
46. Zeldis SM, Levine BJ, Michelson EL, Morganroth J. Cardiovascular complaints: Correlation with cardiac arrhythmias on 24-hour electrocardiographic monitoring. *Chest* 1980; 78:456–62.
47. Kala R, Viitasalo MT, Toivonen L, Eisalo A. Ambulatory ECG recording in patients referred because of syncope or dizziness. *Acta Med Scand* 1982; 668(Suppl):13–19.
48. Gibson TC, Heitzman MR. Diagnostic efficacy of 24-hour electrocardiographic monitoring for syncope. *Am J Cardiol* 1984; 53:1013–17.
49. Bass EB, Curtiss EI, Arena VC, et al. The duration of Holter monitoring in patients with syncope: is 24 hours enough? *Arch Int Med* 1990; 150:1073–1078.
50. Linzer M, Pritchett ELC, Pontinen M, McCarthy E, Divine GW. Incremental diagnostic yield of loop electrocardiographic recorders in unexplained syncope. *Am J Cardiol* 1990; 66:214–219.
51. DiMarco JP, Garan H, Harthorne JW, Ruskin JN. Intracardiac electrophysiology techniques in recurrent syncope of unknown cause. *Ann Intern Med* 1981; 95:542–548.
52. Gulamhusein S, Naccarelli GV, Ko PT, Prystowsky EN, Zipes DP, Varness HJM, Heger JJ, Klein GJ. Value and limitations of clinical electrophysiologic study in assessment of patients with unexplained syncope. *Am J Med* 1982; 73:700–705.
53. Hess DS, Morady F, Scheirman MM. Electrophysiologic testing in the evaluation of patients with syncope of undetermined origin. *Am J Cardiol* 1982; 50:1309–1315.
54. Akhtar M, Shenasa M, Denker S, Gilbert CJ, Rizwi N. Role of cardiac electrophysiologic studies in patients with unexplained recurrent syncope. *PACE* 1983; 6:192–201.
55. Olshansky B, Mazuz M, Martins JB. Significance of inducible tachycardia in patients with syncope of unknown origin: a long-term follow-up. *J Am Coll Cardiol* 1985; 5:216–233.
56. Doherty JU, Pembrook-Rogers D, Grogan EW, Falcone RA, Buxton AE, Marchlinski FE, Cassidy DM, Kienzle MG, Almendral JM, Josephson ME. Electrophysiologic evaluation and follow-up characteristics of patients with recurrent unexplained syncope and presyncope. *Am J Cardiol* 1985; 55:703–708.
57. Teichman SL, Felder SD, Matos JA, Kim SG, Waspe LE, Fisher JD. The value of electrophysiologic studies in syncope of undetermined origin: report of 150 cases. *Am Heart J* 1985; 110:469–479.
58. Denes P, Vretz E, Ezri MD, Borbola J. Clinical predictors of electrophysiology findings in patients with syncope of unknown origin. *Arch Intern Med* 1988; 148:1922–1928.
59. Bass EB, Elson JJ, Fogoros RN, Peterson J, Arena VC, Kapoor WN. Long-term prognosis of patients undergoing electrophysiologic studies for syncope of unknown origin. *Am J Cardiol* 1988; 62:1186–1191.

60. Krol RB, Morady F, Flaker GC, DiCarol LA, Baerman JM, Hewitt J, de Buitleir M. Electrophysiologic testing in patients with unexplained syncope: clinical and noninvasive predictors of outcome. *J Am Coll Cardiol* 1987; 10:358–363.
61. Kapoor WN, Hammill SC, Gersh BJ. Diagnosis and natural history of syncope and the role of invasive electrophysiologic testing. *Am J Cardiol* 1989; 63:730–734.
62. Click RL, Gersh BJ, Sugrue DD, et al. Role of invasive electrophysiologic testing in patients with symptomatic bundle branch block. *Am J Cardiol* 1987; 59(1):817–23.
63. Nelson SD, Kou WH, DeBuitleir M, et al. Value of programmed ventricular stimulation in presumed carotid sinus syndrome. *Am J Cardiol* 1987; 60(13):1073–7.
64. McLaran CJ, Gersh BJ, Osborn MJ, Wood DL, Sugrue DD, Holmes DR, Hammill SC. Increased vagal tone as an isolated finding in patients undergoing electrophysiologic testing for recurrent syncope: response to long-term anticholinergic agents. *Br Heart J* 1986; 55:53–57.
65. Hammill SC, Holmes DR, Wood DL, Osborn MJ, McLaran CJ, Sugrue DD, Gersh BJ. Electrophysiologic testing in the upright position: improved evaluation of patients with rhythm disturbances using a tilt table. *J Am Coll Cardiol* 1984; 4:65–71.
66. Sugrue DD, Holmes DR, Gersh BJ, Wood DL, Osborn MJ, Hammill SC. Impact of intracardiac electrophysiologic testing on the management of elderly patients with recurrent or near syncope. *JAGS* 1987; 35:1079–1083.
67. Morady F, Scheinman MM. The role and limitations of electrophysiologic testing in patients with unexplained syncope. *Int J Cardiol* 1983; 4:229–234.
68. Fujimura O, Yee R, Klein GJ, et al. The diagnostic sensitivity of electrophysiologic testing in patients with syncope caused by transient bradycardia. *N Engl J Med* 1989; 321:1703.
69. DiMarco JP. Electrophysiologic studies in patients with unexplained syncope. *Circulation* 1987; 75(Suppl. III):140–43.
70. McAnulty JH. Syncope of unknown origin: the role of electrophysiologic studies. *Circulation* 1987; 75(Suppl. III):144–145.
71. DiMarco JP, Garan H, Ruskin JN. Complications in patients undergoing cardiac electrophysiologic procedure. *Ann Intern Med* 1982; 97:490–493.
72. Gang ES, Peter T, Rosenthal ME, et al. Detection of late potentials on the surface electrocardiogram in unexplained syncope. *Am J Cardiol* 1986; 58(10):1014–20.
73. Winters SL, Stewart D, Gomes JA. Signal averaging of the surface QRS complex predicts inducibility of ventricular tachycardia in patients with syncope of unknown origin: a prospective study. *J Am Coll Cardiol* 1987; 10(4):775–81.
74. Mark AL. The Bezold-Jarisch Reflex Revisisted: Clinical implications of inhibitory reflexed originating in the heart. *J Am Coll Cardiol* 1983; 1:90–92.
75. Abboud FM. Ventricular syncope. *N Engl J Med* 1989; 32:390–2.
76. Kenny RA, Ingram A, Bayliss J, Sutton R. Head-up tilt: A useful test for investigating unexplained syncope. *Lancet* 1986; 1:1352–5.
77. Fitzpatrick AP, Theodorakis G, Vardas P, Sutton R. Methodology of head-up tilt testing in patients with unexplained syncope. *J Am Coll Cardiol* 1991; 17:125–30.
78. Strasberg B, Rechavia E, Sagie A, et al. The head-up tilt table test in patients with syncope of unknown origin. *Am Heart J* 1989; 118(5 Pt 1):923–7.

79. Raviele A, Gasparini G, DiPede F, et al. Usefulness of head-up tilt test in evaluating patients with syncope of unknown origin and negative electrophysiologic study. *Am J Cardiol* 1990; 65:1322–1327.
80. Abi-Samra FM, Maloney JD, Fouad-Tarazi EM, et al. The usefulness of head-up tilt testing and hemodynamic investigations in the work-up of syncope of unknown origin. *PACE* 1987; 10:406.
81. Brignole M, Menozzi C, Gianfranchi L, Oddone D, Lolli G, Bertulla A. Carotid sinus massage, eyeball compression, and head-up tilt test in patients with syncope of uncertain origin and in healthy control subjects. *Am Heart J* 1991; 122:1664–1651.
82. Almquist A, Goldenberg IF, Milstein S, et al. Provocation of bradycardia and hypotension by isoproterenol and upright posture in patients with unexplained syncope. *N Engl J Med* 1989; 320:346–351.
83. Sra JS, Anderson AJ, Sheikh SH, Avitall B, Tchou PJ, Troup PJ, Gilbert CJ, Akhtar M, Jazayers MR. Unexplained syncope evaluated by electrophysiologic studies and head-up tilt testing. *Ann Intern Med* 1991; 114:1013–1019.
84. Grubb BP, Temesy-Armos P, Hahn H, Elliott L. Utility of upright tilt table testing in the evaluation and management of syncope of unknown origin. *Am J Med* 1991; 90:6–10.
85. Pongigline G, Fish FA, Strasburger JF, et al. Heart rate and blood pressure response to upright tilt in young patients with unexplained syncope. *J Am Coll Cardiol* 1990; 16:165–170.
86. Kapoor WN, Brant NL. Evaluation of syncope by upright tilt testing with isoproterenol. A nonspecific test. *Ann Intern Med* 1992; 116:358–363.
87. Waxman MB, Yao L, Cameron DA, et al. Isoproterenol induction of vasodepressor-type reaction in vasodepressor-prone patients. *Am J Cardiol* 1989; 63(1):58–65.
88. Hackel A, Linzer M, Anderson N, Williams R. Cardiovascular and catecholamine responses to head-up tilt in the diagnosis of recurrent unexplained syncope in the elderly patients. *JAGS* 1991; 39:663–669.
89. Milstein S, Buetikofer J, Dunnigan A, et al. Usefulness of disopyramide for prevention of upright tilt-induced hypotension-bradycardia. *Am J Cardiol* 1990; 65:1339–1344.
90. Benditt DG, Benson W, Kreitt J, et al. Electrophysiologic effects of theophylline in young patients with recurrent symptomatic bradyarrhythmias. *Am J Cardiol* 1983; 52:1223–1229.
91. Nelson SD, Stanley MR, Love CJ, et al. Chronic oral theophylline for the management of vasodepressor syncope. *Circulation* 1990; 82:707 (abstract).
92. Fitzpatrick A, Theodorakis G, Ahmed R, Williams T, Sutton T. Dual chamber pacing aborts vasovagal syncope induced by head-up 60° tilt. *PACE* 1991; 14:13–19.
93. Kapoor W, Karpf M, Maher Y, Miller R, Levey G. Syncope of unknown origin: The need for a more cost-effective approach to its diagnostic evaluation. *JAMA* 1982; 247:2687–2691.
94. Davis TL, Freeman FR. Electroencephalography should not be routine in the evaluation of syncope in adults. *Arch Intern Med* 1990; 150:2027–2029.

# 25

# Diagnosis of Acute Pulmonary Embolism in the Elderly

**Paul D. Stein**
*Henry Ford Heart and Vascular Institute, Detroit, Michigan*

## INTRODUCTION

It has been suggested that the clinical diagnosis of acute pulmonary embolism (PE) among elderly patients is less reliable than in younger patients. This impression relates partially to the impression that elderly patients may be inattentive to new symptoms, such as shortness of breath (1), or the impression that common symptoms of PE may be absent (2). Ventilation-perfusion lung scans are often nonspecific in the presence of associated cardiac or pulmonary disease (3,4), and elderly patients are expected to have associated cardiorespiratory problems. Intuitively, angiography seems to be more dangerous in older patients and, therefore, rarely indicated (5). At first glance, it therefore seems that elderly patients may present an even greater difficulty in correctly reaching a diagnosis of acute PE than younger adults. A recent investigation among elderly patients, however, showed that the clinical manifestations and diagnostic problems are comparable among elderly patients and younger patients (6).

Among 72 patients $\geqslant$ 70 years of age, immobilization was the most frequent predisposing factor, as it was among other age groups (6,7). Among elderly patients 67% were immobilized before the PE. Surgery preceded the PE in 44%. Comparable percentages of patients in the younger age groups were immobilized or underwent surgery before the PE. Malignancy was more frequent among the patients $\geqslant$ 70 years than among patients $<$ 40 years (26 versus 2%). Estrogen therapy was infrequent among elderly female patients, 5%, but its use among patients under 40 years preceded PE in 35%.

## SYNDROMES OF ACUTE PULMONARY EMBOLISM

It is useful to consider PE in terms of its presenting syndromes (8): (1) the syndrome of pulmonary infarction or hemorrhage, (2) the syndrome of circulatory collapse, and (3) the syndrome of unexplained dyspnea not accompanied by pulmonary infarction, hemorrhage, or circulatory collapse. The vast majority of elderly patients presented with one of these syndromes, irrespective of age. The syndrome of pulmonary infarction or hemorrage was most common in patients ⩾ 70 years (51%), as it is among younger patients. Dyspnea unaccompanied by pulmonary infarction or circulatory collapse occurred in 28%, and circulatory collapse was the presenting syndrome in 10%. The frequency of occurrence of these presenting syndromes was comparable to that seen in patients < 40 years of age (6). In contrast to younger patients, PE among 11% of elderly patients was identified on the basis of unexplained radiographic findings of atelectasis, pleural effusion, or pleural-based opacities, often accompanied by tachypnea or a history of thrombophlebitis.

Dyspnea and pleuritic pain were the most frequent symptoms of acute PE, irrespective of age (6,7). Dyspnea occurred in 78% and pleuritic pain in 51% of elderly patients (Table 1). All symptoms occurred with comparable frequency among all age groups, with the exception of hemoptysis. Hemoptysis occurred in only 8% of patients ⩾ 70 years, although it was observed in 32% of patients < 40 years (6).

**Table 1** Symptoms of Acute Pulmonary Embolism Among Elderly Patients

| | ⩾70 Years, $n = 72$ (%) |
|---|---|
| Dyspnea | 78 |
| Pleuritic pain | 51 |
| Cough | 35 |
| Leg swelling | 35 |
| Leg pain | 31 |
| Palpitations | 13 |
| Wheezing | 10 |
| Anginal pain | 10 |
| Hemoptysis | 8 |

Tachypnea (respiratory rate $\geqslant$ 20/min) was the most frequent sign among the elderly, occurring in 74% (6) (Table 2). Tachycardia (heart rate > 100/min) occurred in 29% of elderly patients. All signs occurred with a comparable frequency among all age groups (6,7).

## CHEST RADIOGRAPH

Atelectasis and/or pulmonary parenchymal abnormalities were the most frequent radiographic abnormalities among elderly patients as well as younger patients (6,7,9). All radiographic abnormalities occurred with a comparable frequency among all age groups (6). The chest radiograph was normal in only 4% of patients $\geqslant$ 70 years (Table 3).

## COMBINATIONS OF SYMPTOMS, SIGNS, AND RADIOGRAPHIC ABNORMALITIES

Dyspnea or tachypnea (respiratory rate $\geqslant$ 20) occurred in 92% of elderly patients with acute PE (Table 4) (6). Dyspnea or tachypnea or pleuritic pain occurred in 94%. Dyspnea or tachypnea or radiographic evidence of atelectasis or a parenchymal abnormality occurred in 100%. The prevalence of these combinations of manifestations was comparable among all age groups (6,10).

**Table 2** Signs of Acute Pulmonary Embolism Among Elderly Patients

| | $\geqslant$70 Years, $n$ = 72 (%) |
|---|---|
| Tachypnea $\geqslant$ 20/min | 74 |
| Rales (crackles) | 65 |
| Tachycardia > 100/min | 29 |
| Increased $P_2$ | 15 |
| Deep venous thrombosis | 15 |
| Diaphoresis | 8 |
| Wheezes | 8 |
| Temperature > 38.5°C | 7 |
| Third heart sound | 7 |
| Pleural friction rub | 6 |
| Homan's sign | 4 |
| Cyanosis | 3 |

**Table 3** Chest Radiograph in Acute Pulmonary Embolism Among Elderly Patients

| | ⩾70 Years, $n = 72$ (%) |
|---|---|
| Normal | 4 |
| Atelectasis or pulmonary parenchymal abnormality | 71 |
| Pleural effusion | 57 |
| Pleural-based opacity | 42 |
| Prominent central pulmonary artery | 29 |
| Elevated diaphragm | 28 |
| Cardiomegaly | 22 |
| Decreased pulmonary vascularity | 19 |
| Pulmonary edema | 13 |
| Westermark's sign[a] | 7 |

[a] Prominent central pulmonary artery and decreased pulmonary vascularity.

**Table 4** Combinations of Signs and Symptoms Among Elderly Patients with Acute Pulmonary Embolism

| | ⩾70 Years, $n = 72$ (%) |
|---|---|
| Dyspnea or tachypnea[a] | 92 |
| Dyspnea or tachypnea or hemoptysis | 92 |
| Dyspnea or tachypnea or signs of deep venous thrombosis | 92 |
| Dyspnea or tachypnea or pleuritic pain[b] | 94 |
| Dyspnea or tachypnea or pleuritic pain or signs of deep venous thrombosis[b] | 94 |
| Dyspnea or tachypnea or radiographic atelectasis or parenchymal abnormality | 100 |
| Dyspnea or tachypnea or pleuritic pain or radiographic atelectasis or parenchymal abnormality[b] | 100 |

[a] Tachypnea = respiratory ratio ⩾ 20/min.
[b] The addition of hemoptysis did not improve the sensitivity of the combination for the detection of pulmonary embolism.

## ELECTROCARDIOGRAMS

Nonspecific ST segment or T wave changes were the most common abnormalities, either or both occurring in 56% of patients ⩾ 70 years and with the same frequency in younger patients (Table 5) (3,6,11). With the exception of left anterior hemiblock (left axis deviation) among patients ⩾ 70 years, other electrocardiographic abnormalities occurred in 12% or fewer patients in all age groups. No differences in the frequency of occurrence of any electrocardiographic abnormalities were apparent between patients ⩾ 70 years and younger patients, although incomplete right bundle branch block was less frequent among patients 40–69 years than among patients < 40 years.

## CLINICAL ASSESSMENT

When physicians were 80–100% confident that PE was present based upon clinical judgment and laboratory tests with the exception of ventilation-perfusion scans, they were correct in about 90% of patients ⩾ 70 years, although the sample was small, 10 patients. When they thought that there was only a small (<20%) likelihood of PE, PE was present in only 19% of 69 patients. In most patients, physicians were uncertain of the diagnosis, believing that there was a 20–79% chance of PE. In these patients ⩾ 70 years, PE was present in 37%. The accuracy of clinical assessment was comparable among patients in all age groups (6,12).

**Table 5** Electrocardiographic Findings in Elderly Patients with Acute Pulmonary Embolism

| | ⩾70 Years, $n$ = 57 (%) |
|---|---|
| Normal | 21 |
| ST segment or T wave changes | 56 |
| Left axis deviation | 18 |
| Left ventricular hypertrophy | 12 |
| Acute myocardial infarction pattern | 12 |
| Low-voltage QRS | 9 |
| Complete right bundle branch block | 7 |
| Right ventricular hypertrophy | 4 |
| Right axis deviation | 2 |
| Right atrial enlargement | 2 |
| Incomplete right bundle branch block | 2 |

## VENTILATION-PERFUSION SCANS

Among patients ⩾ 70 years with high-probability ventilation-perfusion scans, 94% had PE (Table 6). The positive predictive value of all probabilities of ventilation-perfusion scans was comparable in all age groups (6).

The sensitivity of high-probability ventilation-perfusion scans among patients ⩾ 70 years, 47%, did not differ significantly from the sensitivity of high-probability ventilation-perfusion scans among younger age groups (6). The specificity of high-probability ventilation-perfusion scans among patients ⩾ 70 years, 99%, was also similar among younger patients.

## COMPLICATIONS OF PULMONARY ANGIOGRAPHY

Neither major nor minor complications of pulmonary angiography were more frequent among patients ⩾ 70 years than among the younger age patients (6,13). Major complications among patients ⩾ 70 years occurred in 1.0%. There was one fatal complication in an 87-year-old woman who suffered ventricular tachycardia followed by hypotension and respiratory arrest. She died 12 h after the procedure.

The most frequent complication of angiography among 200 elderly patients was renal failure, either major or minor, which occurred in 3.0% and was more frequent than in patients ⩽ 69 years, 0.7% ($p < 0.05$). The "minor" complications of renal failure were important complications, although dialysis was not required. These patients either showed an elevation of the serum creatinine from previously normal levels to ⩾2.1 mg per 100 ml (range 2.1–3.5 mg per 100 ml) or increased a previously abnormal serum creatinine ⩾ 2 mg per 100 ml. All but 1 of the patients who developed renal failure after angiography were older than 60 years. Among the 10 patients who developed renal failure, 3 required dialysis.

**Table 6** Ventilation-Perfusion Scans in Elderly Patients with Acute Pulmonary Embolism (PE)

| | ⩾70 Years | |
|---|---|---|
| | Number of patients | % |
| High | 34/36 | 94 |
| Intermediate | 27/100 | 27 |
| Low | 10/71 | 14 |
| Near normal/normal | 1/8 | 13 |

Minor complications included urticaria, pulmonary edema requiring only diuretics, nausea and vomiting, non–life-threatening arrhythmias, hematomas, interstitial staining with contrast material, and narcotic overdose. Minor complications among patients ⩾ 70 years occurred in 7.0%. The rate of occurrence of minor complications was similar among younger patients.

Prospective investigation showed that most clinical manifestations occurred with a comparable prevalence among patients ⩾ 70 years of age and younger patients (6). The usual syndromes of pulmonary embolism, characterized by (1) pleuritic pain or hemoptysis, (2) isolated dyspnea, or (3) circulatory collapse, were observed with comparable frequency among elderly patients and younger patients. However, 11% of patients ⩾ 70 years of age, in contrast to younger patients, did not show these syndromes. They were identified on the basis of unexpected radiographic abnormalities, which may have been accompanied by tachypnea or a history of thrombophlebitis. Unexplained radiographic abnormalities may be an important clue to the diagnosis of PE, particularly among elderly patients, in whom the expected signs and symptoms are absent, as has previously been observed (2). Nevertheless, even among patients ⩾ 70 years, a combination of nonspecific symptoms and signs that typically occurs with PE was present in the great majority. Only a small percentage of patients ⩾ 70 years of age with PE did not have dyspnea, tachypnea, or pleuritic pain.

The utility of ventilation-perfusion scans among patients ⩾ 70 years was comparable to that in younger patients (6,12). Pulmonary angiography was not more hazardous among the elderly, although renal failure was a more frequent sequela among patients ⩾ 70 years than among younger patients (6,13). All the patients who developed renal failure were over 60 years of age, with the exception of a 52-year-old woman who had chronic renal failure before angiography. The definitions of major complications were intentionally conservative. The frequency of major complications may therefore tend to be an overestimate.

In conclusion, the nonspecific manifestations of PE, even among patients ⩾ 70 years, occur with sufficient frequency to suggest the possibility of PE in the differential diagnosis. The typical signs and symptoms known to occur among younger patients were common, even among elderly patients, although occasional exceptions were observed. Unexplained radiographic abnormalities in the absence of these signs and symptoms are important diagnostic clues, particularly among the elderly. When the diagnosis of PE is uncertain, pulmonary angiography can be performed in elderly patients with no greater overall risk than in younger patients, although renal failure was a problem among elderly patients.

## REFERENCES

1. Morrell MT. The incidence of pulmonary embolism in the elderly. *Geriatrics* 1970; 25:138–153.

2. Taubman LB, Silverstone FA. Autopsy proven pulmonary embolism among the institutionalized elderly. *J Am Geriatr Soc* 1986; 34:752–756.
3. Stein PD, Coleman RE, Gottschalk A, Saltzman HA, Terrin ML, Weg JG. Diagnostic utility of ventilation/perfusion lung scans in acute pulmonary embolism is not diminished by pre-existing cardiac or pulmonary disease. *Chest* 1991; 100:604–606.
4. Lesser BA, Leeper KV, Stein PD, et al. The diagnosis of pulmonary embolism in patients with chronic obstructive pulmonary disease. *Chest* 1992; 102:17–22.
5. Busby W, Bayer A, Pathy J. Pulmonary embolism in the elderly. *Age Aging* 1988; 17:205–209.
6. Stein PD, Gottschalk A, Hales CA, Saltzman HA, Terrin ML. Diagnosis of acute pulmonary embolism in the elderly. *J Am Coll Cardiol* 1991; 18:1452–1457.
7. Stein PD, Terrin ML, Hales CA, et al. Clinical, laboratory, roentgenographic and electrocardiographic findings in patients with acute pulmonary embolism and no pre-existing cardiac or pulmonary disease. *Chest* 1991; 100:598–603.
8. Stein PD, Willis PW III, DeMets DL. History and physical examination in acute pulmonary embolism in patients without pre-existing cardiac or pulmonary disease. *Am J Cardiol* 1981; 47:218–223.
9. Stein PD, Willis PW III, DeMets DL, Greenspan RH. Plain chest roentgenogram in patients with acute pulmonary embolism and no pre-existing cardiac or pulmonary disease. *Am J Noninvas Cardiol* 1987; 1:171–176.
10. Stein PD, Saltzman HA, Weg JG. Clinical characteristics of patients with acute pulmonary embolism. *Am J Cardiol* 1991; 68:1723–1724.
11. Stein PD, Dalen JE, McIntyre KM, Sasahara AA, Wenger NK, Willis PW III. The electrocardiogram in acute pulmonary embolism. *Prog Cardiovasc Dis* 1975; 17:247–257.
12. PIOPED Investigators. Value of the ventilation/perfusion scan in acute pulmonary embolism: results of the Prospective Investigation of Pulmonary Embolism Diagnosis (PIOPED). *JAMA* 1990; 263:2753–2759.
13. Stein PD, Athanasoulis C, Alavi A, et al. Complications and validity of pulmonary angiography in acute pulmonary embolism. *Circulation* 1992; 85:462–465.

# 26

# Peripheral Vascular Disease in the Elderly

**Ross T. Lyon, Steven P. Rivers, and Frank J. Veith**
*Albert Einstein College of Medicine and Montefiore Medical Center, Bronx, New York*

## DEFINING THE PROBLEM

The geriatric patient with significant peripheral vascular disease poses a dilemma because of reluctance to intervene but the need to prevent life- and limb-threatening catastrophies. Delay in treatment can be devastating, resulting in stroke, limb loss, or premature death. Overly aggressive intervention can also be harmful in a patient with little systemic reserve. Care of these patients is challenging and requires a thoughtful and intensive effort by individuals familiar with the particular problems and issues presented by this group of patients.

Vascular disease is for the most part a disease of the elderly, with its incidence proportional to increasing age. Although atherosclerotic occlusive disease occurs in middle-aged individuals, it is usually not symptomatic unless known risk factors, such as hypercholesterolemia, diabetes, hypertension, or smoking, are present. In the elderly population, however, its presence is nearly universal even in the absence of such risk factors. Aneurysmal disease, arterial embolism, and venous thromboembolic disease are likewise seen occasionally in younger patients but are considerably more common in the geriatric population.

Arterial occlusive disease is the most frequent cause of death in the elderly population with stroke and heart attack the direct cause of death in more than two-thirds of all people over 65 years of age (1). Aneurysm rupture and pulmonary embolism are more common than is generally appreciated and are in addition to this figure.

More than many other health problems, vascular disease dramatically affects the functional capabilities of the elderly. Stroke is the most common disabling event in this group of patients. Ischemic limb loss, although less common, also makes the elderly patient nearly totally dependent on others, because successful rehabilitation with a prosthetic limb is unusual in this age group.

The high rate of disability and death from peripheral vascular illnesses underscores the importance of preventive and therapeutic treatments for these problems. Yet, if intervention is to be justified in this fragile group, it must be effective and have acceptably low morbidity and mortality rates. Additionally, the longevity of these patients should be sufficient to allow them to enjoy the associated benefits of treatment. It is therefore important to consider that although the average life expectancy at birth is currently approximately 76 years of age, a 75-year-old person usually lives another 10 years and the average 80-year-old another 8 years (2).

Aside from the conservative treatment of venous problems, the mainstay of treatment for advanced peripheral vascular problems involves the use of invasive techniques and surgical procedures. However, advances in diagnosis, anesthesia, operative procedures, and perioperative intensive care have enabled even complex vascular problems to be managed effectively and safely in the elderly population (3).

## COMMON MISCONCEPTIONS ABOUT SURGICAL PROCEDURES IN THE ELDERLY

Unfortunately, there are several fairly common misconceptions about surgical procedures in the elderly that persist and frequently result in delay or denial of treatment, with an attendant increase in morbidity and mortality from the underlying disease or from intervention in a more compromised patient (Table 1). In fact, the results of surgical intervention for both vascular and nonvascular problems in patients 75 years of age or older reveal surprisingly low mortality rates

**Table 1** Misconceptions About Surgical Procedures in the Elderly

| |
|---|
| Elderly patients are too frail to have surgery |
| Life expectancy too short to justify surgical intervention |
| Surgery should only be done in emergency situations |
| All operative procedures in the elderly have a high mortality |
| Coexisting illnesses prohibit vascular surgical procedures |

if operations are done on a nonemergency basis (3–5). If intervention is reserved until emergency surgery is needed, however, then mortality rises considerably. These findings are the basis for the rational treatment of peripheral vascular problems in elderly patients.

## SPECIAL CONSIDERATIONS IN THE GERIATRIC PATIENT

There is often little correlation between chronological age and the physiological condition of elderly patients. In general, though, elderly patients are more physiologically fragile and require a more thorough approach with attention to many details that are not as important in younger patients. Their care is therefore much more labor intensive and requires significant additional dedication and commitment from all the personnel involved, including physicians, nurses, therapists, dietitians, social workers, and family members. Even when there is no mental impairment, such problems as hearing loss, impaired vision, pain, temporary confusion because of illness, and advanced age itself are often mistaken for senility. Thus even usually simple tasks, such as obtaining a medical history, for example, may be difficult or impossible without help from a family member, an attendant, or from medical records. Further complicating their care is the problem that their diseases are often at an advanced stage at the time of presentation. Additionally, most of these patients have other superimposed chronic medical illnesses (Table 2), and their ability to participate in their own care is frequently limited.

Other physiological differences also impact on the care that is required. Such problems as lack of cardiopulmonary reserve, poor balance, reduced muscle strength, fragile skin, bones, and other tissues, poor healing, predisposition to hyponatremia, predilection for arrhythmias, and altered responses to medications (especially anxiolytics, narcotics, and warfarin) must be taken into account

**Table 2** Frequent Coexisting Medical Illnesses

| |
|---|
| Diabetes |
| Hypertension |
| Coronary artery occlusive disease |
| Congestive heart failure |
| COPD |
| Chronic renal insufficiency |
| Previous stroke |
| Malnutrition |
| Depression |

in the care of these patients. These problems can influence everything from the administration of intravenous fluids and simple medications to operative approaches, anesthetics, duration of postoperative mechanical ventilation, and rehabilitation.

## DECIDING WHETHER TO OPERATE

Making the decision to proceed with surgery should involve the input of multiple variables, including but not limited to the severity of the illness and the likelihood of disease progression, the relative risks both with or without surgery, expected quality of life, likelihood of success of the surgery, life expectancy following the procedure, and the desires of the patient and trusted relatives. Every attempt should be made, if possible, to arrive at a decision before the need for urgent or emergency intervention and its accompanying high risks.

Deciding to withhold an otherwise indicated surgical procedure is difficult, and the reasons must be clearly defined, especially in potential limb- and life-threatening situations. Avoid the trap of choosing not to operate electively for lower extremity revascularization, for example, only to find it necessary later to approve an amputation that carries an equivalent or greater perioperative risk, or of postponing aneurysm surgery and allowing the operative and nonoperative risks to increase over time (6,7). Almost always, other chronic medical problems can be successfully managed perioperatively by thoughtful, vigilant care.

Absolute contraindications to most vascular surgical procedures include situations in which the patient is in a chronic vegetative state, the life expectancy of the patient is severely limited because of other active noncorrectable problems, such as metastatic cancer, or when the patient refuses surgical intervention despite the associated nonoperative risk.

## PREOPERATIVE PREPARATION

Careful preoperative evaluation and care can often anticipate, identify, and minimize problems in the perioperative period. Medical care in this situation should consist of optimization rather than medical "clearance." The first step in this process is to identify relevant problem areas, such as ongoing infection of the respiratory or urinary systems and existing deficits in fluid status, blood components, and nutrition, and to correct these when possible. Organ system dysfunction of the respiratory tract, heart, and kidneys should be defined and function maximized (8).

### Respiratory Tract Assessment and Care

Most patients with peripheral vascular occlusive disease have been avid smokers and have some degree of pulmonary dysfunction. However, simple but important findings on examination, such as tachypnea at rest, purse string lips during expiration, a prolonged expiratory phase, or the use of accessory muscles, suggest profound pulmonary compromise and deserve special consideration. Standard tests for evaluating the respiratory tract are usually satisfactory and include a preoperative chest x-ray, pulmonary function tests, and a room air blood gas. Pre- and postoperative pulmonary toilet, use of bronchodilators, a retroperitoneal or extraanatomical surgical approach for abdominal aortic problems, and epidural administration of analgesics can do wonders in these instances.

## Cardiac Issues

It is difficult to place too much emphasis on the importance of a careful cardiac evaluation in the patient with symptomatic peripheral vascular occlusive disease. Patients with overt extremity or carotid occlusive disease usually have some degree of coronary artery disease as well (9). Although it is natural to focus on the acute problem at hand, failure to take into consideration the likelihood of asymptomatic but significant coronary artery disease can be a costly error.

Controversy exists about how extensive the cardiac evaluation of an asymptomatic patient should be (10). If there is no history of myocardial compromise, the operative procedure does not involve an intraabdominal or intrathoracic approach or aortic clamping, and the electrocardiogram is without evidence of ischemic changes, further cardiac testing is not usually recommended.

If the patient is symptomatic, if there is a history of cardiac events or dysfunction, or if an intraabdominal or intrathoracic procedure is planned, then further cardiac evaluation is advised before elective procedures. The most useful additional tests are a dipyridamole-thallium stress test and echocardiography (11,12). These studies localize myocardial tissue with both fixed and reversible ischemic changes, as well as identify significant cardiac dysfunction or other abnormalities, such as pericardial effusion, ventricular aneurysm, or mural thrombi. If evidence of reversibly ischemic myocardium is found, coronary angiography should be done to determine the presence of coronary occlusive lesions. Symptomatic coronary artery disease, valvular lesions, or cardiac rhythm problems should be treated before nonemergency peripheral vascular reconstructive procedures, using standard medical, angioplasty, or surgical techniques. For those patients in whom significant cardiac compromise persists despite these measures, surgical intervention should be modified if possible to avoid the need for intrathoracic or intraabdominal procedures.

Coronary artery angioplasty has become a valuable modality for the perioperative management of patients with significant coronary artery disease that requires vascular surgical intervention (13). Coronary artery bypass is not appropriate for most patients with urgent vascular problems or with otherwise well-controlled coronary artery disease, but coronary artery angioplasty is a relatively safe, effective, and timely means of treating patients who have severe coronary artery disease and require vascular surgical procedures.

For patients truly requiring emergency intervention because of an acute life- or limb-threatening vascular problem, surgery should not be denied, even in the setting of an acute myocardial infarction, unless there is significant hemodynamic instability of cardiac origin (14,15). Untreated, the physiological stress of these problems (i.e., ruptured aneurysm, acutely ischemic leg, and mesenteric ischemia) is usually manyfold greater than effective surgical care. Diagnostic studies before intervention in this group must be carefully chosen and not overdone. Specialists involved in the primary care of the patient (both physician and nurse) should be present during these procedures because radiologists often have little knowledge of patient care issues.

### Renal Insufficiency

Efforts should be directed toward protecting against a decline in renal dysfunction in the perioperative period. Intravascular volume deficits, nephrotoxic antibiotics, and intravascular contrast agents can have a devastating effect on renal function, especially in those patients who already have nephropathy as the result of their underlying hypertension, diabetes, or congestive heart failure. Unfortunately, duplex ultrasound (US), and magnetic resonance imaging (MRI) angiography are not developed sufficiently to eliminate the need for intravenous contrast angiography. Yet, when used in conjunction with selective angiography, detailed information about the presence or absence of vascular pathology can occasionally be obtained, allowing a reduction in the amount of intravenous contrast agents used. Liberal intravenous hydration, use of nonionic contrast agents, and administration of mannitol and low-dose dopamine in special instances can further reduce the risk of angiography (16). In patients with coexisting renal dysfunction and congestive heart failure, a Swan-Ganz catheter should be placed before angiography to allow simultaneous fluid administration, diuresis, and management of cardiac hemodynamics. Transient reduction of renal function is common in patients with underlying renal insufficiency, but the insult rarely leads to permanent loss of renal function.

## INTRAOPERATIVE CONSIDERATIONS

### Anesthetic Management

Although much concern has been focused on the type of anesthesia for a given procedure, the intraoperative control of hemodynamics is much more critical but is dependent more on the skill and experience of the anesthesiologist than on the particular anesthetic (17). A carefully administered balanced general anesthetic technique is much less of a cardiac risk than a spinal or epidural anesthetic, with which hypotension and tachycardia are allowed to develop. Epidural anesthesia, however, is especially attractive for lower extremity revascularization procedures because of its long duration of action, avoidance of endotracheal intubation, relatively minor hemodynamic consequences, lower incidence of pulmonary complications, and option of providing postoperative analgesia.

### Intraoperative Monitoring

Because of the high frequency of coexisting cardiac, pulmonary, and renal dysfunction and the lack of functional reserve, elderly patients must be intensively monitored during vascular surgical procedures in which volume changes, cardiac hemodynamics and the level of anesthetic medications are changing simultaneously on a minute-to-minute basis. This should be the case regardless of the type of anesthesia used. Use of an indwelling urinary catheter, arterial line, Swan-Ganz catheter, temperature probes, and in selective cases transesophageal echocardiography are helpful in achieving low morbidity rates.

### Surgical Technique

Special attention must be paid to the careful handling of tissues, such as the avoidance of retraction injuries, in elderly patients in whom the tissue are often quite delicate. Extra dissection or other procedures that may unnecessarily prolong the operation should be avoided. A retroperitoneal approach for aortic reconstructions is preferred when there has been previous abdominal surgery, chronic obstructive pulmonary disease (COPD), or marked obesity. Minimize exposed tissues and skin surfaces to avoid heat loss. Interact with the anesthesiologist to avoid delays in replacement of volume deficits, need for transfusion, anticoagulation, and cross clamping and release of major vascular structures.

## POSTOPERATIVE CARE

### Postoperative Monitoring

Essentially the same monitoring devices used intraoperatively should be continued as needed in the immediate postoperative period in an intensive care unit (ICU) setting. Particular attention should continue to be given to protect against problems that can increase the risk of myocardial compromise, such as volume deficits and associated hemodynamic changes, hypertension, tachycardia, and hypoxia. As the patient's condition stabilizes, the invasive monitors should be removed rapidly, usually beginning on the first postoperative day. Extending the use of invasive monitors without a specific reason subjects the patient to unnecessary risks, prohibits mobilization, and interferes with the patient's recovery.

## Pain Control

The most frequently mismanaged part of postoperative care in the elderly is the administration, or not, of analgesics. The highly variable response, low therapeutic-toxic ratio, inability of elderly patients to effectively ask or demand to be given medication, and fear of physicians and nurses of overmedicating the elderly patient all contribute to the problem. Indeed, overmedication with narcotics can result in atelectasis, hypoventilation, and even respiratory arrest. Undermedication, on the other hand, may result in similar problems plus anxiety, hypertension, and tachycardia. Both errors can increase the risk of myocardial events, such as infarction or arrhythmia. Constipation, pneumonia, and disorientation are some of the other common problems caused or aggravated by the improper administration of analgesics. Unfortunately, there is no single simple solution to these problems and what works for one patient may well be inappropriate in another. Frequent reassessment of the patient and adjustment of the dose and frequency of the medications is the most successful strategy for safe and effective pain control. If the patient is alert and capable, patient-controlled analgesia is an effective option. Epidural administration of narcotics is an especially attractive alternative in elderly patients who have had abdominal or thoracic procedures, because excellent analgesia can be achieved with minimal respiratory depression. A bladder catheter must be left in place in these instances to prevent urinary retention.

## Other Considerations

Elderly patients are particularly prone to developing decubitus ulcers in the perioperative period. The most common sites are sacral and heel locations. Prevention should begin preoperatively, but special efforts should also be made intraoperatively and immediately postoperatively, when patients are unable to move themselves to avoid injury to pressure points. It is tragic to have an elderly patient undergo a limb salvage procedure only to find that the opposite extremity was not adequately protected and a decubitus ulcer on the heel now threatens the opposite limb. Frequent repositioning, use of an air mattress, and placement of a pillow transversely under the calfs to keep the heels from resting directly on the surface of the bed go far toward preventing the headaches associated with the development of a decubitus ulcer.

Bladder and bowel dysfunction are common in the elderly, especially in the postoperative period. Stool softeners and liberal use of cathartics and bladder catherization are routine. Preoperative bowel preparation and evacuation should be considered even for nonabdominal operations because of nearly universal postoperative constipation and potential soiling of recent incision sites and wounds.

Early mobilization is important in many respects for recuperation from surgical procedures. It improves pulmonary toilet, reduces the risk of deep venous thrombosis and decubitus ulcers, maintains muscle strength, and improves mental status and outlook. It must be an active aggressive process in the elderly and involve the nursing staff, physical therapists, and family members.

## SPECIFIC VASCULAR PROBLEMS AND SURGICAL PROCEDURES

### Carotid Occlusive Disease

Probably the most common and most devastating peripheral vascular problem in the elderly is also the most frequently ignored. Carotid occlusive disease has been suspected as one of the common causes of thrombotic stroke for most of this century; however, until the development of angiography in the 1930s and 1940s, the diagnosis was not able to be made antemortem. Soon thereafter, carotid endarterectomy, a proposed treatment of this problem, was reported in 1954 by Eastcott et al. (18). However, the evolution of an effective treatment for carotid occlusive disease preceded a clear understanding of the natural history of these lesions. Retrospective reviews subsequently supported the belief that carotid endarterectomy could reduce the risk of stroke in patients with symptomatic and perhaps even asymptomatic lesions (19–21). Yet, because of overliberalized indications, highly variable results, and the rising cost of reimbursement, the operation fell into disfavor and then subsequently to disrepute. Several years of controversy regarding the appropriate role of carotid endarterectomy ensued, with highly emotionally charged opinions taking the place of scientific evidence. Recently, however, several prospective randomized trials designed to address this issue have shown a dramatic advantage of carotid endarterectomy, compared to the best nonsurgical treatment, for patients with high-grade carotid stenosis and hemispheric symptoms. The North American Symptomatic Carotid Endarterectomy Trial study revealed that patients with a carotid stenosis of 70% or greater and hemispheric symptoms (transient ischemic attacks or stroke) had nearly a threefold higher incidence of subsequent stroke when managed with antiplatelet therapy compared to those treated by endarterectomy (22). This difference in stroke risk was found after only 2 years and resulted in the early termination of this portion of the study. The European Carotid Surgery Trial had similar findings with surgery in symptomatic patients with a stenosis of 70% or greater having a distinct advantage in reducing stroke compared to nonoperative treatment (23). Studies to further define the role of carotid endarterectomy in asymptomatic patients and in symptomatic patients with lesser degrees of stenosis are in progress (24,25).

Several studies have retrospectively shown that carotid endarterectomy can be done in elderly patients ($> 75$ years of age) with low perioperative morbidity (combined perioperative stroke and death $< 5\%$), even in selected high-risk patients (26–28).

Newer radiological imaging techniques have decreased the risk of cerebral angiography, and in selected instances, carotid endarterectomy can be done based on noninvasive studies alone, thus further lowering the associated incidence of stroke (29).

Postoperative management should include continuous blood pressure monitoring, in an ICU setting, with strict avoidance of postendarterectomy hypertension, avoidance of sedatives, and monitoring of neurological status.

Carotid endarterectomy should be postponed for approximately 4–6 weeks following a major stroke because of the risk of cerebral hemorrhage.

## Abdominal Aortic Aneurysm

Most abdominal aortic aneurysms are asymptomatic until they rupture. Unfortunately, rupture is a catastrophic event that is often lethal, even with all the advances of modern medical transport and care. However, elective surgical repair in the over-80 group can be accomplished with a mortality rate of less than 5% because of improvements in anesthetic management, operative techniques, and intensive postoperative care (30–34). Therefore, age alone should not be a contraindication for repair of this otherwise lethal problem. Deferring repair of an aneurysm that is 5 cm in diameter or larger not only risks rupture but also obligates the physician to arrange for a careful surveillance regimen to check for expansion and allows further progression of other chronic medical illnesses (7). If the patient's functional status is good and longevity is not severely limited by another noncorrectable problem, aneurysm repair should be considered.

## Arterial Embolism

Sudden onset of severe ischemic symptoms in the previously asymptomatic person is the most common presentation of a patient with arterial embolism. Alert patients are usually able to identify precisely the exact time of onset of their symptoms. The majority of arterial emboli originate from the heart, as a result of arrhythmia, mural wall thrombus following myocardial infarction, ventricular aneurysm, valvular heart disease, or cardiac myxoma (35,36). Noncardiac sources include arterial aneurysms, complicated atherosclerotic lesions, and iatrogenic emboli following arterial catheterization procedures. In patients with a patent foramen ovale, paradoxical emboli from a venous source are also possible.

Once the diagnosis of arterial embolism is suspected, systemic anticoagulation with heparin should be started immediately to prevent propagation of thrombus and worsening ischemia and to decrease the likelihood of additional embolic events. Additional diagnostic evaluation and treatment should be done expeditiously to limit the extent of ischemic damage to the affected tissues.

The most common location for emboli to lodge is at the femoral artery bifurcation, but any vascular bed distal to the source is at risk.

Because most of these patients have significant preexisting atherosclerotic arterial occlusive disease and because acute ischemia can be caused by other mechanisms, such as thrombosis, arterial dissection, and cardiogenic shock superimposed upon chronic disease, angiography is almost always needed before further intervention or treatment.

Definitive treatment consists of prompt surgical embolectomy and restoration of arterial perfusion to the affected tissues. Arterial bypass may also be needed in patients with severe preexisting arterial occlusive disease. If the embolization has been to an extremity vessel and there has been more than 5 h of severe ischemia, then fasciotomy should be considered at the time of revascularization. Anticoagulation should be continued permanently unless the source has been eliminated.

When the ischemic symptoms are not severe or there has been a considerable delay between the time of onset of symptoms and presentation of the patient (>24 h), but no evidence of tissue necrosis, then urokinase lysis can be attempted as an alternative treatment in selected cases (37).

In the moribund patient, high-dose anticoagulation alone is an acceptable alternative treatment (38).

Other causes of acute arterial ischemia include spontaneous thrombosis of an aneurysm, aortic dissection, low-flow states superimposed upon chronic arterial occlusive disease, thrombosis of a diseased vessel or of a previously placed arterial bypass, or thrombosis secondary to hypercoagulable states.

## Atheroembolization

Complicated atherosclerotic lesions often have necrotic centers that contain cellular debris and cholesterol crystals (39). Spontaneous or iatrogenically induced plaque ulceration or rupture (secondary to arterial catheterization procedures or surgical manipulation) can result in distal embolization of this material. Essentially all downstream organs are vulnerable, but because atherosclerotic lesions resulting in embolization are usually most advanced in the region of the aortic bifurcation, the lower extremities are the most frequently affected sites. The embolized particles are usually quite small, and they consequently lodge in small arterioles or capillaries less than 200 μm in size (40). This situation results in ischemic lesions at these locations despite the presence of apparent arterial inflow. In the legs this usually results in localized pain and a spectrum of ischemic changes, such as livedo reticularis (irregular, mottled appearance of the skin), cyanosis, or gangrenous changes of the toes or forefoot despite the presence of palpable pedal pulses. The changes seen clinically in the foot are referred to as "blue toe syndrome" (41). Continued embolization and superimposed small-vessel thrombosis can result in tissue necrosis and a threatened extremity or other end organ (42–44). Identifying the responsible lesion can be difficult and often requires biplanar angiography (45). Treatment consists of temporary heparinization until either endarterectomy or bypass of the offending lesion can be accomplished. Iatrogenically induced episodes are often self-limiting, and a single episode can occasionally be tolerated without the need for surgical intervention (46).

## Aortoiliac Occlusive Disease

Absent femoral artery pulses and lower extremity ischemic symptoms indicate clinically significant aortoiliac artery occlusive disease. However, the classic triad of buttock claudication, absent femoral artery pulses, and impotence known as the Leriche syndrome is often absent in the elderly because of a less active life-style. Lumbosacral spine problems, including disk herniation, osteoarthritic narrowing of the spinal nerve foramen, spinal stenosis, and hip arthritis may all cause hip and thigh discomfort with ambulation and thus mimic claudication of vascular origin (47,48). A carefully elicited history and pertinent examination usually help distinguish these problems, but x-rays of the hip and a computed tomographic or MRI scan of the lower back are sometimes necessary to help make the distinction.

In addition to atherosclerotic occlusive disease, other events, such as arterial embolism, thrombosis of an abdominal aortic aneurysm, and aortic dissection, can also prevent as aortoiliac artery occlusive disease. Angiography is crucial in confirming the diagnosis, establishing the etiology, and planning intervention.

In good-risk patients, aortobifemoral artery bypass is the procedure of choice for severe aortic or bilateral iliac artery occlusive disease. In frail elderly patients, axillobifemoral artery bypass, a subcutaneous operation, can be done with few systemic consequences. Unilateral iliac stenosis can often be treated successfully by percutaneous balloon angioplasty (49,50). When angioplasty is unsuccessful, femorofemoral artery bypass can be done, if necessary under local anesthesia. In general, severe aortoiliac occlusive lesions should be treated before treatment of more distal lesions.

## Lower Extremity Arterial Occlusive Disease

Multilevel occlusive disease is usually present by the time a patient with chronic lower extremity arterial occlusive disease progresses to limb-threatening ischemia. However, a typical history of intermittent claudication progressing to nocturnal ischemic rest pain is often absent in the elderly person who walks only short distances because of other limitations. The combination of toe or foot pain and no palpable pedal pulses is an ischemic problem until proven otherwise. Localization of the pain and tenderness to the first metatarsal head and the presence of dependent rubor of the foot should not be mistakenly assumed to be signs of gout or cellulitis. If the patient has a significant neuropathy, however, rest pain might not develop even with advanced ischemia or gangrene. If symptoms are sudden in onset, arterial embolism should be considered; otherwise, chronic progressive atherosclerotic arterial occlusive disease is the most likely cause.

Diagnostic tests to confirm the presence and severity of occlusive disease should include segmental arterial occlusion pressures, Doppler waveforms, or segmental arterial pulse volume recordings. Angiography should be reserved for those instances in which revascularization procedures are planned and in most cases should include evaluation from the infrarenal aorta down to and including the foot vessels.

Extremity revascularization is preferred to amputation even if the patient is nonambulatory. Preservation of even a single functional limb may facilitate the ability of a patient to transfer from a bed to a chair or wheelchair and even to perform the most simple of functions, such as turning in bed. On the other hand, a nonfunctional limb with a fixed contracture is only an impediment, and amputation of a threatened limb in this setting is preferable.

Intervention in elderly patients with chronic arterial occlusive disease should be timed, if possible, to precede the development of ischemic ulceration or gangrene but should not be done for asymptomatic occlusive lesions or in the absence of a potentially limb-threatening situation. Debridement or amputation should not be done on these patients without a complete vascular assessment.

Balloon angioplasty and atherectomy, at present, have a limited role in the treatment of occlusive lesions below the level of the inguinal ligament and should be used only for short stenotic lesions with the understanding that there is a high rate of recurrent stenosis at these sites (51).

Distal lower extremity arterial bypass as far as the vessels in the foot has become routine even in the elderly (52–55). Perioperative rates of graft thrombosis should be less than 10%. Long-term bypass patency can be augmented by periodic bypass surveillance using a duplex ultrasound scanning technique to detect stenotic lesions before the time of graft occlusion.

Gangrenous foot lesions often require partial foot amputations and repeated debridement procedures following successful limb revascularization.

## Lower Extremity Amputation

Loss of an extremity is a devastating event at any age but is particularly so in the elderly in whom rehabilitation is often difficult. Ambulation with a prosthetic limb in patients having amputations after age 70 is possible and depends mostly on the functional status of the individual before limb loss (56). However, amputation in the frail patient is often equivalent to immobilization. As a result, it is not uncommon for some elderly patients to deteriorate in many aspects following a major amputation. On the other hand, if a patient is already bedridden or limited to the use of a wheelchair, amputation of a painful extremity or one with open wounds or a contracture can be a relief and result in increased mobility and a more pleasant existence.

In alert patients, lower extremity amputation should usually be done as far distal as is compatible with healing of the amputation site, as long as the proximal portion of the leg is functional. In bedridden patients with a nonfunctional extremity or in the presence of a fixed contracture, a below-the-knee amputation is contraindicated because of the likelihood of a joint contracture and subsequent stump decubitus ulcer.

In selected instances, angiography and revascularization procedures should be considered before amputation to allow healing at a lower level. For example, revascularization of a deep femoral artery in a limb without a femoral pulse may allow healing of a below-the-knee amputation; otherwise, the above-the-knee amputation or a hip disarticulation may be required.

Rehabilitation following amputation is an important aspect of the care of amputee patients even if they will not be able to ambulate with a prosthetic limb. Learning how to effectively transfer and to prevent joint contracture following amputation are important skills that impact greatly on each patient's future quality of life.

## Renal Artery Hypertension

Although often thought of as a disease occurring mostly in young females with fibromuscular dysplasia or in the middle-aged person with severe atherosclerotic disease, renal artery stenosis is actually most common in patients over 60 years of age (57). A marked worsening of systemic hypertension is the most common presentation. Patients with renal artery stenosis whose hypertension is poorly controlled on multiple antihypertensive agents or who have worsening renal function with adequate treatment should be considered for treatment with either balloon angioplasty or surgery.

Although the diagnosis can be suspected based upon noninvasive tests (captopril renal scan, duplex US, MRI angiography), contrast angiography is the only reliable method at present to confirm or exclude the diagnosis.

For nonorificial stenosis, balloon angioplasty is often an acceptable treatment and may avoid the need for an operative procedure. Total occlusions or stenosis involving the origin of the renal arteries should be repaired surgically by either endarterectomy or bypass.

## Mesenteric Ischemia

Acute mesenteric ischemia is a catastrophic event that is most common in the elderly patient with underlying cardiac problems and diffuse atherosclerotic occlusive disease. Sudden onset of severe abdominal pain and evacuation of intestinal contents in patients whose abdominal examination is unrevealing are typical of this problem. Early recognition and angiography are the keys to successful management.

Based upon angiographic findings, acute mesenteric ischemia is separated into occlusive and nonocclusive types. The occlusive type is usually the result of an embolus to the superior mesenteric or celiac arteries, but acute thrombosis of these vessels superimposed upon chronic occlusive disease is also occasionally seen. Treatment involves laparotomy, embolectomy, bypass to the mesenteric vessels if needed, and resection of nonviable portions of intestine (58). Use of thrombolytic agents should be avoided in most instances because of the risk of gastrointestinal hemorrhage and because of the need to assess intestinal viability. If the diagnosis is delayed until peritonitis has developed, then expeditious resection of ischemic bowel without preoperative angiography is warranted.

Nonocclusive mesenteric ischemia is the result of low cardiac output usually superimposed upon chronic asymptomatic mesenteric arterial occlusive disease. In these instances laparotomy should be avoided and treatment instead should consist of restoring adequate hemodynamics, intraarterial infusion of papaverine begun at the time of the diagnostic angiography, and treatment of the underlying etiological event (59).

Chronic mesenteric ischemia is characteristic in its presentation of poorly localized postprandial abdominal pain eventually developing into "food fear" and weight loss. Diagnosis is confirmed by angiography. Standard treatment consists of endarterectomy or bypass of occlusive lesions. Balloon angioplasty has been attempted in carefully selected instances for nonoroficial lesions (60); however, most surgeons are reluctant to use this method of treatment because of the severe consequences of a iatrogenic embolism or thrombosis at this location. The results of elective surgical treatment for this problem are excellent, with morbidity mostly dependent on cardiac issues (61).

## Venous Stasis, Insufficiency, and Thrombosis

In the upright position, venous flow is highly dependent upon the pumping action of the muscles of the lower extremity. Without this, the blood pools in the veins of the legs. The consequence is venous engorgement, hypertension, and stasis. Prolonged venous hypertension can lead to leg edema, induration, cellulitis, and ulceration. Venous stasis can lead to thrombosis. This sequence of events is particularly common in the elderly, who often spend several hours at a time sitting in one position with their feet resting in the floor. This circumstance results in venous stasis even in the absence of venous valvular insufficiency or congestive heart failure, which can markedly accentuate the problem.

The diagnosis of venous stasis is suggested by the presence of dependent leg edema, which is relieved by leg elevation, or by more chronic changes, consisting of induration, hyperpigmentation, and ulceration of the skin of the medial aspect of the ankle. Treatment consists of leg elevation and use of venous compression stockings when in the upright position.

Venous valvular insufficiency is a relatively common cause of venous hypertension and stasis and can involve either the deep or superficial venous systems. It is most reliably detected on examination by the presence of venous varicosities and confirmed by the visualization of valvular incompetence during a venous duplex ultrasound examination or by the use of an air plethysmograph, which determines volume changes in the leg as a function of positional changes and calf muscle contraction. Ascending and descending contrast venography are also occasionally used for diagnostic purposes. Treatment in uncomplicated cases is essentially the same as for venous stasis alone and requires periodic leg elevation and use of venous compression stockings when upright. If varicosities of the superficial system are prominent and symptomatic, injection sclerotherapy or vein excision may be helpful provided there is no obstruction in the deep system. The use of an intermittent compression pump is recommended for leg edema that does not easily respond to elevation and stocking use. Surgical correction of symptomatic venous insufficiency of the deep venous system is still largely in the developmental stage and should usually be avoided in the elderly.

For the diagnosis of lower extremity venous thrombosis, duplex ultrasound has nearly replaced contrast venography because it is highly sensitive and specific for this diagnosis and is completely noninvasive (62–64). Treatment of deep venous thrombosis consists of leg elevation and systemic anticoagulation, first with heparin and then warfarin. Placement of a caval filter should be reserved for instances in which there is a strong contraindication for anticoagulation or there has been evidence of pulmonary embolization while on adequate anticoagulation. Use of thrombolytic agents for the treatment of deep venous thrombosis should be avoided in the elderly because of the risk of cerebral hemorrhage. Venous thrombectomy should be reserved for use in cases in whom there has been such extensive venous thrombosis that limb viability is at risk.

Superficial venous thrombosis can be treated with leg elevation and nonsteroidal antiinflammatory agents, such as aspirin or ibuprofen, unless there is extension up to the saphenofemoral junction, in which case systemic anticoagulation or saphenous vein ligation is appropriate.

## Iatrogenic Vascular Injuries

Angiography, angioplasty, atherectomy, intravascular ultrasound, administration of thrombolytic agents, and use of percutaneously placed circulatory assist devices have become commonplace. With the increased utilization of these invasive diagnostic and therapeutic procedures, there has been a corresponding growth in the number of associated iatrogenic arterial injuries. Arterial hemorrhage, thrombosis, dissection, embolization, pseudoaneurysm, and arteriovenous fistula formation are the most frequently associated complications. The incidence of these for each procedure is directly proportional to the size of the catheter or sheath used, the severity of the associated underlying arterial occlusive disease, and the skill of the operator. Fortunately, few of these problems are life threatening, except in the patient with unstable cardiac disease, in whom any adverse event can have potentially devastating consequences.

Arterial thrombosis, clinically apparent embolization, and hemorrhage, not eliminated by localized fingertip pressure, should be dealt with by prompt operative intervention, usually under local anesthesia. The use of sandbags and bulky pressure dressings should be condemned because they are ineffective, prevent observation and examination of the site, give a false sense of security, and delay proper evaluation and care.

Small iatrogenic arterial pseudoaneurysms and asymptomatic arteriovenous fistulas usually resolve spontaneously or with duplex ultrasound-guided pressure, as long as the patient is not kept on systemic anticoagulation (65). Pseudoaneurysms that persist for longer than 2 weeks or are equal or greater than 4 cm in diameter should be repaired electively.

Patients with iatrogenic arterial dissections should be kept on systemic anticoagulation with heparin for approximately 48 h until it is clear that progression toward arterial occlusion is not occurring. Occlusions, if symptomatic, should be treated by thrombectomy and local vessel repair or by arterial bypass.

# ON THE HORIZON

Noninvasive diagnostic capabilities have already transformed the practice of vascular assessment and eventually will eliminate the need for current contrast angiography. Percutaneous therapies are in their infancy at present but will continue to blossom as technological innovations and experience increase. Our ability to control the thrombotic and thrombolytic processes has dramatically improved but is still relatively crude. Vasoactive agents to modify not only vascular tone but also metabolic functions will likely increase. Genetic engineering of arterial endothelium whereby endothelial cells are made to express specific genes has already begun (66). Even if our ability to dramatically modify atherogenesis remains relatively limited, the possible therapeutic implications of these other realistic advances are simultaneously exciting and mind-boggling.

## CONCLUSION

Peripheral vascular diseases are a relatively common cause of death and disability in the elderly population. Fortunately, our ability to successfully diagnose and treat a wide range of these problems in the elderly has dramatically improved as a result of new techniques and procedures, improved monitoring capabilities, and better understanding of the issues of particular importance in this group of patients. Although demanding of time and resources, the results can be gratifying for the patient, physician, and associated health care professionals.

## REFERENCES

1. U.S. Department of Health and Human Services, Health and Prevention Profile, 1989.
2. Vital Statistics of the United States, Washington, D.C., U.S. Department of Health and Human Services, National Center for Health Statistics, 1989.
3. Plecha FR, Bertin VJ, Plecha BS, et al. The early results of vascular surgery in patients 75 years of age and older: an analysis of 3259 cases. *J Vasc Surg* 1985; 2:769–774.
4. Greenburg GA, Saik RP, Coyle JJ, Peskin GW. Mortality and gastrointestinal surgery in the aged. *Arch Surg* 1981; 116:788–791.
5. Koruda MJ, Sheldon GF. Surgery in the aged. *Adv Surg* 1991; 24:293–331.
6. Oriel K, Fiore WM, Geary JE. Limb-threatening ischemia in the medically compromised patient: amputation or revascularization? *Surgery* 1988; 104:667–672.
7. Szilagyi DE, Elliott JP, Smith RF. Clinical fate of the patient with asymptomatic abdominal aortic aneurysm and unfit for surgical treatment. *Arch Surg* 1972; 104:600–606.
8. Older P, Smith R. Experience with the preoperative invasive measurement of hemodynamic, respiratory and renal function in 100 elderly patients scheduled for major abdominal surgery. *Anaesth Intensive Care* 1988; 16:389–395.
9. Hertzer NR, Beven EG, Young JR. Coronary artery disease in peripheral vascular patients: a classification of 1000 coronary angiograms and results of surgical management. *Ann Surg* 1984; 199:223–233.
10. Rutherford RB. Preoperative cardiac evaluation in vascular surgery patients: a selective approach. *Semin Vasc Surg* 1991; 4:106–109.
11. Eagle KA, Singer DE, Brewster DC. Dipyridamole thallium scanning in patients undergoing vascular surgery: optimizing preoperative evaluation of cardiac risk. *JAMA* 1987; 257:2185–2189.
12. Crawford MH. The preoperative cardiac evaluation of the patient with vascular

disease: ejection fraction and stress echocardiography. *Semin Vasc Surg* 1991; 4:77–82.

13. Huber KC, Evans MA, Bresnahan JF, Gibbons RJ, Holmes DR. Outcome of noncardiac operations in patients with severe coronary artery disease successfully treated with coronary angioplasty. *Mayo Clin Proc* 1992; 67:15–21.
14. Rivers SP, Scher LA, Gupta SK, Veith FJ. Safety of peripheral vascular surgery after recent acute myocardial infarction. *J Vasc Surg* 1990; 11:70–76.
15. Thompson JE, Weston AS, Sigler L, Raut PS, Austin DJ, Patman RD. Arterial embolectomy after acute myocardial infarction: a study of 31 patients. *Ann Surg* 1970; 171:979–986.
16. Cohan RH, Dunnick NR. Intravascular contrast media: adverse reactions. *AJR* 1987; 149:665–670.
17. Rivers SP, Scher LA, Veith FJ. Epidural and general anesthesia or infrainguinal arterial reconstruction. *J Vasc Surg* 1991; 14:764–770.
18. Eastcott HHG, Pickering GW, Rob C. Reconstruction of internal carotid artery in a patient with intermittent attacks of hemiplegia. *Lancet* 1954; 2:994–997.
19. Thompson JE, Austin DJ, Patman RD. Carotid endarterectomy for cerebral insufficiency: long-term results in 592 patients followed up to thirteen years. *Ann Surg* 1970; 172:663–669.
20. DeWeese JA, Rob C, Satran R, et al. Results of carotid endarterectomy for transient ischemic attacks, five years later. *Ann Surg* 1973; 178:258–264.
21. Thompson JE, Patman D, Persson AV. Management of asymptomatic carotid bruits. *Ann Surg* 1976; 42:77–80.
22. North American Symptomatic Carotid Endarterectomy Trial Collaborators. Beneficial effect of carotid endarterectomy in symptomatic patients with high-grade carotid stenosis. *N Engl J Med* 1991; 325:445–453.
23. European Carotid Surgery Trialist's Collaborative Group. MRC European carotid surgery trial: interim results for symptomatic patients with severe (70–99%) or with mild (0–29%) carotid stenosis. *Lancet* 1991; 337:1235–1243.
24. Asymptomatic Carotid Artery Stenosis Group. Study design for randomized prospective trial of carotid endarterectomy for asymptomatic atherosclerosis. *Stroke* 1989; 20:844–849.
25. Veterans Administration Cooperative Study. Role of carotid endarterectomy in asymptomatic carotid stenosis. *Stroke* 1986; 17:534–549.
26. Meyer FB, Meissner I, Fode NC, Losasso TJ. Carotid endarterectomy in elderly patients. *Mayo Clin Proc* 1991; 66:464–469.
27. Oriel K, Penn TE, Ricotta JJ, May AG, Green RM, DeWeese JA. Carotid endarterectomy in the elderly patient. *Surg Gynecol Obstet* 1986; 162:334–336.
28. Rosenthal D, Rudderman RH, Jones DH, et al. Carotid endarterectomy in the octogenarian: is it appropriate? *J Vasc Surg* 1986; 3:782–785.
29. Gertler JP, Cambria RP, Kistler JP, et al. Carotid surgery without arteriography: noninvasive selection of patients. *Ann Vasc Surg* 1991; 5:253–256.
30. Robson AK, Currie IC, Poskitt KR, Scott DJA, Baird RN, Horrocks M. Abdominal aortic aneurysm repair in the over eighties. *Br J Surg* 1989; 76:1018–1020.
31. Treiman RL, Levine KA, Cohen JL, Cossman DV, Foran RF, Levin PM. Aneu-

rysmectomy in the octogenarian: a study of morbidity and quality of survival. *Am J Surg* 1982; 144:1018–1020.
32. Petracek MR, Lawson JA, Rhea WG, Richie RE, Dean RH. Resection of abdominal aortic aneurysm in the over 80 age group. *South Med J* 1980; 73:579–581.
33. Ammar CD. Mortality of elective abdominal aortic surgery in octogenarians. *Kansas Med* 1987; 5:154–158.
34. O'Donnell TF, Darling CR, Linton RR. Is 80 years too old for aneurysmectomy? *Arch Surg* 1976; 111:1250–1256.
35. Panetta T, Thompson JE, Talkington CM, Wilson VG, Smith BL. Arterial embolectomy: a thirty-four year experience with 400 cases. *Surg Clin North Am* 1986; 66:339–353.
36. Tawes RL, Harris EJ, Brown WH. Arterial thromboembolism: a 20-year perspective. *Arch Surg* 1985; 120:595–599.
37. Camerota AJ, Rubin RN, Tyson RR. Intra-arterial thrombolytic therapy in peripheral vascular disease. *Surg Gynecol Obstet* 1987; 165:1–7.
38. Blaisdell WF, Steele M, Allen RE. Management of acute lower extremity arterial ischemia due to embolism and thrombosis. *Surgery* 1978; 84:822–834.
39. Glagov S, Newman WP, Schaffer SA. Pathobiology of the Human Atherosclerotic Plaque. New York: Springer-Verlag, 1990.
40. Anderson WR, Richard AM. Evaluation of lower extremity muscle biopsies in the diagnosis of atheroembolism. *Arch Pathol* 1968; 86:535–54.
41. Karmody AM, Powers SR, Monaco VJ. "Blue toe" syndrome: an indication for limb salvage surgery. *Arch Surg* 1976; 111:1263–1268.
42. Kempczinski RF. Lower-extremity arterial emboli from ulcerating atherosclerotic plaques. *JAMA* 1979; 241:807–810.
43. Lee BY, Brancato RF, Thoden WR, Madden JL. Blue digit syndrome: urgent indication for limb salvage. *Am J Surg* 1984; 147:428–422.
44. Kaufman JL, Stark K, Brolin RE. Disseminated atheroembolism from extensive degenerative atherosclerosis of the aorta. *Surgery* 1987; 102:63–70.
45. Fisher DF, Clagett GP, Brigham RA. Dilemmas in dealing with the blue toe syndrome: aortic versus peripheral source. *Am J Surg* 1984; 148:836–840.
46. Colt HG, Begg RJ, Saporito JJ, Cooper WM, Shapiro AP. Cholesterol emboli after cardiac catheterization. *Medicine (Baltimore)* 1988; 67:389–400.
47. Arnoldi CC, Brodsky AE, Cauchoix J. Lumbar spinal stenosis syndromes and nerve entrapment syndromes. *Clin Orthop* 1976; 115:4–5.
48. Johansson JE, Barringtin TW, Ameli M. Combined vascular and neurogenic claudication. *Spine* 1982; 7:150–158.
49. Kadir S, White RI Jr, Daufman S, et al. Long-term results of aortoiliac angioplasty. *Surgery* 1983; 94:10–14.
50. Spence R, Freiman D, Gatenby R, et al. Long-term results of transluminal angioplasty of the iliac and femoral arteries. *Arch Surg* 1981; 116:1377–1386.
51. Rush DS, Gewertz BL, Lu CT, et al. Limb salvage in poor-risk patients using transluminal angioplasty. *Arch Surg* 1983; 118:1209–1212.
52. Scher LA, Veith FJ, Ascer E, et al. Limb salvage in octogenarians and nonagenarians. *Surgery* 1986; 99:160–165.

53. Ascer E, Veith FJ, Gupta SK. Bypasses to plantar arteries and other tibial branches: an extended approach to limb salvage. *J Vasc Surg* 1988; 8:434–441.
54. Andros G, Harris RW, Salles-Cunha SX. Bypass grafts to the ankle and foot. *J Vasc Surg* 1988; 7:785–794.
55. Shah DM, Darling RC, Chang BB, Kaufman JL, Fitzgerald KM, Leather RP. Is long vein bypass from the groin to ankle a durable procedure? An analysis of a ten year experience. *J Vasc Surg* 1992; 15:402–408.
56. Steinberg FU, Sunwoo I, Roettger RF. Prosthetic rehabilitation of geriatric amputee patients: a follow-up study. *Arch Phys Med Rehabil* 1985; 66:742–745.
57. Stanley JC. Pathologic basis of macrovascular renal artery disease. In: Stanley JC, Ernst CB, Fry WJ, eds. Renovascular Hypertension. Philadelphia: W. B. Saunders, 1984:46–74.
58. Boley SJ, Bergan JJ, Williams LF. Symposium on acute mesenteric vascular occlusion. *Cont Surg* 1983; 22:125–164.
59. Williams LF. Nonocclusive mesenteric ischemia. In: Current Therapy in Vascular Surgery. Philadelphia: B. C. Decker, 1991:750–756.
60. Golden DA, Ring EJ, McLean GK, et al. Percutaneous transluminal angioplasty in the treatment of abdominal angina. *AJR* 1982; 139:247.
61. Stoney RJ, Ehrenfeld WK, Wylie EJ. Revascularization in chronic visceral ischemia caused by atherosclerosis. *Ann Surg* 1977; 186:468–475.
62. Comerota AJ, Katz ML, Grossi RJ, et al. The comparative value of noninvasive testing for diagnosis and surveillance of deep vein thrombosis. *J Vasc Surg* 1988; 7:40–49.
63. Lensing WA, Prandoni P, Brandjes D, et al. Detection of deep vein thrombosis by real time B-mode ultrasonography. *N Engl J Med* 1989; 320:342–345.
64. Barnes R, Nix M, Ferris E, et al. Perioperative asymptomatic venous thrombosis: role of duplex scanning versus venography. *J Vasc Surg* 1989; 9:251–260.
65. Rivers SP, Slass EL, Lyon RT, Monrad S, Veith FJ. Successful conservative management of iatrogenic arterial trauma. *Ann Vasc Surg* 1992; 6:45–49.
66. Nabel EG, Plautz G, Boyce FM, Stanley JC, Nabel GJ. Recombinant gene expression in vivo within endothelial cells of the arterial wall. *Science* 1989; 244:1342–1344.

# Index

# About the Editors

DONALD D. TRESCH is Professor of Medicine and Director of the Cardiology Fellowship Program at the Medical College of Wisconsin, Milwaukee, and Adjunct Professor in the College of Letters and Science at the University of Wisconsin—Milwaukee. The author or coauthor of over 145 professional papers, book chapters, and abstracts, he is a Fellow of the American Heart Association, the American College of Cardiology, and the Council on Geriatric Cardiology (member, Board of Directors), and a member of the American Geriatrics Society as well as an editorial board member of the Journal of the American Geriatrics Society. Dr. Tresch received the M.D. degree (1966) from the University of Illinois, Urbana.

WILBERT S. ARONOW is Medical Director of Hebrew Hospital Home, Bronx, New York, and Adjunct Professor in the Department of Geriatrics and Adult Development at Mount Sinai School of Medicine, New York, New York. A Fellow of the American College of Physicians, the American College of Cardiology, the Council on Clinical Cardiology of the American Heart Association, the American College of Chest Physicians, the American Geriatrics Society (Founding Fellow of Western Division), the Council on Geriatric Cardiology (Founding Fellow), and the American College of Angiology, among other organizations, he is the author or coauthor of over 450 professional papers and book chapters. Dr. Aronow received the M.D. degree (1957) from Harvard Medical School, Boston, Massachusetts.